NMS *Obstetrics and Gynecology*

NMS *Obstetrics and Gynecology*

6th EDITION

Editor

Samantha M. Pfeifer, MD

Associate Professor
Obstetrics and Gynecology
Division of Reproductive Endocrinology and Infertility
University of Pennsylvania Medical School
Philadelphia, Pennsylvania

Wolters Kluwer | Lippincott Williams & Wilkins
Health

Philadelphia • Baltimore • New York • London
Buenos Aires • Hong Kong • Sydney • Tokyo

Senior Acquisitions Editor: Donna M. Balado
Associate Managing Editor: Liz Stalnaker
Production Editor: Beth Martz
Marketing Manager: Jennifer Kuklinski
Design Coordinator: Holly Reid McLaughlin
Compositor: International Typesetting and Composition

6th Edition
© 2008 by Lippincott Williams & Wilkins, a Wolters Kluwer business
530 Walnut Street
Philadelphia, PA 19106
LWW.com

Printed in the People's Republic of China (PRC)

Library of Congress Cataloging-in-Publication Data

Obstetrics and gynecology.—6th ed. / editor, Samantha M. Pfeifer.
   p. ; cm.
  (National medical series for independent study)
  ISBN-13: 978-0-7817-7071-2
  ISBN-10: 0-7817-7071-8
  1. Gynecology—Outlines, syllabi, etc. 2. Obstetrics—Outlines,
syllabi, etc. 3. Gynecology—Examinations, questions, etc.
4. Obstetrics—Examinations, questions, etc. I. Pfeifer, Samantha M.
II. Series.
  [DNLM: 1. Obstetrics—Examination Questions.
2. Obstetrics—Outlines. 3. Gynecology—Examination Questions.
4. Gynecology—Outlines. WQ 18.2 O141 2008]
  RG112.O37 2008
  618.076—dc22

2007017201

This book is dedicated to my mentors Dr. Luigi Mastroianni and the memory of Dr. Celso-Ramon Garcia, who set an example of excellence in teaching and clinical care of patients. I would also like to dedicate this to Alice and Charlotte Rose for their support and encouragement.

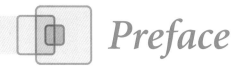 *Preface*

The sixth edition of *NMS Obstetrics and Gynecology* has the same primary goal of the previous edition, and indeed, the entire NMS series: to provide the most up-to-date and relevant information in an easy-to-understand outline format for both students and residents. Basic scientific information is balanced by clinical relevance, and a wealth of more than 200 USMLE-formatted questions allows readers to test their knowledge prior to their board examinations.

This sixth edition represents a collaborative effort between the many contributors who revised existing chapters or wrote new chapters for this edition, and the new editor, Samantha M. Pfeifer, who orchestrated and oversaw the text revision, as well as revamped the USMLE-style questions and online Comprehensive Examination to reflect current Step 2 formats and content areas. The 60 questions in the Comprehensive Examination, available online on The Point (thepoint.lww.com), have been written at a slightly higher level of difficulty than the USMLE-formatted questions in the chapters. Some of the answers, therefore, require a level of knowledge that goes beyond the information presented in the book. The examination thus provides a rigorous and comprehensive review of content.

The content covered in all of the chapters has been thoroughly updated, and two new chapters have been added, one on polycystic ovary syndrome and the other on recurrent pregnancy loss, reflecting the importance these topics have to practitioners and students of obstetrics and gynecology. In addition, the order of the chapters has been slightly rearranged to make the order of presentation more logical, although the chapters can be used in any order. The online case studies, also available on The Point, have been rewritten to reflect current treatment paradigms and incorporate new information that is available and influences the diagnosis and treatment of the specific conditions. In addition, a new case study has been added on the topic of hirsutism.

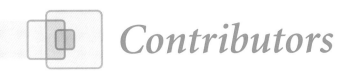

Contributors

Lily Arya, MD
Assistant Professor, Obstetrics and Gynecology
Chief, Division of Gynecologic Urology
University of Pennsylvania School of Medicine
Philadelphia, Pennsylvania

Janice B. Asher, MD
Clinical Assistant Professor, Obstetrics and Gynecology
Clinical Director, Women's Health
Student Health Services
University of Pennsylvania
Philadelphia, Pennsylvania

Kurt Barnhart, MD
Associate Professor, Obstetrics and Gynecology
Director, Women's Health Clinical Research Center
University of Pennsylvania Medical School
Philadelphia, Pennsylvania

Matthew N. Beshara, MD
Assistant Clinical Professor
Obstetrics and Gynecology
University of Pennsylvania School of Medicine
Philadelphia, Pennsylvania

Danielle Burkland, MD
Assistant Clinical Professor
Obstetrics and Gynecology
University of Pennsylvania School of Medicine
Philadelphia, Pennsylvania

Samantha Butts, MD, MSCE
Assistant Professor
Obstetrics and Gynecology
University of Pennsylvania School of Medicine
Philadelphia, Pennsylvania

Sharon Byun, MD
Assistant Clinical Professor
Obstetrics and Gynecology
University of Pennsylvania School of Medicine
Philadelphia, Pennsylvania

Peter Chen, MD
Assistant Clinical Professor
Obstetrics and Gynecology
University of Pennsylvania School of Medicine
Philadelphia, Pennsylvania

Doris Chou, MD
Assistant Professor
Obstetrics and Gynecology
University of Pennsylvania School of Medicine
Philadelphia, Pennsylvania

Christina S. Chu, MD
Assistant Professor
Obstetrics and Gynecology
University of Pennsylvania School of Medicine
Philadelphia, Pennsylvania

Guillermo de la Vega, MD
Obstetrics and Gynecology
University of Pennsylvania Health System
Philadelphia, Pennsylvania

Scott E. Edwards, MD
Assistant Professor
Reproductive Endocrinology and Infertility
University of Pennsylvania School of Medicine
Philadelphia, Pennsylvania

Michal A. Elovitz, MD
Assistant Professor
MFM Fellowship Director
Obstetrics and Gynecology
University of Pennsylvania School of Medicine
Philadelphia, Pennsylvania

Robert Gaiser, MD
Professor
Anesthesiology
University of Pennsylvania School of Medicine
Philadelphia, Pennsylvania

Juan M. Gonzalez, MD
Clinical Fellow
Maternal-Fetal Medicine
Obstetrics and Gynecology
Hospital of the University of Pennsylvania
Philadelphia, Pennsylvania

Clarisa Gracia, MD, MSCE
Assistant Professor
Obstetrics and Gynecology
University of Pennsylvania School of Medicine
Philadelphia, Pennsylvania

Ann Honebrink, MD
Assistant Professor, Obstetrics and Gynecology
Medical Director, Penn Health for Women at Radnor
University of Pennsylvania School of Medicine
Philadelphia, Pennsylvania

Kat Lin, MD
Clinical Fellow
Reproductive Endocrinology and Infertility
Obstetrics and Gynecology
Hospital of the University of Pennsylvania
Philadelphia, Pennsylvania

Jack Ludmir, MD
Professor
Obstetrics and Gynecology
University of Pennsylvania School of Medicine
Philadelphia, Pennsylvania

Monica A. Mainigi, MD
Clinical Fellow
Reproductive Endocrinology and Infertility
Hospital of the University of Pennsylvania
Philadelphia, Pennsylvania

Dominic Marchiano, MD
Assistant Clinical Professor
Obstetrics and Gynecology
University of Pennsylvania School of Medicine
Philadelphia, Pennsylvania

Luigi Mastroianni, Jr., MD
William Goodell Professor of Obstetrics and
   Gynecology
University of Pennsylvania School of Medicine
Philadelphia, Pennsylvania

Jennifer B. Merriman, MD
Clinical Fellow
Maternal-Fetal Medicine
Obstetrics and Gynecology
Hospital of the University of Pennsylvania
Philadelphia, Pennsylvania

Thomas A. Molinaro, MD
Clinical Fellow
Reproductive Endocrinology and Infertility
Obstetrics and Gynecology
Hospital of the University of Pennsylvania
Philadelphia, Pennsylvania

Emmanuelle Paré, MD
Assistant Professor
Obstetrics and Gynecology
University of Pennsylvania School of Medicine
Philadelphia, Pennsylvania

Samuel Parry, MD
Associate Professor, Obstetrics and Gynecology
Chief, Division of Maternal-Fetal Medicine
University of Pennsylvania Medical School
Philadelphia, Pennsylvania

Samantha M. Pfeifer, MD
Associate Professor
Obstetrics and Gynecology
Division of Reproductive Endocrinology and
   Infertility
University of Pennsylvania Medical School
Philadelphia, Pennsylvania

Dahlia M. Sataloff, MD
Clinical Professor of Surgery
Director, Integrated Breast Center
University of Pennsylvania School of Medicine
Philadelphia, Pennsylvania

Courtney A. Schreiber, MD
Assistant Professor
Obstetrics and Gynecology
University of Pennsylvania School of Medicine
Philadelphia, Pennsylvania

Harish M. Sehdev, MD
Assistant Clinical Professor
Obstetrics and Gynecology
University of Pennsylvania School of Medicine
Philadelphia, Pennsylvania

Steven J. Sondheimer, MD
Professor
Obstetrics and Gynecology
University of Pennsylvania School of Medicine
Philadelphia, Pennsylvania

Sindhu K. Srinivas, MD
Clinical Fellow
Maternal-Fetal Medicine
Obstetrics and Gynecology
Hospital of the University of Pennsylvania
Philadelphia, Pennsylvania

Ann L. Steiner, MD
Associate Clinical Professor
Obstetrics and Gynecology
University of Pennsylvania School of Medicine
Philadelphia, Pennsylvania

H. Irene Su, MD
Clinical Fellow
Reproductive Endocrinology and Infertility
Obstetrics and Gynecology
Hospital of the University of Pennsylvania
Philadelphia, Pennsylvania

Richard W. Tureck, MD
Professor
Obstetrics and Gynecology
Division of Reproductive Endocrinology and
   Infertility
University of Pennsylvania Medical School
Philadelphia, Pennsylvania

Serdar Ural, MD
Associate Professor, Obstetrics and Gynecology
Director, Maternal Fetal Medicine
Penn State Milton S. Hershey Medical Center
Hershey, Pennsylvania

Michelle Vichnin, MD
Assistant Clinical Professor
Obstetrics and Gynecology
University of Pennsylvania School of Medicine
Philadelphia, Pennsylvania

Contents

Preface vii

Contributors. ix

1 Endocrinology of Pregnancy 1
SAMUEL PARRY and DOMINIC MARCHIANO
   I.   Introduction 1
   II.   Human Chorionic Gonadotropin 2
   III.   Human Placental Lactogen 3
   IV.   Prolactin 4
   V.   Progesterone 4
   VI.   Estrogens 6

2 Fetal Physiology 11
SERDAR URAL
   I.   Introduction 11
   II.   Placenta 11
   III.   Umbilical Cord 12
   IV.   Amniotic Membranes and Fluid 12
   V.   Fetus 12

3 Normal Pregnancy, the Puerperium, and Lactation 19
PETER CHEN
   I.   Diagnosis of Pregnancy 19
   II.   Pregnancy 20
   III.   Status of the Fetus 22
   IV.   Puerperium 25
   V.   Lactation 27

4 Antepartum Care 32
DANIELLE BURKLAND
   I.   Introduction 32
   II.   Preconception Care 32
   III.   Calculating the Estimated Date of Confinement (EDC) 32
   IV.   Initial Prenatal Visit: History 33
   V.   Initial Prenatal Visit: Physical Examination and Screening 34
   VI.   Aneuploidy Screening 36
   VII. Subsequent Prenatal Visits 36
   VIII. Nutrition 37
   IX.   Lifestyle Modifications 38

5 Identification of the High-Risk Pregnant Patient 42
JACK LUDMIR and GUILLERMO DE LA VEGA
   I.   Introduction 42
   II.   Maternal and Perinatal Mortality 42

III.   Preconception Care 43

IV.   Initial Prenatal Visit 43

V.   Physical Examination 48

VI.   Laboratory Studies 49

VII.   Risk Assessment and Management of Risk in Pregnancy 51

6   Prenatal Diagnosis and Obstetric Ultrasound 56
EMMANUELLE PARÉ

I.   Introduction 56

II.   Indications for Prenatal Diagnosis 56

III.   Genetic Screening 58

IV.   Techniques of Prenatal Diagnosis 60

7   Teratology 67
JENNIFER B. MERRIMAN and DORIS CHOU

I.   Introduction 67

II.   Teratogenic Agents 68

8   Substance Abuse in Pregnancy 81
SERDAR URAL and EMMANUELLE PARÉ

I.   Introduction 81

II.   Definition 81

III.   Signs and Symptoms of Substance Abuse 82

IV.   Psychoactive Substances 82

V.   Alcohol Use in Pregnancy 82

VI.   Cocaine Use in Pregnancy 83

VII.   Other Substances Abused in Pregnancy 85

VIII   Substance Abuse and Prenatal Care 85

9   Antepartum Bleeding 89
DANIELLE BURKLAND

I.   Introduction 89

II.   Placenta Previa 89

III.   Abruptio Placentae (Placental Abruption) 92

IV.   Other Causes of Third-Trimester Bleeding 93

10   Labor and Delivery 98
PETER CHEN

I.   Theories of the Causes of Labor 98

II.   Definition and Characteristics of Labor 98

III.   Normal Labor in the Occiput Presentation 101

IV.   Conduct of Labor 104

11   Intrapartum Fetal Monitoring 111
MATTHEW N. BESHARA

I.   Introduction 111

II.   Pathophysiology of Fetal Hypoxia 111

III.   Types of Fetal Heart Rate Monitoring 112

IV.   Interpretation of Fetal Heart Rate Patterns 112

V.   Fetal Heart Rate Tracings: Assessment and Management in Labor 117

VI.   Other Developments in Intrapartum Monitoring: Fetal Oxygen
        Saturation Monitoring 118

12   Operative Obstetrics 123
        JENNIFER B. MERRIMAN and DORIS CHOU

I.   Cesarean Birth 123

II.   Episiotomy (see Table 10-5) 127

III.   Operative Vaginal Delivery: Forceps and Vacuum-Extractor Operations 127

IV.   Cervical Cerclage 130

V.   Abortion 132

13   Obstetric Anesthesia 139
        ROBERT GAISER

I.   Introduction 139

II.   Physiologic Changes of Pregnancy 139

III.   Neuropathways of Obstetric Pain 141

IV.   Analgesia for Labor 141

V.   Anesthesia for Cesarean Section 143

14   Postterm Pregnancy 148
        SHARON BYUN and SINDHU K. SRINIVAS

I.   Introduction 148

II.   Definition 148

III.   Determining Gestational Age 148

IV.   Etiology of Postterm Pregnancy 148

V.   Clinical Significance of Postterm Pregnancy 149

VI.   Management of the Postterm Pregnancy 149

15   Preterm Labor 154
        JUAN M. GONZALEZ and MICHAL A. ELOVITZ

I.   Preterm Birth 154

II.   Risk Factors for Premature Delivery 154

III.   Prevention of Preterm Birth 155

IV.   Evaluation of Patients in Preterm Labor 155

V.   Management of Preterm Labor 156

VI.   Preterm Premature Rupture of Membranes 158

16   Hypertension in Pregnancy 163
        DOMINIC MARCHIANO

I.   Introduction 163

II.   Definitions 163

III.   Chronic Hypertension 164

IV.   Preeclampsia: Epidemiology 165

V.   Preeclampsia: Pathophysiology 165

VI.   Preeclampsia: Clinical Manifestations 167

VII.   Preeclampsia: Management 167

VIII. Preeclampsia: Prevention 169

IX.   Eclampsia 169

X.   Preeclampsia: Prognosis 169

17 Medical Complications of Pregnancy 175
HARISH M. SEHDEV

   I.   **Diabetes** 175

   II.   **Thyroid Disease** 177

   III. **Urinary Tract Infection** 179

   IV. **Anemia** 180

   V.   **Heart Disease** 182

   VI. **Pulmonary Disease** 183

   VII. **Thromboembolic Disease** 186

   VIII. **Seizure Disorders** 188

   IX. **Rh Isoimmunization** 188

18 Gestational Trophoblastic Disease 196
CHRISTINA S. CHU

   I.   **Introduction** 196

   II.   **Hydatidiform Mole (Table 18-2)** 196

   III. **Gestational Trophoblastic Tumor** 199

19 The Menstrual Cycle 205
THOMAS A. MOLINARO and CLARISA GRACIA

   I.   **Introduction** 205

   II.   **Gonadotropin-Releasing Hormone** 206

   III. **Gonadotropins: Follicle-Stimulating Hormone and Luteinizing Hormone** 206

   IV. **Oogenesis** 207

   V.   **Menstruation** 210

   VI. **Clinical Problems Associated with the Menstrual Cycle** 210

20 Amenorrhea 215
CLARISA GRACIA and THOMAS A. MOLINARO

   I.   **Introduction** 215

   II.   **Classification and Etiology of Amenorrhea** 215

   III. **Clinical Evaluation** 219

   IV. **Management** 220

21 Polycystic Ovary Syndrome 227
MONICA A. MAINIGI and SAMANTHA M. PFEIFER

   I.   **Introduction** 227

   II.   **Definition** 227

   III. **Genetics and Etiology of PCOS** 228

   IV. **Pathophysiology** 229

   V.   **Health Consequences** 230

   VI. **Differential Diagnosis** 230

   VII. **Evaluation** 231

   VIII. **Treatment** 234

22 Hirsutism 238
SAMANTHA M. PFEIFER

   I.   **Introduction** 238

   II.   **Androgens** 238

   III. **Diagnosis** 239

   IV. **Treatment** 242

23   Abnormal Uterine Bleeding 247
SAMANTHA BUTTS

    I.   Definitions 247

    II.   Physiology of Normal Menstrual Bleeding 248

    III.   Pathophysiology of Dysfunctional Uterine Bleeding 249

    IV.   Etiology of Abnormal Uterine Bleeding 249

    V.   Evaluation and Diagnosis of Abnormal Uterine Bleeding 251

    VI.   Treatment of Abnormal Uterine Bleeding 252

24   Uterine Leiomyomas 258
MONICA A. MAINIGI and RICHARD W. TURECK

    I.   Introduction 258

    II.   Etiology 258

    III.   Classification and Pathology 259

    IV.   Associated Symptoms and Signs 260

    V.   Treatment 262

25   Endometriosis 269
SCOTT E. EDWARDS and RICHARD W. TURECK

    I.   Introduction 269

    II.   Etiology 269

    III.   Signs and Symptoms 270

    IV.   Diagnosis 271

    V.   Treatment 272

26   Pelvic Pain 278
THOMAS A. MOLINARO and RICHARD W. TURECK

    I.   Introduction 278

    II.   Definition 278

    III.   Anatomy and Physiology of Pelvic Pain 278

    IV.   Evaluation 279

    V.   Differential Diagnosis 279

27   Ectopic Pregnancy 287
KURT BARNHART

    I.   Introduction 287

    II.   Etiology 287

    III.   Signs and Symptoms 288

    IV.   Diagnosis 288

    V.   Treatment 290

    VI.   Prognosis 291

28   The Infertile Couple 295
H. IRENE SU and STEVEN J. SONDHEIMER

    I.   Introduction 295

    II.   Approach to Treatment 295

    III.   Ovulatory Dysfunction 296

    IV.   "Competent Oocyte"/Decreased Ovarian Reserve 298

    V.   Tubal Factor 299

    VI.   Uterine and Vaginal Outflow Tract Abnormalities 299

    VII.   Endometriosis 300

    VIII. Male Factor Infertility 301

    IX. Coital Problems 302

    X. Unexplained Infertility 302

    XI. Assisted Reproductive Technology 303

29 Recurrent Pregnancy Loss 307
KAT LIN and SAMANTHA BUTTS

    I. Definition 307

    II. Incidence 307

    III. Etiology of Miscarriages in the General Reproductive Population 307

    IV. Etiology of Recurrent Pregnancy Loss 308

    V. RPL Evaluation Overview 311

    VI. Treatments for Women with Recurrent Pregnancy Loss 311

30 Pediatric and Adolescent Gynecology 316
SAMANTHA BUTTS, SAMANTHA M. PFEIFER and MICHELLE VICHNIN

    I. Introduction 316

    II. Vulvovaginal Lesions 316

    III. Neoplasms 318

    IV. Congenital Anomalies in the Pediatric Patient 319

    V. Developmental Defects of the External Genitalia (Ambiguous Genitalia) 320

    VI. Normal and Abnormal Pubertal Development 321

    VII. Special Problems of the Adolescent 324

31 Menopause 330
ANN L. STEINER

    I. Definitions 330

    II. Physiology of Perimenopause 330

    III. Physiology of Menopause 331

    IV. Clinical Manifestations of Perimenopause 333

    V. Clinical Manifestations of Menopause 335

    VI. Hormone Therapy 339

    VII. Recommendations for Care of the Menopausal Woman 341

32 Family Planning: Contraception and Complications 346
COURTNEY A. SCHREIBER

    I. Contraceptive Efficacy 346

    II. Barrier Methods 346

    III. Intrauterine Devices 347

    IV. Progestin-Only Methods 349

    V. Combination Oral Contraceptive Pills 350

    VI. Other Combination Hormonal Methods 352

    VII. Emergency Contraception 353

    VIII. Natural Family Planning 354

    IX. Surgical Sterilization 355

33 Sexually Transmitted Diseases 358
ANN HONEBRINK

    I. Introduction 358

    II. Bacterial Sexually Transmitted Diseases 358

    III. Syphilis 363

IV.   Viral Sexually Transmitted Diseases 365

V.   Trichomoniasis 369

VI.   Ectoparasites 370

34   Pelvic Inflammatory Disease 375
ANN HONEBRINK

I.   Introduction 375

II.   Definitions 375

III.   Epidemiology 375

IV.   Bacteriology 376

V.   Pathophysiology 377

VI.   Diagnosis 377

VII.   Treatment 379

VIII. Other Causes of Pelvic Infection 381

35   Intimate Partner Violence and Sexual Assault 386
JANICE B. ASHER

I.   Relationship Violence 386

II.   Violence in Pregnancy 387

III.   Sexual Assault 388

IV.   Acquaintance Rape and Dating Violence 390

36   Benign Breast Disease 394
DAHLIA M. SATALOFF

I.   Introduction 394

II.   Breast Pain 394

III.   Nipple Discharge 395

IV.   Breast Mass 396

37   Vulvovaginitis 400
MICHELLE VICHNIN

I.   Introduction 400

II.   Vulvovaginal Anatomy 400

III.   Vaginal Physiology 402

IV.   Diagnosis 403

V.   Physical Examination 403

VI.   Vulvovaginal Conditions (see Table 37-1) 404

38   Disorders of the Pelvic Floor 414
LILY ARYA

I.   Introduction 414

II.   Pelvic Organ Prolapse (also called pelvic relaxation) 415

III.   Urinary Incontinence 416

IV.   Fecal Incontinence 418

39   Pelvic Malignancies 423
CHRISTINA S. CHU

I.   Cervical Cancer 423

II.   Endometrial Cancer 427

III.   Epithelial Ovarian Cancer 429

IV.   Nonepithelial Ovarian Cancer 432

V.   Vaginal Cancer 434

VI.   Vulvar Carcinoma 435

40 **Medicolegal Considerations in Obstetrics and Gynecology** **440**
LUIGI MASTROIANNI, JR.

I.   Introduction 440

II.   Malpractice 440

III.   Preconception Issues 440

IV.   Genetic Counseling 442

V.   Termination of Pregnancy 443

VI.   Reproductive Technologies 443

VII.   Birth-Related Suits 444

VIII.   Birth Injury 445

IX.   Informed Consent 445

Index **449**

NMS *Obstetrics and Gynecology*

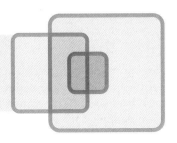

chapter **1**

Endocrinology of Pregnancy

SAMUEL PARRY • DOMINIC MARCHIANO

I INTRODUCTION

Endocrine changes in pregnancy are largely dependent on the concerted production of protein and steroid hormones by the fetoplacental unit. These endocrine changes support the successful establishment, maintenance, and completion of pregnancy.

A Endocrine changes during pregnancy. The most important endocrine changes involve the production of **protein hormones (human chorionic gonadotropin [hCG]** and **human placental lactogen [hPL])** and **steroid hormones (estrogen** and **progesterone).** Levels of hormones in pregnant women differ from those in nonpregnant women because of the presence of:

1. A **placenta,** which has a diverse secretory repertoire that surpasses that of any other endocrine organ.

2. A **fetus,** whose endocrine structures (e.g., pituitary gland, thyroid, adrenal cortex, pancreas, and gonads) function as early as the 11th week of pregnancy.
   a. In the **male fetus,** the testes, in response to placental gonadotropin, produce testosterone, which is necessary for normal male development.
   b. In the **female fetus,** although the ovaries are responsive to placental gonadotropins, normal development is not dependent on the production of fetal ovarian steroids. The ovaries in the fetus produce small but progressively greater amounts of estrogen.

3. **Increased levels of circulating estrogens,** which have the following effects:
   a. To increase the maternal hepatic production of binding proteins such as **thyroid-binding globulin (TBG)** and **cortisol-binding globulin (CBG)**
      (1) These proteins bind **thyroxine** and **cortisol** and raise their total levels in the maternal circulation.
      (2) However, the free fraction changes little. Thus, the metabolic processes that are dependent on these hormones usually are unaltered.
   b. To inhibit maternal pituitary gonadotropin synthesis and release, thus making placental gonadotropins primarily responsible for gonadotropic function
   c. To enhance placental production of **11β-hydroxysteroid dehydrogenase** (11β-HSD), which inactivates maternal cortisol, thereby isolating the fetal pituitary and adrenal from maternal influences

B Significant characteristics of hormones during pregnancy

1. **Chemical nature**
   a. **Protein hormones** (e.g., hCG, hPL, prolactin)
   b. **Steroids** (e.g., progesterone, estrogen, fetal adrenal steroids)

2. **Source**
   a. The **mother** is the exclusive source of certain hormones (such as estrogen and progesterone) early in pregnancy.
   b. By the end of the first trimester, the **fetus** and **placenta** are important sources of sex steroids and protein hormones.
      (1) The **fetus** produces thyroid hormones, pituitary tropic hormones, and gonadal steroids.

(2) The **placenta** secretes large quantities of estrogen and progesterone along with many releasing and inhibiting hormones, including **gonadotropin-releasing hormone (GnRH)**, **corticotropin-releasing hormone (CRH)**, and **thyrotropin-releasing hormone (TRH)**.

c. Occasionally, hormones have multiple sources. For example, the mother, the placenta, and the fetus all produce estradiol.

3. **Secretion patterns.** Recognizing normal patterns of hormone activity throughout pregnancy can help distinguish abnormal pregnancies and fetal compromise.

4. **Biologic functions.** Understanding the function of a particular hormone may illuminate its role in reproductive physiology, particularly in maintaining pregnancy and fetal well-being. For example, it is possible to correct hormone deficiencies that are harmful in pregnancy with the use of exogenous hormones, and the presence of certain hormones may serve as markers for gestational abnormalities. Although deficiencies in estriol or hPL late in gestation have been correlated with fetal growth restriction and fetal demise, obstetricians are advised to use more traditional methods of monitoring to document fetal well-being.

   a. **Unusually high levels of hCG** suggest a trophoblastic neoplasm, because hCG originates in trophoblastic tissue.

   b. **Progesterone deficiency** early in pregnancy suggests corpus luteum insufficiency, because progesterone is produced by the corpus luteum in early pregnancy.

II ▪ HUMAN CHORIONIC GONADOTROPIN

A Chemical nature. hCG is a glycoprotein composed of two subunits, α and β, that are noncovalently linked.

1. The α-subunit of hCG is biochemically identical to the α-subunit in pituitary gonadotropins (follicle-stimulating hormone [FSH] and luteinizing hormone [LH]) and thyroid-stimulating hormone (TSH).

2. The β-subunit of hCG is similar to the β-subunit of LH, differing by only 30 amino acids.

B Source

1. hCG is almost exclusively the product of the trophoblastic tissue, specifically the syncytiotrophoblast.

2. hCG is produced by normal placental tissue as early as 6 to 8 days postconception.

C Secretion patterns

1. Normally, hCG is detected in the maternal serum only after implantation of the pregnancy has occurred, which is approximately 7 days after conception. The level of hCG then rises rapidly, doubling every 2 to 3 days until approximately 6 weeks' gestation, at which point the rate of rise slows. The hCG level reaches a peak at approximately 9 to 10 weeks' gestation, after which the level declines to a plateau and remains detectable throughout the remainder of the pregnancy.

   a. **Significance of abnormally high levels** of hCG
      (1) Multiple placentas (multiple gestation)
      (2) Hydatidiform mole by virtue of trophoblastic proliferation
      (3) Choriocarcinoma
   b. **Significance of abnormally low levels** of hCG
      (1) Ectopic pregnancy
      (2) Miscarriage

2. Detection of hCG in the serum or urine is the basis of **contemporary pregnancy tests**.
   a. **Serum hCG assays** are the most sensitive test and are able to detect pregnancy within 8 to 12 days of ovulation (after the embryo has implanted).
   b. **Urine hCG assays** are not as sensitive, but can still detect hCG within 14 days of ovulation.

3. After delivery at term, hCG can normally be detected in the maternal serum or urine for up to 4 weeks.

4. After first-trimester miscarriage or elective termination of pregnancy, hCG can be detected in the maternal serum or urine for as long as 10 weeks.

D Biologic functions

1. Signals the ovary to **maintain the corpus luteum** and continue progesterone production

2. Regulates **fetal testicular testosterone production**, which is critical in the development of male external genitalia

3. Possesses some TSH-like properties and can cause hyperthyroidism when present in high levels (as in trophoblastic neoplasms)

4. **Clinical uses**
   a. **Assessment of viability of pregnancy**
      (1) Serial quantitative serum hCG levels can be followed in early pregnancy to determine if the pregnancy is progressing normally. If the hCG level plateaus prior to 6 weeks' gestation, then an abnormal pregnancy is suspected.
      (2) Quantitative serum hCG values may be correlated with transvaginal ultrasound findings. When the serum hCG value exceeds 2000 mIU/mL, an intrauterine pregnancy should be visible on transvaginal ultrasound; otherwise, ectopic pregnancy is suspected.
   b. **Multiple marker screen**
      (1) First-trimester screen, in the form of ultrasound for nuchal translucency (NT) plus biochemical markers such as pregnancy-associated plasma protein A (PAPP-A) and free β-HCG, have a detection rate for Down syndrome of 84%.
      (2) In the second trimester, the quadruple screen, consisting of **maternal serum hCG** in conjunction with **α-fetoprotein (αFP**, the primary serum protein in fetuses before midgestation), **inhibin-A** (another peptide produced by the placenta), and unconjugated **estriol**, is used in the prenatal diagnosis of fetal chromosomal abnormalities (see Chapter 4).
         (a) It allows detection of approximately 81% of fetuses with Down syndrome.
         (b) During the second trimester, elevated hCG is the most sensitive serum marker for Down syndrome.
   c. **Observing patients with trophoblastic neoplasia.** hCG determinations are used to follow the course of patients treated for this condition.

III HUMAN PLACENTAL LACTOGEN

A **Chemical nature.** hPL, or **human chorionic somatomammotropin (hCS)**, is a nonglycosylated protein hormone.

B **Source.** hPL is formed by the placenta as early as 3 weeks postconception and is secreted by the syncytiotrophoblast.

C **Secretory patterns.** hPL can be detected in maternal serum as early as 6 weeks postconception. Like most hormones produced by the syncytiotrophoblast, hPL is secreted primarily into the maternal bloodstream. hPL levels rise in maternal serum until 34 weeks' gestation and then plateau.

D Biologic function

1. **Diabetogenic effect of pregnancy.** hPL induces lipolysis and **increases maternal free fatty acids**, ketones, and glycerol, which provide energy for the mother.
   a. In the fed state, free fatty acids **interfere with insulin-directed entry of glucose into cells.**
   b. In the fasting state, ketones can cross the placenta and serve as fuel for the fetus.
   c. However, hPL does not appear to be responsible for acute changes in maternal lipolysis and glycemic control. Therefore, the integrated role of hPL in modulating maternal metabolism is probably chronic.

2. **Increased insulin levels.** hPL **raises plasma insulin** by up-regulating pancreatic islet function.

3. **Clinical use.** Although early studies have shown that low maternal serum levels of hPL are associated with fetal growth restriction and nonreassuring fetal heart rate patterns, subsequent studies have been unable to substantiate the value of hPL monitoring for detecting fetal complications secondary to uteroplacental insufficiency.

IV PROLACTIN

A Chemical nature. Prolactin is a protein hormone that circulates in different molecular sizes.

B Source. The **three potential sources** of prolactin during pregnancy are the:

1. Anterior lobe of the maternal pituitary gland, which is the primary source of elevated maternal serum prolactin levels.

2. Anterior lobe of the fetal pituitary gland.

3. Decidual tissue of the uterus, from which prolactin is secreted primarily into the amniotic fluid but can elevate the maternal serum level.

C Secretory patterns

1. In the nonpregnant state, prolactin levels normally range between 8 and 25 ng/mL.

2. In pregnancy, maternal prolactin levels increase under the influence of estrogen to a maximum of 200 ng/mL in the third trimester.

3. Levels of prolactin in pregnancy should not be interpreted as indicative of pituitary adenoma growth. However, women with prolactin-secreting adenomas who conceive should be monitored by visual field determinations for the possibility of enlargement.

D Biologic function

1. **Preparing the mammary glands for lactation**
   a. Stimulates the growth of mammary tissue.
   b. Stimulates production and secretion of milk into the alveoli. Lactation does not occur during pregnancy because estrogen inhibits the action of prolactin on the breast.

2. Decidual prolactin is thought to be important for fluid and electrolyte regulation of the amniotic fluid.

V PROGESTERONE

A Chemical nature. Progesterone is a **21-carbon steroid** hormone.

B Source. **All steroid hormones are derived from cholesterol.**

1. In **nonpregnant women, progesterone is produced by all steroid-forming glands**, including the ovaries, testes, and adrenal cortex. It serves as an intermediary for other hormones (e.g., aldosterone, cortisol, estrogen, and testosterone) and as an end-product when it is produced by the corpus luteum.

2. In the **pregnant state, progesterone has a dual source**. It is produced by the **corpus luteum** until the seventh to tenth week of pregnancy; then the **placenta** assumes its production until parturition.
   a. This **shift in production** occurs at approximately the **eighth week of pregnancy**, after which the corpus luteum becomes an insignificant source of progesterone.
   b. This point has **clinical significance**, because progesterone produced by the corpus luteum is essential for pregnancy maintenance until the eighth week. Consequently, progesterone suppositories are generally prescribed to women with suspected corpus luteum deficiency for the first 8 to 10 weeks of gestation.

3. The human placenta operates in close communication with the developing fetus (i.e., **fetal adrenal cortex, fetal liver**) in the biosynthesis and actions of all steroid hormones (Fig. 1-1). In the placenta, cholesterol is metabolized to **pregnenolone**, which is converted to progesterone and not metabolized to other steroids.

C Secretory patterns

1. Because progesterone originates initially from the corpus luteum, it is present at ovulation. In a nonconception cycle, the peak production of progesterone reaches 25 mg/day, and levels measure approximately 20 to 25 ng/mL in peripheral blood.

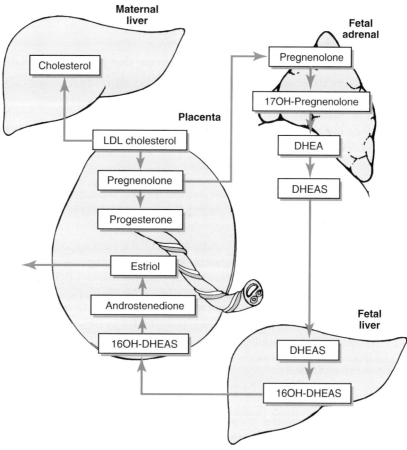

FIGURE 1–1 Schematic representation of estrogen and progesterone synthesis in late pregnancy. DHEA, dehydroepiandrosterone; DHEAS, DHEA sulfate; LDL, low-density lipoprotein.

2. In the late luteal phase in a conception cycle, progesterone levels increase slowly because of hCG stimulation.

3. As placental progesterone supplements corpus luteal progesterone, levels increase more rapidly.

4. Progesterone concentrations in the blood continue to increase up until the time of parturition, at which time the placenta produces 300 mg/day; most of the progesterone produced enters the maternal circulation.

5. Progesterone is produced in larger quantities in the presence of multiple gestation.

D **Biologic functions.** The primary function of progesterone is to **support pregnancy**.

1. It **prepares the endometrium for implantation of the embryo**.

2. It **relaxes the myometrium**.
   a. Progesterone suppresses the calcium–calmodulin–myosin light chain kinase system in smooth muscle.
   b. These effects of progesterone appear to be receptor mediated and can be blocked by the progesterone receptor antagonist **mifepristone (RU486)**, which is used as an abortifacient in the first trimester.

3. It **prevents rejection of the fetus** by the maternal immune system. Specifically, progesterone suppresses lymphocyte production of cytolytic cytokines.

VI ESTROGENS

A Chemical nature

1. Estrogens are **18-carbon steroid hormones that possess an aromatic ring**.
2. Three classic estrogens differ by the number of hydroxyl groups they contain:
    a. **Estrone**, a relatively weak estrogen, has one hydroxyl group.
    b. **Estradiol**, the most potent estrogen, contains two hydroxyl groups.
    c. **Estriol**, a very weak estrogen, contains three hydroxyl groups. Estriol is produced in extremely large quantities by the placenta during pregnancy.

B Source

1. **Role of fetal adrenal glands**. Because the placenta cannot convert pregnenolone to androgens, the fetal adrenal cortex is the primary provider of the immediate **androgen precursors of placental estrogens**.
2. **Production**. Estriol accounts for 80% of the estrogen produced during pregnancy. Its synthesis involves integration of metabolic steps in the mother, the placenta, and the fetus (see Fig. 1-1). Estrogens cannot be produced in the **placenta** due to a lack of the enzyme necessary to convert pregnenolone to androgen precursors. The **fetal adrenal cortex** converts pregnenolone to dehydroepiandrosterone (DHEA) and DHEA sulfate (DHEAS), which is then converted to 16-OH DHEAS in the **fetal liver**. 16-OH DHEAS is then converted to androgen precursors and aromatized to estrogen in the **placenta**.

C Secretory patterns

1. The estrone:estradiol:estriol ratio produced by the placenta is approximately 14:5:81. Estradiol is largely bound to sex hormone–binding globulin in the maternal serum, whereas **estriol remains unbound**. Therefore, estriol is more rapidly excreted in the urine, and maternal serum levels of estriol and estradiol are similar.
2. Early in pregnancy, estradiol is the major form of estrogen produced by the maternal ovaries.
3. Later in pregnancy, estrone and estradiol are produced primarily by the placenta; estriol is produced almost exclusively by the placenta.
4. Significant amounts of estriol are produced early in the second trimester, and levels continue to rise until parturition, increasing 1000-fold over the nonpregnant levels.
5. **Extremely low levels or no estriol** may be associated with:
    a. Fetal demise.
    b. **Anencephaly**. The **limited adrenocorticotropic hormone (ACTH) production** results in atrophy of the fetal zone of the adrenal cortex after 20 weeks' gestation.
    c. Maternal ingestion of corticosteroids. However, placental 11β-HSD limits the transfer of cortisol to the fetus.
    d. **Placental sulfatase deficiency**.

D Biologic activities. Because placental estrogen formation is dependent on androgenic precursors produced by the fetal adrenal cortex, the fetus appears to be ultimately responsible for many of the maternal physiologic effects mediated by estrogen.

1. Estrogen **stimulates** receptor-mediated **low-density lipoprotein (LDL) uptake by the placenta** and placental expression of enzymes that are important in steroidogenesis.
2. Estrogen **increases blood flow to the uterus**.
    a. Effects are mediated in part by prostanoids.
    b. Effects are tonic and do not elicit acute changes in blood flow.
3. **Estrogen regulates end-of-gestation events**.
    a. **Parturition**. Estrogen activates oxytocin secretion and myometrial gap junction formation. Consequently, maternal salivary estriol levels have been used to predict preterm birth. Conversely, **labor and delivery may be delayed in anencephalic fetuses and fetuses with placental sulfatase deficiency**.

    b. Lactation. Estrogen stimulates epithelial cell proliferation in human breast tissue. However, milk release is delayed until estrogen levels decrease after delivery.

4. Because estriol is an index of normal function of the fetus and the placenta, **reduced maternal estriol levels may reflect abnormalities in fetal or placental development.**

    a. Conditions that may occur include fetal demise, hypertensive disease during pregnancy, preeclampsia and eclampsia, and intrauterine growth retardation.

    b. When estriol levels are reduced below normal or fail to increase during pregnancy, fetal and placental well-being may be studied by supplemental tests, including ultrasonography, fetal heart rate testing, and biophysical profile.

Study Questions for Chapter 1

Directions: *Each of the numbered items or incomplete statements in this section is followed by answers or by completions of the statement. Select the ONE lettered answer or completion that is BEST in each case.*

1. A 26-year-old female presents to the emergency room complaining of severe right lower quadrant pain. She is immediately taken to the operating room for presumed appendicitis. At the time of her surgery her appendix is normal. The surgeon sees a large mass on the right ovary and removes the ovary. Frozen section on the mass shows a corpus luteum. Immediately after the surgery her pregnancy test is found to be positive. She is, by dates 6 weeks pregnant. You are called as the consulting gynecologist. Your main concern is the following:

- [A] The hCG level should double over the next 2 days since she is 6 weeks pregnant
- [B] Having one ovary will affect her ability to produce hormones
- [C] Removing the corpus luteum will affect the pregnancy
- [D] Estrogen production will not be affected
- [E] She could still have an ectopic pregnancy

2. A 36-year-old woman, gravida 3, para 2, at 8 weeks' gestation, presents to your clinic reporting painless vaginal bleeding. Her vital signs are as follows: T = 99.9, BP = 162/94, P = 100, and R = 18. Her uterus is consistent with a 14-week pregnancy. Her serum hCG level is 320,000 IU/L. Which of the following endocrine glands is most likely to be affected by hCG?

- [A] Adrenal cortex
- [B] Hypothalamus
- [C] Ovary
- [D] Parathyroid
- [E] Thyroid

3. A 29-year-old woman who is pregnant calls you for advice. She has just found out that her hCG level is elevated. Which of the following is true?

- [A] hCG can stimulate production of TRH, causing hyperthyroidism
- [B] A high level of hCG is indicative of an ectopic pregnancy
- [C] A high level of hCG in the second trimester is indicative of molar pregnancy
- [D] A high level of hCG in the second trimester is the most sensitive marker for Down syndrome
- [E] hCG is part of the quadruple screen in the first trimester

4. Estrogens are produced by the mother, fetus, and placenta. Which one of the following is true?

- [A] Estradiol accounts for 80% of the estrogen produced during pregnancy
- [B] Estriol is produced primarily by the placenta
- [C] Anencephaly is associated with a normal level of estriol
- [D] Estrogen suppresses oxcytocin secretion
- [E] Estrone accounts for 80% of the estrogen produced during pregnancy

QUESTIONS 5–15

For each of the following questions, match the hormone with the description that best fits. Answer choices can be used once, more than once, or not at all.

- [A] hCG
- [B] hPL
- [C] Prolactin
- [D] Progesterone
- [E] Estriol

5. Increases myometrial gap junction formation

6. Suppresses maternal lymphocyte activity

7. Necessary for development of male external genitalia

8. Most sensitive marker for abnormal karyotype

9. Elevates ketone levels

10. Produced by the uterus

11. Inhibits lactation during pregnancy

12. Lack of this hormone can cause spontaneous abortion in the first trimester

13. Lack of this hormone is associated with an enzyme deficiency in the placenta

14. Elevated levels of this hormone are associated with twin pregnancy

15. Anencephaly causes lack of production of this hormone

Answers and Explanations

1. The answer is C [V B 2]. Removing the corpus luteum at this early stage of pregnancy will have an adverse effect on the pregnancy because until 8 weeks of gestation the pregnancy is dependent on the production of progesterone from the corpus luteum for support. Progesterone supplementation should be initiated to support the pregnancy. At this gestation the hCG level no longer doubles every 2 days. The rate of rise slows. It is unlikely that she has an ectopic pregnancy since no abnormalities were seen at laparoscopy. Having one ovary will not affect her hormonal production. Estrogen production from the corpus luteum will be affected since the corpus luteum has been removed.

2. The correct answer is E [II D 3]. The clinical scenario (i.e., vaginal bleeding, early pregnancy-induced hypertension, enlarged uterus, and exaggerated β-hCG levels) is consistent with a molar pregnancy. Because of morphologic similarities between hCG and TSH (the α-subunit is homologous to the α-subunit of TSH), hCG possesses TSH-like properties and can cause hyperthyroidism. The other endocrine glands are not affected by a molar pregnancy.

3. The answer is D [II D 4]. A high level of hCG in the second trimester is the most sensitive marker for Down syndrome. A high level of hCG in the first trimester is suggestive of molar pregnancy. hCG is part of the quadruple screen in the second trimester, not the first trimester. A low level of hCG is suggestive of ectopic pregnancy. hCG stimulates production of TSH, not TRH, leading to hyperthyroidism.

4. The correct answer is B [IV C 3]. Estriol is produced primarily by the placenta. Estriol accounts for 80% of the estrogen produced during pregnancy. Anencephaly is associated with a decreased level of estriol. Estrogen increases oxytocin secretion to allow breastfeeding.

The answers are **5-E** [VI D 3 a], **6-D** [V D 3], **7-A** [II D 2], **8-A** [II D 4c (2)], **9-B** [III D 1 b], **10-C** [IV B 3], **11-E** [IV D 1 b], **12-D** [V B 2 b], **13-E** [VI C 7 d], **14-A** [II C 1 a (1)], **15-E** [VI C 7 b].

Estrogen activates oxytocin secretion and myometrial gap junction formation. Progesterone suppresses production of maternal lymphocytic cytokines, which contribute to immune rejection of the fetus. hCG regulates fetal testicular testosterone production, which is critical for the development of male external genitalia. Elevated hCG is the most sensitive serum marker for Down syndrome. hPL induces lipolysis, which provides energy for the mother in the form of fatty acids. hPL also provides energy for the fetus by elevating ketone levels. Prolactin is produced not only by the decidual tissue of the uterus, but also by the maternal and fetal pituitary glands. Lactation does not occur during pregnancy because estrogen inhibits the action of prolactin on the breast. Progesterone produced by the corpus luteum is essential for pregnancy maintenance until the eighth week. Progesterone suppositories are prescribed during the first 8 weeks of gestation in women with suspected corpus luteum deficiency. Low levels of estriol are associated with placental sulfatase deficiency. Abnormally high levels of hCG are seen in multiple gestation (twins). Anencephaly contributes to lack of ACTH production; therefore, the fetal adrenal cortex is not stimulated properly to convert pregnenolone to DHEA and DHEAS, which are essential in the production of estriol.

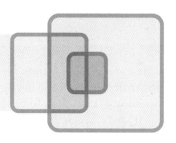

chapter 2

Fetal Physiology

SERDAR URAL

INTRODUCTION

The normal growth and development of the fetus depends on the successful integration of the functions of the placenta, umbilical cord, amniotic fluid, and fetal organ systems.

II   PLACENTA

A Structure

1. **Villi**
   a. These structures, the functioning units of the placenta, are formed by invading placental tissue (trophoblast) and contain the terminal fetal capillaries of the umbilical arteries.
   b. The villi are surrounded by the intervillous space into which maternal blood from the decidual (uterine) arteries is forced by maternal arterial pressure.
   c. Gases and nutrients pass **from the maternal blood** in the intervillous space, across the plasma membrane of the trophoblast to the basement membrane of the fetal capillary, and then through the single endothelial cell layer of the fetal capillary **to the fetal blood**. The fetal capillaries drain into the fetal veins that join to form the umbilical vein. Maternal blood drains from the intervillous space into the maternal veins.

2. **Placental cotyledons (lobes)** are formed from the branching villi supplied by one terminal arterial branch and its partner venous branch of the fetal umbilical vessels. On average, about 20 cotyledons make up the fetal side of the placenta. The maternal side of the placenta is divided by septa into lobes.

B Function.   The placenta transfers nutrition and oxygen from the mother to the fetus, removes metabolic waste products from the fetus to be eliminated by the mother, and synthesizes proteins and hormones that support fetal development and important maternal physiologic changes.

1. **Mother-to-fetus transfer of nutrients**
   a. The essential substances for growth and development move from the mother to the fetus in four ways:
      (1) **Active transport**: amino acids, calcium
      (2) **Facilitated transport**: glucose
      (3) **Endocytosis**: cholesterol, insulin, iron, immunoglobulin G (IgG)
      (4) **Sodium pumps and chloride channels**: ions
   b. Solute size and lipid solubility are also important factors that influence transport.

2. **Gas exchange**. This process involves supplying oxygen to the fetus and removing carbon dioxide from the fetus.

3. **Secretion** of proteins and steroid hormones (see Chapter 1)
   a. **Progesterone** is produced by the placenta from maternal cholesterol, is secreted into the maternal circulation, and is important for maintaining pregnancy.
   b. **Estrogen** is converted from circulating fetal androgens (dehydroepiandrosterone sulfate [DHEAS]) produced in the fetal adrenal glands. Estrogen plays an important role in maternal physiologic changes in pregnancy, labor, and lactation.

   c. Numerous **proteins, peptides,** and **growth factors** are produced in the placenta. They are important for placental growth, fetal growth and development, and the maternal physiologic changes necessary to ensure adequate nutrition to the fetus.

   4. **Immunology**. Invading placental cells express a unique antigen, HLA-G, which is not recognized as a "foreign" antigen by the mother. Other unique antigens and local immune suppression contribute to the prevention of rejection of the fetal–placental unit.

C **Metabolism.** Glucose is the primary substrate for placental aerobic metabolism.

III UMBILICAL CORD

A **Umbilical arteries.** Two umbilical arteries originate from the fetal aorta. They supply fetal blood to all portions of the placenta for gas and solute exchange. A single umbilical artery is associated with low birth weight and chromosomal anomalies in some infants.

B **Umbilical vein.** One umbilical vein returns nutrient-rich, oxygen-rich blood to the fetus.

IV AMNIOTIC MEMBRANES AND FLUID

A **Membranes**

   1. **Amnion**. The amnion is a single layer of epithelial cells surrounding the fetus and containing the amniotic fluid.

   2. **Chorion**. The chorion, which lies adjacent to the uterine endometrium, is exterior and fused to the amnion.

B **Fluid**

   1. Fetal lung fluid appears to be important for the successful development of the bronchial tree, but the amniotic fluid volume derives primarily from the fetal urine.

   2. Early in gestation, the fluid surrounding the embryo is probably transudative. By the second trimester, the fetal lungs and kidneys produce the amniotic fluid. Fluid resorption mainly results from fetal swallowing. Fluid volume increases with increasing gestational age until the middle of the third trimester, after which the volume stays stable and may decrease somewhat at term.

V FETUS

A **Metabolism.** Fetal metabolism is primarily oxidative. Normal metabolism is necessary to maintain the normal function of existing tissue and to support the acquisition of new tissue.

   1. **Requirements**
     a. **Glucose**. The principal sugar in fetal blood is glucose; it is a major nutrient for growth and energy in the fetus. The maternal blood (via the placenta) is the source of fetal glucose, and the fetal glucose level is determined by the maternal level.
     b. **Oxygen**. Fetal oxygen consumption is approximately 8 mL/kg/min compared to an adult oxygen consumption of about 3/mL/kg/min.
     c. **Amino acids**. The fetus synthesizes protein from amino acids from maternal blood.

   2. **Hormones important for fetal growth**. Hormones produced in the fetus, placenta, and mother function together to promote the growth and development of the fetus.
     a. **Human placental lactogen (hPL)** or **human chorionic somatomammotropin (hCS)**. This maternal hormone increases resistance to insulin and blocks the peripheral uptake and use of glucose by maternal tissues, allowing placental transfer of glucose to the fetus.
     b. **Insulin**. The fetus produces its own insulin.
     c. **Insulin-like growth factors I and II, human placental growth hormone, and other growth factors**. Growth factors produced in the placenta are responsible for the regulation of cell proliferation and cell differentiation in the fetus.

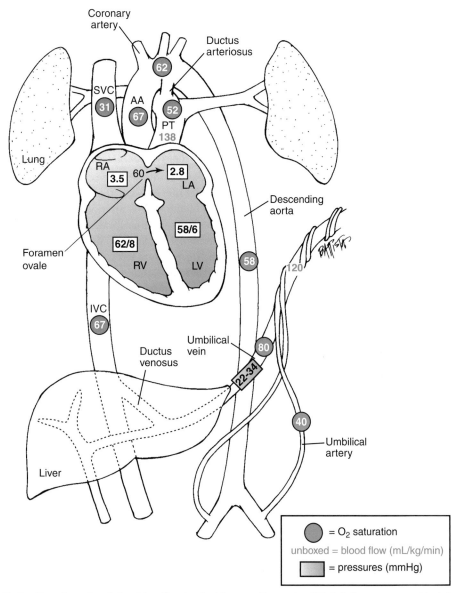

FIGURE 2–1 Hemodynamics of the fetus (in utero). AA, ascending aorta; IVC, inferior vena cava; LA, left atrium; LV, left ventricle; PT, pulmonary trunk; RA, right atrium; RV, right ventricle; SVC, superior vena cava.

B **Organ systems**

1. **Cardiovascular**

   a. **Unique features of the fetal circulation** (Fig. 2-1)

   (1) **Umbilical vein.** The umbilical vein carries oxygenated, nutrient-rich blood from the placenta to the fetus. The umbilical vein gives off branches to the liver and becomes the ductus venosus.

   (2) **Ductus venosus.** The ductus venosus brings oxygenated blood from the placenta to the inferior vena cava. Blood from the portal vein flows into the ductus venosus, thereby decreasing the overall oxygen content of the blood entering the inferior vena cava. Thus, blood flowing into the right ventricle is not as well oxygenated as blood coming directly from the placenta.

   (3) **Foramen ovale.** The foramen ovale is a right-to-left intracardiac (atrial) shunt. Well-oxygenated blood carried by the inferior vena cava from the ductus venosus streams

preferentially across the foramen ovale into the left atrium and then to the left ventricle, brain, and upper body. Less oxygenated blood returning from the systemic circulation also forms a stream in the inferior vena cava that joins blood from the superior vena cava to flow preferentially across the tricuspid valve.

(4) Ductus arteriosus. Blood from the systemic circulation is delivered preferentially to the right ventricle. From the right ventricle, blood flows into the pulmonary artery. The ductus arteriosus connects the left pulmonary artery to the arch of the aorta.

   (a) The high vascular resistance in the fetal lungs is greater than the aortic pressure that diverts blood away from the lungs and into the ductus and the aorta. The umbilical arteries deliver the blood from the aorta to the placenta for gas exchange.

   (b) Prostaglandins, such as prostaglandin E, play a role in maintaining patency of the ductus arteriosus. Prostaglandin inhibitors promote closure of the ductus.

b. Circulatory adjustments to neonatal life. At birth, the lungs expand and pulmonary vascular resistance decreases. With closure of the ductus arteriosus, pulmonary blood flow increases. Right atrial pressure decreases, and the foramen ovale closes. The ductus arteriosus, ductus venosus, and umbilical vein are no longer patent and become known as the ligamentum arteriosum, ligamentum venosum, and ligamentum teres, respectively. The intra-abdominal portion of the umbilical arteries becomes the lateral umbilical ligaments.

c. Heart rate and cardiac output. Cardiac output of the fetal heart is 200 mL/kg/min, which is higher than the cardiac output of the adult (about 70 mL/kg/min). The cardiac output of the right ventricle is greater than that of the left ventricle (60% versus 40%), resulting in a right ventricular dominance. The normal fetal heart rate is 120 to 160 beats per minute.

d. Regulation of blood flow and pressures. The cardiovascular system is controlled by a complex integration of autonomic and hormonal effects. The stimulation of baroreceptors (by changes in blood flow) and chemoreceptors (by changes in oxygenation) is responsible for the initiation of autonomic reflexes and the secretion of hormones to coordinate the regulation of blood flow, pressure, and heart rate in the fetus.

2. Respiratory

a. The fetal lungs play no role in gas exchange. Oxygen and carbon dioxide are exchanged between fetal and maternal blood across the placenta. The partial pressure of oxygen in intervillous blood is lower in the fetus compared with the mother, which favorably influences the transfer of oxygen from maternal to fetal blood. Similarly, physiologic maternal respiratory changes result in a lower partial pressure of carbon dioxide in the maternal circulation, which favors the transfer of carbon dioxide from the fetus to the mother.

b. At about 34 weeks of gestation, the fetal lungs produce **surfactant**, a combination of glycerophospholipids, from the type II pneumocytes. Surfactant is essential for successful respiration because it lowers the surface tension in the alveoli to prevent alveolar collapse.

3. Gastrointestinal/hepatic

a. Although the fetus swallows amniotic fluid, gastrointestinal absorption is not a fetal source of nutrients. The fetal intestine absorbs water from the swallowed amniotic fluid.

b. Meconium is composed of intestinal tract secretions and desquamation of intestinal epithelial cells.

c. The fetal liver is the major source of fetal cholesterol.

d. The majority of unconjugated bilirubin is removed from the fetal circulation by the placenta, where it is transferred to the maternal circulation, conjugated by the maternal liver, and excreted. At term, fetal hepatic conjugation of bilirubin is relatively deficient, and a mild **hyperbilirubinemia** may be seen in the term neonate in the first few days of life.

4. Renal

a. Fetal urine production begins in the first trimester and is important for maintaining amniotic fluid volume as gestation advances.

b. Fetal urine is hypotonic.

c. Most ion exchange occurs in the placenta.

5. Hematologic

a. Hematopoiesis occurs in the yolk sac in the second week of gestation, in the liver and spleen in the fifth week, and in the bone marrow by the 11th week.

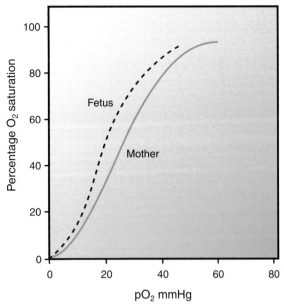

FIGURE 2–2 Comparison of the fetal and maternal hemoglobin dissociation curves. (Redrawn from Gabbe SG. Obstetrics: Normal and Problem Pregnancies. 4th Ed. New York: Churchill Livingstone, 2002:49.)

   b. Hemoglobin
      (1) The hemoglobin concentration is high in the term fetus (16 to 18 g/dL) compared to that in the mother.
      (2) Fetal hemoglobin is composed of two α- and two γ-globin chains. It differs from adult hemoglobin, which is composed of two α- and two β-globin chains.
      (3) Adult hemoglobin is found in the fetus by 12 weeks' gestation and increases with length of gestation. However, at term, 70% of the circulating hemoglobin is fetal hemoglobin.
      (4) Fetal hemoglobin has a high affinity for oxygen, resulting in an oxygen dissociation curve that is shifted to the left compared with that in adults (Fig. 2-2). Because of the high affinity of fetal hemoglobin for oxygen, fetal red blood cells efficiently extract oxygen from the maternal blood in the placenta.
   c. Erythropoietin originates in the fetal liver and is highest in utero.
  6. Endocrine (see Chapter 1)
   a. Thyroid gland. Adequate thyroid function is important for normal neurologic development. Thyroid function is detectable by the end of the first trimester and thyroxine levels steadily increase from midgestation until term.
   b. Adrenal gland. DHEAS is secreted by the fetal zone of the adrenal in response to stimulation by adrenocorticotropic hormone (ACTH) and human chorionic gonadotropin (hCG). The fetal adrenal gland also produces cortisol and catecholamines.

  C | **Immune system**

   1. Although the fetus produces macrophages and granulocytes, the cellular immunity of the fetus and neonate is not as active or efficient as adult cellular immunity. Similarly, the fetus cannot mount adult-level antibody responses to antigen stimulation.

   2. In response to infection, fetal IgM increases. In the absence of infection, fetal levels of IgA and IgM are much lower than adult levels.

   3. The majority of immunoglobulin found in the fetus is IgG and is due to transplacental passage from the mother. IgG is the only immunoglobulin isotype that crosses the placenta.

Study Questions for Chapter 2

Directions: *Each of the numbered items or incomplete statements in this section is followed by answers or by completions of the statement. Select the ONE lettered answer or completion that is BEST in each case.*

1. A 24-year-old woman, gravida 4, para 3, at 18 weeks' gestation dated by her last menstrual period, receives an ultrasound to confirm her "due date" and to evaluate fetal anatomy. Her first pregnancy was complicated by delivery of an infant with spina bifida. Her other two pregnancies were uncomplicated. After confirmation of her gestational age using biparietal diameter, abdominal circumference, and femur length data, you scan the fetal ductus venosus. Using ultrasound, which structure would you see leading <u>into</u> and <u>out of</u> the ductus venosus, respectively?

- A Pulmonary artery; aorta
- B Inferior vena cava; portal vein
- C Umbilical vein; portal vein
- D Portal vein; inferior vena cava
- E Right atrium; left atrium

2. A 37-year-old woman, gravida 1, para 1, just delivered at term a viable male infant weighing 3980 grams with APGARs (American Pediatric Gross Assessment Records) of 9 and 9 at 1 and 5 minutes, respectively. Delivery was via spontaneous vaginal delivery without any complications. After clamping of the umbilical cord, the baby takes his first breath. Which event(s) is/are directly responsible for the most efficient oxygenation of blood inside the lungs?

- A Closure of foramen ovale
- B Closure of ductus arteriosus
- C Closure of foramen ovale and ductus arteriosus
- D Closure of umbilical vein and artery
- E Closure of ligamentum arteriosum and ligamentum teres

3. You are listening to a discussion between two medical students about fetal oxygen consumption and fetal cardiac output. The first student claims that the fetal cardiac output is at least two times that of the adult cardiac output since the average heart rate in the fetus is 140 beats per minutes (two times an adult heart beat). The second student claims that the fetal oxygen consumption is probably half of adult oxygen consumption because fetal hemoglobin has twice the affinity for oxygen than adult hemoglobin. The cardiac output and oxygen consumption in a fetus are approximately what multiple/fraction of that compared with an adult, respectively?

- A 2; 2
- B 3; 3
- C 1/2; 1/2
- D 1/3; 1/3
- E 2; 1/2

4. The most oxygenated blood is found in which part of the fetal circulation?

- A Ductus venosus
- B Portal vein
- C Inferior vena cava
- D Ductus arteriosus
- E Descending aorta

QUESTIONS 5–8

For each substance listed below, select its route of transfer across the placenta. Each answer choice may be used once, more than once, or not at all.

[A] Endocytosis
[B] Facilitated transport
[C] Passive diffusion
[D] Active transport
[E] Ion pumps

5. Glucose

6. Iron

7. Amino acids

8. Carbon dioxide

QUESTIONS 9–13

For each statement below, match the trimester during which the event occurs. Each answer can be used once, more than once, or not at all.

[A] First trimester
[B] Early second trimester (weeks 14 to 21)
[C] Late second trimester (weeks 22 to 28)
[D] Third trimester

9. Highest concentration of hemoglobin containing two α and two β chains

10. Amniotic fluid volume derived from transudation

11. Significant amniotic fluid volume contribution from the lung

12. Production of red blood cells by the spleen

13. Thyroxine levels first detectable in serum

Answers and Explanations

1. The answer is D [V B 1 a (2), 1 a (3)]. Oxygenated blood from the umbilical vein and deoxygenated blood from the portal vein flow into the ductus venosus, which connects to the inferior vena cava through the hepatic veins. From there, blood goes to the right atrium via the inferior vena cava. A large percentage of the oxygenated blood is shunted to the left atrium via the foramen ovale. A small percentage of blood from the inferior vena cava joins the deoxygenated blood from the superior vena cava and flows into the right ventricle. The right ventricle pumps blood via the pulmonary artery through the patent ductus arteriosus into the aorta because the lung is a high-resistance system in the fetus.

2. The answer is C [V B 1 b]. When the baby takes his first breath, resistance in the pulmonary vessel circuit is substantially reduced, and thus blood can flow through the pulmonary artery to the lungs (instead of to the aorta through the ductus arteriosus) to become oxygenated. This event also decreases the pressure in the right atrium, allowing closure of the foramen ovale. Both of these events are necessary for the most efficient oxygenation of blood (closure of the foramen ovale allows all of the blood returning to the heart to be oxygenated). Conditions such as atrial septal defect (ASD) do not allow for the most efficient oxygenation of blood returning to the heart because a small percentage of that deoxygenated blood is shunted to the left atrium and into systemic circulation instead of into the lungs to become oxygenated. The ligamentum arteriosum is the closed (nonpatent) ductus arteriosus, and the ligamentum teres is the closed (nonpatent) umbilical vein.

3. The answer is B [V A 1 b and V B 1 c]. Fetal cardiac output is approximately 200 mL/kg/min, whereas an average adult's cardiac output is 70 mL/kg/min. Fetal oxygen consumption is approximately 8 mL/kg/min, whereas adult oxygen consumption is approximately 3 mL/kg/min.

4. The answer is A [V B 1 a (2)]. The umbilical vein carries the most well-oxygenated blood from the placenta. The ductus venosus carries slightly less oxygen because it mixes with the portal venous blood. The inferior vena cava carries blood from both the ductus venosus and the systemic circulation; it therefore carries less oxygen overall than the ductus venosus. The ductus arteriosus and descending aorta receive blood returning from the systemic circulation and therefore have less oxygen than the other choices.

The answers are **5-B** [II B 1 a (2)], **6-A** [II B 1 a (3)], **7-D** [II B 1 a (1)], **8-C** [II B 2]. Glucose is transported across the placenta via facilitated transport. Iron is transported via endocytosis. Amino acids are transported via active transport. Carbon dioxide passively diffuses across the placenta.

The answers are **9-D** [V B 5 b (2)], **10-A** [IV B 2], **11-B** [IV B 2], **12-A** [V B 5 a], **13-A** [V B 6 a]. The highest concentration of adult hemoglobin is near term. However, even near term, fetal hemoglobin makes up the majority of circulating hemoglobin (almost 70%). Amniotic fluid is a transudative during early pregnancy. In the second trimester, the lung and the kidneys both contribute to amniotic fluid volume. The contribution of the kidney steadily increases until it is the major contributor of amniotic fluid volume by the end of the second trimester and in the third trimester. Hematopoiesis occurs in the yolk sac in the second week of gestation, in the liver and spleen in the fifth week, and in the bone marrow by the 11th week. Thyroid hormones are first detectable in serum near the end of the first trimester.

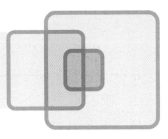

chapter 3

Normal Pregnancy, the Puerperium, and Lactation

PETER CHEN

I DIAGNOSIS OF PREGNANCY

A Presumptive symptoms

1. **Amenorrhea**. Amenorrhea, or the abrupt cessation of spontaneous, cyclic, and predictable menstruation, is strongly suggestive of pregnancy. Because ovulation can be late in any given cycle, the menses should be **at least 10 days late** before their absence is considered a reliable indication.

2. **Breast changes**. In very early pregnancy, women report tenderness and tingling in the breasts. Breast enlargement and nodularity are evident as early as the second month of pregnancy. The nipples and areolae enlarge and become more deeply pigmented.

3. **Nausea (with or without vomiting)**. The so-called **morning sickness of pregnancy** usually begins early in the day and lasts for several hours, although occasionally it persists longer and may occur at other times. Gastrointestinal disturbances begin at 4 to 6 weeks' gestation and usually last no longer than the first trimester. Excessive nausea and vomiting (i.e., **hyperemesis gravidarum**) can result in dehydration, weight loss, electrolyte imbalance, and the need for hospitalization; intravenous hyperalimentation may be indicated in severe cases.

4. **Disturbances in urination**. Early in pregnancy, the enlarging uterus puts pressure on the bladder, causing **frequent urination**. This condition improves as the uterus grows and moves up into the abdomen but returns late in pregnancy when the fetal head settles into the pelvis against the bladder.

5. **Fatigue**. Tiredness is one of the earliest symptoms of pregnancy. Fatigue usually persists into the second trimester; the need for sleep returns to normal by the 16th to 18th week.

6. **Sensation of fetal movement**. Between the 16th and 20th week after the last menstrual period (LMP), a woman begins to feel movement in the lower abdomen, described as a fluttering or gas bubbles. This is known as **quickening**.

B Clinical evidence

1. **Enlargement of the abdomen**. By the end of the 12th week of pregnancy, the uterus can be felt above the symphysis pubis. By the 20th week, the uterus should be at the level of the umbilicus. Between the 20th week and the 37th week, the fundal height in centimeters should correspond, within 2 cm, to the gestational age in weeks (Fig. 3-1).

2. **Uterine and cervical changes**. The uterus enlarges and softens early in pregnancy (at approximately 6 weeks' gestation), and lateral uterine vessel pulsations are palpable on vaginal examination. The softening between the cervix and the uterine fundus causes a sensation of separateness between these two structures (**Hegar sign**). The vaginal mucosa has a bluish color within the first 6 to 8 weeks of pregnancy (**Chadwick sign**).

3. **Endocrine tests for pregnancy**. These tests depend on **human chorionic gonadotropin (hCG)** levels in maternal plasma and excretion of hCG in the urine, which are identified by a number of immunoassays and bioassays. The presence of hCG can be demonstrated in maternal plasma by 8 to 9 days after ovulation.

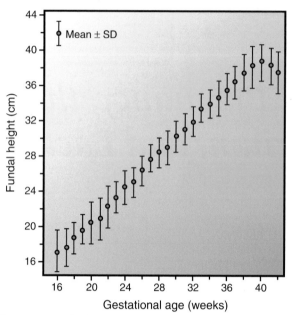

FIGURE 3–1 Fundal height versus gestational age. (Reprinted with permission from Gabbe SG. Obstetrics: Normal and Problem Pregnancies. 3rd Ed. New York: Churchill Livingstone, 1996:181.)

    a. Urine pregnancy tests detect the presence of hCG. This depends on the recognition of hCG or its β-subunit by an antibody to the hCG molecule or the β-subunit.

    b. Serum pregnancy tests detect the presence and quantify the β-subunit of hCG, thus allowing serial determinations to observe increases and decreases in the level of hCG. The serum test is more sensitive than the urine test.

C **Confirming the diagnosis of pregnancy**

    1. Identification of a heartbeat. The diagnosis of pregnancy is confirmed with the identification of the fetal heartbeat, which ranges from 120 to 160 beats per minute. The fetal heart can be identified by the 10th week with an ultrasonic fetal heart Doppler monitor and at 17 to 19 weeks by auscultation with a stethoscope.

    2. Ultrasonographic recognition of the fetus

        a. After 5 weeks of amenorrhea, an early **chorionic (gestational) sac** is visible as a small, fluid-filled structure surrounded by an echogenic rim of tissue on transvaginal ultrasound. The **embryo** is apparent within the gestational sac after 6 weeks of amenorrhea.

        b. Fetal heart activity is seen by real-time ultrasonography after 6 weeks of gestation. The normal heart rate may be as low as 90 beats per minute at 6 weeks and increases during the first trimester.

D **Pregnancy dating.** The **estimated date of confinement (EDC)**, or due date, is based on the assumption that a woman has a 28-day cycle, with ovulation on day 14 or 15. Pregnancy lasts for 280 days (40 weeks) from the LMP. The EDC is therefore 9 calendar months plus 7 days from the start of the LMP; it is customary to estimate the **EDC** by counting back 3 calendar months and adding 7 days to the LMP (**Naegele rule**). Because ovulation does not always occur at midcycle (the postovulatory phase in any cycle lasts for 14 days), the EDC must be adjusted accordingly. For example, ovulation in a woman with a 35-day cycle occurs on approximately day 21; therefore, the EDC in such a woman is later than that predicted by the Naegele rule (see Chapter 6 regarding ultrasound dating).

II   PREGNANCY

A **First trimester.** This period extends from the LMP through the first 12 to 13 weeks of pregnancy.

    1. Signs and symptoms

    a. Nausea
    b. Fatigue
    c. Breast tenderness
    d. Frequent urination
    e. Minimal abdominal enlargement (the uterus is still in the pelvis)

2. Bleeding occurs in the first trimester of approximately 25% of all pregnancies; spontaneous abortion occurs in 25% to 50% of these pregnancies. Uterine cramping with bleeding in the first trimester is more suggestive of impending abortion than either bleeding or cramping alone.

B **Second trimester.** This period extends from 14 weeks of pregnancy through 27 weeks of pregnancy.

1. Signs and symptoms
    a. General well-being. The second trimester is often the most comfortable time for a pregnant woman because the symptoms of the first trimester have disappeared, and the discomfort of the last trimester is not yet present.
    b. Pain. As the uterus grows, a certain amount of pulling and stretching of pelvic structures occurs. Round ligament pain, which results from the stretching of the round ligaments that are attached to the top of the uterus on each side and the corresponding lateral pelvic wall, is common.
    c. Contractions. Palpable uterine contractions (**Braxton Hicks contractions**) that are mild and irregular can begin during the second trimester.

2. Bleeding. A low-lying placenta that causes bleeding at this stage usually moves away from the cervix as the uterus grows.

3. Fetus. The fetus attains a size of almost 1000 g (more than 2 lb) by the 28th week.
    a. Motion. Quickening (see I A 6) begins between the 16th and 20th week.
    b. Viability. Infants born at the end of the second trimester have an 80% to 90% chance of survival. If death occurs, it is usually from respiratory distress due to lung immaturity.

4. Complications of second-trimester pregnancies include an incompetent cervix (i.e., painless dilation of the cervix in the second trimester). Resulting conditions include:
    a. Premature rupture of the membranes (PROM) can occur without labor or with an incompetent cervix and can result in serious bacterial infections in both the mother and fetus.
    b. Premature labor can occur without an incompetent cervix. When dilation or effacement of the cervix occurs, tocolytic agents are necessary to prevent delivery (see Chapter 15).

C **Third trimester.** This period extends from 28 weeks of pregnancy until term, or 40 weeks' gestation.

1. Symptoms
    a. Braxton Hicks contractions (see II B 1 c) become more apparent in the third trimester.
    b. Pain in the lower back and legs is often caused by pressure on muscles and nerves by the uterus and fetal head, which fills the pelvis at this time.
    c. Lightening is the descent of the fetal head to or even through the pelvic inlet due to the development of a well-formed lower uterine segment and a reduction in the volume of amniotic fluid.

2. Fetus
    a. Weight. The fetus gains weight at a rate of approximately 224 g (0.5 lb) per week for the last 4 weeks and weighs an average of 3300 g (7.0 to 7.5 lb) at term.
    b. Motion
        (1) A decrease in fetal motion usually occurs because of the size of the fetus and lack of room within the uterus. However, some decreased fetal activity may indicate fetal compromise due to uteroplacental insufficiency.
        (2) The fetal mortality rate decreases from 44/1000 to 10/1000 as measured by a fetal movement screening method. (This commonly used method [daily fetal kick count] requires maternal perceptions of at least 10 fetal movements in 2 hours daily in the third trimester.)

3. Bleeding
    a. Bloody show, a discharge of a combination of blood and mucus caused by thinning and stretching of the cervix, is a sure sign of the approach of labor.

    b. Heavy bleeding suggests a more serious condition such as **placenta previa** (the placenta developing in the lower uterine segment and completely or partially covering the internal os, usually **painless** bleeding) or **abruptio placentae** (premature separation of the normally implanted placenta, usually **painful** bleeding) (see Chapter 9).

   4. **Rupture of membranes** is either a sudden gush or a slow leak of amniotic fluid that can happen at any time without warning.

    a. Brownish or greenish fluid may represent meconium staining of the fluid, the sign of a **fetal bowel movement** that may or may not represent fetal stress.

    b. At term, **labor** usually begins within 24 hours after rupture of membranes.

    c. At term, **induction of labor** is indicated if there is no labor within 6 to 24 hours of rupture or if there is any evidence of infection (**chorioamnionitis**).

   5. **Labor.** Contractions that occur at decreasing intervals with increasing intensity cause the progressive dilation and effacement of the cervix.

III   STATUS OF THE FETUS

A **Growth and development**

   1. **Weight.** A normal fetus weighs approximately 1000 g (more than 2 lb) at 26 to 28 weeks, 2500 g (5.5 lb) at 36 weeks, and 3300 g (7.0 to 7.5 lb) at 40 weeks.

   2. **Lung maturity.** Fetal lung maturity can be assessed by measuring surface-active lipid components of surfactant (e.g., lecithin and phosphatidylglycerol), which are secreted by the type II pneumocytes of fetal lung alveoli. Fetal lung maturity is essential for normal respiration immediately after birth. These measurements are made by laboratory examination of **amniotic fluid.**

    a. Lecithin-to-sphingomyelin (L/S) ratio. Studies have shown that when the level of lecithin in amniotic fluid increases to at least **twice** that of sphingomyelin (at approximately 35 weeks), the risk of respiratory distress is very low (Fig. 3-2).

    b. Phosphatidylglycerol. The presence of phosphatidylglycerol in the amniotic fluid provides even more definite assurance of lung maturity.

    c. Respiratory distress syndrome (RDS). Infants born before phosphatidylglycerol appears in surfactant, even with an L/S ratio of 2:1, may be at risk for RDS.

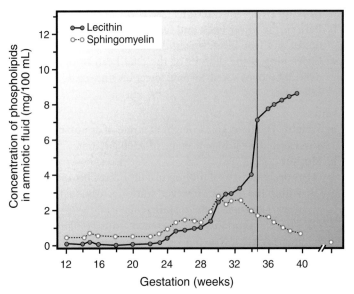

FIGURE 3–2 Changes in mean concentrations of lecithin and sphingomyelin in amniotic fluid during gestation in normal pregnancy. (Reprinted with permission from Cunningham FG, MacDonald PC, Gant NF, et al. Williams Obstetrics. 20th Ed. New York: McGraw-Hill, 1997:970, Figure 42-2.)

    d. Early fetal lung maturation (32 to 35 weeks) is seen with maternal hypertension, PROM, and intrauterine growth retardation, all of which are stressful to the fetus. This stress increases **fetal cortisol secretion**, which in turn accelerates fetal lung maturation.

    e. Glucocorticoids. Administration of glucocorticoids to mothers between the 24th and 34th week of pregnancy effects an increase in the rate of maturation of the human fetal lung and is associated with a reduced rate of respiratory distress in their prematurely born infants.

B **Lie of the fetus** is the relation of the long axis of the fetus to the long axis of the mother and is either longitudinal or transverse.

  1. Longitudinal lie. In most labors (more than 99%) at term, the fetal head is either up or down in a longitudinal lie.

  2. Transverse lie. The fetus is crosswise in the uterus in a transverse lie.

  3. Oblique lie. This indicates an unstable situation that becomes either a longitudinal or transverse lie during the course of labor.

C **Fetal presentation** is determined by the portion of the fetus that can be felt through the cervix.

  1. Cephalic presentations are classified according to the position of the fetal head in relation to the body of the fetus.

    a. Vertex. The head is flexed so that the chin is in contact with the chest, and the occiput of the fetal head presents. A vertex presentation occurs in 95% of all cephalic presentations (Fig. 3-3).

    b. Face. The neck is extended sharply so that the occiput and the back of the fetus are touching, and the face is the presenting part (Fig. 3-4).

    c. Brow. The fetal head is extended partially but converts into a vertex or face presentation during labor (Fig. 3-5).

  2. Breech presentations are classified according to the position of the legs and buttocks, which present first. Breech presentations occur in 3.5% of all pregnancies (Fig. 3-6).

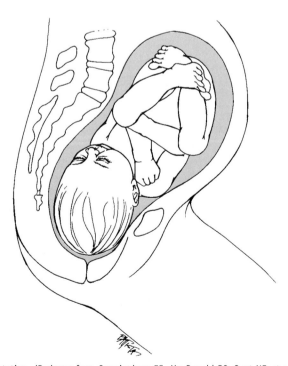

FIGURE 3–3 Vertex presentation. (Redrawn from Cunningham FG, MacDonald PC, Gant NF, et al. Williams Obstetrics. 20th Ed. New York: McGraw-Hill, 1997:320, Figure 12-1 #2.)

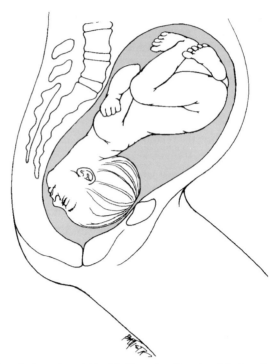

FIGURE 3–4 Face presentation. (Redrawn from Gabbe SG. Obstetrics: Normal and Problem Pregnancies. 3rd Ed. New York: Churchill Livingstone, 1996:473, Figure 16-9.)

  a. In a **complete breech**, both the legs and the hips are flexed.
  b. In an **incomplete breech**, one hip is not flexed, and one foot or knee lies below the breech (i.e., one foot or knee is lowermost in the birth canal).
  c. In a **frank breech**, the hips are flexed and the legs are extended.

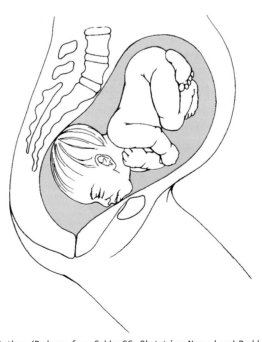

FIGURE 3–5 Brow presentation. (Redrawn from Gabbe SG. Obstetrics: Normal and Problem Pregnancies. 3rd Ed. New York: Churchill Livingstone, 1996:475, Figure 16-10.)

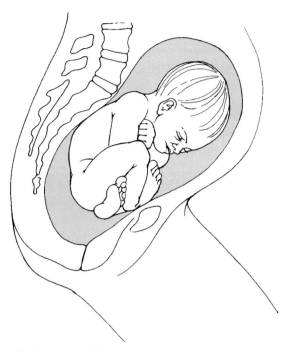

FIGURE 3–6 Breech presentation. (Reprinted with permission from Gabbe SG. Obstetrics: Normal and Problem Pregnancies. 3rd Ed. New York: Churchill Livingstone, 1996:479, Figure 16-14.)

IV   PUERPERIUM

This period of 4 to 6 weeks starts immediately after delivery and ends when the reproductive tract has returned to its nonpregnant condition. Multiple anatomic and physiologic changes occur during this time, and the potential exists for significant complications, such as infection or hemorrhage.

A   Physiology

1. **Involution of the uterus.** The uterus regains its usual nonpregnant size within 5 to 6 weeks, shrinking from 1000 g immediately postpartum to 100 g. This rapid atrophy occurs because of the marked decrease in the size of the muscle cells rather than the decrease in their total number. Breastfeeding accelerates involution of the uterus because stimulation of the nipples releases oxytocin from the neurohypophysis; the resulting contractions of the myometrium facilitate the involution of the uterus.

   a. **Afterpains.** The uterus contracts throughout the period of involution, which produces afterpains, especially in multiparous women and nursing mothers. In primiparous women, the uterus tends to remain contracted tonically, whereas in multiparous women, the uterus contracts vigorously at intervals.

   b. **Lochia.** This uterine discharge follows delivery and lasts for 3 or 4 weeks. Foul-smelling lochia suggests infection.

      (1) **Lochia rubra.** This blood-stained fluid lasts for the first few days.

      (2) **Lochia serosa.** This discharge appears 3 to 4 days after delivery. It is paler than lochia rubra because it is admixed with serum.

      (3) **Lochia alba.** After the 10th day, because of an admixture with leukocytes, the lochia assumes a white or yellow-white color.

2. **Involutional changes of the renal system.** The puerperal bladder has an increased capacity and a relative insensitivity to intravesical fluid pressure.

   a. **Incomplete emptying**, resulting in excessive residual urine, and overdistension may lead to a postpartum urinary tract infection.

   b. **Diuresis** usually occurs between the second and fifth postpartum day.

    c. Anatomic changes, such as the dilation of the calyces, renal pelvis, and ureters, that are characteristic of pregnancy may persist as long as 8 weeks postpartum. Functionally, the increased renal plasma flow, glomerular filtration rate, and creatinine clearance rate associated with pregnancy return to normal by 6 weeks after delivery.

  3. Cardiovascular changes. The changes that occurred during pregnancy (e.g., increases in heart rate, cardiac output, and blood volume) generally return to baseline by approximately 6 weeks postpartum. Peripheral vascular resistance also returns to the prepregnancy level by this time. Most of these parameters return to normal within the first 2 weeks postpartum.

  4. Blood. A marked **leukocytosis** occurs during and after labor. The leukocytosis, primarily a demargination event of granulocytosis, may be as high as 30,000/mm³. Pregnancy-induced changes in **blood coagulation factors** persist for variable periods of time after delivery. Elevated plasma fibrinogen levels are maintained at least through the first week of the puerperium.

  5. Ovulation and menstruation

    a. Nonlactating women. The first menstrual flow usually returns within 6 to 8 weeks after delivery, with ovulation occurring at 2 to 4 weeks postpartum.

    b. Lactating women. Ovulation is much less frequent in women who breast feed compared with those who do not. The first menstrual flow may occur as early as the second month or as late as the 18th month after delivery.

      (1) Amenorrhea during lactation is due to a lack of appropriate ovarian stimulation by pituitary gonadotropins.

      (2) Nevertheless, pregnancy can occur with lactation. Nursing mothers must understand that ovulation and pregnancy can occur even in breastfeeding amenorrheic women.

  6. Family planning. Methods of contraception should be fully reviewed and implemented (see Chapter 24).

    a. Nonlactating mothers may begin using a contraceptive soon after delivery if they wish to avoid becoming pregnant. **Combination oral contraceptives** may be prescribed, or depot medroxyprogesterone acetate can be injected before discharge.

    b. Lactating mothers may begin using progestin-only oral contraceptives as soon as their milk supply is established. **Progesterone-only contraceptives** do not appear to have adverse effects on lactation. Combined oral contraceptives (containing estrogen and progestins) should not be used.

      (1) Intrauterine devices (IUDs) do not interfere with breast milk. However, IUDs are generally not inserted until 4 to 6 weeks postpartum.

      (2) Diaphragms or cervical caps cannot be fitted adequately during the immediate postpartum period, and their use should be delayed until after the 4- to 6-week examination.

      (3) Spermicides and barrier methods have no effect on breastfeeding. Lubricated condoms may offset vaginal dryness secondary to breastfeeding.

    c. Patients for whom the use of oral contraceptives is contraindicated or who prefer other methods of contraception, such as foam or condoms, should also be offered instructions in their use. Fertility awareness methods, such as the rhythm method, are difficult to practice accurately before the resumption of menses and therefore are not recommended.

B **Complications.** The most common complications include hemorrhage, genital tract infections, urinary tract infections, and mastitis.

  1. Postpartum hemorrhage is defined as a blood loss in excess of 500 mL during the first 24 hours after delivery.

    a. Causes

      (1) Failure of compression of blood vessels at the implantation site of the placenta because of:

        (a) An **atonic uterus** due to general anesthesia; overdistension of the uterus from a large fetus, hydramnios (excess amniotic fluid), or multiple fetuses; prolonged labor; very rapid labor; high parity; or a labor vigorously stimulated with oxytocin. **The most common cause of postpartum hemorrhage is uterine atony.**

        (b) Retention of placental tissue, as seen in placenta accreta, a succenturiate placental lobe, or a fragmented placenta

    (2) Trauma to the genital tract because of:

        (a) Episiotomy

        (b) Lacerations of the cervix, vagina, or perineum

        (c) Rupture of the uterus

    (3) Coagulation defects, either congenital or acquired, as seen in hypofibrinogenemia or thrombocytopenia

  b. Management should be directed at the underlying cause(s)

    (1) Vigorous massage of the uterine fundus for uterine atony

    (2) Use of uterine contracting agents for uterine atony

        (a) Oxytocin 20 U in 1000 mL of lactated Ringer's solution intravenously

        (b) Methylergonovine 0.2 mg intramuscularly or intravenously. Because methylergonovine may cause hypertension, it should be avoided in patients with preeclampsia.

        (c) Prostaglandin F$_{2\alpha}$ 0.25 mg intramuscularly up to eight doses at 20-minute intervals. Contraindications include severe asthma.

    (3) Manual exploration of the uterine cavity for retained placental fragments or uterine rupture

    (4) Inspection of the cervix and vagina for lacerations

    (5) Curettage of the uterine cavity

    (6) Hypogastric artery **ligation; embolization** of the uterine vessels; and, rarely, **hysterectomy**

2. Puerperal infection is defined as any infection of the genitourinary tract during the puerperium accompanied by a temperature of **100.4°F (38°C) or higher** that occurs for at least 2 of the first 10 days postpartum, **exclusive of the first 24 hours.** Prolonged rupture of the membranes accompanied by multiple vaginal examinations during labor is a major predisposing cause of puerperal infection.

  a. Pelvic infections

    (1) Endometritis (childbed fever), the most common form of puerperal infection, involves primarily the endometrium and the adjacent myometrium.

    (2) Parametritis, infection of the retroperitoneal fibroareolar pelvic connective tissue, may occur by:

        (a) Lymphatic transmission of organisms

        (b) Cervical lacerations that extend into the connective tissue

        (c) Extension of pelvic thrombophlebitis

    (3) Thrombophlebitis results from an extension of puerperal infection along pelvic veins.

  b. Urinary tract infections are common during the puerperium because of:

    (1) Trauma to the bladder from a normal vaginal delivery

    (2) A **hypotonic bladder** from conduction anesthesia

    (3) Catheterization

  c. Management. Precise identification of bacteria specifically responsible for any puerperal infection can be difficult. Historically, genital tract cultures were obtained; however, they are now of little clinical utility because many of the same pathogens were also found in the uterine cavity in clinically healthy puerperal women. Blood and urine cultures may be useful to identify some of these pathogens, especially in women who have undergone cesarean section.

    (1) Antibiotics should be administered according to the sensitivity of the infecting organism to the drug. Broad-spectrum antibiotics, which include anaerobic coverage, are recommended for those pelvic infections in which identification of the offending organism is impossible. **Common organisms include:**

        (a) Aerobic (group B streptococcus, *Enterococcus,* and *Escherichia coli*)

        (b) Anaerobic (*Peptococcus, Peptostreptococcus, Bacteroides,* and *Clostridium*)

    (2) Heparin should be administered when thrombophlebitis is suspected and a spiking temperature does not respond to intravenous antibiotics.

V LACTATION

A Physiology. Progesterone, estrogen, placental lactogen, prolactin, cortisol, and insulin act together in stimulating the growth and development of the breast's milk-secreting apparatus.

1. **Prolactin**, which is released from the anterior pituitary gland, **stimulates milk production**.
   a. **Initiation of lactation**. The delivery of the placenta causes a sharp decrease in the levels of estrogens and progesterone, which, in turn, leads to the release of prolactin and the consequent stimulation of milk production.
   b. **Continued prolactin production**. A stimulus from the breast (e.g., a suckling infant) curtails the release of prolactin-inhibiting factor from the hypothalamus, thus inducing a transiently increased secretion of prolactin.

2. **Oxytocin** is responsible for the **let-down reflex** and the subsequent release of breast milk. Stimulation of the nipples during nursing causes oxytocin to be released from the posterior pituitary gland.

B **Nursing.** Breast milk is ideal for the newborn because it provides a balanced diet. It contains protective maternal antibodies, and the maternal lymphocytes in breast milk may be important to the infant's immunologic processes. Most drugs given to the mother are secreted in low concentrations in the breast milk. Water-soluble drugs are excreted in high concentrations into colostrum, whereas lipid-soluble drugs are excreted in high concentrations into breast milk.

C **Mastitis.** This parenchymatous inflammation of the mammary glands seldom appears before the end of the first week postpartum and not until the third or fourth week postpartum.

1. **Symptoms.** Engorgement of the breasts is accompanied by a temperature increase, chills, and a hard, red tender area on the breast.

2. **Etiology.** The most common offending organism is *Staphylococcus aureus* from the infant's nose and throat, which usually enters the breast through the nipple at the site of a fissure or abrasion during nursing.

3. **Therapy**
   a. **Gram-positive antibiotic coverage** (e.g., dicloxacillin) is recommended; erythromycin is recommended for penicillin-allergic patients.
   b. **Heat** should be applied to the breast.
   c. **Nursing** from the affected breast should continue to decrease engorgement.
   d. **The abscess should be drained** if the mastitis has progressed to suppuration.

4. **Prevention**. The use of an emollient cream is recommended to help prevent cracking of the nipple.

Study Questions for Chapter 3

Directions: *Each of the numbered items or incomplete statements in this section is followed by answers or by completions of the statement. Select the ONE lettered answer or completion that is BEST in each case.*

1. A 23-year-old primigravida woman just delivered an infant weighing 4350 g by spontaneous vaginal delivery. After 5 minutes of gentle traction on the umbilical cord, you deliver the placenta, which appears to be intact. You begin massaging the uterine fundus and ask the nurse to run 20 U of oxytocin in 1000 mL of lactated Ringer's solution as fast as possible. After careful inspection of the genital tract, you notice a second-degree laceration and a 2-cm left lateral vaginal wall laceration, which you attempt to repair. Suturing is difficult because of brisk bleeding from above the site of laceration. Physical examination reveals a soft, boggy uterine fundus. Her vitals are as follows: T = 98.9, BP = 164/92, P = 130, R = 18. Which of the following is the next best step in management?

- A Oxytocin 10 U direct IV infusion
- B Methylergonovine 0.2 mg IM
- C Prostaglandin $F_{2\alpha}$ 0.25 mg IM
- D Manual exploration
- E Curettage

2. Forty hours ago, a 19-year-old primigravida delivered a viable female infant weighing 3600 g. The baby's APGARs (American Pediatric Gross Assessment Records) were 9 and 9 at 1 and 5 minutes, respectively. The patient is breastfeeding and reports minimal lochia. Review of her labor records reveals that her membranes were ruptured 7 hours before delivery of her infant. Her vital signs before discharge from the hospital are as follows: T = 100.8, P = 105, BP = 110/70, R = 16. Her physical examination is remarkable for slight tenderness in the area of the uterus; nonerythematous, nontender firm breasts; and nontender calves. Which of the following is the best initial step before treatment with antibiotics?

- A Urinalysis and culture
- B Genital tract culture
- C Blood culture
- D Incentive spirometry
- E Uterine curettage

3. A 27-year-old woman, gravida 2, para 1, presents for her first prenatal visit after testing positive on a home pregnancy test. She reports regular cycles every 35 days. She denies use of birth control pills, Depo-Provera, or other contraceptive in the last 7 months. The first day of her last menstrual period was April 1, 2007, and the last day was April 5, 2007. She says her periods always last 4 to 5 days. What is the best estimate of her due date?

- A January 1, 2008
- B January 8, 2008
- C January 12, 2008
- D January 15, 2008
- E June 23, 2008

4. A 16-year-old primigravida presents to labor and delivery with reports of abdominal pain. Her pain is constant and located in both the right lower quadrant and the left lower quadrant. There is no radiation and no associated symptoms other than constipation. The patient ate lunch a few hours ago without any problems. Her vital signs are as follows: T = 97.8, BP = 108/74, P = 96, R = 14. Physical examination of the abdomen reveals bilateral tenderness in the lower abdomen. There is no rebound tenderness or guarding, and costovertebral angles are nontender. Her cervix is closed and uneffaced, and fetal vertex is high. Urinalysis reveals +1 protein, 0 leukocytes, 0 nitrites, 0 bacteria, and 0-1 blood. Amylase, lipase, and liver enzymes are within the normal range except for elevated alkaline phosphatase. Her complete blood cell count is within normal range except for a white blood cell count of 14,000/mm³. Which of the following is the best explanation for her abdominal pain?

- A Braxton Hicks
- B Round ligament
- C Urinary tract infection
- D Uterine leiomyoma
- E Liver disease

5. A 20-year-old woman presents to labor and delivery in labor. She has not had any prenatal care. On examination of her cervix, you palpate a bulging membrane but no fetal parts. The cervix is 4 cm dilated. Ultrasound demonstrates that the fetal head is in the fundus, the fetal spine is parallel to the mother's spine, and the knees and hips are flexed. Both arms are flexed at the elbows. Which of the following is the best description of fetal lie?

- A Complete breech
- B Incomplete breech
- C Frank breech
- D Vertex
- E Longitudinal

Answers and Explanations

1. The answer is C [IV B 1 b (2) (c)]. Uterine atony is the most common cause of postpartum hemorrhage. Because vigorous massage and dilute oxytocin have not been successful in ceasing her bleeding (i.e., uterus is soft and boggy), the next best step is to add another uterotonic agent. Methylergonovine is contraindicated because this patient is hypertensive despite brisk blood loss. The next best agent is prostaglandin F$_{2\alpha}$. Infusion of undiluted oxytocin 10 U intravenously would cause severe hypotension. Manual exploration would be appropriate if you suspect laceration as the cause of bleeding. Here the diagnosis is most likely uterine atony. Curettage is appropriate for delayed postpartum bleeding when you suspect retained products of conception.

2. The answer is A [IV B 2 b and c]. Incomplete emptying results in excessive residual urine, overdistension, and stasis, and intermittent or Foley catheterization during labor. The postpartum bladder is therefore prone to infections. Slight uterine tenderness can be normal in a postpartum uterus, and one should not automatically assume postpartum endomyometritis. Even when endomyometritis is suspected, genital tract cultures have little usefulness because the same organisms can be found in clinically healthy puerperal women. Blood culture is appropriate in the workup of postpartum fevers, but it is not the initial step. Incentive spirometry is used for immediate postoperative patients to promote lung expansion and decrease atelectasis and initial postoperative temperature elevation. Uterine curettage is used to treat postpartum hemorrhage.

3. The answer is D [I D]. The calculated due date of 9 months plus 7 days from the last menstrual period is based on the assumption that a woman has 28-day cycles and that ovulation occurs on day 14 (thus no recent contraception that may change pattern of ovulation). Using Naegele's rule, count back 3 months (April minus 3 months = January) and add 7 days to the first day (not the last day) of the last menstrual period (1 plus 7 = 8). So far, you have January 8. However, this date is based on a 28-day cycle. Because this patient has 35-day cycles and because the luteal phase of the menstrual cycle is always constant (14 days), ovulation occurred on day 21 rather than day 14 (7 days later than you predicted). Therefore, her due date is January 15.

4. The answer is B [II B 1 b]. Round ligament pain is common during the second trimester. It results from stretching of the round ligaments that are attached to the top of the uterus on each side and the corresponding lateral pelvic wall. Braxton Hicks contractions can begin during the second trimester but are more common later in pregnancy. Braxton Hicks contractions usually are not described as a "constant" type of pain. Urinary tract infection is unlikely given that her urinalysis was normal. Uterine leiomyoma that degenerates can cause severe pain, but the pain is usually not bilateral. The history or physical examination would be suggestive of that diagnosis. Liver disease is not likely because all of her liver enzymes are normal. An elevated alkaline phosphatase would be expected during normal pregnancy because of placental production of this enzyme.

5. The answer is A [III C 2]. Lie of the fetus is the relation of the long axis of the fetus to the long axis of the mother. The presentation described in this question is a complete breech. Vertex is a subtype of cephalic presentation.

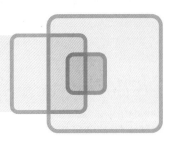

chapter **4**

Antepartum Care

DANIELLE BURKLAND

I INTRODUCTION

Prenatal care begins with preconceptual counseling when a woman is contemplating pregnancy and continues with a comprehensive medical and psychosocial evaluation throughout the antepartum period. The goal of comprehensive prenatal care is to maintain maternal health and deliver a healthy baby while minimizing poor obstetric and fetal outcomes.

II PRECONCEPTION CARE

A Annual gynecologic visits should include evaluation of a woman's interest in starting a family. If planning to conceive, the following should be considered:

1. The health history of the mother and father needs to be assessed. Medical problems that could affect the health of the mother or fetus during pregnancy should be addressed. Medications should be reviewed and those contraindicated in pregnancy stopped. For those with significant medical issues (e.g., significant cardiac disease, cystic fibrosis, hypertension, etc.), referral to a maternal–fetal medicine specialist for preconceptional counseling should be considered.

2. Prenatal vitamins and folic acid supplementation to reduce the incidence of neural tube defects.

3. Rubella immune status; immunize if not immune.

4. Varicella immune status if patient does not recall having the chickenpox; immunize if not immune.

5. Offer cystic fibrosis carrier screening. The incidence of carrying the abnormal gene is 1 in 25 Caucasians. The incidence in African Americans and Asians is low and routine screening may not be indicated.

6. Depending upon ethnic background, the following tests may be ordered to screen for genetic diseases:
   a. Patients of Eastern European Jewish descent: Tay-Sachs, Canavan, Niemann-Pick, Fanconi anemia, Bloom syndrome, Gaucher, and familial dysautonomia
   b. African Americans: sickle cell disease
   c. Mediterranean: thalassemias (α and β)
   d. If family history is significant for other inherited diseases, genetic counseling for screening for diseases such as fragile X and Duchenne muscular dystrophy may be offered (Table 4-1).

III CALCULATING THE ESTIMATED DATE OF CONFINEMENT (EDC)

A The mean duration of pregnancy is 280 days or 40 weeks.

1. Calculation of the EDC is most accurate when a woman has regular menses.

2. It is important to recognize that the first half of the menstrual cycle (follicular phase) is *variable* in length, while the secretory or luteal phase is always 12 to 16 days.

3. Calculating the EDC assumes that a woman's menstrual cycle is approximately 28 days with ovulation occurring on day 14. However, if her cycle is 35 days, then she probably ovulates on cycle day 21. This would change her EDC.

4. Accurate dating of pregnancy is essential as clinical decisions are based on the specific gestational age.

TABLE 4–1 Summary of Antepartum and Peripartum Tests

Test	1st Visit	16–20 Weeks	20–24 Weeks	24–28 Weeks	28–32 Weeks	35–37 Weeks
Pap smear	X					
CBC	X				X	
Urine analysis and culture	X					
Type and screen	X			X Rh-negative patients		
Rubella	X					
Syphilis	X				X*	
HIV	X					
Hepatitis	X					
Gonorrhea and chlamydia	X				X*	
Hemoglobin electrophoresis**	X					
PPD	X					
Triple marker		X				
Amniocentesis***		X				
Ultrasound		X				
1-hour glucose tolerance test	X*			X		
RhoGAM, if antibody negative					X	
Group B streptococcus screen						X
Fetal kick count						X

CBC, complete blood count; PPD, purified protein derivative.
* As indicated or in high-risk populations.
** Offered to African American patients; must consider in Asians.
*** Offered to women over 35 years old at delivery and patients with increased risk of chromosomal defects on triple marker.

B Naegele's rule. The EDC is determined by subtracting 3 months and adding 7 days to the first day of the last menstrual period (LMP). For example, if the LMP is July 15, then the EDC is April 22. This assumes a 28-day menstrual cycle with ovulation occurring on day 14.

C Ultrasound may be used to confirm or identify an EDC when the LMP is uncertain.

1. Transvaginal ultrasound allows for early identification of an embryo and accurate dating of pregnancy by measurement of the crown–rump length.

2. In general, in the first trimester if the EDC by the LMP differs by more than 7 to 10 days based on ultrasound, then the EDC should be adjusted based on ultrasound dating.

3. Subsequently, in the second trimester, if the EDC by the LMP differs by more than 14 days based on ultrasound, then the EDC should be adjusted based on ultrasound dating.

4. Finally, in the third trimester, there is more variation in the size of the fetus, so the EDC should only be adjusted by ultrasound if the EDC varies by more than 21 days and there is no earlier ultrasound confirming the EDC.

IV INITIAL PRENATAL VISIT: HISTORY

A Complete obstetric history

1. Definitions:
   a. **Gravida**: describes the number of pregnancies
   b. **Nulligravida**: describes a woman who is not now and never has been pregnant
   c. **Parity**: describes a woman who has delivered a fetus
   d. **Nulliparous**: describes a woman who has never delivered a fetus
   e. **Primipara**: describes a woman who has delivered only once
   f. **Multipara**: describes a woman who has delivered more than once

2. Standard nomenclature of prior pregnancies

    a. G_P_ _ _ _

    b. G_: total number of pregnancies including the current pregnancy

    c. P_ _ _ _: Referred to as the TPAL system of nomenclature. The first number represents the *total* number of full-term deliveries. The second number represents the total number of *pre*term deliveries at 20 weeks or greater. The third number represents the total number of spontaneous or therapeutic *a*bortions as well as ectopic pregnancies occurring before 20 weeks of gestation. The fourth number represents the total number of *living* children.

B For **each prior pregnancy**, the following information should be obtained:

1. Estimated gestational age (EGA) at the time of delivery

2. Weight of infant

3. Anesthesia

4. Mode of delivery

    a. SVD: spontaneous vaginal delivery

    b. VAVD: vacuum-assisted vaginal delivery

    c. FAVD: forceps-assisted vaginal delivery

    d. Cesarean section, including indication and type of uterine incision

        (1) Low transverse: incision in lower uterine segment in transverse fashion

        (2) Classical: vertical incision through the muscular portion of the uterus

C Identification of prior pregnancy complications

1. History of cervical insufficiency: will require counseling about prophylactic cerclage placement

2. History of prior preterm birth or preterm premature rupture of membranes: will require counseling about 17α-hydroxyprogesterone injections

3. History of gestational diabetes, preeclampsia, shoulder dystocia

D Complete medical, surgical, and gynecologic history

1. Women with medical diseases such as pregestational diabetes and chronic hypertension require additional counseling, laboratory evaluation, and fetal surveillance.

2. A history of any medications taken and any possible exposures in the first trimester should be obtained.

E Thorough family history of both parents

F Social history including screening for substance abuse and domestic violence

V   INITIAL PRENATAL VISIT: PHYSICAL EXAMINATION AND SCREENING

A A complete physical examination should be performed at the initial visit.

1. Height, weight, and blood pressure should be recorded.

2. A systolic flow murmur may be heard at the left sternal border, which is normal in pregnancy.

3. Pelvic examination should include evaluation for abnormal vaginal discharge, performance of cervical cultures and Pap smear, assessment of cervix and uterine size, and assessment of the bony pelvis.

    a. Normal vaginal discharge is a moderate amount of white mucous.

    b. Abnormal vaginal discharge

        (1) Foamy white liquid with a strawberry discoloration of the cervix suggests ***Trichhmonas***.

        (2) White curdy discharge suggests ***Candida***.

        (3) Foul-smelling, gray discharge may indicate **bacterial vaginosis**. It is important to identify patients who may be infected because untreated patients may have a higher incidence of PROM and preterm delivery.

    c. Chadwick sign is a bluish-red hue of the cervix seen in the first trimester.

B Clinical pelvimetry (Fig. 4-1): a pelvis with a diagonal conjugate greater than 11.5 cm is considered to be adequate for delivery of a normal-sized fetus.

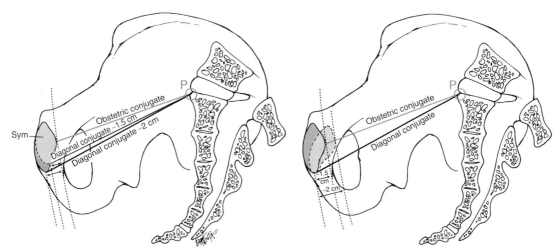

FIGURE 4–1 Variations in length of diagonal conjugate dependent on height and inclination of the symphysis pubis. P, sacral promontory; Sym, pelvic symphysis. (Reprinted with permission from Cunningham FG, MacDonald PC, Gant NF. Williams Obstetrics. 21st Ed. New York: McGraw-Hill, 2001:59, Figure 3-29.)

1. **Diagonal conjugate** is a measure from the sacral promontory to the anterior inferior pubic symphysis, which can be measured on pelvic examination.

2. **Obstetric conjugate** is the length from the sacral promontory to the posterior pubic symphysis. This measurement is determined by subtracting 1.5 to 2 cm from the diagonal conjugate. *The obstetric conjugate is the shortest anterior posterior diameter through which the fetal head must pass.*

C **Pelvic types** (Fig. 4-2)

1. **Gynecoid**: most common type (50%); overall shape is round; the posterior sagittal diameter of

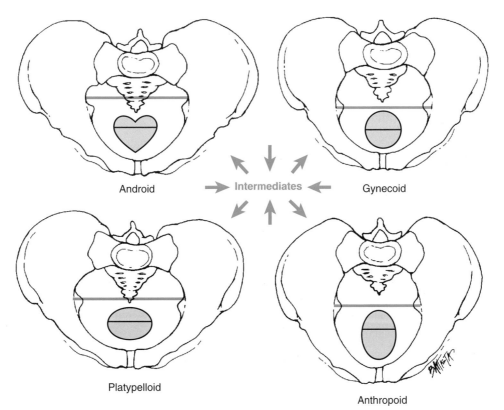

FIGURE 4–2 The four parent pelvic types of the Caldwell-Moloy classification. A line passing through the widest diameter divides the inlet into posterior and anterior segments. (Reprinted with permission from Cunningham FG, MacDonald PC, Gant NF. Williams Obstetrics. 21st Ed. New York: McGraw-Hill, 2001:57, Figure 3-27.)

the inlet is only slightly shorter than the anterior sagittal diameter; ischial spines are not prominent; a wide pubic arch

2. **Android**: seen in about one-third of white women and one-sixth of nonwhite women; overall shape is heart-like; the posterior sagittal diameter of the inlet is much shorter than anterior sagittal, limiting the posterior space for the fetal head; ischial spines are prominent; a narrow pubic arch

3. **Anthropoid**: seen in about one-fourth of white women and one-half of nonwhite women; overall shape is long and oval; the anteroposterior diameter is greater than the transverse; prominent ischial spines; narrow pubic arch

4. **Platypelloid**: least frequent, seen in less than 3% of women; flattened shape with short anteroposterior diameter and wide transverse diameter

D Initial prenatal blood work

1. Blood type and antibody screen, complete blood count (CBC), hemoglobin electrophoresis, rubella status, syphilis screen, hepatitis B surface antigen, HIV status, urinalysis, and urine culture

2. All patients should be offered cystic fibrosis screening.

3. Based on family history and ethnic background, may offer specific genetic screening for certain diseases (see II 6)

4. Cervical culture for gonorrhea and chlamydia

5. Pap smear

6. Purified protein derivative (PPD) for exposed women or for women from endemic areas

7. Early 1-hour glucose tolerance test for women with a history of gestational diabetes or a prior macrosomic infant (more than 4000 g)

VI ANEUPLOIDY SCREENING

A General considerations.   All patients should be offered genetic screening for trisomies and neural tube defects. Women over the age of 35 at the time of delivery should be *offered* diagnostic testing by either chorionic villous sampling or amniocentesis.

B Screening options have expanded in recent years.

1. **First-trimester screening (FTS)** is performed between 10 weeks, 3 days and 13 weeks, 6 days.
   a. FTS involves measurement of nuchal translucency by ultrasound and two serum analytes: pregnancy-associated plasma protein A (PAPP-A) and free β-human chorionic gonadotropin (β-hCG).
   b. FTS permits earlier diagnostic testing for positive tests.
   c. FTS does not screen for neural tube defects.

2. **QUAD screening** is performed in the second trimester, 15 to 21 weeks.
   a. QUAD screening involves four serum analytes: α-fetoprotein (AFP), hCG, unconjugated estriol, and inhibin-A.
   b. Trisomy 21 is associated with decreased levels of AFP and estriol and increased levels of hCG and inhibin.
   c. Trisomy 18 is associated with decreased levels of AFP, hCG, and estriol.

3. **Integrated and sequential screens**. In this algorithm a combination of both first-trimester and second-trimester screens are performed.
   a. In **sequential screening**, the result of the first-trimester screen is released to the patient and provider.
   b. In **integrated screening**, the result of the first-trimester test is withheld and incorporated into a final overall risk assessment.

VII SUBSEQUENT PRENATAL VISITS

A Frequency

1. In uncomplicated pregnancies, visits occur every 4 weeks until 24 to 28 weeks, and then the frequency increases to every 2 to 3 weeks. After 36 weeks, visits occur every week until delivery.

2. Complicated pregnancies require closer surveillance.

B Each visit includes maternal weight, blood pressure, urine dip for glucose and protein, assessment of uterine size, and fetal heart tones.

C Milestones

1. By 20 weeks: complete genetic screening if desired and level II ultrasound for fetal anatomic evaluation.

2. Between 24 and 28 weeks: complete 1-hour glucose tolerance test to screen for gestational diabetes and a third-trimester CBC. If patient is Rh negative, RhoGAM should be administered.

3. Between 35 and 37 weeks: group B streptococcus swab should be performed. Leopold maneuvers should be used to determine fetal presentation.

4. After 41 weeks: nonstress test should be performed twice weekly.

D Patients should be reminded of concerning signs to look out for throughout the pregnancy.

1. After 20 weeks, preterm labor precautions should be given to the patient.

2. After 28 weeks, patients should be instructed to do fetal kick counts. Normal fetal movement is 10 fetal movements in 2 hours.

3. After 35 weeks, patients should be given warning signs of preeclampsia and term labor instructions.

VIII NUTRITION

A Weight gain

1. The recommended weight gain during pregnancy depends on the prepregnancy weight and health of the woman.
   a. For a woman with a normal body mass index (BMI): 25 to 35 lb
   b. For a woman with a BMI less than 19 kg/m^2: 28 to 40 lb
   c. For a woman with a BMI greater than 29 kg/m^2: 15 lb

2. Pregnancy-induced changes account for about 9 to 10 kg (20 to 22 lb) of the weight gain in normal conditions in the following approximate distributions:
   a. Fetus: 3.4 kg (7.5 lb)
   b. Placenta plus membranes: 0.7 kg (1.5 lb)
   c. Amniotic fluid: 0.9 kg (2 lb)
   d. Increase in weight of the uterus: 1.1 kg (2.5 lb)
   e. Increase in blood volume: 1.6 kg (3.5 lb)
   f. Breasts: 0.45 kg (1 lb)
   g. Lower extremity fluid: 1.1 kg (2.5 lb)

B Calories.   Recommended diet should be 2500 kcal/day for pregnant women, about 300 kcal more than prepregnancy needs.

C Dietary composition

1. Protein: requirement is about 60 g/day.
   a. Protein is required for fetal growth.
   b. Best sources are from animal sources such as meat, milk, eggs, poultry, and cheese.

2. Iron: recommended intake is 30 to 30 mg elemental iron per day.
   a. Even in a well-balanced diet, it is hard to maintain adequate iron stores during pregnancy.
   b. Most women need supplemental iron supplementation, which is usually found in prenatal vitamins.
   c. Some women may require still more iron supplementation.

3. Calcium: recommended intake is 1200 mg daily from diet or with addition of calcium supplement.

4. Folic acid: recommended intake is 400 to 1000 μg/day to prevent neural tube defects.
   a. For women with a history of an infant with a neural tube defect, recommended intake is 4 mg/day.

5. Avoid unpasteurized cheeses, raw shellfish, and fish that have high mercury levels.

IX LIFESTYLE MODIFICATIONS

A **Exercise.** It is not necessary to limit exercise, although the level of intensity should not be increased during pregnancy. Restriction may occur if complications of pregnancy such as preterm labor occur.

B **Travel.** Travel does not have harmful effects on pregnancy. Pregnant women on long flights should be advised to move around the cabin every 2 hours to prevent deep vein thrombosis.

C **Coitus.** In uncomplicated pregnancies, sexual intercourse does not pose harm to the pregnancy.

D **Smoking.** Smoking has been associated with low-birth-weight infants, preterm birth, placental abruption, and sudden infant death syndrome (SIDS).

E **Alcohol.** Fetal abnormalities associated with fetal alcohol syndrome include craniofacial defects, growth restriction, and mental retardation.

F **Caffeine.** Caffeine has not been associated with teratogenic effects. Caffeine has only been associated with spontaneous abortion at very high levels (more than 5 cups per day).

G **Flu shot.** The Centers for Disease Control and Prevention (CDC) recommends that all pregnant women have a flu shot.

H **Medications.** Most drugs administered during pregnancy cross the placenta and reach the fetus. Exceptions are large organic ions such as heparin and insulin. The Food and Drug Administration (FDA) created five categories based on risk to the fetus. Package inserts that include FDA classification should be consulted when prescribing medication in pregnancy.

1. **Category A** (e.g., levothyroxine, folic acid). Well-controlled studies in pregnant women show no risk to the fetus in any trimester of pregnancy.

2. **Category B** (e.g., ondansetron, penicillins). Well-controlled studies in pregnant women have shown no increased risk of fetal abnormalities despite adverse findings in animals. Drugs are also placed in this category if, in the absence of adequate human studies, animal studies show no fetal risk. The chance of fetal harm is remote but possible.

3. **Category C** (e.g., prochlorperazine, trimethoprim-sulfamethoxazole). Well-controlled human studies are lacking, and animal studies are lacking as well or have shown a risk to the fetus. There is a **chance of fetal harm if the drug is administered in pregnancy**. However, the potential benefits may outweigh the potential risks.

4. **Category D** (e.g., phenytoin, carbamazepine). Studies in humans have demonstrated a risk to the fetus; therefore, the **drug should not be administered during pregnancy**. However, the potential benefits may be acceptable in cases of a life-threatening situation or serious disease for which a safer drug cannot be used or has proven ineffective.

5. **Category X** (e.g., diethylstilbestrol, thalidomide, Accutane). Studies in animals or human have demonstrated **evidence of fetal abnormalities or risk** that clearly outweigh any possible benefit to the patient.

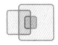

Study Questions for Chapter 4

Directions: *Each of the numbered items or incomplete statements in this section is followed by answers or by completions of the statement. Select the ONE lettered answer or completion that is BEST in each case.*

1. A woman presents to your office for prenatal care. She has had two abortions, two second-trimester miscarriages, one ectopic pregnancy, a fetal demise at 37 weeks' gestation, and two live births. Her son, who is now 13 years old, was delivered at 34 weeks' gestation by spontaneous vaginal delivery. Her daughter, who is now 10 years old, was delivered at 38 weeks' gestation by cesarean section secondary to fetal distress during labor. What are her "Gs and Ps" by simple notation and by TPAL notation, respectively?

- A $G_8 P_2$; $G_8 P_{1142}$
- B $G_8 P_3$; $G_8 P_{2142}$
- C $G_9 P_3$; $G_9 P_{2142}$
- D $G_8 P_3$; $G_8 P_{1142}$
- E $G_9 P_3$; $G_9 P_{2152}$

2. A 34-year-old woman, gravida 2, para 1, at 32 weeks' gestation, presents to your office for routine prenatal care. She delivered her daughter vaginally at 39 weeks without any complications. Her past medical history is unremarkable, and her current pregnancy has been uncomplicated other than occasional Braxton Hicks and increasing vaginal discharge that is nonpruritic, is the same color as her cervical mucus, and has been present during most of her pregnancy. Her BP is 108/73, her temperature is 96.8°F, her fundus measures at 33 weeks, she is 5 feet 4 inches tall, her prepregnancy weight was 120 lb, and she now weighs 135 lb. She is rubella nonimmune, hepatitis B surface antigen negative, O + / antibody −, Venereal Disease Research Laboratory nonreactive, and gonorrhea culture/chlamydia negative. What is the next best step in management?

- A Rubella antibody test
- B 50-g glucose tolerance test
- C 300-µg anti-D immune globulin
- D Follow-up in 2 weeks
- E Counseling about appropriate weight gain

3. A 28-year-old woman, gravida 3, para 2, at 5 weeks' gestation, presents to you for confirmation of pregnancy and possible prenatal care. Her first pregnancy resulted in vaginal delivery of a viable female infant weighing 3900 g at term. Her daughter has a bilateral hearing deficit. Her second pregnancy resulted in cesarean-section delivery of a viable male infant weighing 2900 g at 34 weeks because of pregnancy-induced hypertension. Her son was born with mild myelomeningocele. She denies family history of any diseases or problems. She tells you that she is a lacto-ovo vegetarian. What is the most appropriate advice during this prenatal session?

- A Supplement your diet with additional iron
- B Supplement your diet with additional vitamin B_{12}
- C Increase your folic acid intake to 10 times your prepregnancy amount
- D Eat plenty of green, leafy vegetables
- E Increase your calcium intake to 1200 mg/day

4. You discover two medical students in the low-risk obstetric clinic debating over the recommended weight gain in normal pregnancy and the two largest contributions to weight gain during a normal pregnancy. You agree that the recommended weight gain during normal pregnancy is about 30 lb give or take a few pounds depending on the prepregnancy weight. Aside from the weight of the fetus, what is the largest contributor to weight gain during pregnancy?

- A Blood volume
- B Uterus
- C Placenta
- D Amniotic fluid
- E Breasts

5. A 24-year-old woman, gravida 2, para 1, at 27 weeks' gestation, presents to you for routine prenatal care. She reports plenty of fetal movement and denies spotting or regular contractions. She does report increasing vaginal discharge that is white to yellow in color and has a distinct odor. Her temperature today is 98.2°F and her BP is 100/60. The fundus measures 28 cm above the symphysis pubis. Her last pregnancy was uncomplicated. She has no known drug allergy. Her past medical history is remarkable for asthma (about two wheezing episodes per week and symptom free at nights). You perform a sterile speculum examination and you notice homogenous, adherent, white-yellow discharge in the posterior fornix and the cervix, but the mucosa does not appear inflamed. The pH of the discharge is 5.5. Wet mount displays 30% clue cells. The potassium hydrochloride (KOH) prep is nondiagnostic but has a strong odor. Which of the following is the best diagnosis and treatment combination, respectively?

A   Normal discharge and follow-up in 4 weeks
B   *Trichomonas* and metronidazole
C   Bacterial vaginosis and clindamycin
D   *Chlamydia* and erythromycin
E   *Candida* and fluconazole

Answers and Explanations

1. **The answer is C** [IV A 1–2]. Remember that "parity" refers to the number of pregnancies that reached viability (23 or more weeks of gestation) and not the number of pregnancies resulting in a live-born infant. Additionally, the route of delivery (vaginal versus cesarean section) does not change the parity. In this question's scenario, the woman has been pregnant nine times (her current pregnancy = 1, two abortions = 2, two miscarriages = 2, one ectopic = 1, one fetal demise = 1, and two live births = 2; $1 + 2 + 2 + 1 + 1 + 2 = 9$). Only three pregnancies reached viability (fetal demise at 37 weeks, her preterm delivery at 34 weeks, and her term delivery at 38 weeks). For the **TPAL** notation, **T** refers to the number of term infants delivered regardless of outcome (fetal demise at 37 weeks and term delivery at 38 weeks = 2); **P** stands for preterm (preterm delivery at 34 weeks = 1); **A** stands for abortions, either elective or miscarriages (it does not include ectopic pregnancies) (2 abortions + 2 miscarriages = 4); and **L** refers to number of living offspring (son and daughter = 2). With multiple-gestation pregnancies, the parity does not increase by the number of babies delivered (e.g., a patient who has been pregnant once and delivered twins at 38 weeks would be noted as G_1P_1 and G_1P_{1002}).

2. **The answer is D** [VII A–D, VIII]. In an uncomplicated pregnancy, as in this case, a woman should be seen every 4 weeks for the first 28 weeks, every 2 weeks until 36 weeks, and weekly thereafter until delivery. Although this patient is rubella nonimmune, no action needs to be taken until after she delivers. You can assume that by 32 weeks of gestation, she should have already had a 50-g glucose tolerance test because the recommended time to perform the screening is between 24 and 28 weeks of gestation. This patient does not need anti-D immune globulin because she is Rh positive. For her height and prepregnancy weight, it is appropriate to have gained 15 lb up to this point in the pregnancy.

3. **The answer is C** [VIII A–C]. The most appropriate advice during this session is to remind the patient to increase her folic acid intake to 4 mg/day because she has a history of delivering a child with a neural tube defect. Although it is appropriate to counsel every pregnant patient to supplement with iron, to increase her intake of green leafy vegetables, and to try to consume 1200 mg of calcium per day, these are not the most important to convey in this first prenatal counseling session (you can counsel her about these during the next visit, along with reinforcing folic acid supplementation). Strict vegans (not lacto-ovo vegetarians) are at risk for vitamin B_{12} deficiency.

4. **The answer is A** [VIII A 2]. The top four contributors to weight gain during pregnancy are as follows: #1, fetus (7.5 lb); #2, blood volume (3.5 lb); #3, uterus and lower extremity edema (2.5 lb); and #4, amniotic fluid (2 lb). The placenta contributes only about 1.5 lb, and the breasts contribute only 1 lb.

5. **The answer is C** [V A 3]. A foul-smelling discharge that is grayish in color (sometimes), whose pH is less than 4.5, with more than 15% clue cells on wet mount field, and a positive whiff test (KOH on discharge has fishy odor) is most likely bacterial vaginosis. This condition can be treated with either metronidazole (first choice) or clindamycin. There is no way of diagnosing chlamydia without a culture or test such as ligase chain reaction or an enzyme immunoassay. All the other answers listed (normal vagina, *Candida*, and *Trichomonas*) have a vaginal pH of 4.5 or less.

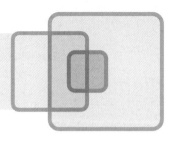

chapter **5**

Identification of the High-Risk Pregnant Patient

JACK LUDMIR · GUILLERMO DE LA VEGA

I   INTRODUCTION

For the majority of women, pregnancy and childbirth are a normal physiologic process that result in the delivery of a healthy infant; however, certain circumstances may place a mother or infant at risk for morbidity. A pregnancy is defined as **high risk** when the likelihood of an adverse outcome is greater than in the general pregnant population. A program of routine prenatal care may optimize pregnancy outcome by achieving the following goals:

A Providing **advice, reassurance, education**, and **support** for the woman and her family

B Managing the **minor ailments** of pregnancy

C Providing a **screening** program to confirm that a woman continues to be at low risk

D **Preventing, detecting**, and **managing** factors that adversely affect the health of the mother and infant

II   MATERNAL AND PERINATAL MORTALITY

A Definitions

1. **Maternal death** occurs either during pregnancy or within 42 days of the termination of pregnancy.

2. The **maternal mortality ratio** is the number of maternal deaths per 100,000 live births. Maternal mortality in the United States has decreased substantially in the past few decades—from 582 per 100,000 live births in 1935 to 8.9 per 100,000 live births in 2002. The maternal mortality rate for blacks has also declined, but it remains **four times higher** than white women (24.9 versus 5.6 per 100,000 live births); this disparity has widened since 2000. According to the National Center for Health Statistics, the risk of maternal death increases for women over age 30, regardless of race. Women aged 35 to 39 years have over three times the risk of maternal death as women aged 20 to 24 years. Major causes of maternal death in nonabortive pregnancies (excluding ectopic pregnancies) are, in descending order, **pulmonary embolism**, hypertensive disorders of pregnancy, obstetric hemorrhage, and sepsis.

3. **Perinatal mortality** is the combination of fetal deaths (after 20 weeks or weighing more than 500 g) and neonatal deaths (up to 28 days after birth) per 1000 live births. The perinatal mortality rate has fallen drastically in the last 30 years, from about 29 per 1000 in 1970 to less than 10 per 1000 in 2000. However, blacks have double the rate of perinatal mortality compared to whites (10.8 versus 5.4 per 1000 live births). The factors responsible for this significant discrepancy remain to be elucidated. In general, women without prenatal care have higher rates of perinatal mortality.

III PRECONCEPTION CARE

A Preconception care involves identifying those conditions that could affect a future pregnancy but may be ameliorated by early intervention, such as hypertension, diabetes mellitus, or other metabolic and inherited disorders.

B Women (and their partners) who are contemplating pregnancy should be evaluated for conditions that may affect a future pregnancy. Reproductive, family, genetic, and medical histories should be reviewed (see below).

IV INITIAL PRENATAL VISIT

A General history

1. **Socioeconomic status. Low socioeconomic status** increases the risk of perinatal morbidity and mortality.
2. **Age** is an identifiable risk factor.
    a. **Maternal age younger than 20 years of age** increases the risk of the following conditions:
        (1) Premature births
        (2) Late prenatal care
        (3) Low birth weight
        (4) Uterine dysfunction
        (5) Fetal deaths
        (6) Neonatal deaths
    b. **Maternal age older than 35 years of age** increases the risk of the following conditions:
        (1) **First-trimester miscarriage**. The miscarriage rate for women older than 40 years is three times higher than for women younger than 30 years.
        (2) **Genetically abnormal concepti**. The risk for fetal chromosomal anomalies increases in direct proportion to maternal age. (This increase may also explain, in part, the increase in first-trimester miscarriages.) **Trisomy 21** represents 90% of the chromosomal abnormalities, but the incidence of other autosomal trisomies (i.e., 13 and 18) and sex chromosomal anomalies also increases with advancing age.
        (3) **Medical complications**
            (a) **Hypertension**
            (b) **Diabetes**
            (c) **Preeclampsia**. The incidence of preeclampsia increases with age; it is 6% at 25 years of age, 9% at 35 years of age, and 15% at 40 years of age.
        (4) **Multiple gestation**. The incidence of multiple gestation increases with age. The rate of dizygotic twins is 3 per 1000 live births in women younger than 21 years of age, and it increases to 14 per 1000 live births in women 35 to 40 years of age.
        (5) **Higher rate of cesarean section**. Part of the increase may be attributed to a greater incidence of placenta previa, abnormal presentations, multiple gestation, and medical complications.
        (6) **Fetal morbidity and mortality**. Women older than 40 years of age have higher rates of stillbirth and low birth weight compared with younger women.
3. **Substance abuse** (see Chapter 8)
    a. **Tobacco**. A dose-response relationship exists between heavy cigarette smoking and increased fetal morbidity and mortality.
    b. **Drugs**. The maternal and fetal consequences of drug addiction in pregnancy depend on the drug ingested. Many (e.g., cocaine, opioids, or marijuana) are associated with low birth weight, and drugs such as cocaine and opioids are associated with neonatal withdrawal. Cocaine is also associated with premature labor, abruptio placentae, fetal demise, and maternal complications such as stroke, seizures, cardiomyopathy, and myocardial infarction.
    c. **Alcohol**. Fifteen percent of pregnant women drink alcohol and 2% drink at least 7 drinks per week. Not only does alcohol abuse undermine maternal health, but also a pattern of

---

TABLE 5–1   Alcohol Abuse Screening: The T-ACE Questionnaire

T: Tolerance; how many drinks does it take to make you feel "high"? Or how many drinks can you hold?
(A positive response is two or more drinks.)

A Have people annoyed you by criticizing your drinking?

C Have you ever felt you ought to cut down on your drinking?

E Have you ever had a drink first thing in the morning to steady your nerves or to get rid of a hangover (*eye-opener*)?

Scoring: The tolerance question carries substantially more weight (2 points) than the three other questions (1 point each). These questions were found to be significant identifiers of risk of drinking in pregnancy (i.e., alcohol intake potentially sufficient to damage the embryo/fetus).

From Sokol RJ, Martier SS, Ager JW. The T-ACE questions: practical prenatal detection of risk-drinking. *Am J Obstet Gynecol* 1989;160:863.

---

abnormalities known as the **fetal alcohol syndrome** manifests in varying degrees of severity in the fetus (facial anomalies, low-set ears, microphthalmia, congenital heart malformations, micrognathia, microcephaly, and mental retardation), complicating 1 in 1000 live births. Regular screening for alcohol abuse should be carried out using tools such as the T-ACE questionnaire (Table 5-1).

   d. **Caffeine.** Caffeine-containing beverages, including coffee, are frequently consumed by pregnant women. There is no increased risk of congenital anomalies; however, a recent study suggested higher rates of spontaneous abortion with caffeine intake.

4. **Environmental risks**
   a. **Noxious chemicals** may cause unpleasant symptoms in the mother (i.e., headache, nausea, and lightheadedness). There is no evidence of increased rate for birth defects.
   b. **Radiation and radioactive compounds** have been associated with spontaneous abortion, birth defects, and childhood leukemia.

5. **Domestic violence.** Victims of domestic violence are more likely to be abused while pregnant. Such assaults may lead to placental abruption; fetal fractures; rupture of the uterus, spleen, or liver; and preterm labor. It estimated that 8% of obstetric patients are physically assaulted while pregnant. Questions on personal safety and violence should be addressed during the prenatal period (Table 5-2).

B **Obstetric history.**   Previous obstetric and reproductive history is essential to care in subsequent pregnancy.

1. **Parity**
   a. **Nullipara.** Nulliparous women are at high risk for development of specific problems, including pregnancy-induced hypertension and possible complications caused by relative lack of knowledge of the pregnancy state.
   b. **Multipara.** Grand multiparous women (five or more pregnancies resulting in viable fetuses) appear to be at increased risk for placenta previa, postpartum hemorrhage secondary to uterine atony, and increased incidence of dizygotic twins (which may occur because grand multiparas are usually of advanced age).

2. **Ectopic pregnancy.** A woman with a history of ectopic pregnancy has an increased risk of another ectopic pregnancy. It is imperative that she be evaluated by quantitative β-human chorionic gonadotropin (β-hCG) and transvaginal ultrasound once the level is above the discriminatory zone to detect an intrauterine pregnancy (see Chapter 27).

3. **Preterm delivery.** The incidence of preterm delivery (delivery before 37 completed weeks' gestation) correlates well with past reproductive performance and increases with each subsequent preterm delivery. The recurrence rate for preterm delivery is as high as 50%. A short cervical length (less than 2.5 cm), as determined by ultrasound at 20 to 24 weeks, has been associated with increased risk of preterm birth. Patents with a history of preterm delivery may benefit from weekly 17-hydroxyprogesterone injections starting in the midtrimester.

4. **Second-trimester pregnancy loss.** Such loss could be the result of an abnormality in the fetus (chromosomal or infectious) or manifestation of a recurrent condition in the mother, such as

TABLE 5–2 **Determination of Frequency and Severity of Physical Abuse during Pregnancy**

Abuse Assessment Screen (Circle YES or NO for each question)
1. Have you ever been emotionally or physically abused by your partner or someone important to you?
   YES   NO
2. Within the last year, have you been hit, slapped, kicked, or otherwise physically hurt by someone?
   YES   NO

If YES, by whom? (Circle all that apply)
Husband   Ex-husband   Boyfriend   Stranger   Other Multiple

Total number of times:
3. Since you've been pregnant, have you been hit, slapped, kicked, or otherwise physically hurt by someone?
   YES   NO

If YES, by whom? (Circle all that apply)
Husband   Ex-husband   Boyfriend   Stranger   Other Multiple

Score each incident according to the following scale:
   1 = Threats of abuse, including the use of a weapon
   2 = Slapping, pushing; no injuries and/or lasting pain
   3 = Punching, kicking, bruises, cuts, and/or continuing pain
   4 = Beaten up, severe contusions, burns, broken bones
   5 = Head, internal, and/or permanent injury
   6 = Use of weapon, wound from weapon
   (If any of the descriptions for the higher number apply, use the higher number)

4. Within the last year, has anyone forced you to have sexual activities?
   YES   NO

If YES, by whom? (Circle all that apply)
Husband   Ex-husband   Boyfriend   Stranger   Other Multiple

Total number of times:
5. Are you afraid of your partner or anyone you listed above?
   YES   NO

From McFarlane J, Parker B, Solken K, et al. Assessing for abuse during pregnancy. *JAMA* 1992;267[23]:3176–3178. Copyright 1992, American Medical Association.

cervical insufficiency, uterine abnormality, or thrombophilia. Cervical insufficiency is characterized by premature delivery associated with painless cervical dilation. Ultrasound evaluation of the cervix during gestation is an objective way to identify the patient at risk for this condition. These patients may benefit from therapeutic interventions, such as cervical cerclage. Congenital structural uterine abnormalities have also been associated with an increased incidence of reproductive loss. Women with septate or bicornuate uteri have higher rates of preterm delivery than do those with didelphys or unicornuate uteri.

5. **Large infant (more than 4000 g).** Large size may indicate previously undetected or uncontrolled glucose intolerance and may be associated with subsequent intrapartum complications, such as:
   a. Difficult vaginal delivery caused by shoulder dystocia
   b. Cesarean section for arrest of dilation or descent
   c. Postpartum complications for the neonate, such as hypoglycemia (see Chapter 17 regarding gestational diabetes)

6. **Perinatal death (stillborn or neonatal).** A pregnancy that follows a perinatal death should be observed closely to avoid a similar outcome. Perinatal death may indicate an underlying problem that may or may not have been detected previously, such as:
   a. Glucose intolerance
   b. Collagen vascular disease
   c. Congenital anomalies
   d. Chromosomal abnormality
   e. Preterm labor

    f. Hemolytic disease

    g. Abnormal labor

    h. Antiphospholipid syndrome (APS)

    i. Thrombophilia

7. Cesarean section

    a. A woman who has had a **previous cesarean section** may attempt a vaginal delivery with a subsequent pregnancy, provided there are no medical or surgical contraindications, such as:

        (1) Classical uterine incision. A trial of labor is contraindicated in patients with a previous incision into the body of the uterus (classical) because of the high risk of uterine rupture (6% to 8%).

        (2) An **active herpes infection** at term

        (3) Myomectomy with penetration into the endometrium

        (4) Placenta previa

    b. Labor in a successive pregnancy is usually safe in patients with one prior transverse scar. The chance of uterine rupture with labor is less than 1%. Currently, not enough data are available to establish the safety of a trial of labor in women with two or more transverse uterine scars.

    c. Women with a history of prior cesarean section are at greater risk for placental abnormalities such as placenta previa and placenta accreta. They are also at greater risk for hemorrhage and hysterectomy. The risk increases with the number of prior cesarean sections.

8. Pregnancy-induced hypertension (preeclampsia and eclampsia)

    a. There appears to be a familial tendency (higher rate for women with affected sisters, mothers, and grandmothers).

    b. Women with a history of severe preeclampsia early in pregnancy may have an increased risk for development of preeclampsia in subsequent pregnancies.

    c. Patients with a history of severe preeclampsia should be followed closely in subsequent gestations. Unfortunately, to date, no intervention has been proven to reduce the risk.

9. History of infertility. In vitro fertilization (IVF) pregnancies have been associated with a higher risk of preterm deliveries, low birth weight, placenta previa, preeclampsia, and cesarean section. The risk of congenital malformations appears to be similar to spontaneous pregnancies, although uncontrolled studies have suggested a slightly greater risk.

C ▪ **Medical history**

1. Chronic hypertension (higher than 140/90 mmHg). Patients with chronic hypertension are at risk of the following conditions:

    a. Superimposed preeclampsia

    b. Abruptio placentae

    c. Perinatal loss

    d. Maternal mortality

    e. Myocardial infarction

    f. Uteroplacental insufficiency

    g. Cerebrovascular accident

2. Cardiac disease. Cardiac disorders have both maternal and fetal implications.

    a. Heart disease may develop or worsen in pregnant women. Because of the hemodynamic changes associated with pregnancy, some cardiac lesions are particularly dangerous, such as Eisenmenger syndrome, primary pulmonary hypertension, Marfan syndrome, and hemodynamically significant mitral or aortic stenosis.

    b. Fetal growth and development depend on an adequate supply of well-oxygenated blood. If this supply is limited, as it appears to be with certain cardiac lesions, then the fetus is at risk of abnormal development and even death.

    c. Offspring of parents with cardiac disease have an increased risk of developing cardiac disease in their lifetimes. This is sometimes identified in utero with fetal echocardiography after 20 weeks.

3. Pulmonary disease. Maternal respiratory function and gas exchange are affected by the associated biochemical and mechanical alterations that occur in a normal pregnancy. The effect of pregnancy on pulmonary disease is often unpredictable. Diseases such as asthma should be managed as they would be normally. When pulmonary disease affects maternal well-being or compromises the supply of well-oxygenated blood to the fetus, there is need for concern.

4. **Renal disease**
   a. In a normal pregnancy, the renal system undergoes certain potentially stressful physiologic, anatomic, and functional changes; therefore, **continuous assessment is necessary** in patients with preexisting or developing renal disease.
   b. With proper medical supervision and control of blood pressure, most women with underlying renal disease can have an **uneventful pregnancy** without adverse effects on either the primary disease or the ultimate prognosis, **provided that the woman's creatinine level is below 1.5 mg/100 mL.**
   c. Pregnancy in patients with history of renal transplant should be followed in conjunction with a nephrologist. About 1 in 50 women of childbearing age with a functioning renal transplant becomes pregnant. More than 90% of pregnancies that continue past the first trimester end successfully.

5. **Diabetes**. The cornerstone of management for women with diabetes is rigid metabolic control to make patients as consistently euglycemic as possible. Ideally, these efforts should begin before conception and continue throughout the pregnancy. The following fetal problems may complicate the pregnancy of a woman with diabetes:
   a. **Congenital anomalies** (two to three times higher than in individuals without diabetes)
   b. **Fetal mortality**
   c. **Neonatal morbidity**, including:
      (1) Respiratory distress syndrome
      (2) Macrosomia
      (3) Hypoglycemia
      (4) Hyperbilirubinemia
      (5) Hypocalcemia
      (6) Polycythemia

6. **Thyroid disease**. Untreated hypothyroidism or hyperthyroidism may profoundly alter pregnancy outcome. The fetal thyroid is autonomous and is unaffected by maternal thyroid hormone; however, treatment of thyroid disease during pregnancy can be complicated because the fetal thyroid responds to the same pharmacologic agents as does the maternal thyroid.

7. **Thromboembolic disease**. Pregnancy is associated with increased production of clotting factors by the liver; this places patients at risk for thromboembolic disease. Patients with prior history of thromboembolism or thrombophilia may benefit from prophylactic or therapeutic anticoagulation during gestation and puerperium.

8. **Systemic lupus erythematosus**. This condition increases the risk of placental abruption, growth restriction, superimposed preeclampsia, and neonatal lupus. The presence of Rho or La antibodies has been associated with greater risk of congenital heart block.

9. **Genetic disorders**
   a. **Genetic disorders in the mother**, such as phenylketonuria, increase the risk of fetal malformation. Proper maternal diet during conception and pregnancy reduces the risk.
   b. **Historical factors** may help identify the at-risk pregnancy.
      (1) **Consanguinity**. Marriage between close relatives results in a large pool of identical genes, thereby increasing the possibility of sharing similar mutant genes, resulting in an:
         (a) Increased risk of miscarriage
         (b) Increased risk of rare recessive genetic disease in offspring
      (2) **Ethnicity**. Specific ethnic groups are more prone to specific diseases.
         (a) **Tay-Sachs disease** (Ashkenazi Jews, French Canadians)
         (b) **Canavan disease** (Ashkenazi Jews)
         (c) **Thalassemias** (Mediterranean, Southeast Asian, Indian, or African people)
         (d) **Sickle cell anemia** (African, Mediterranean, Caribbean, Latin American, or Indian people)
         (e) **Cystic fibrosis** (Caucasians)

10. **Infectious diseases**. In addition to rubella and syphilis, for which pregnant women are routinely screened, the following infections during pregnancy place the mother and infant at high risk for

potential morbidity and mortality. The **TORCH** syndrome refers to an infection developing in a fetus or newborn caused by **to**xoplasmosis, **r**ubella, **c**ytomegalovirus, or **h**erpes simplex.

a. **Cytomegalovirus (CMV)** results in **increased risk of congenital anomalies** with primary infection during gestation and risk of a small-for-gestational-age infant and congenital hearing loss.

b. **Herpes simplex virus** may result in **increased risk of neonatal infection** if active viral lesions are present at birth and the infant is born vaginally.

c. **Toxoplasmosis** leads to **increased risk of congenital anomalies** in the fetus if infection occurs early in pregnancy.

d. **Parvovirus infection** may cause severe anemia in the fetus, resulting in **hydrops** and **death.**

e. **Varicella zoster virus infection** is associated with a **small risk of** fetal sequelae, such as cutaneous scars and limb hypoplasia, if infection occurs early in the pregnancy. The risk of neonatal infection is greater if infection is present within 5 days of delivery.

f. **Hepatitis B virus (HBV)** is associated with **no increased risk of congenital anomalies** but is associated with risk of vertical transmission and neonatal infection (see VI K).

g. **HIV** (see VI M)

11. **Autoimmune disorders**, including **antiphospholipid syndrome (APS)**, an autoimmune syndrome caused by the lupus anticoagulant and the anticardiolipin antibody. APS may be expressed as one or more of the following:

a. Recurrent fetal loss, such as miscarriage or stillbirth

b. Placental infarction

c. Preeclampsia early in gestation

d. Arterial or venous thrombosis, including neurologic disease

e. Autoimmune thrombocytopenia

12. **Depression**. Approximately 1 in 10 women will have depression at any point in pregnancy and the postpartum period. Selective serotonin reuptake inhibitors (SSRIs) are commonly used to treat depression, and their use during pregnancy has been well documented. Recently, the use of the SSRI paroxetine (Paxil) has been associated with a greater risk for fetal cardiac malformations. Furthermore, exposure to SSRIs late in pregnancy has been associated with neonatal complications, including jitteriness, weak cry, poor tone, neonatal respiratory distress, and persistent pulmonary hypertension. Because of the great risk of relapse of depression if SSRIs are discontinued, decisions to take them should be individualized, balancing the risks versus benefits of taking the medication.

D **Medications.** Various medications have adverse effects on the fetus, and it is imperative that the risks and benefits to the mother and fetus be evaluated and discussed with the patient before starting, continuing, or stopping the use of medications. When counseling patients about such risks and benefits, a baseline malformation rate of 2% to 3% in the general population should always be used (see Chapter 8).

V PHYSICAL EXAMINATION

Obstetric patients should undergo a thorough physical examination to assess their general health.

A **General examination.** Maternal size, which may reflect socioeconomic and nutritional status, has become an important predictive index.

1. A pregnant woman who is **short** or **underweight** is at increased risk for:

a. Perinatal morbidity and mortality

b. Delivering a low-birth-weight infant

c. Preterm delivery

2. **Obesity**. Defined as a body mass index (BMI) of 30 or greater, obesity presents a medical hazard to the pregnant woman and her fetus. This problem is greater among non-Hispanic black women (49%) compared with Mexican American women (38%) and non-Hispanic white women (31%). Complications that are more likely to develop in an obese woman include:

a. Hypertension

b. Diabetes

c. Fetal macrosomia and shoulder dystocia

d. Aspiration of gastric contents during the administration of anesthesia

    e. Wound complications

    f. Thromboembolism

B **Pelvic examination**

1. The **perineum, vulva, vagina, cervix**, and **adnexa** should be examined and any abnormalities noted that may affect future management (e.g., adnexal masses, cervical lesions, or diethylstilboestrol [DES] cervical stigmata). A Papanicolaou (Pap) smear should be obtained.

2. **Clinical pelvimetry** should be performed to assess adequacy of the maternal pelvis to facilitate vaginal delivery (see Chapter 4).

C **Evaluation of the uterus.** The size of the uterus is evaluated continuously throughout the pregnancy. The estimated date of delivery should be established at the first prenatal visit so that subsequent discrepancies can be evaluated properly. A strong correlation exists between fundal height in centimeters measured from the symphysis pubis and gestational age in weeks beyond 20 weeks. Size greater or lesser than dates should be evaluated by ultrasound to determine accurate pregnancy dating, presence or absence of multiple gestation, fetal growth abnormalities, and/or amniotic fluid disorders. Reproductive tract abnormalities that may be problematic include:

1. **Leiomyomata (fibroids).** The location and size of the myomas are important in determining possible future sequelae. In general, the pregnancy has an increased risk of being complicated by:
   a. Abortion
   b. Premature labor
   c. Dysfunctional labor
   d. Postpartum hemorrhage
   e. Obstruction of labor by cervical or lower uterine segment myomas
   f. Unstable fetal lie or compound presentation
   g. Pain caused by degeneration

2. **Cervical insufficiency.** Characterized by premature cervical dilation in the second trimester, with minimal labor contractions. This is most often identified on physical examination, although ultrasound may aid in the diagnosis.

3. **Uterine anomalies** of the bicornuate or septate type may increase the patient's risk of spontaneous miscarriage and adverse pregnancy outcome.

VI   LABORATORY STUDIES

Routine laboratory studies may help to identify a high-risk pregnancy.

A **Blood type, including antibody screen**

1. **Rh sensitization** may have profound consequences for the fetus and the management of the pregnancy. If maternal sensitization of an Rh-negative woman to red blood cell antigens has occurred (e.g., prior transfusions or prior pregnancies), the resultant antibodies can be transferred to the fetus and cause hemolytic disease in the Rh-positive fetus.

2. The **antibody screen** is also essential for Rh-positive women because other blood group antigens (e.g., Kell, Kidd, or Duffy) can produce severe hemolytic disease in the fetus.

B **Syphilis test (Venereal Disease Research Laboratory [VDRL]).** Syphilis involves several different stages, and the evaluation of each stage is important in assessing fetal risk. Pregnancy complicated by preexisting or newly acquired syphilis may result in:

1. An uninfected live infant

2. A late abortion (after the fourth month of pregnancy)

3. A stillbirth

4. A congenitally infected infant

C **Gonorrhea culture.** Screening may be either universal or selective, depending on the prevalence of the disease in the patient population. Gonorrhea during pregnancy may be associated with:

1. Intrauterine infection, with premature rupture of membranes and preterm delivery

   2. Histologic evidence of chorioamnionitis

   3. Neonatal eye infection (ophthalmia neonatorum)

   4. Clinical diagnosis of sepsis in the neonate

   5. Associated maternal arthritis, rash, or peripartum fever

D **Chlamydia testing.** Screening is recommended for all high-risk or symptomatic patients. Infection during pregnancy may result in:

   1. Ophthalmia neonatorum

   2. Neonatal pneumonia

   3. Postpartum endometritis

E **Rubella titer**

   1. The **clinical course** of rubella is no more severe or complicated in the pregnant woman than in the nonpregnant woman of comparable age. However, active maternal infection does carry risk for the fetus, including:
   a. First-trimester abortion
   b. Fetal infection, resulting in severe congenital anomalies

   2. **Maternal infection in the first trimester** carries with it the greatest risk to the fetus.

   3. **Immunization**. If a patient is diagnosed as having a rubella titer of less than 1:8, she should be immunized postpartum.
   a. The rubella vaccine is not given during pregnancy because it is a live attenuated vaccine.
   b. There have been no reported cases of congenital rubella from inadvertent administration of the vaccine to pregnant women.

F **Complete blood count**   with red blood cell indices and platelet count

   1. **Anemia**. If present, anemia should be evaluated further and treated. **Microcytosis** without anemia may represent a thalassemia and should also be investigated.

   2. **Leukocytosis**. A mild leukocytosis is normal in pregnancy; however, a grossly abnormal value needs to be evaluated.

G **Urinalysis and culture**

   1. **Asymptomatic bacteriuria** is prevalent in 3% to 5% of pregnant women. Early detection, treatment, and close follow-up must be instituted.

   2. **Acute systemic pyelonephritis**. Asymptomatic bacteriuria predisposes the pregnant woman to the development of acute systemic pyelonephritis, which has serious complications for the mother and fetus and has been associated with premature labor and delivery. Systemic pyelonephritis develops in approximately 20% to 40% of pregnant women with untreated **asymptomatic bacteriuria**.

H **Pap smear.**   Baseline cervical cytology should be established. If abnormalities are noted, institute proper evaluation.

I **Gestational diabetes screen.**   Screening for this condition should be performed at 24 to 28 weeks' gestation using a 1-hour, 50-g glucose test (see Chapter 17).

J **Screening for neural tube defects**

   1. **Elevated maternal serum α-fetoprotein (MSAFP)** in the second trimester is seen in 80% to 90% of pregnancies in which a fetal **neural tube defect** is present (e.g., anencephaly and spina bifida). In the presence of an elevated MSAFP, a targeted ultrasound should be performed to rule out:
   a. Incorrect dates (i.e., pregnancy further along than anticipated)
   b. Multiple gestation
   c. Fetal demise
   d. Abruptio placentae
   e. Other fetal congenital defects (e.g., omphalocele, gastroschisis, and congenital nephrosis)

   2. An unexplained elevated MSAFP may be associated with third-trimester complications such as preeclampsia and placental insufficiency.

K Screening for aneuploidy. The American College of Obstetricians and Gynecologists (ACOG) has recently recommended that screening for Down syndrome should be offered to all pregnant women regardless of their age. First-trimester screen in the form of ultrasound for nuchal translucency (NT) plus biochemical markers such as pregnancy-associated plasma protein A (PAPP-A) and free β-hCG have a detection rate for Down syndrome of 84%. Second-trimester screen consisting of multiple marker screen (quadruple screen) consists of MSAFP, unconjugated estriol, hCG, and inhibin A. This screen has a detection rate of 81%. Pregnancies affected with Down syndrome usually have a low MSAFP, low estriol, high HCG, and high inhibin A. Individualized counseling should be offered to patients to determine the best screening strategy and the need for further invasive testing in the form of chorionic villi sampling (CVS) or genetic amniocentesis.

L HBV testing

1. Identification of pregnant women who are positive for HBV surface antigen (HBsAg) is essential because vertical transmission of HBV is an important cause of acute and chronic hepatitis.
   a. **First-trimester screening programs** should be instituted to identify seropositive women (0.01% to 5% of pregnant patients are seropositive). The neonates of women who test positive can then be treated with passive and active immunoprophylaxis.
   b. **Groups at high risk** for HBV seropositivity include intravenous drug users, HIV-positive women, and Southeast Asian women.
2. **Universal immunization** of **all** neonates, even those of HBsAg-negative mothers, has been recommended by the American Academy of Pediatrics. Immunizations should be given at birth, 1 month of age, and 6 months of age.

M HIV testing. HIV testing and counseling of all pregnant women are now recommended by the Centers for Disease Control and Prevention (CDC).

1. The rate of **mother-to-infant transmission** has been estimated to be 20% to 30%, regardless of maternal symptoms. Babies can be infected in utero, at the time of delivery, and postpartum via contaminated breast milk.
2. **Zidovudine (AZT)** given to HIV-positive women during pregnancy has been shown to reduce perinatal transmission from 25% to 8.3%.
3. **Elective cesarean section** at 38 weeks' gestation may further reduce the rate of vertical transmission, particularly in patients with higher viral loads.

N Sickle-cell screen. This screen is indicated in all patients of African descent. It should also be considered for those of Indo-Pakistani, Caribbean, Mediterranean, Southeast Asian, or Latin American descent.

O Group B streptococcus (GBS). The CDC recommends universal screening of all pregnant patients at 35 weeks' gestation with a vaginal-rectal culture for GBS. Patients with positive cultures should receive intrapartum antibiotic prophylaxis with penicillin to reduce the risk of GBS sepsis in the newborn.

VII RISK ASSESSMENT AND MANAGEMENT OF RISK IN PREGNANCY

Risk is determined based on the patient's history, physical examination, and results of laboratory studies on the first prenatal visit or subsequent visits.

A Once an at-risk patient has been identified, a management plan is implemented to prevent adverse outcome; this plan may be empiric or schematic.

1. **Empiric plan**. The obstetrician decides on the specific management plan on a patient-by-patient basis.
2. **Schematic**. The obstetrician implements a specific, predetermined management scheme every time a risk factor is identified. Table 5-3 represents an example of a schematic risk factor management protocol based on past obstetric history.

B To date, no studies compare empiric versus schematic risk factor management with regard to outcome, although a schematic approach is arguably more scientific.

TABLE 5–3   Schematic Risk Factor Management: Past Obstetric History

Risk Factor	Maternal/Fetal Risk	Management
Previous ectopic pregnancy	Recurrence, maternal anxiety	Early ultrasound to confirm intrauterine pregnancy
Previous stillbirth or early neonatal death	Risk depends on cause (not all are recurrent)	Try to establish cause; early review and specific management
Infant weight		
≤ 2 SD	IUGR	Comprehensive fetal ultrasound Ultrasound for weight
≥2 SD	Gestational diabetes Another large fetus	Random glucose at 28 and 32 weeks Vigilance in labor
Congenital anomaly	Possible recurrence	Obtain details/diagnosis, possible prenatal diagnosis
Blood antibodies	Hemolytic disease	Specific protocol
Preeclampsia	Recurrence	Assess renal function Obtain comprehensive fetal ultrasound Carefully check blood pressure
Preterm delivery	Recurrence	Specific plan depending on cause
Uterine scar	Uterine rupture, cesarean section	Review of mode of delivery at 36 weeks
Short labor	Recurrence and neonatal problems (e.g., trauma, asphyxia, hypothermia)	Specific management plan at 36 weeks
Postpartum hemorrhage	Recurrence	Specific plan at 36 weeks

IUGR, intrauterine growth retardation; SD, standard deviation above the mean for gestation.

Modified from James D. Organization of prenatal care and identification of risk. In James DK, Steer PJ, Weiner CP, et al., eds. High Risk Pregnancy Management Options. Philadelphia: WB Saunders, 1994.

Study Questions for Chapter 5

Directions: *Each of the numbered items or incomplete statements in this section is followed by answers or by completions of the statement. Select the ONE lettered answer or completion that is BEST in each case.*

1. A 39-year-old woman, gravida 3, para 3, is contemplating pregnancy. She delivered three healthy boys by vaginal delivery at ages 17, 23, and 27 years. Her first pregnancy was complicated by low birth weight. Her second pregnancy was unremarkable. She incurred a third-degree laceration after extension of a midline episiotomy upon delivery of her third boy. Her past medical history is unremarkable other than three to four asthma exacerbations every month. What is she at highest risk for in her subsequent pregnancy?

- A Asthma exacerbation
- B Fourth-degree laceration
- C Low-birth-weight infant
- D Twins
- E Uterine dysfunction

2. A 34-year-old primiparous woman is seeing you because she is considering a second pregnancy. She tells you she is afraid to get pregnant given the outcome of her first pregnancy. At 32 years of age, she delivered a term infant with Down syndrome. During that gestation, a serum screen for aneuploidy was not performed. Had a second-trimester multiple marker screen been performed, which of the following results would have been helpful?

- A Low MSAFP, low estriol, low hCG, low inhibin A
- B Low MSAFP, high estriol, low hCG, high inhibin A
- C Low MSAFP, low estriol, high hCG, high inhibin A
- D High MSAFP, high estriol, low hCG, low inhibin A
- E High MSAFP, low estriol, low hCG, low inhibin A

3. A 28-year-old woman, gravida 6, para 1, presents to your office because she tested positive on her home pregnancy test. Her last menstrual period occurred 40 days ago. She normally has regular, 28-day cycles and her periods last 3 to 4 days. She delivered a preterm infant with her very first pregnancy at the age of 17 years. Her subsequent pregnancies have been complicated by three miscarriages and an ectopic pregnancy. She denies any medical problems but admits contracting chlamydia during her late teens (which she sought treatment for). Which of the following is the most important initial step in the management of this patient?

- A Qualitative serum β-hCG
- B Quadruple screen (MSAFP, estriol, hCG, inhibin A)
- C Anticardiolipin antibodies
- D Chlamydia antibody levels
- E Transvaginal ultrasound

4. A 33-year-old woman, gravida 3, para 2, at 32 weeks' gestation, presents to you for her routine prenatal care. She delivered her first baby by cesarean section due to nonreassuring fetal heart rate pattern on the fetal monitor. Her second baby was delivered by cesarean section also because she did not want a trial of labor. Both infants weighed less than 4000 g and are doing fine now. You obtain operative records of her cesarean sections, which show a Pfannenstiel skin incision and low classical type of incision of the uterus. Currently, she is interested in vaginal delivery. What is the best advice you can give her?

- A Vaginal delivery is not recommended because the risk of uterine rupture approaches 8%
- B Vaginal delivery is recommended because the risk of uterine rupture is less than 1%
- C Vaginal delivery is not contraindicated with a history of two previous cesarean sections
- D Vaginal delivery is a possibility, but risk of rupture is between 0.5% and 4%
- E Vaginal delivery is a possibility, but risk of uterine rupture is 8%

5. A 41-year-old woman, gravida 8, para 4, at 18 weeks' gestation, presents to you for her first prenatal visit. She has a history of three therapeutic abortions as a teenager. She has four healthy children—the first two delivered at 32 weeks' gestation, and her third and fourth children delivered at 37 weeks' gestation. Her past medical history is significant for two episodes of pyelonephritis with her first two pregnancies, as well as a partial bicornuate uterus. What in her history places her at greatest risk for preterm delivery with this pregnancy?

[A] Age
[B] Delivery history
[C] Therapeutic abortions
[D] Pyelonephritis
[E] Uterine anomaly

6. A 25-year-old woman, gravida 2, para 1, at 8 weeks' gestation, presents to the high-risk clinic for prenatal care. Her first pregnancy was complicated by delivery of a premature infant with respiratory problems. Her past medical history is remarkable for severe asthma (more than 20 exacerbations per week) for which she uses albuterol and steroid inhalers. She has type II diabetes mellitus that was treated with oral hypoglycemic agents before pregnancy. She also tells you she acquired hepatitis C a few years ago when she used to inject intravenous heroine. She is 5 feet 5 inches tall and weighs 90 lb. Her blood pressure is 180/98, and her urine dipstick is negative. Which of the following predisposes her to delivery of an infant with congenital anomalies?

[A] Weight
[B] Liver disease
[C] Diabetes mellitus
[D] Hypertension
[E] Intravenous drug history

Answers and Explanations

1. The answer is D [IV A 2 b (4)]. Maternal age older than 35 years is a risk factor for multiple gestation, especially dizygotic. The effect of pregnancy on lung diseases is unpredictable; therefore, you cannot assume that her mild asthma will worsen. A third-degree laceration does not necessarily lead to a fourth-degree laceration in a subsequent pregnancy. Laceration degrees depend on obstetric factors, such as size of the baby and length of a midline episiotomy. Teenage pregnancies are at risk for delivery of low-birth-weight infants and uterine dysfunction.

2. The answer is C [VI K]. Trisomy 21 is associated with low MSAFP, low estriol, high hCG, and high inhibin A. It is a screening test that can identify up to 80% of pregnancies with Down syndrome. Multiple marker screens with high MSAFP are associated with neural tube defects.

3. The answer is E [IV B 2]. The most important initial step in a patient with a history of an ectopic pregnancy and possible pelvic inflammatory disease history (history of chlamydial infection) who may be pregnant is to perform a transvaginal ultrasound to rule out another ectopic pregnancy and to rule in an intrauterine pregnancy. A qualitative serum β-hCG will just confirm that the patient is pregnant. Given that the patient has had a positive home pregnancy test, an in-office, ultrasensitive urine hCG is sufficient to confirm pregnancy. A quantitative serum β-hCG is useful to determine when an intrauterine gestation will be visible on transvaginal ultrasound. In this patient who has regular cycles and is 12 days late, an intrauterine gestation should be visible on transvaginal ultrasound. If not, then serum β-hCG is required. The quadruple screen is not useful when performed before 16 weeks' gestation. Anticardiolipin antibodies may be helpful in the future along with other parameters if the patient is interested in delineating the cause of her recurrent spontaneous abortions. Chlamydia antibody levels are not necessary because you already know that the patient has had a chlamydial infection in the past.

4. The answer is A [IV B 7 a (1) and 7 b]. A classical uterine incision (vertical uterine incision through the muscular portion of the uterus) is a contraindication to a trial of labor and vaginal delivery with a subsequent pregnancy. Women with one previous cesarean section are candidates for a vaginal delivery with a subsequent pregnancy, especially if the reason for having the initial cesarean section is nonrepetitive (i.e., breech). Currently, not enough data are available to establish the safety of a trial of labor with two or more previous transverse uterine scars.

5. The answer is B [IV B 3]. A history of two previous preterm deliveries is the strongest risk factor for spontaneous preterm delivery with a subsequent pregnancy. Premature birth is a risk factor with teenage pregnancies, not advanced maternal age pregnancies. Therapeutic abortions, pyelonephritis, and uterine anomalies are all significant risk factors for spontaneous preterm delivery.

6. The answer is C [IV C 5 a]. Pregestational diabetes may increase the risk of birth defects by a factor of three. Anomalies of the heart and central nervous system are the most common problems. The patient with diabetes should be counseled extensively with the aim of achieving good sugar control prior to conception in an attempt to reduce the number of birth defects. Being below ideal body weight does not increase the risk of congenital anomalies. A previous history of intravenous drug use is not significant enough to contribute to congenital anomalies during a current pregnancy. Asthma, hypertension, and liver disease do not increase baseline malformation rate.

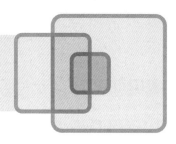

chapter **6**

Prenatal Diagnosis and Obstetric Ultrasound

EMMANUELLE PARÉ

I INTRODUCTION

A **Genetic counseling** assesses the risks of having a child with a genetic condition or a congenital birth defect, interprets the risk, and assists the parents in making a decision regarding contraception, sterilization, adoption, assisted reproductive techniques, disease carrier state detection, referrals to agencies concerned with children with disabilities, prenatal screening and diagnosis, and options regarding pregnancy termination.

B Prenatal diagnosis and screening
   1. The noninvasive diagnostic procedures widely available include ultrasound and fetal echocardiography.
   2. The invasive diagnostic procedures available include preimplantation diagnosis, chorionic villus sampling (CVS), amniocentesis, and percutaneous umbilical blood sampling (PUBS).
   3. Prenatal screening modalities include carrier screening for autosomal recessive conditions and various combinations of serum markers in the first and/or second trimester with or without nuchal translucency for aneuploidy.

C The baseline rate of congenital malformations in the general population is 2% to 3%
   1. Ultrasound for detection of congenital anomalies is offered to most pregnant women.
   2. Fetal echocardiography is recommended when a risk factor for congenital heart defect is present.
   3. In general, invasive prenatal diagnosis is offered when the risk of having an affected offspring exceeds the risks of the procedure.
   4. Carrier screening for autosomal recessive conditions is offered to all women (cystic fibrosis) or only women of certain ethnic backgrounds (e.g., Tay-Sachs to women of Ashkenazi Jewish descent).
   5. Screening for aneuploidy should be offered to all women prior to 20 weeks.

II INDICATIONS FOR PRENATAL DIAGNOSIS

A Chromosomal abnormalities
   1. Positive screening for fetal aneuploidy (see III A)
   2. Advanced maternal age (i.e., at least 35 years at the time of delivery) (Table 6-1). However, in addition to invasive testing, these women should also be offered noninvasive screening.
   3. A previously affected child
   4. Either parent has a chromosomal translocation or inversion
   5. Abnormal ultrasound findings

TABLE 6–1 Incidence of Trisomy 21 According to Maternal Age

Maternal Age	Incidence/Live Births
15–19	1/1250
20–24	1/1400
25–29	1/1100
30	1/900
35	1/350
40	1/100
45+	1/25

   a. Congenital malformations involving a major organ or system

   b. Markers for aneuploidy, ultrasound findings that can be seen in normal fetuses but are observed with an increased frequency in fetuses with chromosomal abnormalities

     (1) Increased nuchal thickness, even isolated, is an indication for invasive prenatal diagnosis.

     (2) Pyelectasis, echogenic bowel, short femur, and short humerus warrant a detailed ultrasound examination to search for anomalies and other markers but may not require invasive prenatal diagnosis if they are an isolated finding.

B Congenital malformations

   1. Congenital heart defects are the most common congenital malformation and occur in 8 per 1000 live births.

   a. They have a multifactorial inheritance pattern.

   b. Risk factors include familial history of congenital heart defects, pregestational maternal diabetes, maternal rubella infection during the first trimester, and exposure to teratogens such as alcohol and some antiepileptic medications.

   2. Neural tube defects (NTDs) are one of the most common congenital malformations and occur in 1 to 2 per 1000 live births.

   a. They have a multifactorial inheritance pattern.

   b. Risks factors include familial history of NTDs, pregestational maternal diabetes, maternal seizure disorder, and maternal intake of some antiseizure medications.

   c. NTD incidence can be reduced by maternal folic acid supplementation at least 3 months prior to conception and during the first 3 months of pregnancy.

     (1) A 0.4-mg dose daily will reduce the incidence of NTDs in the general population by 50%.

     (2) A 4-mg dose daily will reduce the recurrence risk in women with a previous affected child by 70%.

C Mendelian abnormalities

   1. Inborn errors of metabolism

   a. Mucopolysaccharidoses

   b. Mucolipidoses

   c. Lipidoses

   d. Amino acid disorders

   e. Miscellaneous biochemical disorders

   2. Abnormalities in DNA structure. Examples include congenital adrenal hyperplasia; Gaucher disease; Ehlers-Danlos types IV, VI, and VII; Niemann-Pick disease; osteogenesis imperfecta congenita; and xeroderma pigmentosum.

D Abnormal maternal serum α-fetoprotein (MSAFP)

E Fragile X syndrome is the most common cause of inherited mental retardation.

   1. It has an **X-linked recessive** inheritance pattern.

   2. Women who have a child with or a familial history of mental retardation or developmental delay should be tested to see if they carry the premutation and should be offered prenatal diagnosis if they do.

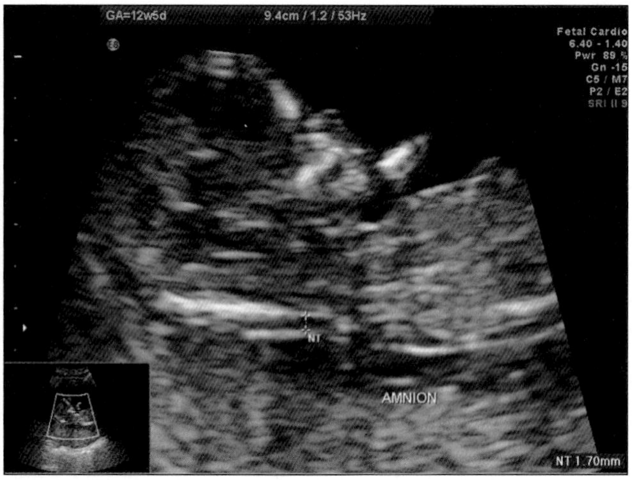

FIGURE 6–1 Ultrasound showing measurement of the fetal crown–rump length during the first trimester.

   3. Women who carry the premutation are at risk for developing premature ovarian failure and may therefore have difficulties conceiving.

III **GENETIC SCREENING**

In the United States, universal screening for fetal aneuploidy should be offered to all women who present for prenatal care before 20 weeks of gestation. Neural tube defect screening should also be offered; this may include second-trimester serum AFP screening or ultrasound. Carrier screening for cystic fibrosis should be made available to all patients. Finally, selective screening for specific disorders should be offered based on ethnicity or familial history. The most common selectively screened genetic disorders are Tay-Sachs disease, sickle cell anemia, and the thalassemias.

A Screening for fetal aneuploidy

   1. Several options for screening for aneuploidy (mostly for Down syndrome and trisomy 18) are now available and include different combinations of five maternal serum markers and one ultrasound marker (nuchal translucency).

   a. First-trimester markers include **nuchal translucency** (NT), which is the measurement of the size of the fluid collection at the back of the fetal neck (Fig. 6-1); **maternal serum β-human chorionic gonadotropin** (β-hCG); and **pregnancy-associated plasma protein A** (PAPP-A). NT measurement is valid from 10 4/7 weeks to 13 6/7 weeks' gestation, and the serum markers are drawn at the same time the NT is measured.

   b. Second-trimester markers include **MSAFP, hCG, estriol, and inhibin A**. Serum markers are drawn between 15 and 22 weeks' gestation.

   2. The values are adjusted for gestational age for the serum markers, and for crown–rump length (CRL) for the NT, and are used in conjunction with the maternal age to calculate the risk for Down syndrome and trisomy 18.

   3. Invasive testing (CVS in the first trimester and amniocentesis in the second trimester) is offered when the risk for those chromosomal anomalies after the screening test is higher than the risk of the procedure.

   4. Combinations of these markers are used as screening tests:

   a. First-trimester tests include:

   (1) NT measurement alone

   (2) Combined first-trimester screen (NT, PAPP-A, and β-hCG)

   b. Second-trimester tests include:

   (1) Triple screen (MSAFP, hCG, and estriol)

   (2) Quadruple screen (MSAFP, hCG, estriol, and inhibin A)

   (3) These are the only options available to women who present for prenatal care after 14 weeks.

    c. Screening tests integrating first- and second-trimester markers: results are disclosed to women only **after the second-trimester portion** of the test is completed.

      (1) Integrated screen (NT, PAPP-A, and quad screen)

      (2) Serum integrated screen (PAPP-A and quad screen)

    d. Screening tests integrating first- and second-trimester markers: invasive testing (CVS) is offered **after the first-trimester portion** is completed if the risk of aneuploidy is high. The final risk assessment incorporates first- and second-trimester results.

      (1) Stepwise sequential screen

      (2) Contingent sequential screen

5. With a 5% screen-positive rate, the sensitivity (or detection rate) is:

    a. Over 85% for the integrated, stepwise sequential, and contingent sequential screens.

    b. Eighty to eighty-five percent for the combined first-trimester screen and quad screen.

    c. Approximately 70% for NT alone and triple screen.

6. Profile of markers associated with aneuploidy

    a. Risk for Down syndrome is increased with **NT** ↑, **free β-hCG** ↑, **PAPP-A** ↓, **AFP** ↓, **hCG** ↑, **estriol** ↓, **and inhibin A** ↑.

    b. Risk for trisomy 18 is increased with **NT** ↑, **AFP** ↓, **hCG** ↓, **and estriol** ↑. **β-hCG , PAPP-A, and inhibin A** are not used in the calculation for trisomy 18.

7. Women who are 35 years or older at the time of delivery should be offered noninvasive screening but should have the option of foregoing noninvasive screening and having an invasive diagnostic procedure (CVS or amniocentesis).

8. For multiple gestations, NT measurements alone may be the only screening option for fetal aneuploidy. Maternal serum marker screening is not as accurate for twins and is unavailable for triplets.

B Screening for neural tube defects

1. NTD screening can include second-trimester MSAFP and/or ultrasound.

2. Both have sensitivity (detection rate) of 80% to 90% for open neural tube defects.

3. NTD screening should be offered to women who elected to have first-trimester screening only, had a CVS, or declined screening for aneuploidy.

4. **MSAFP** can be performed from 15 to 22 weeks' gestation.

    a. An **elevated value** is indicative of an increased risk for a neural tube defect and other disorders (Table 6-2).

    b. A **low value** is indicative of an increased risk for Down syndrome.

C **Cystic fibrosis** is the most common inherited disorder in Caucasians.

1. The carrier rate is 1 in 25 non-Hispanic Caucasians.

2. Screening should be offered when familial history is positive for cystic fibrosis and to all couples when both partners are of Caucasian ethnicity.

3. The most common mutation is the delta F508, which accounts for approximately 70% of mutations found in Caucasians.

4. Most laboratories screen for 23 mutations, which account for 80% of mutations found in Caucasians.

TABLE 6–2 Conditions Characterized by Elevated α-Fetoprotein

Multiple gestation	Fetal death
Bladder exstrophy	Cystic hygroma
Congenital nephrosis	Aneuploidy
Fetal bowel obstruction	Sacrococcygeal teratoma
Underestimated gestational age	
Abdominal wall defects (omphalocele and gastroschisis)	

5. It has an **autosomal recessive** inheritance pattern. Prenatal diagnosis should be offered if both parents are carriers.

D **Hemoglobinopathies**

1. There are approximately 2 million to 2.5 million people in the United States with inherited abnormalities of hemoglobin.

2. Normal hemoglobin is composed of three types of hemoglobin.
   a. Hemoglobin A has two α-chains and two β-chains and makes up 95% of adult hemoglobin.
   b. Hemoglobin A₂ has two α-chains and two δ-chains and makes up 2% to 3.5% of adult hemoglobin.
   c. Hemoglobin F has two α-chains and two γ-chains and makes up the remainder of adult hemoglobin.

3. Sickle cell screening. All people of African descent should undergo carrier screening for sickle cell with a hemoglobin electrophoresis.
   a. Sickle cell disease has an **autosomal recessive** inheritance pattern. Prenatal diagnosis should be offered if both parents are carriers of either sickle cell trait or another hemoglobinopathy such as hemoglobin C trait or β-thalassemia.
   b. The frequency of sickle cell trait in the African American population is approximately 1 in 12.
   c. Sickle hemoglobin (Hb S) results from a substitution from glutamic acid to valine at the sixth position in the β-globin chain.
   d. Hb S functions normally in the oxygenated state. In the deoxygenated state, hydrophobic bonds are formed, which cause red blood cell distortion, or sickling. This leads to vaso-occlusion, tissue infarction, and anemia.

4. Thalassemias. Patients of Southeast Asian or Mediterranean descent should be offered carrier screening with a complete blood count. When the mean corpuscular volume (MCV) is low (less than 80 fL) with normal iron studies, a hemoglobin electrophoresis should be performed.
   a. α-Thalassemia
      (1) Groups at risk are from Southeast Asian, West Indian, Mediterranean, and African descent.
      (2) Production of the α-globin chains is decreased.
      (3) DNA-based testing is needed to detect α-globin gene deletion (when MCV is low, iron studies are normal and Hb electrophoresis is not consistent with β-thalassemia trait).

   b. β-Thalassemia
      (1) Groups at risk are from Mediterranean, Asian, Middle Eastern, Hispanic, and West Indian descent.
      (2) Production of the β-globin chains is decreased.
      (3) Elevated Hb A₂ (more than 3.5%) on Hb electrophoresis is suggestive of β-thalassemia.

E **Tay-Sachs disease** is the congenital absence of the enzyme **hexosaminidase A**, which results in an overaccumulation of GM₂ gangliosides, leading to severe progressive neurologic disease causing death in early childhood.

1. It has an **autosomal recessive** inheritance pattern. Prenatal diagnosis should be offered if both parents are carriers.

2. The carrier rate is 1 in 30 in Ashkenazi Jews and 1 in 300 in those of non-Jewish descent.

3. Carrier screening should be offered if there is a positive familial history, to couples where both members are of Ashkenazi Jewish, French-Canadian, or Cajun descent, and in some cases when only one member is from high-risk descent.

IV TECHNIQUES OF PRENATAL DIAGNOSIS

A **Ultrasound** is the most commonly used method of pregnancy assessment and is a valuable tool in the prenatal diagnosis of congenital anomalies.

1. Ultrasound is **low-energy high-frequency sound waves.** Transabdominal ultrasounds performed for prenatal diagnosis operate at frequencies between 3.5 and 5 MHz.

2. **Safety**
   a. Epidemiologic studies in pregnant women have failed to reveal any association of ultrasound with congenital anomalies or adverse pregnancy outcome.
   b. Most instruments used for diagnosis produce energies far lower than what is considered a safe level of ultrasound exposure to tissues.

3. **Indications for ultrasound during pregnancy**
   a. Evaluation of gestational age
   b. Assessment of fetal viability
   c. Evaluation of multiple gestation
   d. Screening for fetal anomalies, especially in the presence of an abnormal multiple marker screen or MSAFP
   e. Evaluation and follow-up of fetal growth and size
   f. Vaginal bleeding of undetermined etiology
   g. Evaluation of cervical length
   h. Suspected oligohydramnios or polyhydramnios
   i. Assessment of fetal well-being (i.e., biophysical profile)
   j. Determination of fetal presentation
   k. Guidance during procedures: amniocentesis, CVS, version, PUBS
   l. Evaluation for ectopic pregnancy and molar pregnancy
   m. Pelvic mass

4. Ultrasound examinations will provide different information according to the gestational age at which they are done.
   a. **Fetal anatomy** is best evaluated during the **second trimester**, and most routine ultrasounds are performed at that time.
   b. Accurate determination of gestational age is best obtained with a **first-trimester** ultrasound examination.
   c. **Third-trimester** ultrasound examinations are ordered on a routine basis (for fetal weight estimation and detection of **growth** abnormalities), but most are performed for specific indications.

5. **First-trimester ultrasound** can be done transvaginally or transabdominally and should:
   a. Document location of the gestational sac. An intrauterine sac is visible transvaginally as early as 5 weeks' gestation.
   b. Document fetal number.
   c. Confirm fetal viability. Fetal cardiac activity can be detected transvaginally when the embryo is 5 mm or greater in length (approximately 6 weeks' gestation).
   d. Evaluate gestational age. Measurement of the fetal crown–rump length between 6 to 13 weeks' gestation can estimate fetal age within 5 days (Fig. 6-2).
   e. Evaluate the uterus and adnexal structures.
   f. Measure NT when done as part of screening for aneuploidy and only after adequate counseling.

6. **Second-trimester ultrasound** is usually performed transabdominally. It is routinely performed between 18 and 20 weeks' gestation for evaluation of fetal anatomy, gestational age, placental location, and amniotic fluid volume. Measurement of cervical length should be done by transvaginal ultrasound.
   a. The **fetal anatomic survey** should include, but not to be limited to:
      (1) **Intracranial anatomy** with visualization of the lateral ventricles, choroids plexus, thalamus, cerebellum, and cisterna magna.
      (2) Sagittal and transverse views of the cervical, thoracic, lumbar, and sacral **spine**.
      (3) Thorax, diaphragm, and four-chamber view of the **heart**, as well as the outflow tracts when possible.
      (4) Visualization of the **stomach**.
      (5) Visualization of the **kidneys** and **bladder**.
      (6) **Umbilical cord** insertion on an **intact abdominal wall** and determination of the number of **vessels** of the umbilical cord (normal: two small arteries and one large vein).
      (7) Upper and lower **extremities**.

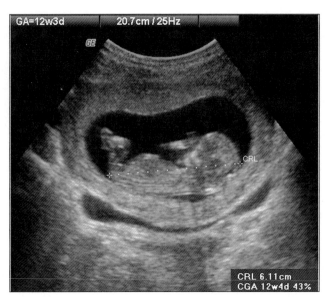

FIGURE 6–2 Ultrasound showing nuchal translucency, which is the measurement of the size of the fluid collection at the back of the fetal neck.

b. Fetal **biometry** includes:

    (1) The **biparietal diameter** is measured at the level of the thalamus and the cavum septum pellucidum. The biparietal diameter is the most accurate measurement of gestational age between 12 and 18 weeks' gestation. The correlation of the biparietal diameter measurement with gestational age decreases as the pregnancy advances because the biologic variability of fetal head size increases dramatically.

    (2) The **head circumference** is measured at the same level as the biparietal diameter.

    (3) The **abdominal circumference** is measured on a true transverse view at the level of the umbilical vein entering the liver.

    (4) The long axis of the femur shaft is measured for the **femur length**.

    (5) **Fetal weight** may be estimated by composite measurement of the biparietal diameter, head circumference, femur length, and abdominal circumference.

c. Placental location should be documented. Placenta previa, a marginal placenta, or a low-lying placenta diagnosed in the second trimester needs to be reevaluated in the third trimester, as many of those will resolve.

d. Amniotic fluid volume can be assessed by semi-quantitative methods:

    (1) Measurement of the **deepest single pocket of amniotic fluid**

        (a) There is **oligohydramnios** if the pocket is less than 2 cm vertically.

        (b) The amniotic fluid volume is **adequate** if the pocket measures 2 to 8 cm vertically.

        (c) There is **polyhydramnios** if a pocket measures more than 8 cm vertically. Polyhydramnios is associated with a higher incidence of congenital abnormalities (Table 6-3).

    (2) The **amniotic fluid index** is calculated by adding together the measurements of the vertical depths of amniotic fluid in the four quadrants of the uterus. Normal values are between 5 cm and 25 cm.

e. Maternal anatomy. Evaluate the uterus and adnexal structures.

7. Third-trimester ultrasound is approached transabdominally. The indications for third-trimester ultrasound are multiple and include estimation of fetal weight and follow-up of fetal growth, evaluation of the amniotic fluid volume, follow-up of a fetal anomaly, determination of fetal presentation, and evaluation of fetal well-being.

a. Fetal weight is estimated as previously described (see IV A 6 b). The margin of error is about 15% and can be even higher in term fetuses.

    (1) If the estimated fetal weight is below the 10th percentile for the gestational age, the fetus is small for gestational age (SGA) and intrauterine growth restriction (IUGR) is suspected.

    (2) If the estimated fetal weight is above the 90th percentile for the gestational age, the fetus is large for gestational age (LGA) and macrosomia is suspected.

TABLE 6–3 Fetal Malformations Associated with Polyhydramnios

Central nervous system	Respiratory system
Anencephaly	Cystic adenomatoid malformation of the lung
Hydrocephaly	Chylothorax
Encephalocele	
Gastrointestinal system	**Musculoskeletal system**
Gastroschisis	Myotonic dystrophy
Omphalocele	Skeletal dysplasia
Esophageal atresia	
Duodenal atresia	
Diaphragmatic hernia	

b. Amniotic fluid volume is assessed as previously described (see IV A 6 c).

c. Fetal well-being can be assessed with the **biophysical profile**.

  (1) The biophysical profile evaluates five components:

   (a) Amniotic fluid volume

   (b) Fetal tone

   (c) Fetal movements

   (d) Fetal breathing

   (e) Nonstress test

  (2) Scoring is as follows:

   (a) A score of 2 (normal) or 0 (abnormal) is assigned to each component.

   (b) A total score of 8 or 10 is normal.

   (c) A total score less than 8 is abnormal and is managed according to the gestational age and the clinical situation.

B **Fetal echocardiography** is a detailed ultrasound examination of the heart. It is of value in detection, diagnosis, and follow-up of congenital heart defects (CHDs) and fetal arrhythmias. It is usually performed between 20 and 22 weeks' gestation and its indications include:

1. Risk factors for CHD (familial history of CHD, maternal diabetes, exposure to cardiac teratogens)

2. Suspected CHDs on regular ultrasound examination

3. Suspected fetal arrhythmia on ultrasound examination or heard on Doptone

4. Other congenital anomalies detected on regular ultrasound examination

5. Nonimmune hydrops fetalis

C **Amniocentesis** is a transabdominal, fine-needle aspiration of amniotic fluid (usually 10 to 30 mL). It should be performed under ultrasound guidance. It is imperative that Rh-negative women who are not sensitized receive **Rho(D) immune globulin** after the procedure. The amniotic fluid contains fetal cells, which can be cultured and evaluated for chromosomal abnormalities and molecular testing. Specific markers can also be dosed in the amniotic fluid.

1. Genetic amniocentesis is usually performed from 15 to 18 weeks' gestation, at which time ample fluid is present, diagnostic tests can be performed, and elective termination, if desired by the patient, is still possible.

  a. The **risk of fetal loss** from a second-trimester amniocentesis is **0.25% to 0.5%**.

  b. Amniotic fluid can be assessed for α-fetoprotein and acetylcholinesterase levels in the evaluation of neural tube defects.

2. Chromosomal abnormalities such as Down syndrome (trisomy 21), trisomy 18, trisomy 13, triploidy, Turner syndrome (45, XO), and Klinefelter (47, XXY) can be identified.

  a. Karyotype is obtained from cultured cells, and chromosomes are counted and analyzed for structural alterations.

  b. Fluorescence in situ hybridization (**FISH**) can be used for more rapid identification of additional or missing chromosomes.

      c. DNA of the fetus can be retrieved and tested for specific diseases.

        (1) If the precise molecular basis of the disease is known (e.g., mutation from adenine to guanine in the codon for the sixth amino acid in the gene coding for (β-globin), then specific probes can be used.

        (2) If the precise molecular basis of the disease is not known, prenatal diagnosis is still possible in a given family using **restriction fragment length polymorphisms**. This method can be used for Huntington chorea, adult-onset polycystic kidneys, adrenal 21-hydroxylase deficiency, and some forms of Duchenne muscular dystrophy, hemophilia A or B, and β-thalassemia.

   3. Amniocentesis can also be done later in pregnancy for other indications.

      a. The level of **bilirubin** in the amniotic fluid can be assessed by spectophotometry, which reflects fetal hemolysis and indirectly evaluates the degree of fetal anemia. It is used in the management of alloimmunization.

      b. Evaluation of **fetal lung maturity** is performed using the lecithin-to-sphingomyelin (L/S) ratio and presence of phosphatidyl glycerol (PG).

      c. Diagnosis of in utero **infections** can be done if maternal infection has been documented or fetal infection is suspected on ultrasound examination.

      d. The risk of preterm delivery from a third-trimester amniocentesis is **1% to 2%**.

D **Chorionic villus sampling** is usually performed at 10 to 12 weeks' gestation. Fetal cells can be obtained either by a transabdominal or transcervical approach. The major benefit of this procedure is earlier prenatal diagnosis.

   1. The **risk of fetal loss** from the procedure is **1%**.

   2. The accuracy is comparable to that of amniocentesis.

   3. Chromosomal analysis and fetal DNA analysis are possible; however, amniotic fluid levels of markers such as AFP cannot be measured with this method.

   4. Limb reduction defects have been associated with this procedure.

   5. Rh-negative women must receive **Rho(D) immune globulin** after the procedure.

E **Other techniques**

   1. Percutaneous umbilical blood sampling or cordocentesis is used to sample fetal blood for karyotype, DNA-based analysis, hemoglobin electrophoresis, and diagnosis of fetal infection, anemia, or thrombocytopenia.

      a. It must be performed under ultrasound guidance.

      b. The **risk of fetal loss** from the procedure is reported as **1% to 3%**, but varies greatly according to the indication.

      c. Rh-negative women must receive **Rho(D) immune globulin** after the procedure.

   2. Preimplantation diagnosis requires the use of in vitro fertilization techniques and is performed on one or two embryo cells at a very early stage.

   3. Fetal skin sampling can be performed to obtain fetal cells.

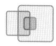

Study Questions for Chapter 6

Directions: *Each of the numbered items or incomplete statements in this section is followed by answers or by completions of the statement. Select the ONE lettered answer or completion that is BEST in each case.*

1. Which combination of markers is suggestive of Down syndrome?

- [A] AFP ↑, hCG ↑, estriol ↑, inhibin A ↑
- [B] AFP ↓, hCG ↓, estriol ↓, inhibin A ↓
- [C] AFP ↑, hCG ↓, estriol ↑, inhibin A ↑
- [D] AFP ↓, hCG ↑, estriol ↓, inhibin A ↑
- [E] AFP ↑, hCG ↓, estriol ↓, and inhibin A ↓

2. Which of the following cannot be detected on a second-trimester ultrasound examination?

- [A] Anencephaly
- [B] Renal agenesis
- [C] Tay-Sachs disease
- [D] Two-vessel cord
- [E] Tetralogy of Fallot

3. A 32-year-old woman, gravida 1, para 1, comes to see you for genetic counseling. Her first child was born with sickle cell disease. She has since remarried, and is requesting prenatal testing. Which of the following is appropriate to offer the patient first?

- [A] Percutaneous umbilical blood sampling at the appropriate gestational age
- [B] Fetal chromosome analysis
- [C] Maternal hemoglobin electrophoresis
- [D] Paternal hemoglobin electrophoresis
- [E] Multiple markers screening

4. Which of the following procedures poses the lowest risk for fetal loss?

- [A] Chorionic villus sampling
- [B] Fetal echocardiography
- [C] Percutaneous umbilical blood sampling
- [D] Fetal biopsy
- [E] Amniocentesis

5. Which of the following is NOT an indication for prenatal diagnosis?

- [A] Paternal age 45 years
- [B] Elevated MSAFP
- [C] Previous child with cystic fibrosis
- [D] Maternal ventricular septal defect (VSD)
- [E] Omphalocele detected on second-trimester ultrasound

Answers and Explanations

1. The answer is D [III A 5 a]. The risk for Down syndrome is increased when AFP and estriol levels are lower than normal and hCG and inhibin A levels are higher than normal. The risk for trisomy 18 is increased when AFP, hCG, and estriol levels are all lower than normal; inhibin A is not used in the calculation for trisomy 18 risk. Other combinations of markers have not been associated with specific chromosomal anomalies.

2. The answer is C [IV A 6 a]. The fetal anatomic survey should include views of the head, spine, thorax, heart, stomach, kidney, bladder, umbilical cord, abdominal wall, and extremities. It can thus detect anomalies such as anencephaly, congenital heart defects, renal agenesis, or two-vessel cord. Prenatal diagnosis of Tay-Sachs disease can only be performed using invasive methods (CVS or amniocentesis) to obtain fetal DNA.

3. The answer is D [III D 3]. Because this patient has already had an affected child and is asymptomatic, she must be a heterozygous carrier. Her previous husband must also be a carrier. Because the father in this case is different, he should undergo hemoglobin electrophoresis to evaluate his carrier status. Fetal chromosome analysis will not detect a fetus affected with sickle cell disease.

4. The answer is B [IV A–D]. Fetal echocardiography is a noninvasive diagnostic procedure and thus does not carry any fetal loss risk. Amniocentesis has a 0.25% to 0.5% fetal loss rate. CVS has a 1% fetal loss rate. Percutaneous umbilical blood sampling carries a 1% to 3% loss rate. Fetal biopsy is an invasive procedure.

5. The answer is A [II A–E]. Paternal age has minimal effect on chromosomal anomalies and congenital malformations risk and is not an indication for prenatal diagnosis. Elevated MSAFP indicates an increased risk for NTDs and other anomalies and further testing should be offered. With a previous child affected with cystic fibrosis, the recurrence risk is 25%. Familial history of CHDs is a risk factor for CHDs, and fetal echocardiography should be offered. Omphalocele is associated with chromosomal anomalies and other congenital malformations.

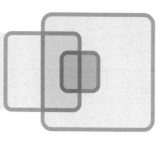

chapter 7

Teratology

JENNIFER B. MERRIMAN · DORIS CHOU

I   INTRODUCTION

Teratology is the **study of abnormal fetal development**. Major birth defects occur in approximately 3% of all deliveries. A teratogenic agent, which can be identified in less than 50% of the cases, is any chemical (drug), infection, physical condition, or deficiency that, on fetal exposure, can alter fetal morphology or subsequent function. Teratogenicity appears to be related to genetic predisposition (both maternal and embryonic), the developmental stage of the fetus at the time of exposure, and the route and length of administration of the teratogen. Because any woman in her reproductive years may be pregnant, all women should be warned of any teratogenic potential associated with a drug. In cases of known teratogens, women and their physicians have a responsibility to effectively prevent pregnancy.

A Genetic susceptibility. Species differences in response to teratogens have been demonstrated. Human newborns exposed to the tranquilizer thalidomide in utero demonstrated major malformation of the arms (phocomelia), whereas laboratory animals (rats) showed no effect at similar doses. Animal studies, although helpful, do not always reliably predict the response in humans.

B Developmental stage at time of exposure (Fig. 7-1). Susceptibility of the conceptus to teratogenic agents depends on the developmental stage at the time of exposure.

   1. Resistant period. From day 0 to day 11 of gestation (postovulation), the fetus exhibits the "all or none" phenomenon with regard to major anomalies; that is, it will either be killed by the insult or survive unaffected. This is the period of predifferentiation when the aggregate of totipotential cells can recover from an injury and continue to multiply.

   2. Maximum susceptibility (embryonic period). From days 11 to 57 of gestation, the fetus is undergoing organ differentiation and, at this time, is most susceptible to the adverse effects of teratogens. The particular malformation depends on the time of exposure. After a certain time in organogenesis, it is thought that abnormal embryogenesis can no longer occur. For example, because the neural tube closes between days 22 and 28 postconception (5 weeks after the last menstrual period), a teratogen must be active before or during this period to initiate development of a neural tube defect (e.g., spina bifida or anencephaly).

   3. Lowered susceptibility (fetal period). After 57 days (8 weeks) of gestation, the organs have formed and are increasing in size. A teratogen at this stage may cause a reduction in cell size and number, which is manifested by:
   a. Growth retardation
   b. Reduction of organ size
   c. Functional derangements of organ systems

C Administration of teratogen. The route and length of administration of a teratogen alter the type and severity of the malformation produced. Abnormal developments increase in frequency and degree as the dosage increases. Agents may be less teratogenic if systemic blood levels are reduced by the route of administration (e.g., poor gastrointestinal antibiotic absorption may account for lower blood levels in pregnancy).

D Definition. Teratogenicity of an agent or factor is defined by the following criteria:

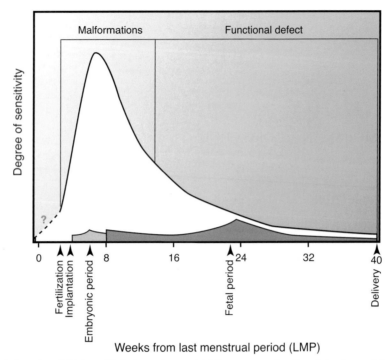

FIGURE 7–1 Embryonic and fetal sensitivity to environmental influences as a function of developmental state. (Reprinted with permission from Creasy RK, Resnik R. Maternal–Fetal Medicine: Principles and Practice. Philadelphia: WB Saunders, 1984:95.)

1. **Presence of the agent during the critical period of development when the anomaly is likely to appear**. Malformations are caused by intrinsic problems within the developing tissues at a specific time in organogenesis.

2. **Production of the anomaly in experimental animals when the agent is administered during a stage of organogenesis similar to that of humans.** Teratogenicity may not become apparent for several years; for example, in utero exposure to diethylstilbestrol is known to cause genital tract abnormalities, such as adenosis and carcinoma, but these abnormalities may not become apparent until the reproductive years.

3. **Ability of the agent to act on the embryo or fetus either directly or indirectly through the placenta.** For example, heparin is not teratogenic because, unlike warfarin, it cannot cross the placenta because of its large molecular weight.

E Structural defects. These defects have been categorized into three groups (Fig. 7-2).

1. **Malformations** are morphologic defects of an organ or other part of the body resulting from an abnormality in the process of development in the first trimester. This leads to incomplete or aberrant morphogenesis (e.g., ventricular septal defect).

2. **Deformations** are abnormal forms, shapes, or positions of a body part caused by constraint within the uterus, usually occurring in the second or third trimester. An example is clubfeet from oligohydramnios.

3. **Disruptions** are defects from interference with a normally developing organ system, usually occurring later in gestation (i.e., in the second or third trimester, after organogenesis). An example is amniotic band syndrome.

II **TERATOGENIC AGENTS**

A Ionizing radiation

1. **Acute high dose (more than 250 rad)**. The dose of radiation and the gestational age during exposure are predictive of the adverse neonatal effects: microcephaly, mental retardation, and

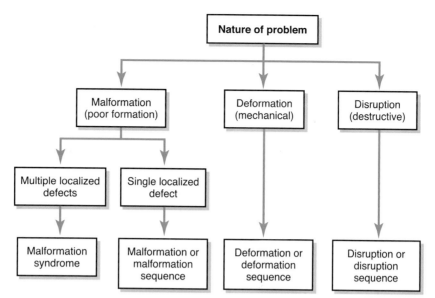

FIGURE 7–2 Categories of structural defects. (Adapted from Graham JM Jr. Smith's Recognizable Patterns of Human Deformation. Philadelphia: WB Saunders, 1988:4.)

growth retardation. For example, the in utero victims of the atomic explosions in Hiroshima and Nagasaki have suffered from both birth defects and leukemia. However, follow-up studies have shown that most children with these adverse effects were those exposed before 15 weeks' gestation, during the period of organogenesis, whereas most of the children exposed during the third trimester had growth retardation but normal intelligence.

  a. Time of exposure. Fetal effects depend on the gestational age (postovulation) at the time of exposure.

   (1) At 2 to 4 weeks, either the fetus is normal or a spontaneous abortion occurs.

   (2) At 4 to 12 weeks, microcephaly, mental retardation, cataracts, growth retardation, or microphthalmia may occur.

   (3) At 12 to 16 weeks, mental retardation or growth retardation occurs.

   (4) After 20 weeks, the effects are the same as with postnatal exposure and include hair loss, skin lesions, and bone marrow suppression.

  b. Dose effect

   (1) After exposure to less than 5 rad, and probably less than 10 rad, an adverse fetal outcome is unlikely to result.

   (2) After exposure to 10 to 25 rad, some adverse fetal effects may result.

   (3) After exposure to more than 25 rad, classic fetal effects, including growth retardation, structural malformations, and fetal resorption, may be detected. At this level of exposure, elective abortion should be offered as an option.

 2. Chronic low dose

  a. In **diagnostic radiation,** the dose to the conceptus should be calculated by the hospital's radiation biologist (Table 7-1). Such a dose rarely adds up to significant exposure, even if several radiographic studies are performed.

  b. Associated risk of teratogenicity

   (1) The mutagenic effects of radiation, if present, have proved to be very small. The estimated risk of leukemia for children exposed in utero to radiation during maternal radiographic pelvimetry increases from 1 in 3000 among unexposed children to 1 in 2000.

   (2) The results of several studies provide no conclusive evidence linking preconception low-dose radiation exposure with an increased risk of delivering an infant with a chromosomal abnormality.

 3. Radioactive iodine. Radiation exposure from radioisotopes administered internally for organ visualization is roughly equal to that of radiographic procedures; however, after the 10th week of gestation, fetal thyroid development can be retarded in addition to any adverse effects of radiation.

TABLE 7–1   Doses to the Uterus and Embryo for Common Radiologic Procedures

Study	View	Dose/View (mrad)	Films/Study	Dose/Study (mrad)
Skull	AP, PA	<0.01		
	Lat	<0.01	4.1	<0.05
Chest	AP, PA	0.01–0.05	1.5	0.02–0.07
	Lat	0.01–0.03		
Mammogram	CC	0.1–0.5	4.0	
	Lat	3–5		7–20
Lumbar spine	AP (7″ × 17″)	30–58	2.9	51–126
	14″ × 17″			
	Lat	33–65		
		11–32		
Lumbosacral	AP	92–187	3.4	168–359
spine	PA	40–97		
	Lat	12–33		
Abdomen	AP	80–163	1.7	122–245
	PA	23–55		
	Lat	29–82		
Intravenous pyelogram	AP	130–264	5.5	686–1398
	PA	43–104		
	Lat	13–37		
Retrograde pyelogram	AP	109–220	1.0	
Hip	AP	72–140	2.0	103–213
	Lat	18–51		

AP, anteroposterior; CC, cranial-caudal; Lat, lateral; PA, posteroanterior.

B **Drugs and medications.**   In the United States, surveys show that 45% to 95% of pregnant women ingest either over-the-counter or prescription drugs other than iron and vitamins during their pregnancy. Many are taken before a woman realizes that she is pregnant or are taken without the advice of a physician. The prohibition of all medications during pregnancy is impossible and is likely to be more harmful to the patient. However, the issue of whether a medication is harmful to the fetus is raised in most pregnancies. Physicians caring for women of childbearing age should be aware of potential teratogenicity of medications and should be able to address questions arising from the accidental or intentional ingestion of drugs during pregnancy.

1. Approximately 3% to 5% of newborns have **congenital malformations** caused by a host of environmental and genetic factors, most of which are unable to be identified. Drugs and medications account for less than 1% of these malformations.

2. **Access to the fetoplacental unit** is critical in the causation of developmental anomalies. Factors affecting access of the drug or medication to the fetus include:
   a. Maternal absorption
   b. Drug metabolism
   c. Protein binding and storage
   d. Molecular size (molecules with a molecular weight of more than 1000 daltons do not cross the placenta easily)
   e. Electrical charge
   f. Lipid solubility

3. **Animal research** can help identify teratogenic potential, but results may be misleading because of species variation.
   a. The most striking example is **thalidomide**, in which exposure in the animals tested (mice and rats) failed to produce limb defects but caused severe limb reduction defects in humans, monkeys, and rabbits. Although the thalidomide-associated embryopathy led to the belief that human teratogenicity could not be predicted by animal studies, it is erroneous.
   b. **Every drug found to be teratogenic in humans has subsequently been shown to cause similar defects in animals**, although species variation exists. It is worth noting that drugs that cause

teratogenesis in animals often do so at much higher doses than used clinically in humans, where similar outcomes are not seen. Of the 1600 drugs that have been tested in animals, about one-half cause congenital anomalies; however, there are only 30 documented human teratogens.

4. **Human research**. Case reports once suggested that drugs such as warfarin, diethylstilbestrol, and isotretinoin were teratogenic. Other studies have led to the "mislabeling" of safe drugs (e.g., Bendectin). Pharmaceutical companies also play a role in the identification of teratogens by participating in postmarketing surveillance studies. To learn more about the teratogenic effects of certain drugs, women can call centers that monitor exposure to prescription and over-the-counter medications.

   a. **Formal epidemiologic studies** are designed to assess whether mothers who took a drug during pregnancy have larger numbers of malformed children than those who did not (cohort studies) or whether mothers of children with a specific malformation took the drug more often than mothers of children without the malformation (case-control studies). Long-term studies are also important; it is becoming increasingly clear that adverse effects of drugs on neurodevelopmental behavior may be more serious than structural defects.

   b. Difficulties occur with the study of teratogens. Because most malformations occur rarely, large sample sizes of exposed individuals are necessary. Maternal illnesses that require the use of medications may be a confounding factor in the study of the teratogenicity of any drug used to treat that disorder. Recall bias also confounds the study of drugs and their potential teratogenic affects, because women whose children have abnormalities are much more likely to recall an exposure (especially in case-control studies).

5. **Risk factors for adverse fetal effects** have been assigned to all drugs based on the teratogenic risk that the drug poses to the fetus. The Food and Drug Administration has proposed the following classification scheme, which is generally accepted by manufacturers and authors (see chapter 4).

6. **Known teratogenic drugs**. The list of proven teratogens is surprisingly short. Certain commonly used agents should be avoided even while a patient is trying to conceive. These include the vitamin A isomer isotretinoin or doses of vitamin A higher than 8000 IU daily; alcohol; excess caffeine; and some of the sex steroids. The live virus vaccines, such as rubella, should never be prescribed if a patient is possibly pregnant or planning to conceive within 1 month. However, if the aforementioned drugs are inadvertently given, the outcome is still usually favorable.

7. A **dose threshold** is a theoretic dose for each teratogen below which no adverse effects have been noted.

8. **"Recreational" drugs** (see Chapter 8). Because most recreational drugs are taken with other agents, such as alcohol or tranquilizers, the precise effect is difficult to ascertain. Listed below are commonly used drugs and their potential effects.

   a. **Alcohol**. Consumption of alcohol in pregnancy is the most common known teratogenic cause of mental retardation. Both abortion and stillbirth are increased in heavy drinkers. **Fetal alcohol syndrome**, which manifests as mental retardation, growth retardation, abnormal facies, ocular and joint anomalies, and cardiac defects, has been associated with the ingestion of 1 oz or more of absolute alcohol per day.

      (1) The **threshold dose** of alcohol (the point at which congenital anomalies are induced) is unknown; therefore, alcohol consumption in pregnancy can never be regarded as "safe."

      (2) **Early exposure**. The critical period for facial dysmorphology has been found to be around the time of conception.

      (3) **Late exposure**. Exposure late in gestation or in small quantities may result in isolated effects, such as learning or behavioral disorders.

      (4) **Heavy alcohol consumption** (more than 3 oz of absolute alcohol or six drinks daily) is associated with some or all of the features of fetal alcohol syndrome, including:

         (a) **Prenatal or postnatal growth retardation**. Growth retardation is usually prenatal in onset, but postnatal catch-up generally does not occur. It is manifested by decreased birth weight, length, and head circumference.

         (b) **Central nervous system (CNS) involvement** includes small brain size and brain malformations. Functional deficits, such as moderate mental retardation, delayed motor development, poor coordination, tremulousness, hyperactivity, and poor attention spans, have been noted.

(c) **Characteristic facial dysmorphology** includes a shortened palpebral fissure (observed in more than 90% of affected children); a short, upturned nose; a hypoplastic maxilla; and a thinned upper lip. One study linked craniofacial abnormalities with prenatal alcohol exposure in a dose-response manner.

(5) **Risk of fetal alcohol syndrome.** A large number of children whose mothers drank moderately or heavily during pregnancy may exhibit features of prenatal alcohol exposure, such as developmental delay, but not the full-blown syndrome.

(a) Approximately 30% of children born to chronic alcoholic women have fetal alcohol syndrome.

(b) The risk of major or minor congenital anomalies in infants of mothers who ingest excessive amounts of alcohol but do not meet the criteria for chronic alcoholism is around 32%.

(c) Intrauterine fetal growth retardation is increased 2.7 times in pregnant women who drink excessively.

b. **Marijuana.** There is no evidence that smoking marijuana is teratogenic, although the adverse effects of smoking in pregnancy should not be overlooked (see Chapter 8).

c. **Heroin** has not been shown to cause birth defects, but the drugs that are often taken with heroin are associated with congenital anomalies. The principal adverse fetal effect in heroin addicts is severe neonatal withdrawal, causing death in 3% to 5% of neonates. Methadone is used to replace heroin, and, although it is not teratogenic, it is associated with severe neonatal withdrawal.

d. **Phencyclidine (PCP),** or "angel dust," is a hallucinogenic agent associated with facial abnormalities in a small percentage of exposed infants.

e. **Cocaine** is rapidly becoming the most abused drug in pregnancy, second only to alcohol. One study showed an increased risk of congenital malformations, stillbirths, and low-birth-weight infants in cocaine users. A clear causal relationship exists between cocaine use and abruptio placentae because of the drug's vasoconstrictive properties (see Chapter 9).

9. **Cancer chemotherapy.** Although there is a high incidence of fetal loss, including spontaneous abortion and stillbirth, the incidence of congenital malformations is surprisingly low.

a. When cancer chemotherapy is administered during the first trimester of pregnancy, there are varied and unpredictable effects, ranging from severe deformity to no abnormality. The fetal heart, neural tube, and limbs are affected during early organogenesis, with the palate and ears being susceptible later in organogenesis.

b. After the period of organogenesis (weeks 2 to 8 postconception), there is less teratogenic risk from chemotherapy in pregnancy, though intrauterine growth restriction, stillbirth, preterm delivery, and low-birth-weight infants are possible with second- and/or third-trimester exposure. Even after organogenesis, the fetal eyes, genitalia, hematopoietic system, and CNS remain vulnerable to continued exposure (Cardonick E, Iacobucci A. Use of chemotherapy during human pregnancy. *Lancet Oncol.* 2004 May; 5(5):283–91).

C **Hyperthermia.** Studies suggest that sustained maternal hyperthermia (body temperature of more than 102°F [38.9°C] for more than 24 hours between 4 and 14 weeks' gestation), rather than spiking fevers, is teratogenic. Malformations noted in infants of mothers who were febrile from infectious agents or who frequented saunas in the first trimester include the following:

1. Growth restriction

2. CNS defects, such as mental deficiency, microcephaly, hypotonia, and anencephaly, and increased risk of neural tube defects

3. Facial anomalies, including midfacial hypoplasia, cleft lip and palate, microphthalmia, micrognathia, and external ear anomalies

4. Minor limb anomalies, such as syndactyly

D **Maternal medical disorders.** Women with medical disorders should be counseled about the teratogenic risks both from the condition being treated and from the treatment. In some cases, the untreated medical disorder poses greater risks to the fetus than the teratogenic potential of the specific drug therapy.

1. **Diabetes mellitus.** Infants of insulin-dependent diabetic mothers have up to a 22% incidence of cardiac, renal, gastrointestinal, CNS, and skeletal malformations. Most of the malformations

occur between the third and sixth week postconception and are increased if there is hyperglycemia during that stage of gestation.

 a. The level of risk may be estimated by obtaining glycosylated hemoglobin (hemoglobin A_{Ic}) in the first trimester. Levels greater than 8% (depending on the laboratory) have been associated with a significantly increased risk. Strict glucose control preconceptually has been shown to decrease the frequency of malformations.

 b. Two particular **malformations** are found in infants of diabetic mothers:

  (1) Caudal regression syndrome with hypoplasia of the caudal spine and lower extremities.

  (2) Congenital heart disease, most commonly ventricular septal defects.

 c. Because neural tube defects occur more frequently in infants of diabetic mothers, maternal serum α-fetoprotein (MSAFP) screening should be performed at 16 weeks' gestation. An extensive anatomic survey by ultrasound at 18 to 22 weeks' gestation should identify most of the major anomalies (i.e., cardiac and spinal defects) in an affected fetus.

2. Hypothyroidism. This endocrine disorder has been associated with a twofold increase in stillbirths and congenital anomalies. Cretinism is the result of maternal, fetal, and neonatal thyroid hormone deficiency in iodine-poor areas. Severe cretinism is characterized by mental retardation, deaf mutism, spasticity, strabismus, and abnormal sexual maturation. Congenital hypothyroidism occurs in severely iodine-deficient areas. Maternal subclinical hypothyroidism has recently been observed to increase the risk of first-trimester miscarriage and possibly decrease several points of IQ scores in their offspring.

3. Phenylketonuria (PKU). This genetic disorder is characterized by a deficiency of phenylalanine hydroxylase, a liver enzyme that catalyzes the conversion of phenylalanine to tyrosine. The resulting high levels of phenylalanine in maternal serum result in high levels in the fetus. A special diet low in phenylalanine beginning before conception can prevent the adverse effects (mental retardation) of this disorder. Children born to mothers with PKU who have neglected their special diets are at risk for the following conditions:

 a. Mental retardation (92% incidence)

 b. Microcephaly (73% incidence)

 c. Congenital heart disease (12% incidence)

 d. Low birth weight (40% incidence)

4. Virilizing tumors (arrhenoblastoma). This condition can have masculinizing effects on the mother and produce pseudohermaphroditic changes in the female fetus, including fusion of the labia and clitorimegaly.

5. Epilepsy. This condition is a classic example of the contribution of a disease process and its treatment to an increase in birth defects. Management of epilepsy is complicated by the fear that anticonvulsants may cause fetal abnormalities.

 a. In general, infants born to epileptic mothers have a **6% to 7% incidence of major and minor congenital abnormalities.** Unfortunately, all the major anticonvulsants have some level of teratogenic risk.

 b. The **most commonly observed malformations** in infants of mothers who take anticonvulsants are **cleft lip, cleft palate, and congenital heart disease.** Valproic acid carries a 1% to 2% risk of neural tube defects.

 c. Some studies have suggested that increased seizure frequency leads to higher incidence of malformations. Other research has indicated that malformations may also be inherent to the seizure disorder itself; mothers who take phenytoin for indications other than epilepsy did not have a higher incidence of malformations. The highest fetal malformation rate occurs when mothers are taking multiple anticonvulsants.

 d. Several new antiepileptic medications have been used recently, some as monotherapy. All of these have limited experience in human pregnancy; therefore, an online pregnancy registry is available for enrollment to patients and physicians.

  (1) Lamotrigine. May be associated with a lower risk of teratogenicity. The frequency of major birth defects in the registry is 2.9%, which is encouraging. Of note, women exposed to both lamotrigine and valproate have an increased risk of major fetal malformations.

  (2) Topiramate

  (3) Gabapentin

6. **Psychotropic drug use in pregnancy**. Most psychotropic medications readily cross the placenta. Although no psychotropic drug has yet been specifically approved for use in pregnancy, continued use of the agent may prevent maternal relapse of psychiatric disease. Studies of patients taking antipsychotic medications show that the rate of malformation in exposed patients is similar to that in unexposed patients; however, the rate is still approximately two times that in the general population. This suggests that some other factor may be responsible for the higher incidence of malformations.

   a. Lithium has been associated with 10 to 20 times the normal rate of Ebstein anomaly after first-trimester exposure.

   b. Benzodiazepines are associated with a very small (less than 1%) risk of associated cleft anomalies.

7. **Thrombophilic disorders**. These disorders predispose persons to clot inappropriately. Thromboembolism is the number one cause of death during pregnancy. Several thrombophilias can be inherited such as with protein C/S or antithrombin III deficiency, factor V Leiden, and prothrombin G20210A mutation carriers. Other affected individuals have a precipitating medical diagnosis such as a mechanical heart value, atrial fibrillation, trauma, or even pregnancy.

   a. Most pregnant individuals are treated with heparin anticoagulation during pregnancy as heparin does not traverse the placenta. Commonly, patients are treated with low-molecular-weight heparin (enoxaparin or Lovenox) as opposed to unfractionated heparin given the longer half-life, improved bioavailability, and increased absorption from subcutaneous dosing.

   b. There are some possible indications where oral warfarin therapy may have a role (i.e., patients with mechanical heart valves), or patients may become pregnant while taking such medications. Exposure to warfarin during the sixth to ninth weeks of gestation can lead to a constellation of malformations known as fetal warfarin syndrome. The characteristics of fetal warfarin syndrome can include the following:

    (1) Flattened nasal bridge

    (2) Stippled bony epiphyses

    (3) Birth weight less than 10th percentile for gestational age

    (4) Ocular defects

    (5) Extremity hypoplasia

    (6) Developmental retardation

    (7) Seizures

    (8) Scoliosis

    (9) Deafness/hearing loss

    (10) Congenital heart disease

    (11) Death

   c. Fondaparinux is a synthetic analog of the antithrombin-binding pentasaccharide sequence found in heparin. Fondaparinux is approved for the treatment of venous thromboembolism. Fondaparinux does not cross the human placenta. The risk to the fetus appears to be low, though data in pregnancy are scarce.

   d. Argatroban is a parenteral direct thrombin inhibitor approved for treatment of persons with heparin-induced thrombocytopenia (HIT). It is metabolized in the liver; therefore, it must be used with caution in patients with liver dysfunction. There are no data in human pregnancy. It is not known whether argatroban crosses the placenta, and to date, animal studies have been encouraging.

   e. Hirudin/bivalirudin are also parenteral direct thrombin inhibitors approved for treatment of persons with HIT. Hirudin was originally isolated from the salivary glands of the medicinal leech. Recombinant hirudin (lepirudin) is now available, though data in human pregnancy are quite limited. It does appear to be able to cross the placenta, because it is able to cross the rat placenta.

  E | **Infections.** Exposure to viral infections during gestation has been recognized as a significant cause of birth defects. Most infants, if infected during the first trimester, suffer from a syndrome of congenital malformations and are small for gestational age.

1. **Rubella virus (German measles)**. When rubella infections occur in the first month of pregnancy, there is a 50% chance of anomalous development. This chance decreases to 22% in the second

month and to 6% to 10% in the third to fourth month. The timing of infection is important. If infection occurs during week 6, cataracts may form. Deafness occurs when infection takes place between weeks 7 and 8. If a mother is infected at the time of delivery, the newborn may contract pneumonitis or encephalitis. **Congenital rubella syndrome** includes the following symptoms:

  a. Neuropathologic changes
  (1) Microcephaly
  (2) Mental and motor retardation
  (3) Meningoencephalitis

  b. Cardiovascular lesions
  (1) Persistent patent ductus arteriosus
  (2) Pulmonary artery stenosis
  (3) Atrioventricular septal defects

  c. Ocular defects
  (1) Cataracts
  (2) Microphthalmia
  (3) Retinal changes
  (4) Blindness

  d. Inner ear problems, resulting in sensorineural deafness

  e. Symmetric **intrauterine growth retardation**

2. **Cytomegalovirus (CMV).** This ubiquitous virus infects 1% to 2% of all infants in utero. Between 1 in 5000 and 20,000 infants suffer severe problems that are recognizable at birth.

  a. The risk of severe complications is much greater for infants of mothers who had a primary infection in pregnancy compared with those who had a recurrent infection.
  (1) Seronegative mothers infected with primary CMV transmit the infection to the fetus in 30% to 40% of cases. Of those infected, 2% to 4% are severely symptomatic at birth.
  (2) Seropositive mothers who have a recurrent infection transmit the infection to the fetus in only 1% of cases, and 99% of these infants appear normal at birth. Later in life, these affected infants may suffer from delayed speech development and learning difficulties due to sensorineural hearing loss. A small group has chorioretinitis.

  b. A specific relation between time of exposure and subsequent deficit has not been demonstrated, although the most damage seems to occur early in pregnancy. Gestational age at the time of exposure does not appear to influence the rate of fetal infection. The neonatal effects of fetal CMV infection include the following:
  (1) Microcephaly and hydrocephaly
  (2) Chorioretinitis
  (3) Hepatosplenomegaly
  (4) Cerebral calcification
  (5) Mental retardation
  (6) Heart block
  (7) Petechiae

3. **Herpes simplex virus type 2 (HSV-2).** Although mucocutaneous herpetic infection is common, less than 1 in 7500 infants suffer from perinatal transmission of HSV-2. Fetal transmission occurs by hematogenous spread during a maternal viremia or by direct contact during passage through an infected birth canal; however, congenital infection, which causes fetal malformations, is rare. It is thought that fetal infection during the first trimester results in miscarriage. In a few cases, a syndrome was described that resembled other infants with viral infections during the first trimester, including the following fetal anomalies:
  a. Growth retardation
  b. Microcephaly
  c. Chorioretinitis
  d. Cerebral calcification
  e. Microphthalmia encephalitis

4. **Toxoplasmosis.** This disease, which is caused by a protozoan, *Toxoplasma gondii*, may be transmitted from mother to fetus antepartum. Although infection is most common outside the United States (e.g., in Sweden), the incidence of congenital infection in the United States ranges

from 1 to 6 cases per 1000 live births. Approximately 30% of infected women transmit the disease to their unborn children. The disease can be contracted by changing infected cat litter or eating poorly cooked meat. In a population of 550 French women who acquired toxoplasmosis during pregnancy, 61% of the neonates had evidence of congenital infection; of these neonates, 6% died, 5% had severe clinical illness, 9% had mild disease, and 41% had subclinical disease.

    a. Fetal infection early in pregnancy increases the severity of infection.

        (1) The pregnancy may result in a spontaneous abortion, perinatal death, severe congenital anomalies, abnormal growth, and residual handicaps.

        (2) In severe disease, the characteristic triad of anomalies includes chorioretinitis; hydrocephaly or microcephaly; and cerebral calcification, resulting in psychomotor retardation.

    b. Transmission to the fetus is more likely later in pregnancy, although the neonatal handicap is much more benign and, in fact, is often subclinical.

5. Syphilis (*Treponema pallidum*). The incidence of syphilis in pregnant women is increasing. The rise in congenital syphilis has paralleled the increase in primary and secondary syphilis in adults. Several hundred cases of congenital syphilis are diagnosed each year; half of these infants are born to women with no prenatal care. *T. pallidum* appears to be able to cross the placenta at any time during pregnancy. Because the fetus has an immature immune system, it is rarely infected before 16 to 18 weeks' gestation. Before this time, antibiotic therapy is highly successful.

    a. The incidence of congenital infection is inversely proportional to the duration of maternal infection and to the degree of spirochetemia.

        (1) Recent or secondary infection in the mother confers the greatest risk of fetal infection. All infants born to women with primary and secondary infection are infected, but 50% are asymptomatic.

        (2) Only 40% of infants born to women with early latent disease are infected, and the incidence drops to 5% to 15% for late latent infection.

    b. In utero infection may result in:

        (1) Preterm delivery or miscarriage

        (2) Stillbirth

        (3) Neonatal death in up to 50% of affected infants

        (4) Congenital infection (asymptomatic or symptomatic), which, when symptomatic, can manifest as:

            (a) Hepatosplenomegaly

            (b) Joint swelling

            (c) Skin rash

            (d) Anemia

            (e) Jaundice

            (f) Snuffles

            (g) Metaphyseal dystrophy

            (h) Periostitis

            (i) Cerebrospinal fluid changes

    c. Adequate antibiotic therapy for the pregnant woman is generally thought to provide adequate therapy for the unborn child. However, several case reports have described congenitally infected infants born to mothers treated with benzathine penicillin G. The risk of treatment failure appears to be greater for women who are treated for secondary syphilis or who are in the last trimester of pregnancy.

6. Varicella zoster virus (VZV). This condition, which can take the form of **chickenpox** and, later, **herpes zoster**, is an uncommon virus, occurring in 1 to 7 of 10,000 pregnancies. The infection is much more severe in adults than in children, and pregnancy does not seem to alter this risk. Transplacental transmission of VZV is now well documented and occurs in about 24% of cases after maternal varicella in the last month of pregnancy and in 0% of cases of maternal zoster (see II E 6 c). The frequency of fetal infection in the first trimester is less than 5%.

    a. Inconclusive reports have described an increased risk of leukemia in infants born with gestational varicella. One case also describes chromosome breaks in the leukocytes of a child whose mother had varicella in pregnancy.

b. Multiple cases of congenital malformations may occur in the offspring of women who have chickenpox during the first 20 weeks of pregnancy. These include abnormalities of several organ systems.

    (1) Cutaneous

        (a) Cicatricial skin scarring with denuded skin and limb hypoplasia

        (b) Vesicular rash (hemorrhagic rash) if infection occurs in the last 3 weeks of pregnancy

    (2) Musculoskeletal

        (a) Limb hypoplasia (unilateral) involving the arm, mandible, or hemithorax

        (b) Rudimentary digits

        (c) Clubfoot

    (3) Neurologic

        (a) Microcephaly

        (b) Cortical and cerebellar atrophy

        (c) Seizures

        (d) Psychomotor retardation

        (e) Focal brain calcifications

        (f) Autonomic dysfunction, such as loss of bowel and bladder control, dysphagia, and Horner syndrome

        (g) Ocular abnormalities, such as microphthalmia, optic atrophy, cataracts, and chorioretinitis

    (4) Other

        (a) Symmetric intrauterine growth retardation

        (b) Fever, vesicular rash, pneumonia, and widespread necrotic lesions of the viscera, leading to death if infection occurs in the last 3 weeks of pregnancy

c. No good evidence proves that **herpes zoster** causes congenital anomalies. A few case reports have described microcephaly, microphthalmia, cataracts, and talipes equinovarus in infants born to mothers suffering from zoster during pregnancy; however, these cases may represent chance occurrences.

7. Mumps. Mumps infection is not strictly teratogenic; however, after maternal exposure, neonates have been born with endocardial fibroelastosis, ear and eye malformations, or urogenital abnormalities.

8. Enteroviruses (Coxsackie B). Serious or fatal illness (40%) in the fetus results from maternal exposure to Coxsackie B virus. Surviving infants may exhibit cardiac malformations; hepatitis, pneumonitis, or pancreatitis; or adrenal necrosis.

9. Parvovirus B19 is the cause of erythema infectiosum, otherwise known as "fifth disease" or "slapped cheek" disease. This virus can trigger fetal aplastic anemia, which can lead to congenital heart failure and hydrops fetalis.

Study Questions for Chapter 7

Directions: *Each of the numbered items or incomplete statements in this section is followed by answers or by completions of the statement. Select the ONE lettered answer or completion that is BEST in each case.*

1. A 23-year-old woman who was seen in the emergency department yesterday for a superficial gunshot wound to the wrist tested positive on a routine serum β-hCG screen. Her cycles have always been regular and occur every 28 days and are 4 days in duration. She believes she is on day 23 of her current cycle. She denies past medical history. She does not smoke or consume any alcohol. She does take mega doses of vitamins, which include 20,000 IU of vitamin A daily. Above which dose of vitamin A has teratogenicity been noted?

- A 5000 IU
- B 8000 IU
- C 10,000 IU
- D 12,000 IU
- E 20,000 IU

2. A 28-year-old woman, gravida 2, para 1, at 11 weeks of gestation, who just moved from another state is seeing you for her first prenatal visit. She has an idiopathic respiratory disease that predisposes her to recurrent lung infections. She tells you that she can't even count how many radiographs she has received in the last 2 months. You contact her previous hospital's radiation biologist, who calculates her radiation exposure at approximately 260 mrad. Which of the following is the likely possible outcome of this pregnancy?

- A No adverse outcome
- B Growth retardation
- C Spontaneous abortion
- D Bone marrow suppression
- E Mental retardation

3. A 28-year-old woman just tested positive on a home pregnancy test even though she and her husband use condoms regularly. Her last menstrual period was 36 days ago. Her periods usually occur every 30 days. Her past medical history is unremarkable and she denies use of tobacco, alcohol, or drugs. Her only concern is that 3 weeks ago she received a rubella vaccine and was told by her doctor to not become pregnant for the next 1 month after administration of the vaccine. Which of the following is the best advice?

- A You should schedule an elective termination as soon as possible
- B You have the option of having a therapeutic abortion within the first trimester
- C Rubella vaccine is not harmful to your fetus
- D Pregnancy outcome is usually favorable even after exposure to this vaccine
- E Live viral vaccines are associated with a fourfold increased risk of malformation

4. A 19-year-old woman, gravida 1, para 0, presents to you at 7 weeks of gestation by her last menstrual period for prenatal care. Her history and physical examination are completely unremarkable. You educate her about nutrition and exercise during pregnancy and perform an in-office transvaginal ultrasound to confirm her gestational age. You then order routine prenatal labs. While chatting with her, you discover that she has a stressful job and likes to use the hot tub at least several times a day in excess of 4 hours. What is the best advice to give to this patient?

- A You should not use hot tubs during pregnancy
- B Hot tub use in pregnancy is associated with fetal growth restriction
- C Minimize hot tub use in the first trimester because it may cause malformations
- D Hot tub use during pregnancy is acceptable as long as it is in short intervals
- E Hot tub use is acceptable as long as water temperature is below 102.5°F

QUESTIONS 5–9

Match the statement below with the teratogenic agent that best describes it. Each answer may be used once, more than once, or not at all.

[A] Rubella
[B] Parvovirus
[C] Herpes simplex
[D] Varicella zoster
[E] Mumps

5. Persistent patent ductus arteriosus

6. Endocardial fibroelastosis

7. Triad of heart, eye, and ear defects or malformations

8. Skin scarring and shortened limbs

9. Aplastic anemia

QUESTIONS 10–15

Match each description below with the number that most closely pertains to it. Each answer may be used once, more than once, or not at all.

[A] 3
[B] 6
[C] 10
[D] 30
[E] 50

10. Exposure to ___ rad may have some adverse fetal effects

11. After week ___, exposure to radioactive iodine may affect fetal thyroid development

12. Baseline risk of major congenital anomaly is _____

13. Intrauterine fetal growth retardation is increased ___ times in excessive drinkers

14. Infants born to epileptic mothers have ___% incidence of congenital abnormalities

15. Rate of congenital anomalies in pregnant women taking antipsychotic medications is _____

Answers and Explanations

1. The correct answer is B [I B 1 and II B 6]. It is known that consuming the vitamin A isomer isotretinoin or doses of vitamin A higher than 8000 IU daily can be teratogenic to a developing fetus. If this woman became pregnant around cycle day 14, then the pregnancy does not exceed 11 days. Therefore, exposure to the teratogen occurred within the resistant period. The possible outcomes are either fetal death or continuation of pregnancy.

2. The correct answer is A [II A 1 b (1)]. Exposure to 260 mrad (260×10^{-3} rads) at 11 weeks of gestation is unlikely to result in any problems—exposure to radiation of 5 rad or less has not been associated with adverse fetal outcomes. Large-dose radiation (more than 250 rads) during weeks 4 through 12 may cause mental retardation or cataracts. Spontaneous abortion may occur if the fetus is exposed to more than 250 rad during weeks 2 through 4. Growth retardation may occur if the fetus is exposed to large-dose radiation during weeks 12 through 16. Bone marrow suppression is seen when the fetus is exposed to large-dose radiation after 20 weeks of gestation or postnatally.

3. The correct answer is D [II B 6]. Even if known teratogenic agents, such as live viral vaccines (rubella), excess caffeine, alcohol, isotretinoin, and excess vitamin A, are inadvertently taken during pregnancy, the outcome is still usually favorable. Simple exposure to a live viral vaccine is not an indication for therapeutic abortion. The rubella vaccine can be harmful to the fetus. The risk for congenital malformations is different between various live viral vaccines (rubella, mumps, measles, etc.).

4. The correct answer is C [II C]. Sustained maternal hyperthermia (over 102°F) for more than 24 hours during the first trimester is associated with growth restriction and CNS defects, such as microcephaly, anencephaly, and mental deficiency. As her physician, you should not prohibit use of saunas if they are important to her for stress relief. Simply telling the patient that "hot tub use is associated with fetal growth restriction" is not the best advice even though it is a true statement. Answer choices D and E are not the best answers. Simply revealing the parameters (over 102°F, more than 24 hours, short intervals rather than sustained hyperthermia) of studies that have shown an association between sustained maternal hyperthermia and pregnancy outcomes is not the best advice.

5. The answers are 5-A [II E 1 b (1)], **6-E** [II E 7], **7-A** [II E 1 b, 1 c, 1 d], **8-D** [II E 6 b 1, b 2], **9-B** [II E 1]. Congenital rubella infection can cause a triad of ocular defects (cataracts, blindness), inner ear problems (sensorineural deafness), and cardiovascular lesions, such as persistent patent ductus arteriosus, pulmonary artery stenosis, and atrioventricular septal defects. Maternal infection with rubella at the time of delivery can result in newborn pneumonia and encephalitis. Although rare, after maternal exposure to mumps, neonates have been born with endocardial fibroelastosis, ear and eye malformations, or urogenital abnormalities. Infection with chickenpox during first 20 weeks of gestation may result in congenital malformations, such as cicatricial skin scarring and limb hypoplasia. Parvovirus B19 infection during pregnancy can lead to fetal aplastic anemia, which can progress to fetal nonimmune hydrops if undetected.

6. The answers are 10-C [II A 1 b (2)], **11-C** [II A 3], **12-A** [I], **13-A** [II B 8 a 5 (c)], **14-B** [II D 4 a], **15-B** [II D 5]. Exposure to less then 5 rad (and probably less than 10 rad) is unlikely to cause an adverse outcome. However, exposure to 10 to 25 rads may have some adverse fetal effects. After the 10th week of gestation, fetal thyroid development can be retarded in addition to any adverse effects of radiation. Major birth defects occur in approximately 3% of all deliveries. Intrauterine growth retardation is increased 2.7 times in pregnant women who drink excessively. Infants born to epileptic mothers have a 6% incidence of congenital malformations. The rate of congenital anomalies in pregnant women taking antipsychotic medications is two times that in the general population (which is 3%).

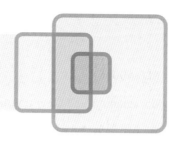

chapter 8

Substance Abuse in Pregnancy

SERDAR URAL • EMMANUELLE PARÉ

I   INTRODUCTION

Substance abuse during pregnancy is currently a significant problem in modern obstetrics. It is common to abuse more than one substance at a time.

A Frequency of occurrence.   Use of illicit substances in the general population has become so prevalent that the obstetrician and neonatologist are faced daily with the effects of these drugs on their patients. The true prevalence of drug use in pregnancy is difficult to determine. In the United States, prevalence based on urine toxicology is a minimum of 10%. This number is probably much higher because the urine test is valid for recently used drugs only, and its sensitivity is low.

B Substances most likely to be abused. Alcohol and cocaine   have become the leading abused substances, with alcohol being the most common potentially teratogenic substance in pregnancy. Although other substances are abused in pregnancy, these two substances are examples of how a significant social problem can affect obstetric practice.

C Problems related to substance abuse.   Women who abuse substances while pregnant tend to have other related problems, including sexually transmitted diseases, poor nutrition, and poor prenatal care.

II   DEFINITION

Substance abuse is divided into three stages: use, abuse, and dependence.

A Use   involves taking low, infrequent doses of illicit substances for experimentation or social reasons. Damaging consequences are rare or minor.

B Abuse   is the persistent or repeated use of a psychoactive substance for more than 1 month, despite the persistence or recurrence of adverse social, occupational, psychological, or physical effects.

C Dependence   is present if **three or more of the following criteria** are met continuously for 1 month or repeatedly in a given year:

1. Abandonment of social, occupational, or recreational activities
2. Continued substance use despite knowledge of social, psychological, or physical problems exacerbated by drug use
3. Substance is taken to relieve or avoid withdrawal symptoms
4. Withdrawal symptoms
5. Persistent desire or one or more unsuccessful attempts to control substance use
6. Substance taken in larger amounts or over a longer period than intended
7. Frequent intoxication or withdrawal symptoms occur when the individual is expected to fulfill obligations at work, school, or home
8. Significant time spent obtaining or taking the substance or recovering from the effects of its use

III **SIGNS AND SYMPTOMS OF SUBSTANCE ABUSE**

A Disorientation, euphoria, sedation, agitation, and other unusual behavior

B Hallucinations, hypertension, tachycardia, inflamed nasal mucosa, track marks, and pupil abnormalities

C Unusual infections, such as cellulitis and hepatitis

IV **PSYCHOACTIVE SUBSTANCES**

A Opiates

1. **Examples** include heroin, morphine, methadone, and codeine.
2. **Effects** include euphoria, relaxation, mood elevation, drowsiness, and respiratory depression.

B Depressants

1. **Examples** include barbiturates, methaqualone, and diazepam.
2. **Effects** include euphoria, relaxation, mood elevation, drowsiness, mood volatility, respiratory depression, and impaired coordination.

C Stimulants

1. **Examples** include cocaine and amphetamine.
2. **Effects** include euphoria, alertness, sense of well-being, suppression of fatigue and hunger, increased sexual arousal, increased pulse and blood pressure, tremor, insomnia, paranoia, psychosis, cardiac arrest, abruptio placentae, and fetal growth retardation.

D Hallucinogens

1. **Examples** include lysergic acid diethylamide (LSD), mescaline, and psilocybin.
2. **Effects** include altered perception, detachment, increased blood pressure, tremor, impaired judgment, and panic.

E Phencyclidine (PCP) and related compounds

1. One **example** is ketamine hydrochloride. Street names include angel dust and crystal.
2. **Effects** include detachment, mental numbness, distorted perception, anxiety, and impaired coordination.

F Cannabinoids

1. **Examples** include marijuana and hashish.
2. **Effects** include euphoria, relaxation, altered perception, sexual arousal, increased appetite, disorientation, impaired judgment, incoordination, and paranoia.

V **ALCOHOL USE IN PREGNANCY**

A Alcohol use is the leading cause of teratogenesis by drugs or environmental agents (see Chapter 7). Ethanol crosses the placenta and the fetal blood–brain barrier freely. It is thought to cause toxicity both directly and indirectly by its metabolites.

B Women who drink during pregnancy are often older and have higher rates of other illicit drug use, less education, and lower social status.

1. **Fetal alcohol syndrome** is a congenital syndrome involving a triad of growth retardation, facial abnormalities, and central nervous system (CNS) dysfunction. The **most common abnormalities** are:
   a. Prenatal and postnatal growth deficiency
   b. Mental retardation
   c. Behavioral disturbances

      d. Atypical facial appearance: short palpebral fissure, epicanthal folds, flat midface, and hypoplastic philtrum

      e. Congenital heart defects

    2. In the United States, the incidence is 1 in 500 to 1000 deliveries.

C **Threshold of alcohol abuse.** There is **no safe level of alcohol use in pregnancy**. Patients should be advised that it is safest not to consume any alcohol during pregnancy. The daily consumption of 1 to 2 oz of absolute alcohol (moderate to heavy drinking) may result in infants who show characteristics of fetal alcohol syndrome. Use of smaller amounts of alcohol has also been related to fetal alcohol syndrome. Alcohol is excreted in breast milk. There is evidence that drinking alcohol during breastfeeding may have a detrimental effect on the baby's motor development.

VI COCAINE USE IN PREGNANCY

The rise in the use of cocaine among the general population has spawned a rise in use among pregnant women, thus making the maternal and fetal complications associated with cocaine use more common. In addition, the increase in rates of exchanging sex for crack cocaine has increased the number of cocaine-complicated pregnancies.

A **Use in general population.** Cocaine use has increased among the general population because of the availability of inexpensive **"crack"** cocaine, a highly purified form of cocaine that is named for the cracking or popping sound made when the crystals are heated in a test tube. Cocaine can be smoked as crack, taken intranasally, or injected intravenously.

B **Pharmacologic effects**

    1. Cocaine produces **complex cardiovascular effects** that depend on an intact sympathetic nervous system and direct stimulation of the myocardium and vasculature.

    2. Cocaine **blocks dopamine and norepinephrine reuptake at the postsynaptic junction**, thereby increasing CNS irritability.

    3. This leads to **maternal and fetal vasoconstriction and tachycardia**, as well as **stimulation of uterine contractions**.

C **Maternal complications**

    1. Neurologic

      a. Seizures

      b. Rupture of intracranial aneurysm

      c. Postpartum intracerebral hemorrhage

      d. Cerebral infarction

    2. Cardiovascular

      a. Myocardial infarction

      b. Hypertension

      c. Arrhythmias

      d. Rupture of the ascending aorta

      e. Sudden death

    3. Infectious

      a. Intravenous use predisposes the patient to bacterial endocarditis, hepatitis, and HIV exposure.

      b. Sexually transmitted diseases, such as gonorrhea, chlamydia, human papillomavirus, and syphilis, are common, frequently because of the exchange of sex for drugs or sex for money to buy drugs.

    4. Obstetric

      a. Possible increase in spontaneous abortions

      b. Increased incidence of preterm labor and delivery

      c. Increased incidence of premature rupture of membranes (PROM)

      d. Intrauterine growth restriction

      e. Abruptio placentae

    f. Increased risk of intrauterine fetal demise

    g. Increased risk of fetal distress

    h. Congenital anomalies

        (1) Fetal microcephaly

        (2) Nonduodenal intestinal atresia–infarction

        (3) Limb reduction defects

        (4) Genitourinary tract anomalies

        (5) Cerebral infarctions in utero

    i. Neonatal and infant behavioral disturbances (e.g., sudden infant death syndrome)

    j. Meconium-stained amniotic fluid

D **Management**

1. Detection

    a. Consider drug abuse in the differential diagnosis.

    b. Educate patients about drug use and its effects on the mother and developing infant.

    c. Ask patients directly about types of psychoactive substances used.

    d. Examine patients for **inflammation of nasal passages and intravenous injection sites**, especially in patients who do not keep prenatal appointments or who show signs of anemia, fetal growth retardation, or preterm labor.

    e. Consider **urine toxicology screening**. Although this can be used as a method of monitoring and instructing pregnant women about drug use, some states require that these results be reported to government authorities.

        (1) A **patient–physician alliance** can be best forged through directly confronting a patient about the suspected drug abuse. At that time, the physician can impress on the patient the need to treat the problem in the interest of both herself and the developing infant.

        (2) **Urine screening** can then be obtained through reasoned persuasion rather than deception.

2. Treatment

    a. Refer the patient to a chemical dependency treatment center. Ideally, treatment center options should include individual and group counseling, intensive day treatment, and residential treatment. Optimally, residential treatment should include obstetric facilities.

    b. Use the assistance of social services to coordinate a management plan, because a patient's hostile home and social environment (e.g., pervasive poverty, easy access to drugs, or positive opinion of drug culture) can lead to conditions that compound complications caused by cocaine use (e.g., lack of prenatal care and poor nutrition). Dealing effectively with the patient's environment may determine the success or failure of any medical intervention.

    c. Prevent premature labor and intrauterine growth retardation using education, nutrition counseling, ultrasound, and fetal testing. Choose magnesium sulfate rather than β-mimetics to treat preterm labor, because magnesium sulfate does not have stimulating effects on the heart muscle.

    d. With **symptoms of abdominal pain**, differentiate between abruptio placentae, appendicitis, and bowel ischemia. Laboratory evaluation and fetal monitoring clarify the diagnosis and point to the best treatment option (see Chapter 9). Drug screening is essential.

    e. With **cocaine overdose**, control seizures, hyperthermia, and hypertension by reducing CNS irritability and sympathetic nervous system overactivity. In addition, evaluate the patient's cardiovascular system.

        (1) Obtain a urine toxicology screen, a complete blood count, and coagulation studies, and measure cardiac and liver enzymes, electrolytes, and arterial blood gas.

        (2) Administer oxygen and consider intubation for intractable seizures.

        (3) Monitor urine output, vital signs, and fetal heart rate.

        (4) Use ice baths or cooling blankets to treat hyperthermia.

        (5) Treat seizures with magnesium sulfate or diazepam.

        (6) Maintain normotension and normal heart rate.

    f. Consider hospitalization for detoxification, treatment of psychological disorders, and coordination of further therapy.

    g. Once **abstinence** has been achieved, perform periodic urine screens to monitor continued abstinence.

VII OTHER SUBSTANCES ABUSED IN PREGNANCY

A Marijuana

1. Marijuana is a commonly used illicit substance among pregnant women.

2. There is no evidence that marijuana is associated with congenital anomalies in humans.

3. Maternal smoking level may correlate with increased perinatal mortality, preterm delivery, PROM, and infants of lower birth weight. This correlation may be because marijuana is commonly abused along with other substances.

B Heroin

1. Heroin causes no increase in congenital anomalies.

2. Intrauterine growth retardation, stillbirth, prematurity, and perinatal death are increased.

3. Neonatal withdrawal, behavioral disturbances, and mild developmental delay have been reported.

4. The poor nutritional status of many heroin addicts may be as important as the heroin use.

C Methadone

1. Methadone causes no increase in congenital anomalies.

2. Methadone use is associated with low-birth-weight infants.

D Tobacco (nicotine)

1. Twenty-five percent of reproductive-age women are smokers.

2. Concurrent use with other substances is a likely possibility.

3. Spontaneous abortion, abruptio placentae, PROM, preterm delivery, and lower-birth-weight infants are increased.

4. No increase in congenital anomalies has been seen.

VIII SUBSTANCE ABUSE AND PRENATAL CARE

A Prenatal care may **reduce the adverse effects of substance abuse** for the mother and fetus.

B A **multidisciplinary approach**, including social workers, is essential; substance abusers probably have nonmedical problems that tend to complicate pregnancy.

C Treatment for substance abuse should be offered.

D Intensive **counseling on the risks associated with substance abuse** is essential.

E Laboratory studies, ultrasound examinations, and frequent visits may be necessary; frequency should be determined on a case-by-case basis.

F Counseling on breastfeeding and exposure of the infant to substances used by the mother is important.

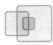

Study Questions for Chapter 8

Directions: *Each of the numbered items or incomplete statements in this section is followed by answers or by completions of the statement. Select the ONE lettered answer or completion that is BEST in each case.*

1. An 18-year-old student enjoys drinking once or twice a week with her college friends. Lately, she has been drinking more than 10 mixed alcoholic beverages each time she goes out. Although she gets a severe "hangover" after each night of drinking, she still enjoys drinking alcohol and doesn't believe it causes any harm to her body. She is an average student at school and is able to keep a part-time job without any difficulty. She has many friends and is well liked. She claims that everybody around her drinks as much as she does. She doesn't have a thirst for alcohol throughout the day, but admits that a month ago she only had to drink four drinks to get the same "buzz" she gets now with six drinks. Her pattern of alcohol consumption is best described as:

- [A] Use
- [B] Abuse
- [C] Tolerance
- [D] Dependence
- [E] Withdrawal

2. A 30-year-old woman, gravida 2, para 1, at 8 weeks of gestation, likes to drink one glass of red wine at night with dinner and doesn't believe it will harm her developing fetus. She drank the same amount throughout her last pregnancy and she delivered a normal healthy neonate weighing 8 lb 4 oz. Her past medical history is unremarkable other than an appendectomy. When performing her ultrasound at 18 weeks of gestation, the ultrasonographer should pay close attention to the anatomy of the baby's:

- [A] Bones
- [B] Brain
- [C] Heart
- [D] Kidneys
- [E] Vertebrae

3. A 20-year-old woman, gravida 4, para 3, presents to you at 22 weeks of gestation for routine prenatal care. She has missed her last two appointments. All of her previous pregnancies were complicated by preterm labor and delivery of small infants with significant respiratory distress. She has a history of a small inferiolateral myocardial infarct from the previous year. In the office she appears anxious. Her vital signs are as follows: T = 99.0, BP = 170/96, P = 135, R = 18. The rest of her physical examination is unremarkable other than what she describes as "stretch marks" on her antecubital fossa. Which of the following obstetric complications is most likely to occur during this pregnancy?

- [A] Cerebral infarction
- [B] Chorioamnionitis
- [C] Placenta previa
- [D] Placental abruption
- [E] Seizures

4. A 25-year-old woman, gravida 1, para 0, at 13 weeks of gestation, presents to you for routine prenatal care. She says her baby moves frequently and keeps her up part of the night. She also reports increasing vaginal discharge that is odorless and otherwise asymptomatic. Upon measuring the fundal height, you smell alcohol on her breath. She fails the finger-to-nose test. The rest of the physical examination is unremarkable. She has no medical history and denies smoking, alcohol, or drug use. What is the initial best step?

- [A] Alcohol and drug screen
- [B] Prescribe metronidazole and follow-up in 4 weeks
- [C] Refer her to a social worker
- [D] Confront her about your findings
- [E] See her back in 4 weeks

5. A 35-year-old woman, gravida 3, para 2, at 20 weeks of gestation, is seeing you for a routine prenatal visit. Today she has no complaints. Her previous pregnancies have been unremarkable. She has chronic hypertension and a history of a cholecystectomy. She has no known drug allergies. She is a successful attorney who admits to smoking marijuana several times a week for relaxation and says she has read several papers that show no increased risk of congenital anomalies. Her vitals are as follows: T = 97.9, BP = 108/68, P = 100, R = 16. Doppler shows fetal heart rate at 156 bpm. What is the best course of action during this prenatal visit?

A Educate her about the possibility of delivering a small infant
B Refuse to see her if she does not stop using marijuana
C Refer her to a social worker for possible substance abuse
D Acknowledge that she is correct about no increased risk of congenital anomalies
E See her back at 24 weeks of gestation

Answers and Explanations

1. The answer is B [II B]. This teenager is abusing alcohol because she consumes alcoholic beverages despite recurrent adverse physical effects (i.e., hangover). Alcohol "use" would imply low, infrequent quantities of consumption. Although she is beginning to build up tolerance (needing six drinks instead of four to get the same effect), "tolerance" is not the best term to describe her entire pattern of alcohol consumption and its effect on her lifestyle. She doesn't meet most of the criteria for alcohol dependence. She does not have problems at work or school, she does not have withdrawal symptoms, and she does not spend excessive time obtaining or drinking alcohol. Alcohol withdrawal can be serious. It involves autonomic hyperactivity, tremor, agitation, insomnia, and even seizures. The student doesn't have these symptoms.

2. The answer is C [V B 1 e]. There is no safe level of alcohol use in pregnancy. Although the chances of congenital anomalies are small with small amounts of alcohol use during pregnancy, there is still a slight possibility of an anomaly. Heavy alcohol use during the early first trimester has been associated with congenital heart defects (especially ventricular septal defect). The anatomy of bone in the developing fetus is not changed; however, its growth velocity is affected by alcohol. Although fetal alcohol syndrome causes mental retardation, brain anatomy is infrequently changed to the point of detection on a routine 18-week ultrasound. Alcohol is rarely associated with kidney and spine anomalies.

3. The answer is D [VI C 4 d]. High blood pressure, anxiety, needle-track marks, and a history of repetitive preterm deliveries and myocardial infarct in a young, healthy woman are suspicious for drug use. Cocaine use is associated with much higher rates of placental abruption than in the general pregnant population. Cerebral infarction and seizures can occur in both the mother and the developing infant because of cocaine use. Neither is, however, an "obstetric" complication; seizures and infarction are both maternal and fetal/neonatal complications. No association exists between cocaine use and placenta previa or chorioamnionitis.

4. The answer is D [VI D 1 e(1)]. A patient–physician alliance can be best forged through directly confronting a patient about the suspected drug abuse. Alcohol and drug screen can be obtained after confronting the patient rather than through deception. This patient's discharge is normal during pregnancy and most likely doesn't require antibiotic treatment. Referring her to a social worker is premature if you have not confronted her about the possibility of alcohol abuse. A multidisciplinary approach is important for long-term treatment and maintenance of abstinence, but is not the initial best step. Seeing her back in 4 weeks without addressing the issue of alcohol use during pregnancy would be inappropriate.

5. The answer is A [VI D 1 b and VII A 3]. Educating patients about drug use and its effects and establishing a strong patient–physician relationship are key to successfully managing substance abuse during pregnancy. This educated patient would benefit from knowing that her newborn may be of lower birth weight because of her use of marijuana during pregnancy. Refusing to see a patient without at least a 30-day notice and referral to another physician sets grounds for a lawsuit. A social worker consult may be helpful later but not at this initial visit. Acknowledging that she is correct about her facts without addressing the consequence on low birth weight with marijuana use is not the best course of action. It is not proper to see her back in 4 weeks without addressing the issue of illicit substance use.

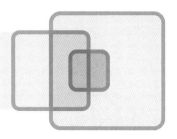

chapter 9

Antepartum Bleeding

DANIELLE BURKLAND

I INTRODUCTION

Obstetric hemorrhage remains a direct cause of maternal death in nearly 30% of cases. First-trimester bleeding is associated with spontaneous abortion, ectopic pregnancy, and molar pregnancy (see Chapters 18, 27, and 29). In the third trimester, bleeding is most often associated with placental abnormalities.

II PLACENTA PREVIA

A Definition. **Placenta previa is defined as the implantation of the placenta over the cervical os.** There are three types of placenta previa (Fig. 9-1):

1. **Total or complete placenta previa**. The placenta completely covers the internal os. Complete previa presents the greatest maternal risk and is associated with the largest amount of blood loss.

2. **Partial previa**. The placenta partially covers the internal os.

3. **Marginal previa**. The placenta extends to the margin of the internal cervical os.

B Incidence. Placenta previa occurs in approximately **1 in 200 live births (0.5%)**. Ultrasound performed in the second trimester may show a placenta previa in 5% to 15% of cases. However, as the lower uterine segment develops, over 90% of these previas will resolve. A repeat ultrasound should be performed at 28 weeks to confirm the presence of a placenta previa.

C Etiology. Little is known about the cause of placenta previa. Several epidemiologic risk factors have been identified.

1. Previous placenta previa

2. **Previous cesarean section**. The incidence of placenta previa increases with an increasing number of cesarean sections; it is between 1% and 4% with one previous cesarean section. In patients with four prior cesarean sections, the risk of a previa is 10%.

3. **Multiparity**. Approximately 80% of cases of placenta previa occur in multiparous patients.

4. **Advanced maternal age**
   a. Age older than 35 years: relative risk of 4.7
   b. Age older than 40 years: relative risk of 9

5. **Smoking**

6. **Asian and African ethnic background**

7. **Previous dilation and curettage (D and C)**

D Clinical presentation. **Painless vaginal bleeding** in the third trimester is the most characteristic sign. Bleeding may occur in the following circumstances:

1. During rest or activity (70% of bleeding occurs during rest)

2. After trauma, coitus, or pelvic examination

3. During labor, when the lower uterine segment begins to efface and dilate. The tearing of the placental attachments at or near the internal cervical os causes the bleeding.

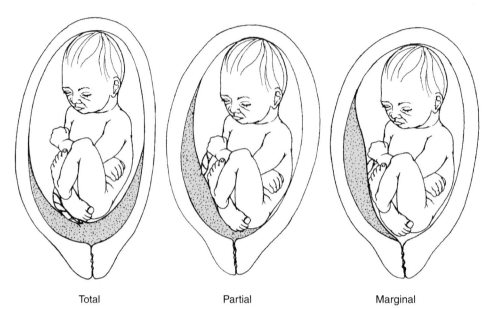

| Total | Partial | Marginal |

FIGURE 9-1 Variations of placenta previa. (From Niebyl JR, Simpson JL, Gabbe SG. Obstetrics: Normal and Problem Pregnancies. 4th Ed. London: Churchill Livingstone, 2001.)

E Diagnosis. Placenta previa should be suspected in all patients who present with vaginal bleeding after 24 weeks. Women suspected of having a placenta previa should undergo an **ultrasound** to determine the position of the placenta. Digital and pelvic examination is deferred until the diagnosis of placenta previa is excluded by ultrasound.

1. **Ultrasound. Transabdominal ultrasound has up to a 7% false-negative rate. Transvaginal ultrasound** may also be performed when the diagnosis is still in question.

2. **Examination.** Prior to the availability of ultrasound nearly 24 hours a day, cervical examination was performed. Definitive diagnosis of placenta previa can be made by clinical palpation of placenta tissue though the cervical os and should only be attempted during a **double set-up** examination (i.e., the patient is in the delivery room prepared for a vaginal examination and an emergent cesarean section), as it may precipitate a hemorrhage. Therefore, it is performed only when:
   a. Delivery is contemplated at the time of the examination.
   b. The examination is performed in the operating room with the patient prepped for surgery, an anesthesiologist present, the surgeon scrubbed, and blood cross-matched and available.
   c. The pregnancy is at or near term.

F Management. Treatment depends on gestational age, amount of vaginal bleeding, maternal hemodynamic status, and fetal condition.

1. **Expectant management.** This approach is justifiable if the fetus is preterm (less than 37 weeks) and can benefit from further intrauterine development. Expectant management should proceed as follows:
   a. Hospitalization until bleeding subsides. The patient may be discharged after the bleeding lessens and a physician judges that the fetus is healthy.
   b. Daily fetal monitoring strips
   c. Steroids for fetal lung maturity if gestational age is less than 34 weeks
   d. Tocolysis (see Chapter 15) may be safely undertaken in patients with placenta previa before 34 weeks. The agent of choice is magnesium sulfate because it is associated with fewer hemodynamic alterations.

2. **Delivery.** Decisions concerning delivery are made based on the gestational age of the fetus, the amount of vaginal bleeding, and maternal hemodynamic status. Indications for **cesarean section** include:

    a. Elective
      (1) When the gestational age is **37 weeks and**
      (2) When **fetal lung maturity** is demonstrated by amniocentesis
    b. Emergent
      (1) When the amount of bleeding presents a threat to the mother regardless of gestational age or fetal size
      (2) Nonreassuring fetal heart rate tracing

G **Maternal and fetal complications.** Maternal and fetal morbidity can occur from a pregnancy with placenta previa and may be significant.

  1. Maternal morbidity
    a. Maternal shock can result from acute blood loss.
    b. Severe postpartum hemorrhage (PPH) can occur after the delivery because the placental implantation is in the lower uterine segment, which has decreased muscle content. Thus, muscle contraction may be less effective in controlling the bleeding. PPH may lead to the following conditions:
      (1) Renal damage (acute tubular necrosis), which may result from prolonged hypotension
      (2) Pituitary necrosis (Sheehan syndrome) and resulting panhypopituitarism
      (3) Disseminated intravascular coagulation (DIC) due to excessive blood loss and possible death
    c. Placenta accreta (growth of placenta into the myometrium), or any of its variations, due to the absence of decidua basalis. Placenta accreta should always be considered in the presence of placenta previa.
      (1) The incidence of placenta accreta (with placenta previa) is 4%. The incidence of placenta accreta increases to 16% to 25% after a previous cesarean section.
      (2) The presence of a placenta accreta may necessitate a cesarean hysterectomy to control the blood loss. There are three types of placenta accreta (Fig. 9-2):

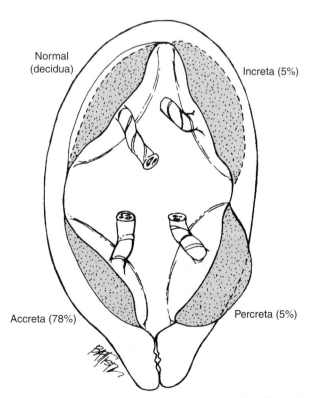

FIGURE 9–2 Uteroplacental relationships found in abnormal placentation. (From Niebyl JR, Simpson JL, Gabbe SG. Obstetrics: Normal and Problem Pregnancies. 4th Ed. London: Churchill Livingstone, 2001.)

(a) **Placenta accreta**. The placenta is attached directly to the myometrium.
(b) **Placenta increta**. The placenta invades the myometrium.
(c) **Placenta percreta**. The placenta penetrates completely through the myometrium.

2. **Fetal morbidity. Preterm delivery** may be necessary secondary to maternal bleeding, and the infant may experience the complications of prematurity (see Chapter 15).

III ABRUPTIO PLACENTAE (PLACENTAL ABRUPTION)

A Definition. Abruptio placentae is **premature separation of a normally implanted placenta** after 20 weeks' gestation.

1. **Pathophysiology**. Initiated by bleeding into the decidua basalis, the bleeding splits the decidua, and the hematoma that forms causes further splitting.
   a. The process may be **self-limited**, with no further complication to the pregnancy.
   b. Bleeding insinuates between the fetal membranes and uterus, which may extravasate or may remain concealed. Concealed abruptions can often be more compromising to maternal hemodynamic status since they are generally underappreciated.

B Incidence

1. The reported incidence of abruptio placentae is about **1 in 75 to 200 births**.
   a. Abruptio placentae severe enough to kill the fetus occurs in **1 in 1500 births**.
   b. It is a direct cause of 12% of all stillbirths.

C Etiology. The primary cause of abruptio placentae is uncertain; several associated conditions have been identified.

1. **Maternal hypertension**, either chronic or pregnancy induced, is most often identified as a risk factor and is associated with a three- to fourfold increase.

2. **Cocaine** use is associated with both an increase in maternal hypertension and vasoconstriction of the placental vasculature. Recent increases in cocaine use have led to an increase in the number of cases of abruptio placentae.

3. **Preterm premature rupture of membranes (PPROM)** has been associated with cases of abruptio placentae. The incidence of abruptio placentae is 5% in pregnancies between 20 and 36 weeks complicated by PPROM.

4. **Maternal trauma** accounts for a small number of cases of abruptio placentae. Clinical evidence of abruption is not always immediately apparent. A period of prolonged monitoring is required to exclude developing abruptio placentae.

5. Either **sudden decompression** of the uterus by rupture of membranes in a patient with polyhydramnios or delivery of a first twin can lead to a shearing effect on the placenta as the uterus contracts, thus causing abruptio placentae.

6. **Cigarette smoking** is associated with decidual necrosis on pathologic examination and an increased risk of abruptio placentae. This risk is increased in patients with chronic hypertension as well.

7. **Uterine fibroids** may contribute to abruptio placentae when the placenta is implanted directly over the submucosal fibroid.

8. **History of abruptio placentae** predisposes patients to subsequent abruptions; the risk is increased 10-fold (0.4% to 4%). Placental abruption is frequently a sudden event and not predicted with antenatal testing.

9. **Thrombophilia**. Both inherited, such as factor V Leiden, and acquired, such as antiphospholipid antibody syndrome, may contribute to abruptio placentae.

D Clinical presentation. The clinical signs of abruption including vaginal bleeding, abdominal pain, and uterine contractions. The severity of the clinical presentation is variable.

1. Partial placental abruption in which no maternal or fetal compromise is noted

2. Complete placental abruption with profuse bleeding, signs of maternal DIC, and a stillbirth

E Diagnosis. The basis of diagnosis consists of history, clinical examination, and a high index of suspicion. The **triad of vaginal bleeding, uterine or back pain, and fetal distress is common**.

1. **Fetal heart rate monitoring** may reveal loss of variability or may have late decelerations. The uterine tone may be increased without periods of relaxation.

2. **Premature contractions** that are unresponsive to tocolytics may suggest either abruptio placentae or intra-amniotic infection.

3. **Ultrasound** is often unhelpful. A retroplacental clot may not be detected unless a very large abruption occurs.

4. **Laboratory tests** are nonspecific but may reveal thrombocytopenia, hypofibrinemia, and anemia. Remember, a normal fibrinogen level in a pregnant woman is higher than normal, around 400 mg/dL.

F Management. Treatment depends on the condition of the mother and fetus and on the gestational age of the fetus.

1. **Maternal hospitalization** with continuous fetal monitoring should be considered.
   a. **Delivery may be delayed** if the fetal heart rate tracing is reassuring and the maternal condition remains stable.
   b. **Immediate delivery is necessary** in the following conditions:
      (1) The fetal heart rate tracing is nonreassuring and the gestational age is greater than 24 weeks.
      (2) The maternal condition deteriorates regardless of gestational age.
   c. **Vaginal delivery is desirable** if the maternal and fetal condition permits.

2. **Tocolytic drugs** (see Chapter 15) may be used if the pregnancy is less than 34 weeks and the status of the mother and fetus is reassuring.
   a. **Magnesium sulfate** is the tocolytic of choice because of its efficacy and side-effect profile.
   b. **β-mimetic tocolytics** should be avoided in cases of suspected abruptio placentae because they may mask maternal hypovolemia by causing tachycardia.
   c. **Prostaglandin inhibitors** should be used with caution because they are associated with a theoretic risk of platelet dysfunction.

3. **Complications**
   a. **Hemorrhagic shock** may occur either from external bleeding or from concealed clots. Treatment includes:
      (1) Aggressive intravenous fluid replacement
      (2) Replacement of blood loss and coagulation factors
      (3) Prompt delivery after maternal stabilization
   b. **Consumptive coagulopathy (DIC)** may occur in 30% of cases of severe abruptio placentae that lead to fetal demise.
   c. **Renal failure**, in the form of acute tubular necrosis, may result from intrarenal vasospasm or from massive hemorrhage and ensuing hypotension.
   d. **Couvelaire uterus** results from extravasation of blood into the myometrium. The hematoma seldom interferes with uterine contractions, and the uterus responds well to uterotonic agents. A Couvelaire uterus is not an indication for hysterectomy.
   e. **Fetal maternal hemorrhage** or the presence of fetal red blood cells in the maternal circulation is more commonly seen with traumatic instances of abruptio placentae. Rh-negative patients should receive RhoGAM (anti-D immune globulin).

IV OTHER CAUSES OF THIRD-TRIMESTER BLEEDING

A Obstetric causes

1. **Bloody show** is a normal part of labor, bleeding is usually minimal, and the blood is mixed with mucus.

2. **Rupture of a vasa previa** is a rare but very serious cause of vaginal bleeding. The bleeding is fetal in origin.
   a. The **cause** of ruptured vasa previa is rupture of a placental vessel with a velamentous cord insertion. This is usually detected antenatally during the level II ultrasound.

      b. Diagnosis is made using the **Apt test**, which involves:
        (1) Collecting blood from the vagina
        (2) Adding a small amount of tap water
        (3) Centrifuging the sample
        (4) Adding the pink supernatant to 1 mL of a sodium hydroxide solution
        (5) "Reading" the treated sample in 2 minutes
          (a) Pink color: presence of fetal hemoglobin
          (b) Yellow-brown color: presence of adult hemoglobin

  3. A **uterine rupture** must be considered if a patient has a history of previous uterine surgery or fetal parts are palpable abdominally.

B Nonobstetric causes

  1. Vaginal lacerations from trauma

  2. Vaginal infections, such as bacterial vaginosis or *Trichomonas*

  3. Cervical pathology, such as gonorrhea, chlamydia, cervical polyps, or cervical cancer

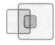

Study Questions for Chapter 9

Directions: *Each of the numbered items or incomplete statements in this section is followed by answers or by completions of the statement. Select the ONE lettered answer or completion that is BEST in each case.*

1. A 25-year-old woman, gravida 2, para 1, at 36 and 4/7 weeks of gestation with a history of prior cesarean section, presents with abdominal pain and vaginal bleeding. She admits to using cocaine. Her vital signs are significant for T = 99.9, HR = 120, BP = 170/100. Fetal heart rate baseline is in the 160s with minimal variability and repetitive late decelerations. Her blood work is significant for a hemoglobin of 7.5, platelets of 110,000, and a fibrinogen level of 250 mg/dL. The most likely diagnosis is:

- [A] Trauma
- [B] Cervical polyp
- [C] Placenta previa
- [D] Placental abruption
- [E] Uterine rupture

2. A 39-year-old woman, gravida 5, para 4004, presents at 38 weeks with complaints of severe headache, abdominal pain, and vaginal bleeding. Her past obstetric history is significant for an emergent cesarean section in the setting of placental abruption with her last pregnancy. Her past medical history is significant for chronic hypertension and tobacco use. Her vital signs are as follows: P = 105, BP = 180/105. Her examination is significant for right upper quadrant tenderness and a tender uterus. Her urinalysis shows 3+ protein. The following are all risk factors for placental abruption *except*:

- [A] Hypertension
- [B] History of previous placental abruption
- [C] Increased maternal age
- [D] History of previous cesarean section
- [E] Multiparity

3. A 20-year-old woman, gravida 1, para 0, at 28 weeks of gestation, arrives to labor and delivery reporting continuous vaginal bleeding and back pain. She denies sexual intercourse within the last 48 hours. She also denies trauma to the abdomen. You perform a pelvic ultrasound and note the fetus in cephalic presentation, amniotic fluid index of 10, and an anterior-fundal placenta. The fetal monitoring strip displays coupled contractions. The fetal heart rate baseline is 130 with moderate variability. Her vitals are as follows: T = 96.8, BP = 110/60, P = 90, R = 16. Examination reveals about 100 mL of blood in the vaginal vault. Her cervix is closed upon examination. Which of the following medications would you definitely administer?

- [A] RhoGAM
- [B] Terbutaline
- [C] Oxytocin
- [D] Betamethasone
- [E] Indocin

4. A 34-year-old woman, gravida 2, para 1, at 34 and 2/7 weeks of gestation, presents to labor and delivery reporting painless vaginal bleeding. You immediately perform a transvaginal ultrasound and note the placenta completely overlying the internal os, a fetus in cephalic presentation, and an amniotic fluid index of 14. The cervical length appears closed on speculum examination. Her blood pressure is 110/78 and her pulse is 106. She has slow, continuous bleeding from her vagina. Fetal monitoring reveals one uterine contraction every 30 minutes, and the fetal heart rate is reactive. What is the next best step in management?

- [A] Magnesium sulfate
- [B] Hospitalization
- [C] Vaginal delivery
- [D] Cesarean section
- [E] Dexamethasone

5. A 28-year-old woman, gravida 3, para 1, at 37 weeks of gestation, presents to labor and delivery for a scheduled repeat cesarean section with possible cesarean hysterectomy. She has a history of two previous low transverse cesarean sections. The first was because of fetal distress during labor, and the second was an elective repeat cesarean section. Her current pregnancy has been complicated with complete placenta previa with occasional spotting and recent hospitalization. Delivery by low transverse cesarean section is complicated by hemorrhage and hypotension. The patient receives 20 units of packed red blood cells (PRBCs). Which of the following organs is most likely to malfunction?

    [A] Adrenal cortex
    [B] Hypothalamus
    [C] Kidney
    [D] Liver
    [E] Heart

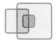 *Answers and Explanations*

1. The answer is D [III C 1–9]. The most likely explanation is placental abruption in the setting of cocaine use and hypertension. Although the patient does have a history of cesarean section and is at risk for uterine rupture, this clinical scenario is most consistent with placental abruption.

2. The answer is D [III C 1–9]. There are several risk factors associated with placental abruption, including tobacco use, prior history, mulitparity, and hypertension. A prior cesarean section has not been shown to increase the risk for placental abruption.

3. The answer is D [III F 2]. The clinical scenario is describing placental abruption. Since the bleeding is significant and the fetus is preterm, administering betamethasone to decrease complications of prematurity should delivery occur would be appropriate. At this point, the mother and fetus need close observation to determine if both are stable for conservative management. It would not be appropriate to give terbutaline because it would increase maternal heart rate and then make it difficult to use heart rate as a measure of maternal stability. Indocin should be avoided given the theoretical risk of platelet dysfunction. RhoGAM would be appropriate if the patient is Rh negative, but this is not known at this time.

4. The answer is B [II F 1–2]. Expectant management is justifiable if the fetus is preterm (less than 37 weeks) and can benefit from further intrauterine development. Hospitalization is appropriate until the bleeding subsides. The patient may be discharged after the bleeding lessens and the physician judges that the fetus is healthy. Tocolysis (magnesium sulfate) is not necessary because the patient is not having significant, regular uterine contractions and the cervix is closed. Vaginal delivery or cesarean section is not necessary at this point because the pregnancy is preterm, the mother's vital signs are stable, and the fetus is stable (reactive on fetal monitoring strip). Steroids (dexamethasone or betamethasone) for advancement of fetal lung maturity are useful only between 24 to 34 weeks of gestation in a pregnancy with intact membranes.

5. The answer is C [II G 1]. After severe hemorrhage (e.g., 20 U PRBCs and severe hypotension during surgery), renal damage in the form of acute tubular necrosis is most likely to occur. This patient is also at risk for Sheehan syndrome, which is pituitary necrosis (not hypothalamus). Injury to the liver, heart, and adrenal glands can occur but is less likely.

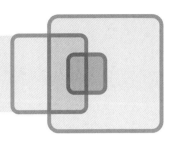

chapter **10**

Labor and Delivery

PETER CHEN

I   THEORIES OF THE CAUSES OF LABOR

The exact mechanism by which labor is initiated spontaneously, at either term or preterm, is not known. Many theories have been proposed.

A   **Oxytocin stimulation.**   Oxytocin is known to cause uterine contractions when administered late in pregnancy; therefore, endogenously produced oxytocin may play a role in the spontaneous onset of labor.

1. Levels of oxytocin in maternal blood in early labor are higher than before the onset of labor, but there is no evidence of a sudden surge.

2. Oxytocin influence must therefore rely on the presence of oxytocin receptors.
   a. Receptors are found in the nonpregnant uterus.
   b. There is a sixfold increase in receptors at 13 to 17 weeks' gestation and an 80-fold increase at term.
   c. In preterm labor, receptor levels are two to three times higher than would be expected at the same gestational age in the absence of labor.

B   **Fetal cortisol levels.**   Fetal cortisol levels and the proper functioning of the fetal adrenal gland may influence the spontaneous onset of labor.

1. In sheep, infusion of either cortisol or adrenocorticotropic hormone into a fetus with an intact adrenal gland causes premature labor. Hypophysectomy, adrenalectomy, or transection of the hypophyseal portal vessels in a sheep fetus results in prolonged gestation.

2. In humans, an anencephalic fetus has a prolonged gestation caused by faulty brain-pituitary-adrenal function.

C   **Progesterone withdrawal.**   Although in rabbits the withdrawal of progesterone is followed by the prompt evacuation of the contents of the pregnant uterus, there is no decrease in the human maternal blood levels of progesterone at term. However, the progesterone level at the placental site may decrease before the onset of labor and assist in the synthesis of prostaglandin.

D   **Prostaglandin release.**   Prostaglandins (PGs), particularly $PGF_{2\alpha}$ and PGE_2, have long been believed to be involved in the spontaneous onset of labor. Recent evidence suggests that this may not be true. Although prostaglandin levels are increased in amniotic fluid during labor, there seems to be **no parturition-related increase prior** to the onset of labor. The normal processes of labor appear to result in **inflammation**, which results in increased prostaglandin synthesis. Prostaglandins produced in myometrial tissue may contribute to the effectiveness of myometrial contractions during labor.

II   DEFINITION AND CHARACTERISTICS OF LABOR

A   **Definition.**   Labor is characterized by contractions that occur with increasing frequency and intensity, causing dilation of the cervix.

B   **Myometrial physiology**

1. **Contraction of uterine smooth muscle** is caused by the interaction of the proteins **actin** and **myosin**.

a. The interaction of actin and myosin is regulated by the enzymatic phosphorylation of myosin light chains.

b. The phosphorylation of myosin light chains is catalyzed by the enzyme myosin light-chain kinase, which is activated by calcium ion (Ca^{2+}).

2. **Gap junctions** are important cell-to-cell contacts that facilitate communication between cells via electrical or metabolic coupling.

a. Myometrial gap junctions, which are virtually absent during pregnancy, increase in size and number before and during labor.

b. Gap junctions facilitate synchronization of the contraction of individual cells, which permits the simultaneous recruitment of large numbers of contractile units during excitation.

c. Progesterone appears to prevent and estrogen appears to promote gap junction formation.

d. Prostaglandins are believed to be important stimulators of gap junction formation. If prostaglandins are inhibited, gap junction formation is inhibited as well.

e. Oxytocin does not stimulate gap junction formation.

3. **Substances that interfere with the physiology of the myometrium** can inhibit contractions.

a. **Tocolysis** or pharmacologic inhibition of uterine activity occurs with the following agents:

(1) **Antiprostaglandin agents**, such as indomethacin and acetylsalicylic acid, inhibit the synthesis of prostaglandin, which, in turn, decreases uterine contractions and inhibits gap junction formation. If the drugs are discontinued by 34 weeks' gestation, premature closure of the fetal ductus arteriosus does not occur.

(2) **Calcium channel blockers** (e.g., nifedipine and magnesium sulfate) inhibit calcium influx.

(3) **β-mimetic agonists** (e.g., terbutaline) stimulate cyclic adenosine monophosphate (cAMP) generation. An increase in intracellular cAMP stimulates calcium uptake in various cellular organelles, including the sarcoplasmic reticulum, thereby lowering intracellular free calcium.

b. **Potential complications associated with tocolytic agents** (Table 10-1)

c. **Contraindications to tocolytic agents in preterm labor** (Table 10-2)

C Stages of labor

1. **First stage.** The first stage of labor entails effacement and dilation. It begins when uterine contractions become sufficiently frequent, intense, and long to initiate obvious effacement and

TABLE 10–1 Potential Complications of Tocolytic Agents

β-Adrenergic Agents	Indomethacin
Hyperglycemia	Hepatitis[b]
Hypokalemia	Renal failure[b]
Hypotension	Gastrointestinal bleeding[b]
Pulmonary edema	
Cardiac insufficiency	
Arrhythmias	
Myocardial ischemia	
Maternal death	
Magnesium Sulfate	Nifedipine
Pulmonary edema	Transient hypotension
Respiratory depression[a]	
Cardiac arrest[a]	
Maternal tetany[a]	
Profound muscular paralysis[a]	
Profound hypotension[a]	

[a]Effect is rare; seen with toxic levels.
[b]Effect is rare; associated with chronic use.
From the American College of Obstetricians and Gynecologists. ACOG Technical Bulletin, No. 206, June 1995:6.

TABLE 10–2   Contraindications to Tocolytic Agents in Preterm Labor[a]

General Contraindications
Acute fetal distress (except intrauterine resuscitation)
Chorioamnionitis
Eclampsia or severe preeclampsia
Fetal demise (singleton)
Fetal maturity
Maternal hemodynamic instability

Contraindications to Specific Tocolytic Agents
β-Mimetic agents
   Maternal cardiac rhythm disturbance or other cardiac disease
   Poorly controlled diabetes, thyrotoxicosis, or hypertension
Magnesium sulfate
   Hypocalcemia
   Myasthenia gravis
   Renal failure
Indomethacin
   Asthma
   Coronary artery disease
   Gastrointestinal bleeding (active or past history)
   Oligohydramnios
   Renal failure
   Suspected fetal cardiac or renal anomaly
Nifedipine
   Maternal liver disease

[a]Relative and absolute contraindications to tocolysis based on clinical circumstances should take into account the risks of continuing the pregnancy versus those of delivery.
From the American College of Obstetricians and Gynecologists. ACOG Technical Bulletin, No. 206, June 1995:5.

dilation of the cervix. The first stage of labor is further divided into a relatively flat latent phase and a rapidly progressive active phase (Fig. 10-1).

2. **Second stage**. The second stage of labor involves the expulsion of the fetus. It begins with the complete dilation of the cervix and ends when the infant is delivered.

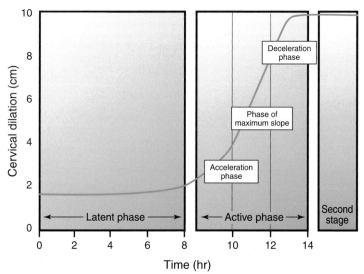

FIGURE 10–1   Composite of the average dilation curve for nulliparous labor. The first stage is divided into a relatively flat latent phase and a rapidly progressive active phase. In the active phase, three identifiable component parts include an acceleration phase, a linear phase of maximum slope, and a deceleration phase. (From Pritchard JA, MacDonald PC, Gant NF. Williams Obstetrics. 21st Ed. New York: McGraw-Hill, 2001:428, Figure 18-4.)

TABLE 10–3   True Versus False Labor

	True Labor	False Labor
Contractions	Regular intervals 2–4 minutes apart; intensity gradually increases and can last for 1 minute	Irregular intervals; no pattern; intensity remains steady
Discomfort	Back and abdomen	Lower abdomen
Dilation	Progressive	No change in cervix
Effect of sedation	Contractions are not affected	Contractions are relieved or stopped

3. **Third stage**. The third stage of labor involves the separation and expulsion of the placenta. It begins with the delivery of the infant and ends with the delivery of the placenta.

D True labor and false labor   are compared in Table 10-3.

E Characteristics of uterine contractions

1. **Effective uterine contractions** last for 30 to 90 seconds, create 20 to 50 mmHg of pressure, and occur every 2 to 4 minutes.

2. The **pain of contractions** is thought to be caused by one or more of the following:
   a. Hypoxia of the contracted myometrium
   b. Compression of nerve ganglia in the cervix and lower uterus by the tightly interlocking muscle bundles
   c. Stretching of the cervix during dilation
   d. Stretching of the peritoneum overlying the uterus

3. During labor, **contractions cause the uterus to differentiate** into two parts.
   a. The **upper segment of the uterus** becomes thicker as labor progresses and contracts down with a force that expels the fetus with each contraction.
   b. The **lower segment of the uterus** passively thins out with the contractions of the upper segment, promoting effacement of the cervix.

F Changes of the cervix before or during labor

1. **Effacement of the cervix** is the shortening of the cervical canal from a structure of approximately 2 cm in length to one in which the canal is replaced by a more circular orifice with almost paper-thin edges. Effacement occurs as the muscle fibers near the internal os are pulled upward into the lower uterine segment.

2. **Dilation of the cervix** involves the gradual widening of the cervical os. For the head of the average fetus at term to be able to pass through the cervix, the canal must dilate to a diameter of approximately 10 cm. When a diameter is reached that is sufficient for the fetal head to pass through, the cervix is said to be **completely or fully dilated**.

III   NORMAL LABOR IN THE OCCIPUT PRESENTATION

A Occiput (vertex) presentations   occur in approximately 95% of all labors (Fig. 10-2). The occiput may present in the transverse, anterior, or posterior position. **Position** refers to the relation of an arbitrarily chosen portion of the fetus (**in this case, the occiput of the fetal head**) to the right or left side of the maternal birth canal. Positions of the occiput presentation include the following:

1. **Occiput transverse**. On vaginal examination, the sagittal suture (in the midline front to back) of the fetal head occupies the transverse diameter of the pelvis more or less midway between the sacrum and the symphysis.
   a. In the **left occiput transverse positions**, the smaller posterior fontanelle is to the left in the maternal pelvis, and the larger anterior fontanelle is directed toward the opposite side.
   b. In the **right occiput transverse positions**, the reverse is true.

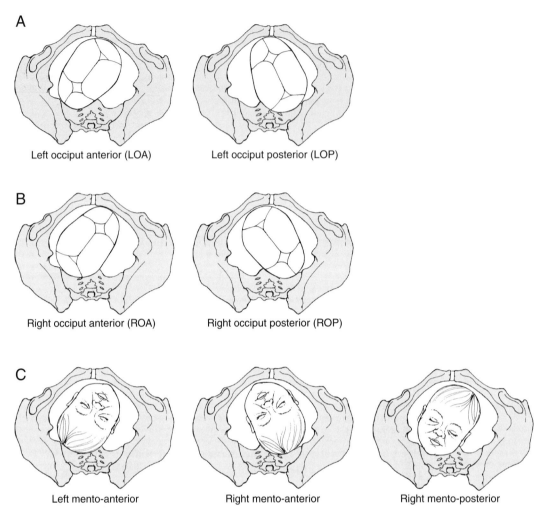

FIGURE 10–2   Occiput and face presentations in labor. **A.** Left positions in occiput presentations, with the fetal head viewed at a cross-section of the pelvis from below. **B.** Right positions in occiput presentations. **C.** Left and right positions in face presentations. (From Pritchard JA, MacDonald PC, Gant NF. Williams Obstetrics. 21st Ed. New York: McGraw-Hill, 2001:294–296.)

2. **Occiput anterior**. The head enters the pelvis with the occiput rotated either 45 degrees anteriorly from the transverse, right occiput anterior, or left occiput anterior position.

3. **Occiput posterior**. The incidence of posterior positions is approximately 10%. The right occiput posterior position is more common than the left occiput posterior position. The posterior positions are often associated with a narrow forepelvis.

   a. In the **right occiput posterior position**, the sagittal suture occupies the right oblique diameter. The small posterior fontanelle is directed posteriorly to the right of the midline, whereas the large anterior fontanelle is directed anteriorly to the left of the midline.

   b. In the **left occiput posterior position**, the reverse is true.

B The mechanism of labor and delivery involves **seven cardinal movements** (Fig. 10-3). A process of positional adaptation of the fetal head to the various segments of the pelvis is required to complete childbirth. These positional changes occur sequentially in the following order:

1. **Engagement**. The biparietal diameter of the fetal head, the greatest transverse diameter of the head in occiput presentations, passes through the pelvic inlet.

   a. **When engagement occurs**, the lowest point of the presenting part is, by definition, at the level of the ischial spines, which is designated as **0 station**. Levels 1, 2, and 3 cm above the spines are designated as **−1, −2** and **−3 stations**, respectively; levels 1, 2, and 3 cm below the spines are designated as **+1, +2** and **+3 stations**, respectively. At +3, the presenting part is on the perineum.

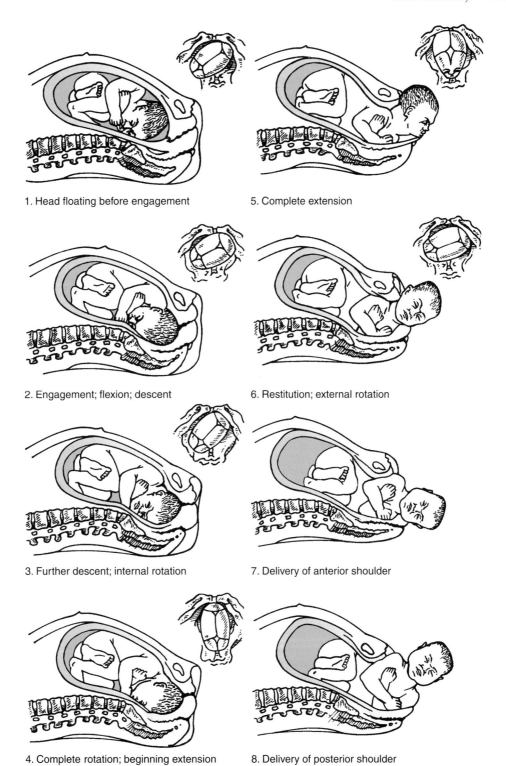

1. Head floating before engagement

2. Engagement; flexion; descent

3. Further descent; internal rotation

4. Complete rotation; beginning extension

5. Complete extension

6. Restitution; external rotation

7. Delivery of anterior shoulder

8. Delivery of posterior shoulder

FIGURE 10–3 Principal movements in labor and delivery, left occiput anterior position. (From Cunningham FG, MacDonald PC, Gant NF. Williams Obstetrics. 21st Ed. New York: McGraw-Hill, 2001:302, Figure 12-13.)

b. **Engagement may take place during the last few weeks of pregnancy, or it may not occur until labor begins.** It is more likely to happen before the onset of labor in a primigravida than in a multigravida.

c. **When the fetal head is not engaged at the onset of labor**, and the fetal head is **freely movable** above the pelvic inlet, the head is said to be **floating.**

2. **Descent**. The first requirement for the birth of an infant is descent. When the fetal head is engaged at the onset of labor in a primigravida, descent may not occur until the start of the second stage. In a multiparous woman, descent usually begins with engagement.

3. **Flexion**. When the descending head meets resistance from either the cervix, the walls of the pelvis, or the pelvic floor, flexion of the fetal head normally occurs.
   a. The chin is brought into close contact with the fetal thorax.
   b. This movement causes a smaller diameter of fetal head to be presented to the pelvis than would occur if the head were not flexed.

4. **Internal rotation**. This movement is always associated with descent of the presenting part and usually is not accomplished until the head has reached the level of the ischial spines (0 station). The movement involves the gradual turning of the occiput from its original position anteriorly toward the symphysis pubis.

5. **Extension of the fetal head**. This extension is essential during the birth process. When the sharply flexed fetal head meets the vulva, the occiput is brought in direct contact with the inferior margin of the symphysis.
   a. Because the vulvar outlet is directed upward and forward, extension must occur for the head to pass through.
   b. The expulsive forces of the uterine contractions and the woman's pushing, along with resistance of the pelvic floor, result in the anterior extension of the vertex in the direction of the vulvar opening.

6. **External rotation**. After delivery of the head, restitution occurs. In this movement, the occiput returns to the oblique position from which it started and then to the transverse position, left or right. This movement corresponds to the rotation of the fetal body, bringing the shoulders into an anteroposterior diameter with the pelvic outlet.

7. **Expulsion**. After external rotation, the anterior shoulder appears under the symphysis and is delivered. The perineum soon becomes distended by the posterior shoulder. After delivery of the shoulders, the rest of the infant's body is extruded quickly.

IV CONDUCT OF LABOR

A Detection of ruptured membranes. Ruptured membranes are signified at any time during pregnancy by either a sudden gush or a steady trickle of clear fluid from the vagina. In a term pregnancy, labor usually follows within 24 hours of membrane rupture. The risk of intrauterine infection (chorioamnionitis) increases if the patient has ruptured membranes for longer than 24 hours, with or without labor.

1. **Pooling**. Upon sterile speculum examination, a pool of amniotic fluid may be present and visible at the vaginal vault.

2. **Nitrazine test**. Nitrazine paper changes color, depending on the pH of the fluid being tested. Amniotic fluid, which is alkaline, turns Nitrazine paper deep blue. This test is also sometimes referred to as the "dye test."

3. **Ferning**. Amniotic fluid, like many body fluids, has a high sodium content, which causes a ferning pattern when the fluid is air-dried on a slide. Other vaginal secretions do not have such a ferning pattern. A positive fern test confirms ruptured membranes because the Nitrazine paper can turn blue with alkaline cervical mucus or blood in the absence of ruptured membranes.

B First stage of labor. On average, the first stage of labor lasts for approximately 12 hours in the primigravida and approximately 7 hours in the multigravida, although there is great patient-to-patient variability. A graph of cervical dilation and descent versus time produces a characteristic sigmoid pattern in normal labor (Fig. 10-4).

1. **Fetal monitoring**. The fetal heart tones should be monitored immediately after a uterine contraction because a sudden drop to less than 120 beats per minute (bpm) or an increase to above 180 bpm may indicate fetal distress.

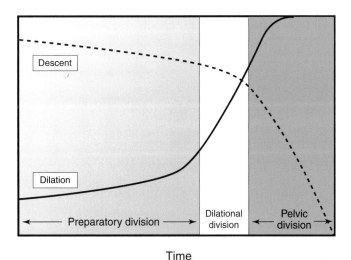

Time

FIGURE 10–4 Graph of cervical dilation and descent versus time. (From Cunningham FG, MacDonald PC, Gant NF. Williams Obstetrics. 21st Ed. New York: McGraw-Hill, 2001:428, Figure 18-2.)

2. **Amniotomy**. Artificial rupture of the membranes reveals the color of the amniotic fluid (whether it is stained by **meconium**, a sticky, dark-green substance found in the intestine of the full-term fetus) and often shortens the length of labor if a woman is already contracting regularly.

3. **Latent phase of labor**. During the latent phase, the uterine contractions typically are infrequent; somewhat uncomfortable; and, in some cases, irregular. However, they generate sufficient force to cause slow dilation and some effacement of the cervix. A prolonged latent phase is more than 20 hours in the primigravida and more than 14 hours in the multigravida.

4. **Active phase of labor**. The active phase, or clinically apparent labor, follows the latent phase and is characterized by progressive cervical dilation. A prolonged active phase is seen in the primigravida who dilates less than 1.2 cm per hour and in the multigravida who dilates less than 1.5 cm per hour.

5. **Dysfunctional labor patterns**. Uterine dysfunction in any phase of cervical dilation is characterized by lack of progress because one of the cardinal features of normal labor is its progression. Abnormal labor patterns, diagnostic criteria, and methods of treatment are summarized in Table 10-4.

C **Second stage of labor.** On average, the second stage lasts for approximately 50 minutes in the primigravida and approximately 20 minutes in the multigravida. However, second stages that last 2 hours, especially in the primigravida, are common. The second stage is characterized by intense pushing on the part of the patient.

1. **Spontaneous vaginal delivery**
   a. **Delivery of the head**. With each contraction, the vulvar opening is dilated by the head. The encirclement of the largest diameter of the fetal head by the vulvar ring is known as **crowning**. The head is then delivered slowly with the base of the occiput rotating around the lower margin of the symphysis pubis.
   b. **Delivery of the shoulders**. In most cases, the shoulders appear at the vulva just after external rotation and are delivered spontaneously. If the shoulders are not delivered spontaneously, gentle traction is used to engage and deliver the anterior and then the posterior shoulders. Excessive traction with extension of the infant's neck can result in temporary or permanent injury to the brachial plexus, known as Erb palsy.

2. **Episiotomy** is the most common operation in obstetrics (Table 10-5). It involves an incision in the perineum that is either in the midline (**median episiotomy**) or begun in the midline but directed laterally away from the rectum (**mediolateral episiotomy**). The episiotomy substitutes a straight, clean surgical incision for the ragged laceration that may otherwise result. An episiotomy is easier to repair and heals better than a tear, shortens the second stage of labor, and spares the infant's head from prolonged pounding against the perineum.

TABLE 10–4   Abnormal Labor Patterns, Diagnostic Criteria, and Methods of Treatment

Labor Pattern	Diagnostic Criteria		Preferred Treatment	Exceptional Treatment
	NULLIPARAS	MULTIPARAS		
Prolongation disorder (prolonged latent phase)	>20 hr	>14 hr	Therapeutic rest	Oxytocin or cesarean delivery for urgent problems
Protraction Disorders				
Protracted active phase dilatation	<1.2 cm/hr	<1.5 cm/hr		
Protracted descent	<1.0 cm/hr	<2 cm/hr	Expectant management and support	With CPD: cesarean delivery
Arrest Disorders				
Prolonged deceleration phase	>3 hr	>1 hr	Without CPD: oxytocin	Rest if exhausted
Secondary arrest of dilatation	>2 hr	>2 hr		
Arrest of descent	>1 hr	>1 hr	With CPD: cesarean delivery	Cesarean delivery
Failure of descent	No descent in deceleration phase of second stage of labor	Cesarean delivery	Cesarean delivery	

CPD, cephalopelvic disproportion.
From Cunningham FG, MacDonald PC, Gant NF. Williams Obstetrics. 21st Ed. New York: McGraw-Hill, 2001:431, Table 18-4.

D **Third stage of labor.**   The placenta usually is delivered within 5 minutes of the delivery of the infant.

1. **Signs of placental separation**
   a. The uterus becomes globular and firm.
   b. There often is a sudden gush of blood.
   c. The uterus rises in the abdomen because the placenta, having separated, passes down into the lower uterine segment and vagina, where its bulk pushes the uterus upward.
   d. The umbilical cord protrudes farther out of the vagina, indicating that the placenta has descended.

2. **Uterine hemostasis**. The mechanism by which hemostasis is achieved at the placental site is **vasoconstriction**, produced by a well-contracted myometrium. Intravenous or intramuscular

TABLE 10–5   Types of Episiotomy

Type	Advantages	Disadvantages
Median	Ease of repair Faulty healing is rare Dyspareunia is rare Good anatomic result Small blood loss	Extension through anal sphincter and into rectum is relatively common
Mediolateral	More space at vaginal outlet for breech or shoulder dystocia Rare extension through anal sphincter	Faulty healing is common Difficulty of repair Occasional dyspareunia Occasional faulty anatomic result Greater blood loss than with median episiotomy

oxytocin (10 U intramuscularly or 20 U in a 1000-mL intravenous bottle), **ergonovine** (0.2 mg intramuscularly or intravenously), or **prostaglandin F$_{2\alpha}$** (0.25 mg intramuscularly and repeated if necessary at 15- to 90-minute intervals up to a maximum of eight doses) helps the uterus contract and decreases blood loss. These medications are administered after the placenta has been delivered.

E **Lacerations of the birth canal.**   There are four types of vaginal or perineal lacerations, all of which are less likely to occur with an appropriate episiotomy.

1. **First-degree lacerations** involve the fourchette, perineal skin, and vaginal mucosa, but not the fascia and muscle.

2. **Second-degree lacerations** involve the skin, mucosa, fascia, and muscles of the perineal body, but not the anal sphincter.

3. **Third-degree lacerations** extend through the skin, mucosa, and perineal body, and involve the anal sphincter.

4. **Fourth-degree lacerations** are extensions of the third-degree tear through the rectal mucosa to expose the lumen of the rectum.

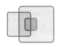

Study Questions for Chapter 10

Directions: *Each of the numbered items or incomplete statements in this section is followed by answers or by completions of the statement. Select the ONE lettered answer or completion that is BEST in each case.*

1. A 26-year-old woman, gravida 2, para 1, at 39 weeks of gestation, is admitted to the hospital in labor with ruptured membranes. Her cervix is dilated 5 cm and is 100% effaced, and fetal vertex is at +1 station. You place a fetal scalp monitor and an intrauterine pressure catheter. Fetal monitoring strip reveals five contractions in 10 minutes, and each contraction produces 50 mmHg of pressure. Three hours later, her cervix is 5 cm dilated and 100% effaced, and fetal vertex is at +1 station. What is the next best step in management?

A Augmentation with oxytocin
B Cesarean section
C Vacuum delivery
D Magnesium sulfate
E Methergine

2. A 22-year-woman, gravida 1, para 0, at 40 weeks of gestation, presents to labor and delivery reporting regular contractions for the last 2 hours. She denies loss of fluid from the vagina and reports good fetal movement. Her cervix is dilated 2 cm and 50% effaced, and fetal vertex is at 0 station. The fetal monitoring strip shows regular uterine contractions every 2 to 3 minutes. The fetal heart rate baseline is 154 bpm without decelerations and is reactive. What is the next step in management?

A Cesarean section
B Oxytocin
C Fundal massage
D Walk for 1 to 2 hours then return to check her cervix
E Meperidine

3. A 29-year-old woman, gravida 2, para 1, at 32 weeks of gestation, presents to labor and delivery reporting flank pain, fever, chills, and cramping. She is having contractions every 3 to 4 minutes, and the fetal heart rate baseline is 180. You check her cervix and discover a dilation of 3 cm and 100% effacement, and you see that the fetal head is floating. From the physical examination and from results of the urinalysis, you conclude that she has pyelonephritis and admit her to the hospital for intravenous antibiotics, magnesium sulfate to try to slow contractions, and steroids. Several hours later, you are paged because she is having trouble breathing. Her vitals are follows: T = 102.1, BP = 110/78, P = 105, R = 28, and oxygen saturation is 96% on room air. Physical examination reveals that her heart is tachycardic but without murmurs. You hear bilateral rales over the lung bases. Her abdomen is soft, gravid, and nontender. She still has costovertebral angle tenderness. There is 2+ pedal edema. Which of the following is the most likely diagnosis?

A Complication of pyelonephritis
B Congestive heart failure
C Pulmonary embolus
D Pulmonary edema
E Respiratory muscle paralysis

4. A 24-year-old woman, gravida 1, para 0, at 39 weeks of gestation, is crowning. The fetal head is not emerging from the vagina after two pushes. You palpate a thick hymenal ring of tissue at the introitus. Fetal monitoring strip shows bradycardia after the third push, so you decide to cut a 3-cm episiotomy that extends through the hymenal ring and vagina and ends laterally in the perineum. What is the advantage of this type of episiotomy?

A Clean surgical incision
B Avoids fourth-degree laceration
C Less dyspareunia
D Commonly used when distance between posterior introitus and anus is large
E Easier to repair

5. A professor of obstetrics is explaining the seven cardinal movements of labor: first—the greatest transverse diameter of the fetal head passes through the pelvic inlet; second—the fetal head descends; third—the fetal chin is brought into close contact with the fetal thorax; fourth—turning of the occiput toward the 12 o'clock position; fifth—the uterine contractions extend the fetal vertex anteriorly. What is the next step?

A Delivery of the head
B Rotation of occiput to transverse position
C Rotation of occiput to posterior position
D Delivery of anterior shoulder
E Expulsion

Answers and Explanations

1. The answer is B [IV B 4; Table 10-4]. This is a clinical scenario where the patient has had arrest of dilation (i.e., there has been no change in dilation in the last 2 hours in this multiparous patient). Augmentation with oxytocin is not necessary because she has adequate contraction frequency (every 2 to 3 minutes) and intensity (50 mmHg) in a 10-minute period. This patient is not a candidate for vacuum delivery. To perform a low vacuum delivery, the cervix must be fully dilated, the station must be +2 or greater, the rotation of the fetal head is unnecessary, and a valid indication for use of vacuum must be present (i.e., fetal distress, prolonged second stage of labor, or maternal disease process [e.g., heart condition or brain aneurysm], which benefit from reduction in pushing during the second stage of labor). There is no need to use a tocolytic to slow down labor. You want to achieve the opposite. Methergine is used for postpartum hemorrhage.

2. The answer is D [II D; Table 10-3]. This patient is in the first stage, the latent phase, of labor. It is difficult to predict when a person will make the transition from the latent phase to active phase of labor. At this point, you cannot tell if this patient is in true labor or if this is false labor. By having the patient walk for 1 to 2 hours and then return so you can check her cervix, you are able to diagnose labor if the cervical dilation changes. For example, if she returns in 2 hours and her cervix is dilated to 4 cm, then you can diagnose labor because her regular uterine contractions have produced cervical change. There is no need to augment her contractions with oxytocin in this stage of labor. She is not a candidate for cesarean section because there are no fetal or maternal indications. A fundal massage is a maneuver useful immediately after delivery of the placenta to help contract the uterus. Meperidine would be useful if the patient had prolongation of the latent phase of labor, that is, if she was having regular, painful uterine contractions for more than 20 hours (in nulliparas = "para 0") and did not have a change in her cervix.

3. The answer is D [Table 10-1]. This patient has many risk factors for noncardiogenic pulmonary edema. She has pyelonephritis and has been given magnesium sulfate (known to have pulmonary edema as a complication). She has bilateral lung rales because of exudation of fluid from the capillaries into the alveoli of the lung bases. There is no reason to think she has a heart problem (she is young, there is no mention of family history, heart examination is normal, and pedal edema is found in normal pregnancy). Pulmonary embolism is always a possibility and must be ruled out because she is pregnant and has tachypnea, but it is lower down in the differential diagnosis. Pyelonephritis can lead to sepsis and adult respiratory distress syndrome (ARDS), but again this is lower down in the differential because there is no mention of blood culture results, her blood pressure is stable, oxygen saturation is high, and there is no mention of her level of distress. Respiratory muscle paralysis occurs at very high levels of magnesium sulfate (there is no mention of her serum magnesium level).

4. The answer is B [IV C 2; Table 10-5]. A mediolateral episiotomy is cut if there is not enough space in the introitus for emergence of the fetal head and if there is a short distance between the posterior introitus and anus (because a median episiotomy has a high risk of extending into the anal sphincter and even rectal mucosa). A median episiotomy is easier to repair, has less blood loss, causes less dyspareunia, heals better, and has better anatomic results. Clean surgical incision is obtained with both median and mediolateral episiotomy.

5. The answer is B [III B 6]. The sixth cardinal movement begins with delivery of the fetal head by extension and ends with rotation of the occiput from the anterior position to the oblique and then to the transverse position. Expulsion and delivery of the anterior shoulder is the seventh cardinal movement.

chapter 11

Intrapartum Fetal Monitoring

MATTHEW N. BESHARA

I INTRODUCTION

A **The fetal heart rate (FHR)** is under the control of the autonomic nervous system (ANS). An intact ANS reflects the interplay between the sympathetic and parasympathetic nervous systems. This results in a variability note on the fetal heart rate monitor and is an indication of **normal fetal oxygenation**.

B **Intrapartum FHR monitoring** is used to **assess fetal well-being** during labor. It closely **quantifies and interprets the FHR** to obtain reassurance that fetal oxygenation is normal.

1. A **reassuring FHR pattern** is usually associated with **adequate oxygenation** of the fetus and a newborn that is vigorous at birth. When the FHR pattern is **reassuring**:
   a. A clinician can safely allow labor to proceed.
   b. There is a **low risk of perinatal asphyxia**, which refers to **damaging acidemia, hypoxia, and metabolic acidosis** associated with **neonatal neurologic sequelae** and other organ dysfunction.

2. A **nonreassuring FHR pattern** is a sign of potential **hypoxia**. When the FHR pattern is **nonreassuring**:
   a. A clinician must obtain other reassurance of fetal well-being.
   b. It may be necessary to expedite delivery.

II PATHOPHYSIOLOGY OF FETAL HYPOXIA

A Normal fetal oxygenation

1. **Uterine blood flow, intervillous blood flow**, and **transplacental gaseous exchange are reduced** during normal labor, temporarily resulting in relative fetal hypoxemia.

2. **Transient**, sometimes repetitive, episodes of **hypoxemia and hypoxia**, even at the level of the central nervous system (CNS), are **common during normal labor** and are **usually well tolerated** by the fetus.

3. **Greater fetal oxygen-carrying capacity** allows adequate delivery of oxygen to the fetal tissues despite the low fetal arterial partial pressure of oxygen (PO_2) for the following reasons:
   a. Higher fetal cardiac output
   b. Higher systemic blood flow rate (compared with adults)
   c. Greater affinity of fetal hemoglobin for oxygen

B Fetal hypoxia

1. When uterine or umbilical blood flow is impaired, fetal tissue perfusion is decreased and **oxygen transfer is diminished**.

2. Carbon dioxide accumulates in the fetal circulation, causing a **decline in pH, resulting in acidemia**.

3. Prolonged periods of decreased uterine or placental perfusion lead to **metabolic acidosis** as the fetus becomes dependent on anaerobic glycolysis to meet its energy requirements.

4. As pyruvic and lactic acids accumulate, there is a further drop in fetal pH, eventually resulting in **asphyxia** if unresolved.

III TYPES OF FETAL HEART RATE MONITORING

A Continuous monitoring. The FHR pattern can be continuously evaluated in two ways.

1. An **external ultrasound device** placed on the maternal abdomen emits and receives the reflected **ultrasound signal from the movement of the fetal heart valves.** The reflected sound waves return to the transducer, permitting an assessment of the FHR activity.

2. A **fetal scalp electrode** measures **consecutive R-R wave intervals** of the fetal QRS complex, directly measuring the FHR. The signal is transmitted to a monitor, where it is amplified, counted, and recorded.

B Intermittent FHR auscultation. This method is **equivalent to continuous monitoring** in assessing fetal condition when performed at specific intervals with a 1:1 nurse–patient ratio. However, continuous monitoring is more commonly used in the United States because it is convenient and less expensive.

1. During the **active phase of labor**, auscultation is recorded **at least every 15 minutes** after a contraction.

2. During the **second stage of labor**, auscultation is recorded **every 5 minutes**.

IV INTERPRETATION OF FETAL HEART RATE PATTERNS

When describing the FHR tracing in labor, the clinician evaluates the **baseline FHR, variability, contraction frequency**, and **periodic changes.**

A Baseline FHR. The FHR is the heart rate that occurs between contractions, regardless of accelerations or decelerations.

1. **Normal**
   a. **Normal baseline FHR is 110 to 160 beats per minute (bpm).**
   b. The baseline FHR decreases gradually from 16 weeks' gestation to term as the parasympathetic system develops.

2. **Tachycardia**
   a. **Baseline tachycardia is an FHR greater than 160 bpm** for periods of 10 minutes or more.
   b. Recurrent tachycardia can be associated with the following conditions:
      (1) Hypoxia
      (2) Maternal fever
      (3) Chorioamnionitis
      (4) Prematurity
      (5) Drugs (e.g., terbutaline, atropine)
      (6) Fetal stimulation
      (7) Fetal arrhythmias
      (8) Maternal anxiety
      (9) Maternal thyrotoxicosis

3. **Bradycardia**
   a. **Baseline bradycardia is an FHR less than 110 bpm** for periods of 10 minutes or more.
   b. Recurrent bradycardia can be associated with the following conditions:
      (1) Hypoxia
      (2) Drugs (e.g., mepivacaine, beta-blockers)
      (3) Autonomic mediated reflex (e.g., to pressure on fetal head)
      (4) Arrhythmias
      (5) Hypothermia
      (6) Maternal hypotension

B FHR variability

1. **Baseline variability** is defined as deflections from the baseline FHR resulting from the continuous interaction between fetal sympathetic and parasympathetic nervous systems. **Normal variability** is one of the best indicators of **intact integration** between the fetal CNS and the heart.

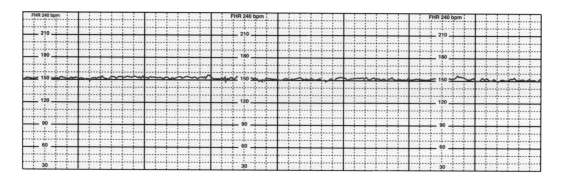
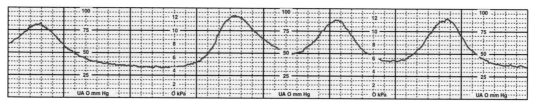

FIGURE 11–1 Minimal variability.

2. Causes of **loss of variability**
   a. **Hypoxia**
   b. Fetal sleep state (sleep cycles of 30 minutes or less)
   c. CNS depressants (e.g., atropine, scopolamine, tranquilizers, narcotics, barbiturates, anesthetics)
   d. Prematurity
   e. Baseline tachycardia
   f. Fetal cardiac abnormalities or arrhythmias
   g. Fetal CNS abnormalities

3. Characterization of variability
   a. **Absent**: undetectable amplitude
   b. **Minimal** (Fig. 11-1): detectable amplitude but less than 5 bpm
   c. **Moderate** (Fig. 11-2): amplitude of 6 to 25 bpm
   d. **Marked**: amplitude of more than 25 bpm

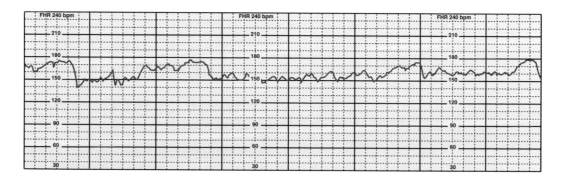
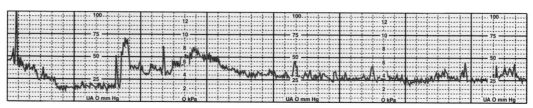

FIGURE 11–2 Moderate variability.

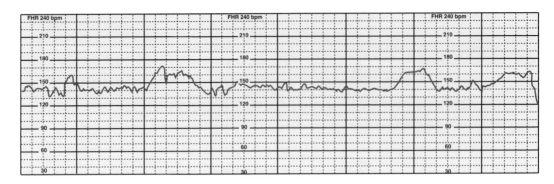

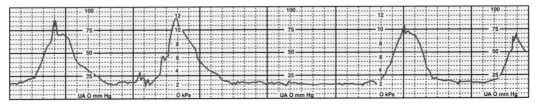

FIGURE 11–3 Accelerations are defined as abrupt increases in baseline fetal heart rate, which peak in less than 30 seconds.

C **Contractions.** Assessment occurs in two ways.

1. **Tocodynamometer**
   a. A pressure-sensitive tocodynamometer is placed around the maternal abdomen.
   b. The tocodynamometer measures **only the frequency of contractions**, not their intensity or strength.

2. **Intrauterine pressure catheter (IUPC).** This method allows internal monitoring of contractions.
   a. After the catheter is introduced into the uterine cavity, it is attached to a strain gauge, which measures the pressure generated by the uterine contractions.
   b. IUPC measures **both the frequency and strength of contractions.**

D **FHR accelerations** (Fig. 11-3) are defined as abrupt increases in baseline FHR (onset to peak FHR in less than 30 seconds).

1. **Before 32 weeks' gestation,** accelerations are defined as having a peak **of at least 10 bpm** above baseline, **lasting for 10 seconds or more.**

2. **After 32 weeks' gestation,** accelerations are defined as having a peak **of at least 15 bpm** above baseline, **lasting between 15 seconds and 2 minutes.**

E **FHR decelerations.** The **three patterns of periodic decelerations** are based on the waveform **configuration** and the **timing of the deceleration in relation to the uterine contraction.**

1. **Early decelerations** (Fig. 11-4)
   a. **Definition.** Early decelerations begin with the onset of uterine contractions, **reach their lowest point (never less than 100 bpm) at the peak of the contraction,** and return to baseline as the contraction ends.
   b. **Mechanism.** Early decelerations are thought to be caused by local changes in cerebral blood flow, which result in stimulation of the **vagal centers,** with acetylcholine release at the sinoatrial node.
   c. **Associated conditions.** Early decelerations can occur when the **fetal head is compressed** as it moves down the birth canal. The decelerations are considered physiologic and are **not associated** with fetal acidemia.

2. **Variable decelerations**
   a. **Definition.** Variable decelerations are **abrupt decreases in FHR** with a rapid return to baseline (onset of deceleration to nadir less than 30 seconds) that may **occur before, during, or after** the onset of uterine contractions.

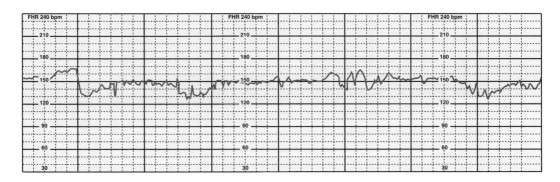

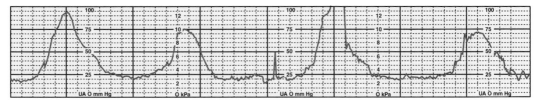

FIGURE 11–4 Early decelerations reach their lowest point at the peak of the contraction.

b. Mechanism. Variable decelerations involve **reflex-mediated changes** in the FHR controlled by the vagus nerve.

c. Associated conditions. Variable decelerations are generally caused by **umbilical cord compression** between fetal parts or between fetal parts and the uterine wall. They can also be seen in patients with **oligohydramnios**.

d. Types of variable decelerations

    (1) Mild (Fig. 11-5)

        (a) Duration of less than 30 seconds

        (b) Minimal clinical significance

    (2) Moderate (Fig. 11-6)

        (a) Two types

            (i) Nadir of 70 to 80 bpm, with duration of more than 60 seconds

            (ii) Nadir of less than 70 bpm, with duration of 30 to 60 seconds

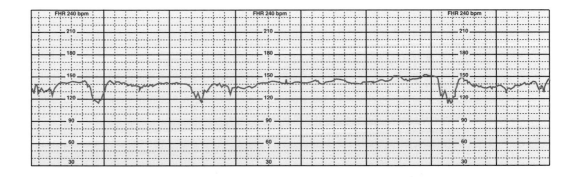

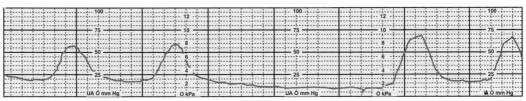

FIGURE 11–5 Mild variable decelerations last less than 30 seconds.

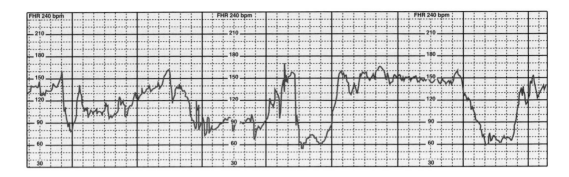

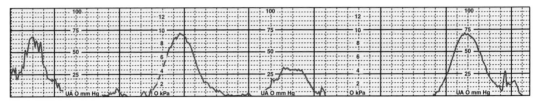

FIGURE 11–6 Moderate and severe variable decelerations.

(b) Persistent moderate variable decelerations can lead to a reduction in fetal oxygenation, resulting in hypoxemia and acidemia.

(3) **Severe** (Fig. 11-6)

(a) Nadir of less than 70 bpm, with duration of more than 60 seconds

(b) Prolonged or severe variable decelerations may lead to a significant reduction in respiratory gas exchange with subsequent fetal hypoxemia and acidemia.

3. **Late decelerations** (Fig. 11-7)

a. **Definition**. Late decelerations are gradual decreases and returns to baseline FHR associated with uterine contractions (onset to nadir is 30 seconds or more). The **nadir occurs after the peak of the contraction**.

b. **Mechanism and associated conditions**

(1) Late decelerations associated with **normal variability** represent reflex responses mediated via the vagus nerve. They may be seen with **mild transient hypoxia**.

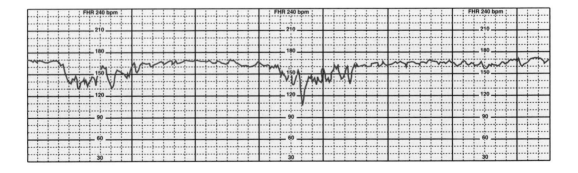

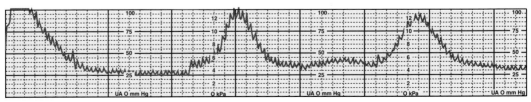

FIGURE 11–7 Late decelerations. The nadir of each deceleration occurs after the peak of the contraction.

      (2) Late decelerations associated with **decreased variability** can result from direct myocardial depression and can be seen with **prolonged hypoxia and acidemia**.

      (3) Uteroplacental insufficiency, which results from decreased uterine perfusion or decreased placental function, can lead to repetitive late decelerations and minimal variability. Conditions that may lead to uteroplacental insufficiency include:

        (a) Postdates pregnancy

        (b) Maternal diabetes mellitus

        (c) Maternal hypertension (chronic or pregnancy induced)

        (d) Abruptio placentae

        (e) Maternal anemia

        (f) Maternal sepsis

        (g) Hypertonia (excessive uterine tone)

        (h) Hyperstimulation (excessive uterine contractions)

4. Prolonged decelerations

    a. Definition. Prolonged decelerations are decreases from baseline of 15 bpm or more that last 2 to 10 minutes.

    b. Mechanism. Prolonged decelerations can result from the following factors:

      (1) Vagus nerve discharge (e.g., head compression during rapid descent)

      (2) Fetal hypoxia caused by mechanisms such as:

        (a) Uterine hyperactivity

        (b) Sympathetic blockade from regional anesthesia

        (c) Supine hypotension

        (d) Unrelieved cord compression

        (e) Maternal respiratory arrest

V   FETAL HEART RATE TRACINGS: ASSESSMENT AND MANAGEMENT IN LABOR

A **Reassuring FHR patterns.** When FHR tracings are reassuring, practitioners allow labor to continue. FHR accelerations contribute to the reassurance of fetal well-being.

B **Nonreassuring FHR patterns**

1. Characteristics

    a. Repetitive decelerations

    b. Abnormal baseline FHR

    c. Absence of accelerations

    d. Loss of variability

    e. Repetitive late decelerations; repetitive, moderate to severe variable decelerations; and absent variability or baseline tachycardia

2. Further evaluation is necessary.

    a. Evaluate for the **potential causes** of the nonreassuring FHR pattern.

    b. Obtain information and reassurance about the fetal well-being.

    c. Perform intrauterine resuscitation to improve placental perfusion and oxygen transfer to the fetus.

C **Management of women with nonreassuring FHR patterns**

1. Change in maternal position

    a. In the **supine position**, the uterus obstructs blood flow through the aorta and the inferior vena cava, potentially leading to decreased placental perfusion.

    b. Placement in a lateral recumbent position during labor causes the uterus to fall away from the great vessels, which should improve fetal oxygenation.

2. Oxygenation. Maternal hyperoxia may increase the maternal–fetal oxygen gradient, potentially improving the FHR pattern. Oxygen should be given by mask.

3. Reversal of anesthetic effects

    a. Sympathetic blockade from epidural anesthesia may result in decreased venous return and cardiac output, maternal hypotension, and decreased uteroplacental perfusion.

b. Administration of intravenous fluids or ephedrine to the mother may improve uterine blood flow and, therefore, the FHR tracing.

4. Regulation of uterine activity

a. Hyperstimulation or multiple uterine contractions from prostaglandin or oxytocin stimulation may lead to incomplete uterine relaxation and possibly decreased fetal oxygenation.

b. Intravenous hydration, **discontinuation of the uterotonic agent,** or uterine relaxation with terbutaline (β-sympathomimetic) may improve the FHR pattern.

5. Correction of cord compression. Variable decelerations, which are caused by **umbilical cord compression,** may be corrected with the following maneuvers:

a. Change in maternal position, which may relieve the compression

b. Placement of an **amnioinfusion,** which is an intrauterine catheter through which saline is infused into the uterine cavity. However, amnioinfusion has been found to be ineffective and is no longer used.

D **Further assessment of fetal well-being.**   After optimization of the maternal position, maternal vital signs, and labor pattern, further evaluation of fetal well-being should take place.

1. Vibroacoustic stimuli (VAS). An artificial larynx is placed on the maternal skin over the fetal head, and the fetus is stimulated by noise for 1 second.

a. The presence of fetal accelerations in response to VAS is considered reassuring.

b. The fetus is restimulated if no accelerations occur within 10 seconds. The VAS test may be repeated up to four times.

2. Scalp stimulation test. The examiner rubs the fetal scalp during a digital examination.

a. An acceleration is usually seen in the FHR tracing of the uncompromised, nonacidotic fetus. The presence of an **acceleration** is associated with an intact ANS and a fetal scalp **blood pH greater than 7.20**.

b. If an acceleration is not obtained after scalp stimulation, fetal scalp blood can be sampled to measure the fetal pH or one can progress to immediate surgical delivery.

3. Fetal scalp blood sampling. The fetal scalp is visualized through the dilated cervix, and blood is collected in heparinized capillary tubes after making a tiny stab on the scalp with a small blade. The capillary tubes are sent to the laboratory for pH measurement. The normal fetal capillary pH is 7.25 to 7.35 in the first stage of labor.

a. A **fetal scalp pH greater than or equal to 7.20** is reassurance that **the fetus is not acidotic.** Labor can proceed for 20 to 30 minutes.

(1) If a nonreassuring FHR pattern persists after 20 to 30 minutes and scalp stimulation is ineffective, the fetal scalp pH may be repeated to obtain reassurance on fetal well-being.

(2) In the case of a nonreassuring FHR pattern, the decision to intervene depends on the clinician's assessment of the likelihood of hypoxia and the estimated time to spontaneous delivery.

b. A **pH of less than 7.20** may represent significant **acidosis.** Delivery is thus indicated by operative (vacuum or forceps assisted) vaginal delivery, if possible, or cesarean delivery. The clinician must decide on the **most expeditious** way to deliver the baby based on the clinical circumstances.

c. In some centers, this test is no longer performed, and if the fetal scalp stimulation test is poor, the baby is delivered immediately by cesarean section.

VI **OTHER DEVELOPMENTS IN INTRAPARTUM MONITORING: FETAL OXYGEN SATURATION MONITORING**

A **Normal fetal oxygen saturation ranges between 35% and 75%,**   with an average level of 55% to 60%. If the fetal oxygen saturation remains **above 30% during labor,** there appears to be **no risk of fetal metabolic acidosis.**

B The U.S. Food and Drug Administration approved the first device for monitoring fetal oxygen saturation.

1. The sensor is slid through the cervix and lodges against the fetal cheek. It is held in place by the pressure created by the fetal cheek and the pelvic sidewall.

2. This method is used at some centers but has not yet been broadly instituted. (Research conducted on pulse oximetry has been suggested to decrease the false-positive rate of nonreassuring fetal heart rate patterns.

3. Some studies described decreased cesarean section rates, but overall the data have not supported this finding. The use of fetal oxygen saturation monitors is not endorsed by the American College of Obstetricians and Gynecologists at this time.

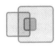

Study Questions for Chapter 11

Directions: *Each of the numbered items or incomplete statements in this section is followed by answers or by completions of the statement. Select the ONE lettered answer or completion that is BEST in each case.*

1. A 25-year-old woman, gravida 1, para 0, at 39 weeks of gestation, has been laboring for a few hours. Her cervix is dilated to 6 cm and 80% effaced, and fetal vertex is at 0 station. Membranes have been ruptured for 20 hours and her labor is being augmented with oxytocin. The intrauterine pressure catheter detects contractions every 1 to 2 minutes at 80 mmHg of pressure and lasting 2 minutes. Fetal heart rate baseline by scalp electrode is 90 bpm for the last 2 minutes (FHR baseline 30 minutes ago was 140 bpm). What is the best next step in management?

- [A] Penicillin
- [B] Cesarean section
- [C] Left lateral position
- [D] Discontinue oxytocin
- [E] Amnioinfusion

2. A 27-year-old woman, gravida 1, para 0, at 40 and 3/7th weeks of gestation, is in the middle of the first stage of labor. Her cervix is dilated to 4 cm and a decision has been made to place an epidural. Prior to placement of the epidural, she receives a 500-mL bolus of lactated Ringer's to prehydrate her, and augmentation with oxytocin is begun. Her vitals are as follows: T = 99.1, BP = 110/74, P = 102, R = 18. The fetal heart rate baseline is 142 bpm with three accelerations every 20 minutes. She is contracting every 3 minutes. After placement of the epidural, fetal heart rate baseline drops to 130 bpm, and no accelerations are seen within a 10-minute period. The fetal heart rate also shows a gradual decline in the middle of each contraction to about 115 bpm and then returns to baseline of 130 bpm. She has contractions every 2 to 3 minutes now. Her vitals at this point are as follows: T = 99.2, BP = 78/56, P = 115, R = 18. What is the best next step in management?

- [A] Tylenol
- [B] Penicillin
- [C] Intravenous hydration
- [D] Ephedrine
- [E] Discontinue oxytocin

3. A 22-year-old woman, gravida 2, para 1, at 41 weeks of gestation, is laboring. Her cervix is dilated to 8 cm and 100% effaced, and fetal vertex is at +1 station. Membranes have been ruptured for more than 24 hours, and labor is being augmented with oxytocin. An amnioinfusion is running because of 3–4+ meconium. Fetal heart rate by scalp electrode has a baseline of 138 bpm with reduced short-term variability and occasional mild variable decelerations. You are suddenly called to evaluate a nonreassuring fetal heart rate. The tocodynamometer shows six contractions in a 10-minute period with a pressure of 70 mmHg, and fetal heart rate is now 70 bpm for more than 3 minutes. She is placed in the left lateral position, oxytocin infusion is stopped, she is given oxygen by mask, and her intravenous fluid rate is increased. Fetal heart rate is now 98 bpm. What is the best next step in management?

- [A] Cesarean section
- [B] Vacuum delivery
- [C] Ephedrine
- [D] Knee–chest position
- [E] Terbutaline

4. A 19-year-old woman, gravida 1, para 0, at 38 weeks of gestation, is in active labor. Her cervix is dilated to 5 cm and fetal vertex is at +1 station. The tocodynamometer displays contractions every 2 to 3 minutes, lasting 1 minute, and producing 50 mmHg of pressure inside the uterus. The fetal heart rate by scalp electrode has a baseline of 140 bpm with random sharp decelerations to 70 bpm that return to baseline in 60 to 80 seconds. When this type of deceleration occurs, what is the best description of the initial acid–base status of the fetus?

  A Respiratory acidosis
  B Metabolic acidosis
  C Uteroplacental insufficiency
  D Asphyxia
  E Increased PCO_2

Answers and Explanations

1. The answer is D [V C 4 a and b]. This clinical scenario is describing hyperstimulation of the uterus caused by excessive stimulation by oxytocin, which has caused a nonreassuring fetal heart rate (in this case, bradycardia). No level of oxytocin is predictive of hyperstimulation because there are variations in response to oxytocin between individuals and different gestational ages. Remember that normal labor contractions last about 1 minute, produce up to 50 mmHg, and occur every 2 to 3 minutes. When the uterus is hyperstimulated, blood vessels are compressed for an extended period (greater than the fetal reserve), the blood flow to the fetus is reduced, and the fetus becomes hypoxic. None of the other answer choices addresses the problem of hyperstimulation, which has caused the nonreassuring fetal heart rate pattern.

2. The answer is D [V C 4 b]. One of the complications with placement of an epidural blockade is hypotension (before the epidural BP = 110/74 and after the epidural BP = 78/56). An epidural blocks sympathetic discharge to vessel walls, and vasoconstriction is inhibited. This causes blood to pool in dependent areas of the body, thus decreasing venous return to the heart. Cardiac output decreases and subsequently results in decreased uteroplacental circulation. To avoid hypotension, anesthesiologists hydrate patients before placement of the epidural and then give ephedrine to keep the BP near its baseline. Although the patient has a low-grade temperature (99.2°F), the fever is not the cause of the nonreassuring fetal heart rate; therefore, neither Tylenol nor penicillin are the best choices. Hyperstimulation is not the problem, so there is no need to discontinue the oxytocin. This patient has already been prehydrated, so additional hydration would not be as efficacious as giving ephedrine.

3. The answer is E [V C 4 b]. This clinical scenario is describing hyperstimulation. Normal labor contractions have the following properties: frequency—every 2 to 3 minutes; duration—45 seconds to a minute; intensity—up to 50 mmHg. In this case, oxytocin has already been stopped, but the non-reassuring fetal heart rate pattern has not resolved because oxytocin is still in the circulation. Thus, before taking the patient for a cesarean section, terbutaline should be tried to reverse the hyperstimulation by tocolysis. This patient is not a candidate for vacuum delivery (she is not even fully dilated yet). Ephedrine is not useful in this case. The knee–chest position is sometimes more useful than the left lateral position when there is a nonreassuring fetal heart rate pattern, especially a severe variable deceleration.

4. The answer is A [II B]. This clinical scenario is that of a severe variable deceleration. As the umbilical cord is compressed, decreased perfusion of fetal tissue occurs. This causes the partial pressure of carbon dioxide to increase and the partial pressure of oxygen to decrease. The increased PCO_2 decreases the pH, resulting in acidemia. The initial event is therefore respiratory acidosis. When there is a prolonged decrease in perfusion, the fetus becomes dependent on anaerobic (not requiring oxygen) glycolysis to meet its energy return and thus produces pyruvic acid and lactic acid. This causes a further drop in the pH, resulting in metabolic acidosis. Eventually, if the acidosis is unresolved, asphyxia occurs. Uteroplacental insufficiency is a term that describes late decelerations. It does not describe the "acid–base" status of the fetus. Although increased PCO_2 (one of the initial occurrences) contributes to respiratory acidosis, it is not the best description of the fetal acid–base status.

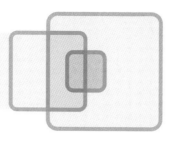

chapter **12**

Operative Obstetrics

JENNIFER B. MERRIMAN · DORIS CHOU

I   CESAREAN BIRTH

Cesarean section is delivery of a viable fetus through an abdominal incision (laparotomy) and uterine incision (hysterotomy). Cesarean section is the most important surgical procedure in obstetrics. It can be traced to 700 BC in Rome, when the procedure was first used to remove infants from women who died late in pregnancy. The first cesarean section was performed on a living patient in 1610. The maternal mortality rate was high up to the end of the 19th century, most often because of hemorrhage and infection. However, advances in surgical and anesthetic techniques, safe blood transfusions, and the discovery of effective antibiotics have led to a dramatic decline in the mortality rate.

A Incidence. The incidence of cesarean sections in the United States has continued to increase over the past 30 years. Cesarean section is now the most common operative procedure performed in many hospitals throughout the country.

1. In the United States, **approximately 29%** of infants were delivered by cesarean birth in 2004, compared to 21% in 1996, 15% in 1970, and 5% in 1960. Several factors contribute to the dramatic increase in cesarean births during this period.
   a. As procedure-related morbidity and mortality rates decreased with advances in anesthetic and operative techniques, the rate of **primary cesarean sections** increased.
      (1) The **widespread use of electronic fetal monitoring** has led to an increased rate of cesarean section for fetal distress.
      (2) The **growing trend of delaying childbirth** in the United States has affected women in labor in two ways. First, a higher proportion of nulliparous women give birth. Second, nulliparity is associated with complications that increase rates of cesarean section, such as dystocia and preeclampsia. The average maternal age has increased in the past 20 years; rates of cesarean section increase with advancing age.
      (3) **Dystocia** or abnormal progress of labor is used more freely as an indication for cesarean section, with a corresponding decline in the rate of forceps deliveries.
      (4) Vaginal **breech** deliveries are not recommended in singleton gestations.
      (5) **Multiple gestation**, an indication for cesarean section, **occurs more frequently**.
   b. As the number of primary cesarean sections increased, previous cesarean section as an indication for a **repeat cesarean section** increased. **Thirty-eight** percent of cesarean sections performed in the United States were repeat cesarean sections in 2004.
2. **Perinatal mortality**. There is little documentation for an association between the increase in rates of cesarean delivery and a decline in perinatal mortality and morbidity. Although increasing rates of cesarean delivery initially led to decreased perinatal mortality, the perinatal mortality rate is not higher in European countries with lower cesarean birth rates. The major causes of perinatal morbidity and mortality continue to be low birth weight and congenital anomalies. In **preterm fetuses weighing greater than 750 g and with malpresentation**, however, cesarean section is believed to **improve** perinatal outcome.

B Indications. Compared with vaginal delivery, a properly performed cesarean section carries no increased risk for the fetus; however, the risk of **maternal morbidity and mortality is higher**. Cesarean birth is preferred when the benefits for the mother, fetus, or both outweigh the risk of the procedure for the mother.

1. **Contraindications to labor**
   a. Placenta previa
   b. Vasa previa
   c. Previous classic cesarean section
   d. Previous myomectomy with entrance into the uterine cavity
   e. Previous uterine reconstruction
   f. Malpresentations of the fetus
   g. Active genital herpes infection
   h. Previous cesarean section and patient declines trial of labor

2. **Dystocia and failed induction of labor**
   a. Cephalopelvic disproportion, failure to descend, or arrest of descent or dilation
   b. Failure to progress in normal-size infant, usually because of fetal malposition or posture
   c. Failed forceps or vacuum extractor delivery
   d. Certain fetal malformations that may obstruct labor (i.e., large hydrocephalus, sacrococcygeal tumor)

3. **Emergent conditions that warrant immediate delivery**
   a. Abruptio placentae with antepartum or intrapartum hemorrhage
   b. Umbilical cord prolapse
   c. Nonreassuring antepartum or intrapartum fetal testing
   d. Intrapartum fetal acidemia, with intrapartum scalp pH of less than 7.20
   e. Uterine rupture
   f. Impending maternal death

C **Types of cesarean operations.** Cesarean operations are classified according to the **orientation (transverse or vertical)** and the **site of placement (lower segment or upper segment)** of the uterine incision.

1. **Low transverse (Kerr).** The low transverse uterine incision is the **preferred** incision and the one **most frequently used** today.
   a. The incision is made in the **noncontractile portion of the uterus**, minimizing chances of rupture or separation in subsequent pregnancies.
   b. The incision requires creation of a bladder flap and lies behind the peritoneal bladder reflection, allowing reperitonealization.
   c. **Uterine closure is accomplished more easily** because of the thin muscle wall of the lower segment, and the **potential for blood loss is lowest** with this type of incision.
   d. This incision may involve potential extension into the uterine vessels laterally and into the cervix and vagina inferiorly.

2. **Low vertical (Sellheim or Krönig).** The vertical incision begins in the noncontractile lower segment but usually extends into the contractile upper segment.
   a. This incision is used **when a transverse incision is not feasible**.
      (1) The lower uterine segment may not be developed if labor has not occurred; the transverse incision may not provide enough room for delivery of the infant.
      (2) Malpresentations of the term or premature infant may necessitate a vertical incision to allow more room for delivery of the infant.
      (3) This incision is sometimes used when an anterior placenta previa is noted to facilitate delivery without cutting through the body of the placenta.
   b. This incision also requires creation of a bladder flap and allows reperitonealization.
   c. The **risk of uterine rupture** in subsequent pregnancies **is increased** when the upper segment of the uterus is entered.
   d. **Uterine closure is more difficult**, and **blood loss is greater** if the upper segment is involved.

3. **Classic incision (Sanger).** The classic incision is a longitudinal incision in the anterior fundus.
   a. This incision is **currently used infrequently** because of the significant **risk of uterine rupture in subsequent pregnancies**, which can occur before labor begins, and higher complication rate.
   b. **Indications for this incision** include invasive carcinoma of the cervix, presence of lesions in the lower segment of the uterus (myomas) that prohibit adequate uterine closure, and transverse lie with the back down (most cases). It is the **simplest and quickest incision** to perform.

c. This incision does not require bladder dissection, and reperitonealization is not performed; the potential for intraperitoneal adhesion formation is greater.

d. Uterine closure is more difficult because of the thick muscular upper segment, and the **potential for blood loss is greater**.

D Procedure

1. **Patient preparation**
   a. The patient should be **well hydrated**.
   b. The **preoperative hematocrit** should be known, and **blood should be readily available** as indicated.
   c. The **bladder should be empty**. Placement of a Foley catheter is typical.
   d. **Prophylactic antibiotics** are usually given after clamping the umbilical cord.
   e. **Antacids** are also given to reduce the acidity of the stomach contents in the event that the patient aspirates material into the lungs.
   f. **Informed consent** should always be obtained.

2. **Anesthesia**. Most often, anesthesia is regional (spinal or epidural), but it can be inhalational (general) as dictated by the individual situation. General anesthesia may result in depression of the infant immediately after delivery, the degree of which increases with the length of time from incision to delivery. For this reason, the patient is prepared before the induction of general anesthesia (i.e., Foley catheter placement, skin "prep," and draping).

3. **Surgical techniques**
   a. **Abdominal incision**
      (1) The abdominal incision may be **midline, paramedian,** or **Pfannenstiel**.
         (a) **Midline**. The infraumbilical vertical midline incision is less bloody and allows more rapid entry into the abdominal cavity.
         (b) **Paramedian**. A vertical incision lateral to the umbilicus. It is rarely used.
         (c) **Pfannenstiel**. This low transverse incision near the symphysis pubis provides the most desired cosmetic effect and is **used most often**. However, it requires more time to perform.
      (2) The incision is made with the patient on the operating table in a **left lateral tilt** to prevent maternal hypotension and uteroplacental insufficiency, which may result from compression of the inferior vena cava by the uterus when the patient is supine.
      (3) The **approach to the uterus** in reference to the peritoneal cavity can be made in one of two ways:
         (a) The **transperitoneal approach** is **used almost exclusively** today. The parietal peritoneum is opened to expose the abdominal contents and uterus.
         (b) The **extraperitoneal approach** is mentioned for historical purposes; it has been virtually abandoned since the advent of effective antibiotics. This approach was devised for cases of amnionitis to avoid seeding the abdominal cavity in attempts to decrease the risk of peritonitis.
   b. **Uterine incision**. The pregnant uterus is palpated and inspected for rotation. The type of uterine incision is selected depending on development of the lower uterine segment, presentation of the infant, and placental location.
      (1) A **bladder flap** is created to approach the lower uterine segment. The reflection of bladder peritoneum is incised and dissected free from the anterior uterine wall, exposing the myometrium. This step is not necessary with a classical incision.
      (2) **Incision of the myometrium** is made as indicated.
   c. **Delivery of the infant**
      (1) The **infant** is delivered with the hand, forceps, vacuum extraction, or breech extraction.
      (2) The **placenta** is delivered spontaneously or can be removed manually.
   d. **Wound closure**
      (1) The **uterus is often exteriorized** to massage the fundus, inspect the adnexa, and facilitate visualization of the wound for repair.
      (2) The **uterine cavity is cleaned**. Oxytocics are administered as indicated to facilitate contraction of the myometrium and hemostasis.

(3) A **transverse uterine incision** is closed in one or two layers. A **vertical incision** usually is closed in three layers because of the myometrial thickness of the upper segment.

(4) The **peritoneum of the bladder reflection** can be either reattached with fine absorbable sutures or, typically, left open.

(5) The **abdominal incision** is closed in the usual manner.

E **Complications.** Common postoperative complications include the following conditions:

1. **Endomyometritis.** Postoperative infection is the most common complication after cesarean section.

   a. The average **incidence of endomyometritis** is 34% to 40%, with a range of 5% to 85%.

   b. **Risk factors** include lower socioeconomic status, prolonged labor, prolonged duration of ruptured membranes, and the **number of vaginal examinations**.

   c. Infection is **polymicrobial** and includes the following organisms: aerobic streptococci, anaerobic Gram-positive cocci, and aerobic and anaerobic Gram-negative bacilli.

   d. Use of **prophylactic antibiotics** at the time of the procedure **decreases incidence**. With the use of modern, broad-spectrum antibiotics, the incidence of serious complications, including sepsis, pelvic abscess, and septic thrombophlebitis, is less than 2%.

2. **Urinary tract infection**

   a. Urinary tract infections are the **second most common infectious complication** following cesarean delivery after endomyometritis. Incidence varies from 2% to 16%.

   b. **Practices that decrease risk** include preparing the patient properly and minimizing duration of catheter.

3. **Wound infection**

   a. The **incidence** of postcesarean wound infection rates ranges from 2.5% to 16%.

   b. **Risk factors** include prolonged labor, ruptured membranes, amnionitis, meconium staining, morbid obesity, anemia, and diabetes mellitus.

   c. **Common isolates** include *Staphylococcus aureus*, *Escherichia coli*, *Proteus mirabilis*, *Bacteroides* sp., and group B streptococci.

4. **Thromboembolic disorders**

   a. The **incidence** is 0.24% of deliveries, and deep vein thromboses are three to five times more common after cesarean delivery.

   b. **Diagnosis and treatment** are the same as for nonpregnant women. Prompt diagnosis and treatment decrease the risk of complicating pulmonary embolus to 4.5% and that of death to 0.7%.

5. **Cesarean hysterectomy**

   a. Hysterectomy after cesarean delivery is an **emergency procedure** that occurs in less than 1% of cesarean sections.

   b. **Indications** include uterine atony (43%), placenta accreta (30%), uterine rupture (13%), extension of a low transverse incision (10%), leiomyoma preventing uterine closure, and cervical cancer.

6. **Uterine rupture in future pregnancies**

   a. The **risk of rupture** of previous cesarean scar **varies with the location of the incision**.

      (1) **Low transverse scar** (one): less than 1%

      (2) **Low vertical scar**: 0.5% to 6.5%

      (3) **Classic scar**: as high as 10%

   b. Separation of the uterine scar can be categorized as **dehiscence or rupture**.

      (1) A **dehiscence** is a frequently asymptomatic separation and is found incidentally at the time of repeat cesarean or on palpation after a vaginal birth.

      (2) **Uterine rupture** is a catastrophic event with sudden separation of the uterine scar and expulsion of the uterine contents into the abdominal cavity. Fetal distress is usually the first sign of rupture, followed by severe abdominal pain and bleeding.

F **Vaginal birth after cesarean section.** Previous cesarean section is no longer a contraindication to subsequent labor and a vaginal birth. All women who are candidates should be counseled adequately and encouraged to attempt a vaginal birth.

1. **Considerations**. The risks of a vaginal birth after cesarean section, when performed in the proper setting, are less than the risks of a repeat cesarean section.
   a. There is a 60% to 80% rate of successful vaginal delivery after previous cesarean section.
      (1) A previous vaginal delivery is the best prognostic indicator for success.
      (2) Women with "nonrecurring" indications (e.g., breech presentation, fetal distress, or hemorrhage) have higher success rates than women with "recurring" indications (e.g., previous cephalopelvic disproportion or failure to progress). However, as many as 50% of women with previous cesarean section for cephalopelvic disproportion have a successful vaginal birth.
   b. One-third of all cesarean births are repeat cesareans, and an effective strategy to decrease the current cesarean section rate is to encourage vaginal births after cesarean section, when safely indicated.

2. **Prerequisites**
   a. No maternal or fetal contraindications to labor
   b. Previous low transverse cesarean section, with documentation of the uterine scar
   c. Informed consent regarding risks and benefits of repeat cesarean and vaginal birth
   d. Personnel able to perform emergency delivery and appropriate facility

3. **Contraindications**. The risk of vaginal birth after cesarean section in multiple gestations and breech presentations has not been determined.
   a. Previous classic uterine incision
   b. Maternal or fetal contraindications to labor
   c. Trial of labor declined by mother
   d. Previous low vertical scar, unless absence of upper segment extension is well documented
   e. History of more than two prior cesarean sections

II   EPISIOTOMY (see Table 10-5)

A   **Definition.** An episiotomy is an incision of the perineum made to enlarge the vaginal outlet to facilitate delivery.

1. It is made at the end of the second stage of labor just before delivery, when indicated.

2. It increases the area of the outlet for the fetal head during delivery, particularly in assisted deliveries with forceps or the vacuum extractor.

B   **Function**

1. An episiotomy is used to prevent major perineal lacerations.

2. Prophylactic episiotomy has been advocated to prevent pelvic relaxation, although this has never been proven.

C   **Types**

1. **Median or medial episiotomy.** This incision should be one-half the length of the distended perineum and is cut vertically in the midline of the perineal body.
   a. **Advantages:** less blood loss, easier to repair, more comfortable during healing
   b. **Disadvantage:** possible occurrence of inadvertent cutting or extension into the anal sphincter and rectum. It is important to recognize and repair this complication during repair of the episiotomy so that rectovaginal fistula does not result.

2. **Mediolateral episiotomy.** This incision of the perineum, at a 45-degree angle to the hymenal ring, extends laterally to the anus onto the inner thigh, allowing more room than a median incision.
   a. **Advantage:** more room with less risk of injury to the rectum and sphincter
   b. **Disadvantages:** more difficult to repair, more blood loss, more discomfort during healing

III   OPERATIVE VAGINAL DELIVERY: FORCEPS AND VACUUM-EXTRACTOR OPERATIONS

A   **Definition.** An operative vaginal delivery is defined as the application of direct traction on the fetal head with forceps or a vacuum.

B **Incidence.** The incidence of operative vaginal delivery is approximately 10% to 15%.

C **Indications.** An operative vaginal delivery is performed to shorten the second stage of labor with certain maternal or fetal indications.

1. **Nonreassuring fetal status** based on heart rate pattern, auscultation, lack of response to scalp stimulation, or scalp pH

2. **Prolonged second stage of labor** secondary to malposition, deflexion, or asynclitism (lateral deflection) of the fetal head. A prolonged second stage is defined as follows:
   a. **Nulliparous patient**: more than 3 hours with a regional anesthetic or more than 2 hours without regional anesthesia
   b. **Multiparous patient**: more than 2 hours with a regional anesthetic or more than 1 hour without regional anesthesia

3. Certain **maternal illnesses** (such as heart disease or pulmonary compromise), which make avoidance of voluntary maternal expulsive efforts desirable

4. **Poor voluntary expulsion efforts** because of exhaustion, analgesia, or neuromuscular disease

D **Prerequisites for instrumental delivery.** The successful results of an instrumental delivery depend largely on the skill and judgment of the obstetrician.

1. The cervix must be fully dilated.

2. The membranes must be ruptured.

3. The position and station must be known, and the head must be engaged (0 station; see Chapter 10).

4. The maternal pelvis must be judged adequate in size for delivery.

5. The bladder should be empty.

6. A skilled operator must be present.

7. Adequate anesthesia is needed before forceps or vacuum application.

E **Contraindications**

1. Nonvertex presentation, except for **Piper forceps in the breech delivery**

2. **Nonengagement** of the presenting part

3. Head that cannot be advanced with ordinary traction when using forceps or the vacuum extractor

4. Prematurity, fetal bleeding disorder, or certain maternal infections (i.e., HIV)

F **Classification of forceps deliveries.** Forceps deliveries are classified according to station and rotation (Fig. 12-1).

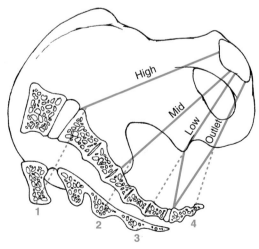

FIGURE 12–1 The four major planes of the pelvis.

1. **Outlet forceps**. To be categorized as an outlet forceps delivery, the following criteria must be satisfied:
   a. Scalp is visible at the introitus without separating the labia.
   b. Fetal skull has reached the pelvic floor.
   c. Sagittal suture is in the anteroposterior diameter or right or left occiput anterior or posterior position.
   d. Fetal head is at or on the perineum.
   e. Rotation does not exceed 45 degrees.

2. **Low forceps**. In low forceps delivery, the leading point of the fetal skull has descended to at least +2 station but has not reached the pelvic floor.

3. **Midforceps**. The station is above +2 but the presenting part is engaged.

G **Types of forceps.** The forceps are two matched blades that articulate and lock. The design of the blades provides standard cephalic and pelvic curves; that is, they conform to the shape of the fetal head and to the vaginal canal, respectively. Each matching part of the forceps has three parts: the blade, the shank, and the handle.

1. **Classic**. These forceps are used primarily for traction when there is to be little or no rotation (Fig. 12-2).

2. **Specialized**. These forceps are designed for rotation or special indications (Fig. 12-3).
   a. **Kielland** (for rotation)
   b. **Barton** (for rotation)
   c. **Piper** (for the aftercoming head in breech deliveries)

H **Vacuum extractors.** There are two types of vacuum extractors, based on the type of cup used for application to the fetal head. Each type has three parts: a cup, a rubber hose, and a vacuum pump.

1. **Malmström vacuum extractor**. This device consists of a metal cup (40 to 60 mm in diameter) that is applied to the fetal scalp. The pump is then used to create a vacuum, not exceeding 0.7 to 0.8 kg/cm^2. Traction is then applied to bring the infant's head through the introitus.

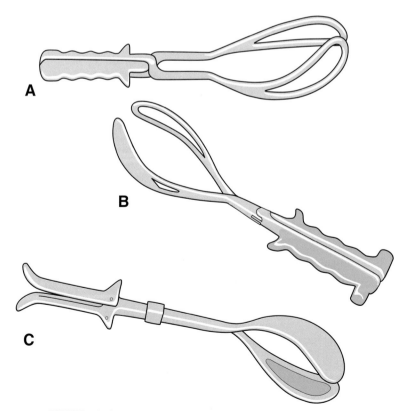

FIGURE 12–2 Classic forceps: **A.** Simpson. **B.** Elliot. **C.** Tucker-McLean.

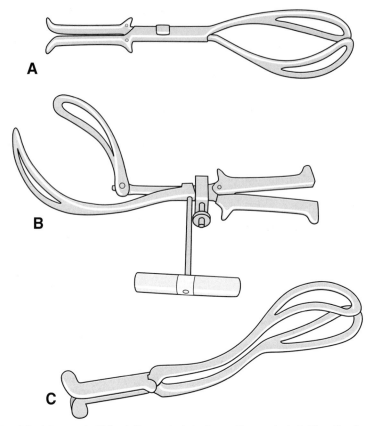

FIGURE 12–3 Specialized forceps: **A.** Kielland (for rotation). **B.** Barton (for rotation). **C.** Piper (for the aftercoming head in breech deliveries).

    2. Plastic cup extractor. This device, which is **more widely used in the United States**, consists of a flexible Silastic cup that is applied to the fetal scalp more easily and with less trauma than the Malmström extractor. The vacuum pressures attained are about the same, but they can be reached more quickly and with less trauma to the fetal scalp.

I Complications

    1. Maternal complications are usually of minor clinical consequence (incidence, 1.4% to 22%) and include lacerations of the cervix, vagina, and perineum; episiotomy extensions; and associated hemorrhage. More serious complications (incidence, 0.1% to 0.3%) include bladder lacerations, pelvic floor injury, pelvic hematoma, and coccygeal fracture.

    2. Neonatal injury
        a. Scalp abrasions or lacerations are the most common injury associated with vacuum extraction.
        b. Soft tissue injury is the most common injury associated with **forceps delivery**.
        c. Cephalohematoma (separation of the fetal scalp from underlying structures) occurs in 0.5% to 2.5% of live births, with an incidence of 14% to 16% in vacuum deliveries and 2% in forceps deliveries.
        d. Subgaleal hemorrhages occur in 26 to 45 in 1000 vacuum deliveries.
        e. Intracranial hemorrhage is a rare complication, occurring in 0.75% of instrumental deliveries.

IV CERVICAL CERCLAGE

    A Definition.   A suture is placed in the cervix to treat **cervical incompetence**.

    1. Cervical incompetence is **characterized** by gradual, progressive, painless dilation of the cervix, usually leading to spontaneous pregnancy loss early in the **second trimester**. A minority (15% to 20%) of second-trimester losses are associated with cervical incompetence.

2. Cervical incompetence may be **acquired or congenital**.

    a. Acquired causes primarily result from obstetric or gynecologic trauma to the cervix (e.g., rapid delivery, use of forceps, trauma, surgical dilation, conization, or breech extraction).

    b. Congenital causes include anomalies caused by diethylstilbestrol (DES) exposure in utero [and other reproductive tract].

3. Cervical incompetence is **diagnosed** by a characteristic history of second-trimester spontaneous losses associated with **painless cervical dilation**. There is still considerable debate about the diagnosis and management of cervical incompetence. Transvaginal ultrasonography has been used to assess cervical length. More studies are needed to confirm whether prophylactic cerclage would decrease the risk of preterm birth in those individuals with short cervical length as measured by ultrasound.

B   **Techniques.**   Cervical cerclage involves placing an encircling suture around the **cervical os** using a heavy, nonabsorbable suture or Mersilene tape. The suturing prevents protrusion of the amniotic sac and consequent rupture by correcting the abnormal dilation of the cervix. **Three techniques** for cervical cerclage are used today.

1. Shirodkar technique. In the more complicated of the two procedures using a vaginal approach, the suture is almost completely buried beneath the vaginal mucosa at the level of the internal os. It can be left in place for subsequent pregnancies if a cesarean section is performed. This procedure requires dissection of the bladder and is associated with an increased blood loss.

2. McDonald technique. This procedure is a simple purse-string suture of the cervix and is simpler, incurring less trauma to the cervix and less blood loss than the Shirodkar procedure (Fig. 12-4).

3. Abdominal placement. This uncommon, permanent procedure is used in women with a short or amputated cervix or in those in whom a vaginal procedure has failed. Cesarean birth is necessary for delivery.

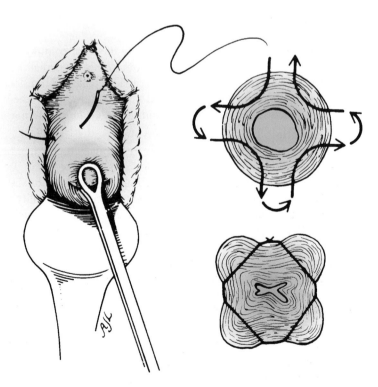

FIGURE 12–4 McDonald cerclage.

C Timing. Cerclage is **usually performed** between the **12th and 16th** weeks of gestation but can be performed as late as the 24th week. The suture is **removed at the 38th week** or earlier if labor begins. **Fetal viability and the absence of anomalies** should be documented **before** performing the procedure.

D Effectiveness. The **success rate of cerclage** has been stated to be as high as 80% to 90%. However, there have been no randomized trials to define the efficacy and benefit of cerclage; this benefit is probably overstated. Except in women with a strong history consistent with cervical incompetence, the benefit of cerclage has not been proven.

E Complications

1. Cervical lacerations occur in 1% to 13% of deliveries after a McDonald cerclage.

2. Cervical dystocia with failure to dilate, requiring a cesarean birth, occurs in 2% to 5% of cases.

3. Displacement of the suture occurs in 3% to 12% of cases. A second cerclage is then attempted, which has a lower success rate.

4. Premature rupture of the membranes complicates cerclage in 1% to 9% of cases.

5. Chorioamnionitis complicates 1% to 7% of cases.

6. Early, elective cerclages have a low rate (1%) of infection; cerclage placement with dilation of the cervix has a much higher risk (30%) of infection.

V ABORTION

The end of a pregnancy before viability, usually designated as 20 weeks' gestation (i.e., before the fetus is capable of surviving outside the uterus), is known as abortion. Abortions can occur spontaneously or intentionally (i.e., induced).

A Spontaneous abortion is expulsion of the products of conception without medical or mechanical intervention.

1. **Incidence**. Spontaneous loss occurs in 15% of clinically recognized pregnancies; the risk increases directly with maternal age, advancing paternal age, minority race, increasing gravidity, and history of previous spontaneous losses.

2. **Etiology**. Chromosomal abnormalities are the most common reason for first-trimester losses, occurring at a 60% frequency. Most chromosomal abnormalities are sporadic defects; in a small percentage of cases, one of the parents carries a balanced translocation. Autosomal trisomies are the most common anomaly, followed by 45,X monosomy (the most common single anomaly seen in abortuses), triploidy, tetraploidy, translocations, and mosaicism.

3. **Classification**. Spontaneous abortions are classified into five types.
   a. **Threatened abortion**. This term is traditionally used when bleeding occurs in the first half of gestation without cervical dilation or passage of tissue. Twenty-five percent of pregnant women experience spotting or bleeding early in gestation; 50% of these proceed to lose the pregnancy. An ultrasound is obtained to document viability after 6 weeks' gestation.
   b. **Inevitable abortion**. This type of pregnancy loss is diagnosed when bleeding or rupture of the membranes occurs with cramping and dilation of the cervix. Suction curettage is performed to evacuate the uterus.
   c. **Incomplete abortion**. This type of pregnancy loss occurs when there has been partial but incomplete expulsion of the products of conception from the uterine cavity. Therapy is evacuation of remaining tissue by suction curettage.
   d. **Missed abortion**. Death of the fetus or embryo may occur without the onset of labor or the passage of tissue for a prolonged period. Suction curettage is used to evacuate the first-trimester uterus. Dilation and evacuation (D&E) and prostaglandin induction of labor are methods used to evacuate the early second-trimester uterus.
   e. **Recurrent pregnancy loss**. In the past, this condition has been called **habitual abortion or recurrent miscarriage** and is defined as three or more spontaneous, consecutive first-trimester losses. This affects 2% of couples. In women with previous liveborn infants who

have had a loss, the risk of a subsequent abortion is 25% to 30% regardless of whether she has had one or more losses. In women with no previous liveborn infants, the recurrence risk is 40% to 45%. Evaluation is indicated after three losses (and sometimes after two losses depending on the age of the woman).

4. Workup for recurrent pregnancy loss
   a. Detailed history and physical examination
   b. Chromosomal evaluation of the couple
   c. Endometrial biopsy or midluteal-phase progesterone level to exclude luteal-phase defect
   d. Thyroid function test
   e. Hysterosalpingogram or hysteroscopy to evaluate uterine cavity
   f. Screening test for lupus anticoagulant and anticardiolipin antibody

B **Induced (elective) abortion.** Abortion became legal in 1973 and can be induced up to approximately 24 weeks' gestation in most states. Forty states and the District of Columbia have laws banning most postviability abortions (i.e., after 24 weeks gestation). Four states have laws affirming a right to abortion before viability, and at any time thereafter if necessary to preserve the life or health of the mother (CT, ME, MD, WA). Legal abortion is one of the most frequently performed surgical procedures in the United States. Therapeutic abortions are terminations of pregnancy that are performed when maternal risk is associated with continuation of the pregnancy or fetal abnormalities are associated with genetic, chromosomal, or structural defects.

1. Techniques of pregnancy termination. Techniques used effectively to empty the uterus of the products of conception fall under the categories of surgical evacuation or induction of labor. The preferred procedure depends on gestational age and, in some cases, operator training.
   a. Surgical evacuation
      (1) Suction curettage. This method of dilation of the cervix and vacuum aspiration of the uterine contents is used for termination of pregnancy at 12 weeks' or less gestational age. Suction curettage is the most common method of pregnancy termination in this country.
         (a) Hygroscopic dilators such as laminaria (stems of a brown seaweed that absorb water) can be used when necessary to facilitate gentle dilation of the cervix 12 to 24 hours prior to the procedure.
         (b) Prophylactic antibiotics administered just before or after the procedure significantly reduce the risk of infection associated with induced abortion.
      (2) Dilation and extraction (D&E). This technique is the preferred method of termination at 13 or more weeks of gestation.
         (a) As the length of gestation increases, wider cervical dilation is necessary to accomplish the procedure successfully. Preoperative cervical laminaria may be used.
         (b) Vacuum aspiration of uterine contents is usually an adequate method of evacuation between 13 and 16 weeks. After 16 weeks, uterine evacuation is accomplished with forceps extraction. Successful completion of this procedure depends largely on operator skill. Evaluation for major fetal parts is an important component of this procedure. Simultaneous ultrasound monitoring can be helpful to decrease risk to the mother and ensure complete evacuation of the uterus.
         (c) Prophylactic antibiotics may be given.
      (3) Other mechanical methods (now **obsolete**). These methods include sharp curettage, hysterotomy, and hysterectomy (used only when there is another indication for this procedure).
   b. Induction of labor. Medical means of inducing abortion include extrauterine and intrauterine administration of abortifacients, such as prostaglandins, urea, hypertonic saline, and oxytocin. These methods are used for second-trimester terminations; frequency of use increases with increasing gestational age.
      (1) Prostaglandins are most commonly administered as vaginal tablets of prostaglandin E_2; 90% of abortions are accomplished within 24 hours. Common side effects include fever, nausea and vomiting, diarrhea, and uterine hyperstimulation.
      (2) Hypertonic solutions of saline or **urea** are injected directly into the amniotic cavity. This procedure requires amniocentesis and care to avoid intravascular injection.

(3) Complication rates are lowest when the uterus is successfully evacuated within 13 to 24 hours. Laminaria to facilitate cervical dilation is useful to shorten the length of induction.

c. Progesterone antagonists. These effective agents for pregnancy termination, used in Europe and other countries and previously unavailable in the United States, are now approved by the U. S. Food and Drug Administration.

(1) Mifepristone (RU486; Mifeprex), taken orally, is highly effective in pregnancies with up to 49 days of amenorrhea. Its effectiveness can be increased with the addition of prostaglandin E.

(2) Side effects are minimal, and complication rates, including hemorrhage and retained tissue, are low.

2. Anesthesia. Sedation with a local paracervical block is usually used for induced abortion. General anesthesia can be used but is accompanied by a higher incidence of hemorrhage, cervical injury, and perforation because general anesthetics render the uterine musculature more relaxed and, thus, easier to penetrate.

3. Complications. The incidence of complications is largely determined by the method of termination and gestational age; incidence varies directly with increasing gestational age.

a. Immediate complications. These complications develop during the procedure or within 3 hours after completion.

(1) Hemorrhage. The incidence of hemorrhage is most accurately determined by the rate of transfusion. Rates vary with method of termination and are reported to be within 0.06% to 1.72%. The lowest rates are seen with suction curettage, and the highest with saline instillation.

(2) Cervical injury. The rates of cervical injury associated with suction curettage are within the range of 0.01% to 1.6%. Factors that decrease the risk of this complication include the use of local anesthetics instead of general anesthesia; use of laminaria; and an experienced operator.

(3) Uterine perforation. The incidence of this potentially serious complication of suction curettage abortions is approximately 0.2%.

(a) Risks. Factors that increase the risk of uterine perforation include multiparity, advanced gestational age, and operator inexperience. The use of laminaria to facilitate cervical dilation decreases the risk.

(b) Complications. Serious consequences of uterine perforation include hemorrhage and damage to intra-abdominal organs. Because of the location of the uterine vessels, lateral perforations may be associated with hemorrhage.

(c) Treatment. Many cases of uterine perforation require only observation. Surgical exploration is indicated when there is evidence of hemorrhage, when injury to abdominal organs is suspected, or when perforation occurs with a suction curette.

(4) Acute hematometra. This complication occurs in 0.1% to 1% of suction curettage procedures and is evidenced by decreased vaginal bleeding and an enlarged, tender uterus. **Treatment** is repeat curettage and administration of an oxytocic agent.

b. Delayed complications

(1) Postabortal infection. This condition is often associated with retained tissue. The incidence of infection varies with the method of termination.

(a) Risks. Factors that increase the risk of infection include the presence of cervical gonococcal or chlamydial infection, advanced gestational age, uterine instillation methods of termination, and the use of local anesthesia instead of general anesthesia. Infection complicates less than 1% of suction curettage procedures, 1.5% of D&E terminations, and 5.3% to 6.2% of induction terminations.

(b) Treatment. Uterine infection is usually polymicrobial, similar to other gynecologic infections, and is treated with broad-spectrum antibiotics and prompt evacuation of retained tissue. The use of prophylactic antibiotics significantly decreases the risk of infectious complications associated with induced abortions.

(2) Retained tissue. This condition complicates less than 1% of suction curettage abortions.

(a) **Associated conditions**. Retained tissue may be associated with infection, hemorrhage, or both.

(b) **Treatment**. Therapy requires repeat curettage and antibiotic administration if infection is present.

(3) **Rh sensitization**. The risk of sensitization increases with advanced gestational age. The Rh status of every pregnant woman should be known, and Rh immune globulin (RhoGAM) should be administered to an Rh-negative woman whenever maternal fetal hemorrhage is a possibility.

(a) The estimated risk of sensitization associated with suction curettage is 1.8% if RhoGAM is not administered appropriately.

(b) The recommended dose for Rh immune globulin prophylaxis is 50 μg up to 12 weeks' gestation, and 300 μg thereafter.

(4) **Future adverse pregnancy outcomes**. The incidences of infertility, spontaneous abortion, and ectopic pregnancy **do not** increase after uncomplicated suction curettage procedures.

4. **Maternal mortality**. The case mortality rate for induced abortion is less than 0.05 per 100,000 procedures. The risk varies with gestational age and method of termination.

a. The leading cause of death associated with induced abortion is anesthetic complications, followed (in frequency) by hemorrhage, embolism, and infection.

b. The risk of death is lowest for suction curettage procedures and highest for instillation procedures. Risk increases with advancing gestational age.

Study Questions for Chapter 12

Directions: *Each of the numbered items or incomplete statements in this section is followed by answers or by completions of the statement. Select the ONE lettered answer or completion that is BEST in each case.*

1. A 26-year-old woman, gravida 2, para 1, at 20 weeks of gestation, sees you in the office for prenatal care. Her fundus measures 18 weeks and you are unable to hear fetal heart tone by Doppler. You perform an ultrasound and confirm lack of fetal heart activity and lack of fetal movement. Her last pregnancy was complicated by severe preeclampsia at 34 weeks that forced her to deliver a preterm baby. She has no medical problems other than mild asthma. Upon further inquiry she tells you she had one episode of spotting 4 weeks ago but did not have cramping nor did she pass any clots or tissue from the vagina. Which of the following is the most descriptive diagnosis?

- [A] Threatened abortion
- [B] Fetal demise
- [C] Incomplete abortion
- [D] Spontaneous abortion
- [E] Missed abortion

2. Chromosomal abnormalities account for the majority of first-trimester spontaneous abortions. If one was to analyze the chromosomal composition of the products of conception that are extruded in a spontaneous abortion, which of the following would be the most common finding?

- [A] Balanced translocation
- [B] 45,X monosomy
- [C] Triploidy
- [D] Trisomy
- [E] Mosaicism

3. A 30-year-old woman, gravida 4, para 3, at 12 weeks of gestation, is seeing you for prenatal care. Her first pregnancy ended with a successful vaginal delivery, at term, of a healthy boy. Her second pregnancy was uncomplicated and resulted in a cesarean section with low transverse incision of uterus for breech presentation after failed external version. Her last pregnancy resulted in the successful "natural" birth of her daughter. What is the best advice you can give this patient regarding vaginal birth after cesarean section (VBAC)?

- [A] You are not a candidate for VBAC
- [B] You are an excellent candidate for VBAC
- [C] You are an average candidate for VBAC
- [D] You should consider a cesarean section given your risk of uterine rupture
- [E] Your risk of uterine rupture is 1 in 80

4. You are an attending obstetrician in charge of a busy hospital. You are monitoring the progress of a woman (gravida 2, para 0) who has been in labor for the past 24 hours; her membranes have been ruptured for 17 hours. Three hours ago, her cervix was 10 cm dilated and 100% effaced. The fetal vertex had reached the pelvic floor and was in the left occiput anterior position. She has an epidural. The fetal heart rate tracing was reassuring, and she began pushing. Now, the fetal vertex has reached +2 station though the fetal vertex feels asynclitic. Given her protracted second stage of labor, you decide to perform a forceps delivery. What step is not necessary prior to proceeding?

- [A] Adequate anesthesia
- [B] Completely dilated cervix
- [C] Ruptured membranes
- [D] An additional obstetrician in the room
- [E] Confirmation of fetal head position

QUESTIONS 5–11

Match the description below with the best range of numbers above. Each answer choice may be used once, more than once, or not at all.

A 0%–10%
B 25%–30%
C 35%–45%
D 60%–70%
E 71%–80%

5. Risk of sensitization in Rh-negative woman after D&E if RhoGAM not given

6. Risk of uterine perforation after D&E

7. After three spontaneous abortions (SABs), risk of SAB if no history of liveborn

8. Annual percent of births by cesarean section in the United States

9. Risk of endomyometritis after cesarean section

10. Uterine atony as the indication for a cesarean hysterectomy

11. Success rate for VBAC after one previous low transverse cesarean section for fetal distress and two previous successful VBACs

Answers and Explanations

1. The answer is E [V A 3 d]. The best term to describe this clinical scenario is "missed" abortion. Death of the fetus or embryo (less than 23 weeks and before viability) occurred without onset of labor or passage of tissue and was unrecognized for 4 weeks. Fetal demise is a "missed abortion" that occurs after fetal viability, or 23 weeks or more of gestation. A threatened abortion is an event that is occurring in the present. The fetus is alive inside the uterus but is threatening to abort by causing spotting from the vagina. An incomplete abortion describes an abortion in progress. This means that the patient recently had bleeding and cramping, and there was partial or incomplete expulsion of the products of conception. The cervical os is open. A spontaneous abortion is too broad a term. Most of the answer choices are subtypes of "spontaneous abortion."

2. The answer is D [V A 2]. The most common chromosomal abnormality found in spontaneous abortions is autosomal trisomies (e.g., trisomy 16 or trisomy 21). The most common single anomaly seen in abortuses is 45,X monosomy or Turner's. Don't confuse triploidy (an extra set of 23 chromosomes in humans) with trisomy (one extra chromosome).

3. The answer is B [I F 2]. This patient is an excellent candidate for VBAC for two reasons: she has had one prior successful VBAC with her third pregnancy and she had a cesarean section with her second pregnancy for a "nonrecurring" reason (breech). One should not dissuade a woman wanting a VBAC if the prerequisites are met (1. No maternal or fetal contraindication; 2. two or fewer previous low transverse cesarean section(s); 3. informed consent regarding risks and benefits; and 4. personnel able to perform emergency delivery). The risk of uterine rupture after one previous low transverse type of cesarean section is less than 1% (i.e., less than 1 in 100).

4. The answer is D [III C, D]. This clinical scenario describes the protracted second stage of labor with regional anesthesia in a primipara, which is an indication for assisted vaginal delivery if the appropriate criteria are met. The fetal asynclitism is likely the cause of the protracted course. Since this patient is fully dilated (10 cm) with ruptured membranes and a known fetal vertex position with the station at +2, it is appropriate to proceed with vaginal delivery. Anesthesia always needs to be assured prior to instrumentation and, likewise, the patient's bladder needs to be emptied. Additional obstetric staff are not necessary unless the obstetrician is not an experienced operator, such as in an academic teaching institution.

5. A [V B 3 b 3], **6.** A [V B 3 a 3], **7.** C [V A 3 e], **8.** B [I A 1], **9.** C [I E 1 a], **10.** C [I E 5 b], **11.** E [I F 1 a]. The estimated risk of sensitization (i.e., formation of antibodies against the Rh antigen on red blood cells) associated with curettage is 1.8% if RhoGAM is not administered. The incidence of uterine perforation after a suction curettage is 0.2%. After three spontaneous abortions, a woman with a previous liveborn infant has a 25% to 35% risk of SAB versus 40% to 45% with no history of any liveborn. Approximately 29% of infants were delivered by cesarean birth in 2004. Postoperative infection is the most common complication after cesarean section, especially endomyometritis (incidence 34% to 40%). The most common indication for cesarean hysterectomy is postpartum hemorrhage caused by uterine atony (incidence 43%). There is a 60% to 80% rate of successful vaginal delivery after previous cesarean section, especially if there is a nonrecurring indication (fetal distress) and previous successful VBAC.

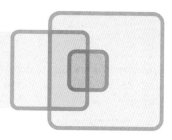

chapter 13

Obstetric Anesthesia

ROBERT GAISER

I   INTRODUCTION

A Obstetric anesthesia involves caring for the parturient. Objectives for the obstetric anesthesiologist include:

1. Pain control during delivery that is safe for both the mother and the fetus

2. Anesthetic management during cesarean delivery that does not affect the fetus or harm the mother

3. Assisting the obstetrician with the management of comorbidities during labor and delivery and with the hemodynamic management

B Most hospitals provide 24-hour anesthesia coverage of the labor and delivery suite. In the United States, approximately 85% of parturients receive some form of analgesia or anesthesia during childbirth.

C Two terms are important to understand. Analgesia refers to pain relief; it does not involve the removal of complete sensation. Anesthesia refers to rendering the patient completely insensate to pain. Anesthesia can be accomplished via two means:

1. General anesthesia, in which the patient is rendered unconscious and the whole body is rendered insensate. Protection of the airway is required as the patient is at risk for aspiration.

2. Regional anesthesia, in which a specific area of the body is rendered insensate to surgical stimuli by the use of local anesthetics injected into specific areas. The parturient maintains her natural airway and is not at risk for aspiration.

D Obstetric anesthesia continues to improve with regard to maternal safety and may represent one of the most impressive accomplishments in health care for the 20th century. From 1991 to 1997, anesthesia accounted for 1.7% of all maternal deaths (as defined as a death occurring during pregnancy or up to 1 year following delivery). This is a significant improvement when compared to a rate of 5% for the previous time period of 1979 to 1986.

E Obstetric anesthesia involves the care of two patients, the mother and the fetus. The mother undergoes various physiologic changes to adapt to the enlarging uterus and to support the growing fetus. These changes must be considered when designing a plan for the patient's analgesia.

II   PHYSIOLOGIC CHANGES OF PREGNANCY

A Cardiac

1. Pregnancy results in an increase in cardiac output to meet the demands of increased oxygen consumption. Cardiac output increases 40% during pregnancy, with most of the increase occurring during the first trimester. The increase in cardiac output allows a 10- to 20-fold increase in uterine blood flow. The increase in cardiac output is multifactorial, resulting from an increase in both stroke volume and heart rate (an increase of 10 to 20 beats per minute [bpm]). Despite the increase in cardiac output, systolic, diastolic, and mean blood pressure decrease.

2. Maternal blood volume increases during pregnancy by 35%. The increase begins early in gestation and continues throughout pregnancy. The increased blood volume during pregnancy

allows parturients to tolerate normal blood loss of delivery (approximately 400 mL during vaginal delivery and 700 mL during cesarean section). Blood volume returns to prepregnancy levels within 7 to 14 days after delivery.

3. Normal parturients are less responsive to vasopressors and chronotropic agents, such as ephedrine or phenylephrine. This decrease in response may be related to down-regulation of α and β receptors. As such, one may need to increase the amount of vasopressor administered to a pregnant patient.

4. In the supine position, up to 15% of pregnant patients develop nausea, hypotension, and vomiting (supine hypotension syndrome). The supine position allows the gravid uterus to compress the inferior vena cava and aorta. Caval compression results in decreased venous return to the right atrium and hence, cardiac output. Anesthetic drugs or techniques that cause venodilation worsen the decrease in blood pressure. A decrease in blood pressure results in a decrease in uterine perfusion. Further decreases in uterine blood flow occur if the uterus compresses the aorta. By tilting the patient to the left, the uterus is displaced off the vena cava and the aorta. As such, pregnant women should not lie supine after 20 weeks' gestation; the uterus should be tilted to the left, by placing a wedge underneath the right hip.

B **Respiratory system**

1. Various changes occur in the maternal airway during gestation. There is vascular engorgement of the airway, resulting in edema of the oral and nasal pharynx, larynx, and trachea. This airway edema can make intubation of the trachea difficult. Exacerbation of these changes may occur in patients with upper respiratory tract infections or preeclampsia. The mucous membranes are also very friable. Manipulation, such as nasal intubation or the insertion of a nasogastric tube, may result in excessive bleeding.

2. The gravid uterus results in a 4-cm elevation of the diaphragm. Despite this elevation, there is little change in total lung capacity as the chest expands in anterior-posterior and traverse diameters to compensate. The diaphragmatic elevation does cause a 20% decrease in functional residual capacity (FRC) at term. This decrease is a result of decreases in both residual volume and expiratory reserve volume. Oxygen consumption increases by 20% due to increased metabolism and increased work of breathing. The parturient compensates for this increased oxygen consumption in two ways: (1) increased alveolar ventilation and (2) shifting the oxyhemoglobin dissociation curve to the right, thus facilitating unloading of oxygen at the cellular level.

3. The decrease in FRC and increased oxygen consumption make parturients very vulnerable to hypoxia. After complete denitrogenation by oxygen breathing, nonpregnant patients tolerate 9 minutes of apnea before oxygen saturation is less than 90%, whereas parturients can only tolerate 2 to 3 minutes.

4. Alveolar ventilation increases by 70%. This increase results primarily from increased tidal volume and secondarily from a small increase in respiratory rate. The $PaCO_2$ decreases to 32 mmHg as a result of increased ventilation and PaO_2 increases 5 to 10 mmHg. Decreased serum bicarbonate from 26 mmHg to 22 mmHg results in a partially compensated respiratory alkalosis.

C **Gastrointestinal changes**

1. The enlarged gravid uterus displaces the stomach cephalad. This displacement changes the angle of gastroesophageal junction, decreasing competence of the gastroesophageal sphincter. The uterus also displaces the pylorus upward and posteriorly, resulting in delayed gastric emptying. Elevated concentrations of progesterone decrease gastrointestinal motility and food absorption. These changes facilitate the occurrence of gastric reflux and heartburn in as many as 70% of pregnant women. These changes also place pregnant women at major risk for regurgitation and aspiration of gastric contents during induction or maintenance of general anesthesia or any other loss of consciousness.

D **Hematologic changes**

1. Plasma volume increases 45% but the red cell mass increases only 20%, leading to the physiologic (dilutional) anemia of pregnancy.

E Renal

1. Renal plasma flow and glomerular filtration rate (GFR) increase during the first trimester to 50% above normal by the fourth month. During the third trimester, both slowly return to normal. The increase in renal plasma flow and glomerular filtration rate results in an increased creatinine clearance, with a decreased blood urea nitrogen (BUN) and creatinine (Cr). BUN decreases 40% to 8 to 9 mg/dL, while creatinine decreases to 0.4 to 0.5 mg/dL.

F Central nervous system

1. The minimum alveolar concentration (MAC) for inhaled anesthetics is decreased up to 40% in pregnancy. The mechanism is unclear, although it may be related to progesterone (which has sedative activity) and endorphins. A concentration of an inhalation agent that may not produce loss of consciousness in nonpregnant patients may render pregnant women unconscious, placing the parturient at risk for aspiration.

2. Pregnant women require less local anesthetic to produce the same level of epidural or spinal block. In the epidural space, it may be partly due to epidural vein engorgement, thus decreasing the volume of the epidural space. However, this decreased requirement is seen in the first trimester, well before significant mechanical changes have occurred.

G Reproductive tract

1. The uterus weighs 50 to 70 g in the nonpregnant state and increases to 1.0 to 1.5 kg in pregnant women at term. Total uterine blood flow increases from 50 mL/min in nonpregnant women to 700 mL/min in pregnant women at term, representing approximately 10% of the cardiac output.

III NEUROPATHWAYS OF OBSTETRIC PAIN

A First stage of labor

1. The pain resulting from the first stage of labor is primarily due to dilation of the cervix with consequent distention and stretching. Although cervical dilation accounts for the majority of pain, there is also uterine contraction pain as the pressure and stretching of the uterine muscles stimulate the high threshold mechanoreceptors.

2. The pain is typically described as a visceral pain, a strong dull pain over the lower abdomen between the umbilicus and symphysis pubis, laterally over the iliac crest in a bandlike distribution, and posteriorly in the skin and soft tissue over the lower lumbar spines.

3. The location of this pain is explained by the innervation of the uterus and cervix and by the concept of referred pain. The sensory nerves, which transmit noxious impulses that produce pain from the uterus and cervix, enter the spinal cord at T10, T11, T12, and L1. These fibers synapse in the spinal cord in the same location as the cutaneous fibers from T10, T11, T12, and L1. The brain interprets the increased firing in this area as originating from the cutaneous fibers and refers the pain to the abdomen, back, and hips.

B Second stage of labor

1. Second-stage pain occurs as the fetus descends through the birth canal. This results in stretching and tearing of fascia, skin, subcutaneous tissue, and other somatic structures.

2. This somatic pain is transmitted primarily through the pudendal nerve, which is derived from the anterior primary divisions of sacral nerves S2, S3, and S4.

3. The woman knows exactly where it hurts, the perineum.

IV ANALGESIA FOR LABOR

A Epidural analgesia

1. Epidural blockade plays a prominent role in obstetrics and obstetric anesthesia. To successfully use epidural blockade, the anesthesiologist must be able to locate the epidural space.

2. Immediately peripheral to the dura mater is the epidural space. It extends from the foramen magnum to the sacral hiatus. The posterior longitudinal ligament forms the anterior boundary

of this space, while the ligamentum flavum forms the posterior boundary. The pedicles and intervertebral foramina form the lateral boundaries.

3. The contents of the epidural space include the nerve roots, fat, lymphatic tissue, and blood vessels.

4. The epidural space is entered with a needle and relies upon the anesthesiologist's sense of feel. Once entered, a catheter is passed and various combinations of local anesthetic and narcotic are administered.

5. Epidural medications
   a. Local anesthetics
      (1) Local anesthetics are a group of drugs that reversibly block nerve conduction.
      (2) All local anesthetics are weak bases that have a three-part structure: a lipophilic aromatic ring, an intermediate chain, and a hydrophilic carbon chain bearing an amino group. The intermediate chain determines to which classification a local anesthetic belongs. The esters have the COO configuration, while amides have the NHCO configuration.
      (3) Local anesthetics prevent impulse generation in the nerve and propagation by gaining access to the sodium channel and blocking permeability to sodium ions.
      (4) Local anesthetics have their major toxic effects in the brain and myocardium. The brain is more susceptible than the heart to the toxic effects. All of the early signs and symptoms of local anesthetic toxicity are related to the central nervous system. Myocardial dysfunction is only seen after central nervous system toxicity.
      (5) Parturients are more sensitive to the neural blocking properties of local anesthetics. The cardiac toxicity is not increased during pregnancy.
      (6) For analgesia, a low concentration of local anesthetic is used. This allows for the preservation of motor function.
   b. Opioids
      (1) Opioids are frequently added to the local anesthetic solution in the epidural space. The opioids provide analgesia and allow for a lower dose of local anesthetic to be used. By using a low dose of opioid and local anesthetic, side effects are reduced.
      (2) By using a low concentration of opioid, the neonate is not exposed to the opioid.
      (3) The most common opioids added to the local anesthetic solution are fentanyl or sufentanil.

6. Risks of epidural analgesia are hypotension and postdural puncture headache. Epidural analgesia does not increase the risk of cesarean section. It may increase the risk of operative vaginal delivery if the patient experiences motor blockade. It may also prolong the duration of labor, with studies reporting a range of 30 minutes to 2 hours.
   a. The hypotension results from sympathetic blockade with venous dilation in the lower extremities. A fluid bolus prior to epidural analgesia will decrease the risk of hypotension.
   b. Hypotension is treated with either intravenous phenylephrine or ephedrine.
   c. Postdural puncture headache results if the dura is punctured with the epidural needle. It is a postural headache that is located in the frontal-occipital area that is treated with an epidural blood patch. A blood patch involves the injection of autologous blood into the epidural space.

B **Combined spinal epidural analgesia**

1. An 18-gauge Tuohy needle is inserted into the epidural space and serves as an introducer for a 24- or 26-gauge long pencil-point spinal needle.

2. A subarachnoid injection is given. The spinal needle is withdrawn, and an epidural catheter passed and secured.
   a. An opioid with a small amount of local anesthetic is administered.
   b. The most common opioids are fentanyl 25 μg or sufentanil 10 μg.
   c. The most common local anesthetic is isobaric bupivacaine 0.25%, 1 mL.

3. The intrathecal injection provides analgesia of rapid onset. The major difference between the combined spinal epidural and traditional epidural analgesia is the speed of onset of the analgesia.

4. Side effects of intrathecal narcotics include pruritus, nausea, and respiratory depression. The hypotension is not a result of sympathetic blockade, but rather the removal of pain. There has been no study that has shown that intrathecal narcotics affect the fetus or uterine blood flow.

C Intravenous analgesia

1. Patients with clotting disorders, thrombocytopenia, or previous spinal surgery may not be candidates for epidural analgesia. Intravenous patient-controlled analgesia (IV-PCA) should be considered for these patients.

2. Fentanyl

   a. Fentanyl is probably the best opioid for IV-PCA. It has less sedation and nausea associated with it. It is also associated with a lower placental transfer.

   b. The loading dose is typically 1 to 2 µg/kg. Patients generally do not receive a continuous infusion, rather a bolus of 50 µg with a lockout of 10 minutes.

3. Morphine

   a. Morphine is used early in labor, usually during a prolonged latent phase with a dose of 10 mg IM or 2 to 5 mg IV.

4. Nalbuphine

   a. Nalbuphine is a synthetic agonist–antagonist (in low doses it acts as an agonist; in higher doses, its antagonist properties prevail).

   b. Given the antagonist properties, respiratory depression is unlikely.

5. Naloxone

   a. Naloxone is capable of reversing the effects of opioids, such as respiratory depression or pruritus. Of note, it also reverses the analgesia of opioids.

6. Intravenous opioids decrease fetal heart rate variability. Even with the low placental transfer, there is approximately a 20% incidence for the need for naloxone in the neonate.

D Other regional blocks

1. Paracervical block

   a. Fibers innervating the uterus and cervix leave the cervix and join the sensory nerves that accompany the sympathetic nerves of T10 to L1.

   b. Paracervical block involves the injection of local anesthetics submucosally into the fornix of the vagina laterally to the cervix (generally at 4 o'clock and 8 o'clock). The somatic sensory fibers of the perineum are not blocked.

   c. Paracervical block is effective only for the first stage of labor, and is associated with a high incidence of fetal bradycardia.

   d. Its major role is in providing analgesia for dilation and curettage.

2. Pudendal bock

   a. Somatic pain of the second stage of labor results from distention of the pelvic floor, vagina, and perineum as the fetus descends through the birth canal. These painful impulses are transmitted primarily through the pudendal nerve, which is derived from the anterior primary divisions of the sacral nerves S2 to S4.

   b. Pudendal block involves the injection of local anesthetic below the ischial spines (the approximate location of the pudendal nerve). This block is administered during the second stage of labor and is useful for vaginal delivery and outlet forceps. It is also helpful for suturing following delivery as it anesthetizes the perineum.

V ANESTHESIA FOR CESAREAN SECTION

A Anesthesia for cesarean section can be divided into two different types: general and regional. The decision regarding the type depends on the urgency of the cesarean section, the comorbidities, and the patient's desires.

B Spinal anesthesia

1. Spinal anesthesia for cesarean section involves the injection of sufficient local anesthetic to achieve a T4 sensory level.

2. Spinal anesthesia is chosen when the length of the procedure is known. If the duration is in question, a continuous technique is preferred.

3. The major risks of spinal anesthesia include postdural puncture headache, bradycardia, hypotension, and limited duration of anesthesia.

4. Compared to epidural anesthesia, umbilical cord pH is lower for spinal anesthesia than for epidural anesthesia.

5. Hypotension from spinal anesthesia may be treated with either phenylephrine 100 μg or ephedrine 10 mg.

C Epidural anesthesia

1. Surgical anesthesia is rapidly achieved in a patient with an epidural catheter placed for labor.

2. The use of 1.5% lidocaine with epinephrine 1:200,000 achieves a T4 level in 4 to 6 minutes.

3. The use of 3% 2-chloroprocaine with sodium bicarbonate can achieve a T4 sensory level in 90 to 120 seconds.

4. The choice of drug depends on the urgency of the situation.

5. Approximately 20 mL of local anesthetic is required to achieve a T4 sensory level. The higher volume places the patient at risk for local anesthetic toxicity if injected intravascularly and high spinal if injected subarachnoid.

D General anesthesia

1. General anesthesia for cesarean delivery is indicated in true emergency situations to reduce delays in delivering the infant, when the mother prefers or requires this method, or when regional anesthesia is contraindicated (thrombocytopenia, coagulopathy).

2. Clear antacids, metoclopramide, and histamine blockers are suggested to reduce the risk of aspiration syndrome if the patient should aspirate during the anesthesia.

3. To secure the airway, thiopental (or propofol) and succinyl choline are administered in rapid sequence with cricoid pressure. For failed intubation, cesarean delivery has been accomplished with the laryngeal mask airway.

4. When general anesthesia is given, neonatal depression (as quantified by reduced APGAR scores in the newborn infant) is worsened by delays between induction and uterine incision and by delays between uterine incision and delivery.

5. Maternal awareness is prevented by maintaining low end-tidal concentrations of volatile agents.

E Postoperative analgesia

1. When cesarean section is performed during regional anesthesia, preservative-free morphine is administered in the epidural intraoperatively. The use of preservative-free morphine provides analgesia of 12 to 24 hours' duration.

2. Administering higher doses of morphine in the epidural or spinal does not improve the duration of analgesia, but rather increases the incidence of side effects. The most common side effect is pruritus. Pruritus is treated with small doses of naloxone. Diphenhydramine is frequently given, although it is not as effective.

3. Postoperative orders should include respiratory monitoring and treatment for respiratory depression or pruritus.

4. When cesarean section is performed during general anesthesia, patient-controlled intravenous analgesia is typically used. The opioid chosen is morphine, as it has the fewest effects on the neonate if the mother is breastfeeding.

Study Questions for Chapter 13

Directions: *Each of the numbered items or incomplete statements in this section is followed by answers or by completions of the statement. Select the ONE lettered answer or completion that is BEST in each case.*

1. A 24-year-old parturient is at 20 weeks' gestation. Her past medical history is notable for mitral stenosis secondary to rheumatic heart disease as a child. What physiologic change places her at risk for the development of heart failure during her pregnancy?

- A Increase in minute ventilation
- B Increase in stroke volume
- C Increase in uterine size
- D Increase in renal plasma flow
- E Increase in red cell mass

2. A parturient at 40 weeks' gestation is scheduled for a magnetic resonance imaging scan to assess for placenta accreta. The radiologist is unable to complete the study due to nausea whenever the patient is supine. What do you recommend to the radiologist?

- A Antiemetic medication
- B Fasting prior to the study
- C Intravenous fluid loading
- D Tilting the patient to the left
- E Supplemental oxygen

3. A 24-year-old parturient with severe preeclampsia requires urgent cesarean delivery for nonreassuring fetal heart rate. The anesthesiologist plans general anesthesia. Which of the following maneuvers would you recommend to increase the safety for airway management in this patient?

- A Place a nasogastric tube prior to the anesthetic
- B Have small-diameter endotracheal tubes available
- C Obtain an arterial blood gas prior to induction
- D Administer a bronchodilator prior to induction
- E Hydrate the patient with 2 L crystalloid

4. A 28-year-old parturient at 40 weeks' gestation requires general anesthesia for cesarean delivery due to umbilical cord prolapse. With induction of anesthesia, there is a rapid decline of the oxygen saturation. This decline is a result of a decrease in which lung volume?

- A Dead space
- B Total lung
- C Tidal
- D Residual
- E Inspiratory reserve

5. The pain of the second stage of labor is conveyed by which nerve?

- A Paracervical
- B Ilioinguinal
- C Pudendal
- D Genitofemoral
- E Iliohypogastric

6. A 25-year-old woman requires cesarean section during epidural anesthesia. Prior to the injection of local anesthetic, the anesthesiologist administers a test dose of 3 mL lidocaine 1.5% with epinephrine 1:200,000. The patient complains of tinnitus and a rapid heart rate. What is the most likely etiology of her symptoms?

- A Anaphylaxis
- B Intravascular injection
- C Intrathecal injection
- D Eclampsia
- E Anxiety

7. A 24-year-old parturient at 40 weeks' gestation is in active labor and requests epidural analgesia. During epidural placement, the dura is punctured. The patient is at increased risk for the development of which of the following complications postoperatively?

- A Leg weakness
- B Backache
- C Headache
- D Hemorrhage
- E Dyspnea

8. A 21-year-old parturient is considering epidural analgesia. Which of the following is increased in patients with epidural analgesia?

- A Prolonged labor
- B Cesarean delivery
- C Impaired breastfeeding
- D Neonatal depression
- E Cerebral palsy

Answers and Explanations

1. The answer is B [II A 1]. During pregnancy, the cardiac output increases. This increase occurs as a result of an increase of both stroke volume and heart rate. A parturient with a fixed cardiac lesion cannot increase her cardiac output to meet the increased demands placed upon her, and as such is at risk for the development of heart failure. An increase in minute ventilation, uterine size, and renal plasma flow will not affect her risk of heart failure. While red cell mass and plasma volume are increased, the increase is generally well tolerated by an individual with cardiac disease.

2. The answer is D [II A 4]. Approximately 15% of patients develop symptoms of nausea when supine. In this position, the gravid uterus compresses the vena cava and decreases venous return. This in turn decreases cardiac preload and hence cardiac output. If these symptoms develop, it is important to tilt the patient to the left or place a wedge under her right hip. Not all patients develop these symptoms because of sympathetic compensation. Patients with anesthesia must be maintained in the left uterine displacement position as they do not possess the ability for sympathetic compensation.

3. The answer is B [II B 1]. Airway edema occurs during pregnancy and may be worsened by preeclampsia. It is important to have small-diameter endotracheal tubes available prior to starting anesthesia in a patient with preeclampsia. If the intubation is hindered by the edema, a smaller-diameter endotracheal tube may allow for the securing of the airway.

4. The answer is D [II B 2]. Pregnancy results in a decrease in both residual and expiratory reserve volume. These volumes comprise the functional residual capacity. Given this decrease, less time is available during periods of apnea for a decline in oxygen saturation to develop. Tidal volume actually increases during pregnancy.

5. The answer is C [III B 2]. Second-stage pain occurs as the fetus descends through the birth canal. This results in stretching and tearing of the fascia, skin, and subcutaneous tissue. This somatic pain is transmitted primarily through the pudendal nerve. The pudendal nerve is derived from the anterior primary divisions of the sacral nerves S2 to S4. This nerve is easily blocked by the obstetrician by the administration of local anesthetic close to the ischial spines. Also, this innervation explains why patients frequently experience pain during the second stage of labor. The sacral nerves are large and not easily blocked. Local anesthetic administered epidurally always travels cephalad more easily than caudad. It is not uncommon for a woman to experience "sacral sparing" of her epidural, resulting in pain during the second stage.

6. The answer is B [IV A 5 a (4)]. These symptoms are classic for intravascular injection. The tinnitus results from intravenous lidocaine and the rapid heart rate from intravenous epinephrine. A test dose is always administered prior to giving the epidural anesthetic. When placing an epidural catheter, there are three places it can be: epidurally, intrathecally, and intravascularly. Prior to injection, a test dose is administered to rule out intrathecal or intravascular injection. An intrathecal injection results in numbness, while an epidural injection does not result in any symptoms.

7. The answer is C [IV A 6]. Postdural puncture headache is a bilateral headache that develops within 7 days after dural puncture and usually disappears 14 days after the dural puncture (longer time periods have been described with larger-gauge needles). It worsens within 15 minutes of assuming the upright position and improves within 30 minutes of resuming a recumbent position. It usually occurs in the frontal, occipital, or both areas. It results from leakage of cerebrospinal fluid through the dural tear into the epidural space.

8. The answer is A [IV A 6]. Epidural analgesia does not increase the risk of cesarean section. The fetus is exposed to minimal medication. As such, it does not interfere with breastfeeding or result in a depressed neonate. Multiple studies indicate that labor is prolonged in patients with epidural analgesia.

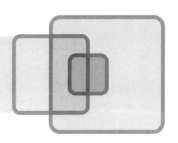

chapter 14

Postterm Pregnancy

SHARON BYUN • SINDHU K. SRINIVAS

I INTRODUCTION

Postterm pregnancy occurs in approximately 10% of all pregnancies. The reason that postterm pregnancy is a concern is that an increase in perinatal mortality and morbidity has been observed in those pregnancies progressing beyond term.

II DEFINITION

Term gestation is defined as a pregnancy between 37 and 42 completed weeks (260 to 294 days) after the first day of the **last menstrual period (LMP)**. Postterm pregnancy begins when 42 completed (menstrual) weeks have elapsed. The first day of the LMP occurs approximately 2 weeks before conception in a 28-day cycle.

III DETERMINING GESTATIONAL AGE

A Naegele's rule uses the first day of the LMP to calculate the **estimated date of confinement (EDC)**. Assuming a 28-day cycle, subtract 3 months and add 7 days to the first day of the LMP to determine the delivery date.

B Quickening is the maternal perception of fetal movement and begins around 16 to 20 weeks of gestation.

C Uterine size increases with gestational age. The uterus is a pelvic organ until 12 weeks, at which time the **fundus** can be palpated at the level of the iliac crests. The uterine fundus is palpable at the umbilicus around 20 weeks. Between 20 and 36 weeks, the measurement of the uterus in centimeters from the symphysis pubis to the fundus approximates the gestational age within 2 weeks.

D An electronic Doppler ultrasound may detect fetal heart tones as early as 10 to 11 weeks' gestation.

E Ultrasound examination in the first trimester provides the most accurate dating. Measurement of the **crown–rump length (CRL)** is accurate to within 5 to 7 days of the actual gestational age. Second- and third-trimester ultrasound uses several parameters for determining gestational age. These parameters include the **biparietal diameter (BPD)**, the **femur length (FL)**, and the **abdominal circumference (AC)**. In the second trimester, the BPD is the most accurate but only to within 14 days of the actual gestational age. Measurements in the third trimester may have an error up to ±21 days of the actual gestational age.

IV ETIOLOGY OF POSTTERM PREGNANCY

The most frequent cause of an apparent postterm pregnancy is error in determining the time of ovulation and conception based on the reported last menstrual period. Frequently encountered problems are the patient's failure to recall the date of her last menstrual period and the variable length of the proliferative phase of the cycle, which allows for variation in the ovulation date. ***When postterm*** *pregnancy truly exists, the cause is usually unknown.* Parturition is a complex process that involves events within the fetal brain, adrenals, placenta, amnion, and chorion; it induces changes in the maternal tissues, including the decidua, myometrium, and cervix. The theorized mechanism of parturition begins with a stimulus in the fetal brain, resulting in **activation of the fetal hypothalamic-pituitary axis. Adrenocorticotropic hormone (ACTH)** production results in stimulation of the **fetal adrenal.** The fetal adrenal increases production of **dehydroepiandrosterone sulfate (DHEAS) and cortisol.** The presence of **placental sulfatase** in the placenta is required so that the placenta can convert the DHEAS to **estradiol.** Estrogen is thought to be important in increasing myometrial activity, and cortisol is thought to be important in stimulating **prostaglandin** output in the placental tissues. Prostaglandins are important for myometrial contractility. Several disorders may result in delayed parturition and postterm pregnancy. These disorders are all similar in that they are associated with low estrogen production. *These rare causes of postterm pregnancy include:*

[A] **Anencephaly** is an absence of the fetal cranium with gross abnormalities associated with the fetal brain. The absence and abnormalities of these structures prevent the normal initiation of parturition and result in prolonged gestation.

[B] **Congenital primary fetal adrenal hypoplasia** has been associated with prolonged gestation. The fetal adrenal is important in the production of cortisol and androgens, which help parturition to occur.

[C] **Placental sulfatase** is required to convert fetal DHEAS to estrogen. Deficiency of placental sulfatase leads to decreased estrogen levels and a subsequent delay in parturition. This is an X-linked disorder that affects male fetuses, occurring in 1 in 2500 newborns.

[D] **Previous postterm pregnancy** and **primiparity** are also associated with postterm pregnancy.

V   CLINICAL SIGNIFICANCE OF POSTTERM PREGNANCY

An increase in the **perinatal mortality rate** has been observed in postterm pregnancies (i.e., after 42 completed weeks of pregnancy). **Postterm pregnancies have been reported to have a higher incidence of meconium and meconium aspiration, oxytocin induction, shoulder dystocia, macrosomia, oligohydramnios, fetal heart rate abnormalities, and cesarean section.**

VI   MANAGEMENT OF THE POSTTERM PREGNANCY

The goal of management of postterm pregnancy is to decrease the risk of an adverse perinatal outcome (including stillbirth). Antenatal testing and induction of labor are the two most widely used strategies for management.

[A] **Antenatal testing** is generally started twice weekly between 41 and 42 weeks' gestation. It can include the **nonstress test (NST)**, the **contraction stress test (CST)**, or the **biophysical profile (BPP)** (see Chapter 6).

   1. The **nonstress test** is a noninvasive test of fetal activity that correlates with fetal well-being. Fetal heart rate (FHR) accelerations are observed during fetal movement. An external monitor is used to record the FHR, and the mother participates by indicating fetal movements.
      a. A **reactive test** requires **two fetal heart rate accelerations** of at least 15 beats' amplitude of 15 seconds' duration in a 20-minute period.
      b. In one study, 99% of oxytocin challenge tests were negative for signs of fetal distress when performed after a reactive NST.
      c. The most common cause for a nonreactive NST is a period of fetal inactivity or sleep. Studies have shown that the longest interval of fetal inactivity in the healthy fetus is 40 minutes.
      d. If the test is nonreactive after 40 minutes, a CST is performed.
      e. Approximately 25% of fetuses that have a nonreactive NST have a positive CST.
   2. The **contraction stress test** is a test of FHR that indirectly measures placental function in response to uterine contractions. An intravenous infusion of oxytocin is used to stimulate

TABLE 14–1 Management Based on Biophysical Profile Score

Score	Interpretation	Management
10	Normal	Repeat testing
8	Normal	Repeat testing
6	Suspect chronic asphyxia	If ≥36 weeks, deliver Repeat testing in 4–6 hours
4	Suspect chronic asphyxia	If ≥32 weeks, deliver Repeat testing in 4–6 hours
0–2	Strongly suspect chronic asphyxia	Extend testing to 120 minutes; if score ≤4, deliver at any gestational age

uterine contractions. The nipple stimulation test is an endogenous means of releasing oxytocin in response to manual stimulation of the patient's nipples. It is a noninvasive CST. A CST is performed when the NST is nonreactive.

a. Criteria for a negative CST consist of three uterine contractions of moderate intensity lasting 40 to 60 seconds over a 10-minute period with no late decelerations in the FHR tracing. A positive CST has late decelerations associated with more than 50% of the uterine contractions. A CST with inconsistent late decelerations is considered suspect.

b. More often, a favorable outcome follows a negative CST, but as many as 25% of fetuses may experience intrapartum fetal distress after a negative CST.

c. CSTs have a **25% false-positive rate**.

d. Studies have shown the incidence of perinatal death within 1 week of a negative CST to be less than 1 in 1000. Most of these deaths are caused by cord accidents or abruptions.

e. A positive CST has been associated with an increased incidence of intrauterine death, late decelerations in labor, low 5-minute APGAR scores, intrauterine growth retardation, and meconium-stained amniotic fluid. The overall perinatal death rate after a positive CST is between 7% and 15%.

f. A suspect CST should be repeated in 24 hours.

3. **Biophysical profile** (see Chapter 6) is a composite of tests utilizing fetal heart rate tracing and ultrasound designed to identify a compromised fetus during the antepartum period (Table 14-1).

a. **Components of the profile**

(1) NST

(2) Fetal breathing

(3) Fetal tone

(4) Fetal motion

(5) Quantity of amniotic fluid

b. **Scoring of the profile**. Each test is given either 2 or 0 points, for a maximum of 10 points. An important feature in the postterm profile is the amniotic fluid profile component. Oligohydramnios is an ominous sign that signifies placental insufficiency and increased risk of poor perinatal outcome.

B **Induction of labor.** Induction of labor may be performed at 41 weeks if the cervix is favorable. If the cervix is unfavorable, then expectant management with antepartum fetal surveillance should be continued. Generally, at 42 weeks' gestation, if the cervix remains unfavorable, prostaglandins are administered to "ripen" the cervix for induction. A cervix is determined to be favorable by its Bishop score (Table 14-2). Induction is usually successful with a score of 9 or greater.

C **Intrapartum management** includes continuous electronic fetal heart rate monitoring.

TABLE 14-2   Bishop Scoring System Used for Assessment of Inducibility

	Dilation	Effacement (%)	Station	Cervical Consistency	Cervical Position
1	Closed	0–30	–3	Firm	Posterior
2	1–2	40–50	–2	Medium	Midposition
3	3–4	60–70	–1.0	Soft	Anterior
4	≥5	≥80	+1, +2	—	—

Reprinted with permission from Cunningham FG, MacDonald PC, Gant NF. Williams Obstetrics. 21st Ed. New York: McGraw-Hill, 2001:471, Table 20-1.

Study Questions for Chapter 14

Directions: *Each of the numbered items or incomplete statements in this section is followed by answers or by completions of the statement. Select the ONE lettered answer or completion that is BEST in each case.*

1. A 33-year-old woman, gravida 2, para 1, who is in the third trimester presents to you for her first prenatal care. She is not sure of her due date because she has been given three different dates by three different doctors. She tells you that her periods are irregular and occur every 21 to 35 days. She has not taken any form of birth control for the past 2 years. The first day of her last menstrual period was July 19, 2006. You obtain a record of an ultrasound performed in the emergency room on September 5, 2007, which showed her to be at 8 0/7 weeks of gestation. You also obtain a record from her last doctor who performed an ultrasound on December 22, 2007, which showed her to be at 24 3/7 weeks of gestation. Which one of the following is the best estimate of her due date? (You can use a pregnancy wheel.)

- [A] April 7, 2008
- [B] April 8, 2008
- [C] April 19, 2008
- [D] April 24, 2008
- [E] April 26, 2008

2. A 22-year-old woman, gravida 1, para 0, at 15 weeks of gestation by her last menstrual period, presents to you for an ultrasound examination to confirm her due date. Which of the following measurements on the fetus is the best at predicting her actual due date?

- [A] Crown–rump length
- [B] Biparietal diameter
- [C] Abdominal circumference
- [D] Femur length
- [E] Head circumference

3. A 25-year-old woman, gravida 3, para 0, at 42 weeks of gestation, presents to your clinic for prenatal care. She has accurate dating and has been receiving twice-weekly NSTs for the last week. Underdevelopment of which structure in the fetus may contribute to prolongation of this woman's gestation?

- [A] Cerebral cortex
- [B] Thalamus
- [C] Thymus
- [D] Adrenal cortex
- [E] Ovary

4. A 34-year-old woman, gravida 3, para 1, abortions 1, at 42 1/7 weeks of gestation by a week-6 ultrasound, presents to your clinic. Her NST is reactive and amniotic fluid volume (AFV) is 8.5. Her cervix is 0.5 cm dilated, 20% effaced, midposition, and firm, and the fetal vertex is at –4 station. Which of the following is the best next step in management?

- [A] Oxytocin
- [B] Prostaglandin analog
- [C] Twice-weekly NST
- [D] Repeat modified BPP (NST and AFV)
- [E] Artificial rupture of membranes (AROM)

Answers and Explanations

1. The answer is C [II, III A]. Because this patient has irregular periods, estimation of her due date by her last menstrual period is inaccurate. Therefore, Naegele's rule cannot be used to determine her EDC because it assumes a regular 28-day cycle (April 26 is incorrect). Thus, the best estimate of her actual due date is provided by the first-trimester ultrasound. Using the pregnancy wheel, if you match September 5 with 8 weeks, then you will see that 40 weeks (due date) corresponds to April 16, 2008, ±1 day (given inherent error between different pregnancy wheels). Because this is a first-trimester ultrasound, there can be a maximum of ±7 days error. Therefore, the due date must fall between April 8 and April 24 (April 16 ± 8 days). April 19 is the best estimate of the actual due date.

2. The answer is B [III E]. In the second trimester (over 13 weeks), BPD is the most accurate at determining actual gestational age. Crown–rump length is the most accurate in the first trimester. None of the other measurements is as useful at estimating gestational age except for the head circumference.

3. The answer is D [IV B]. Fetal adrenal hypoplasia has been associated with prolongation of gestation. Anencephaly, not lack of cerebral cortex or thalamus, has been associated with prolongation of gestation. Anencephaly results in lack of the hypothalamic-pituitary axis, which is theorized to be responsible for the inception of parturition. The ovary is probably not involved in the initiation of labor. However, estrogen produced by placental conversion of DHEAS is thought to increase myometrial activity.

4. The answer is B [IV B]. At 42 weeks of gestation, if the cervix remains unfavorable, as in this case (her Bishop score is $1 + 1 + 1 + 1 + 2 = 6$), prostaglandins will be administered to "ripen" the cervix for induction. Use of oxytocin for induction of an unfavorable cervix results in prolonged labor and increases the possibility of cesarean section. AROM is not a good idea if the fetal vertex is very high (−4 station). You should never send a postterm patient (more than 42 weeks) home to follow up with twice-weekly NSTs because the perinatal mortality rate is very high. There is no reason to repeat the modified BPP because this one is reassuring.

chapter 15

Preterm Labor

JUAN M. GONZALEZ • MICHAL A. ELOVITZ

I PRETERM BIRTH

A **Definition.** Preterm infants are born **before 37 weeks' gestation** (less than 259 days from the date of the last menstrual period). Preterm birth is a major contributor to developmental delay, visual and hearing impairment, chronic lung disease, and cerebral palsy. In the United Sates preterm birth is the leading cause of neonatal mortality (less than 28 days of life) and of African-American infant mortality (less than 365 days of life). Neonates born before 32 weeks have the greatest risk for poor health outcome and death. Those born between 32 and 36 weeks are still at higher risk for health and developmental problems than those born full term.

B **Epidemiology.** Preterm birth now accounts for 12.5% of all births in the United States—an increase of 30% since 1981. Much of the increase is a result of an increase in the number of multiple gestations secondary to fertility treatment. Preterm births account for more than 60% of non–anomaly-related neonatal mortality and morbidity.

1. **"Spontaneous" preterm birth**. Seventy-five percent of preterm births occur spontaneously after preterm labor and preterm premature rupture of membranes (PPROM).

2. **"Indicated" preterm birth**. Twenty to thirty percent of all preterm births occur because of a medical or obstetric disorder that places the mother or fetus at significant risk for serious morbidity or mortality.

3. Neonatal morbidity and mortality increase as the gestational age at delivery decreases.

II RISK FACTORS FOR PREMATURE DELIVERY

A Sociodemographic factors

1. **Low socioeconomic status**. Low income, low level of education, and poor nutrition are associated with preterm delivery.

2. **Ethnicity**. African Americans have a higher preterm delivery rate than other ethnic groups in the United States.

3. **Age**. Maternal age of 18 years or less or of 40 years or more increases the risk of preterm delivery.

4. **Previous premature birth**. The risk in the subsequent pregnancy after prior premature birth is 15% to 56%, depending on the presence of other risk factors.

5. **Tobacco smoking**

6. **Cocaine use**

B Maternal medical and obstetric conditions

1. **Uterine conditions**
   a. **Müllerian malformations**. Women with unicornuate or bicornuate uteri are at increased risk of preterm delivery.
   b. **Cervical insufficiency**. This painless cervical dilation in the second trimester is associated with eventual pregnancy loss. It can be caused by trauma during an obstetric or gynecologic procedure, diethylstilbestrol exposure in utero, or unknown etiology. However, distinguishing patients with cervical insufficiency from early preterm delivery remains difficult.

    c. Uterine overdistention
       (1) Polyhydramnios (amniotic fluid index of more than 25 cm)
       (2) Multiple gestation. Twin intrauterine pregnancies have a preterm labor rate of approximately 40%. Triplet intrauterine pregnancies have a 25% risk of delivery prior to 24 weeks' gestation and a 10% delivery rate from 24 to 28 weeks' gestation.

2. Obstetric conditions
  a. Preeclampsia-eclampsia
  b. Placenta abruptio
  c. Placenta previa
  d. Fetal growth restriction
  e. Prematurely ruptured membranes

3. Other maternal conditions. These disorders include chronic hypertension, diabetes mellitus type 1, renal disease, osteogenesis imperfecta, and collagen vascular disease.

C **Infection.** Significant maternal infections that may cause preterm labor and delivery include:

1. Systemic infections
  a. Pyelonephritis
  b. Pneumonia

2. Local infections
  a. Bacterial vaginosis (This is associated with preterm rupture of membranes, but it remains unclear if there is a mechanistic association.)
  b. Subclinical and clinical intra-amniotic infections
  c. Sexually transmitted diseases (STDs) (very poorly defined relationship with preterm labor)

III   PREVENTION OF PRETERM BIRTH

A **Secondary prevention with progesterone.** In two randomized clinical trials, women with a history of preterm birth treated with supplemental progesterone had a reduced risk of recurrent preterm birth.

1. The American College of Obstetricians and Gynecologists (ACOG) recommends considering the use of 17α-hydroxyprogesterone in patients with a prior *spontaneous* singleton (not medically indicated) preterm birth. The use of this drug for other risk factors for preterm birth has not been adequately studied and should not be used outside the scope of research investigations.

2. Weekly intramuscular injections of 250 mg of 17α-hydroxyprogesterone caproate starting between 16 to 20 weeks of gestation

IV   EVALUATION OF PATIENTS IN PRETERM LABOR

A **History.** **Symptoms** of preterm labor include:

1. Uterine cramping or contractions

2. Rhythmic low back pain

3. Pelvic pressure

4. Increased vaginal discharge

5. Vaginal bleeding (bloody show), which may result from cervical dilation

B **Physical examination**

1. A sterile **speculum examination** is part of the physical examination. The evaluation of fetal membrane status and presence of cervicovaginal infection is determined at this time. If vaginal bleeding is present, an ultrasound must be performed to rule out placenta previa before a digital examination is performed.
  a. Endocervical samples are obtained for gonorrhea and chlamydia testing only if STD suspected.

b. Group B streptococcus cultures are obtained.

c. Premature rupture of membranes (PROM) is ruled out by doing fern and Nitrazine tests.

2. **If there is no evidence of PROM**, a baseline **digital cervical examination** is performed, and follow-up examinations are warranted with continued uterine contractions.

3. A **urine specimen** is sent for culture. While this is routinely performed, there is not well-established evidence for this practice.

4. **Fetal heart rate** and **uterine activity monitoring** are used to assess fetal well-being and patterns of uterine contraction. Uterine contractions without cervical change may not constitute preterm labor.

   a. Intravenous normal saline infusion is started during the initial evaluation.

   b. Parenteral fluids can treat dehydration, which is a cause of uterine irritability. Since most patients with preterm labor are not dehydrated, care should be taken to avoid fluid overload.

C Diagnosis

1. Regular uterine contractions associated with progressive cervical change (i.e., cervical dilation of 2 cm or more or cervical effacement of 80% or more) must be present.

2. The goal is early identification of pregnant women who develop preterm labor and are at risk for delivery. In women who present with the symptoms of preterm labor, the currently used techniques have only an average positive predictive value. These techniques are mainly used for their high negative predictive values. They are also used to reduce the overdiagnosis of preterm labor.

   a. **Cervical length**. This value can be measured accurately by a transvaginal ultrasound in a woman with an empty bladder. A cervical length of less than 25 mm in a patient with a history of preterm birth at less than 32 weeks has a positive predictive value of 55%. This measurement should be done in the second trimester. However, the clinical utility of this measurement is limited until effective treatment options are identified. There are insufficient data on the utility of cervical length in patients with active preterm labor.

   b. **Fetal fibronectin**. This extracellular matrix glycoprotein found in fetal membranes plays an active role in intercellular adhesion. Fibronectin found in the cervicovaginal fluid in the late second and early third trimesters has been associated with preterm birth. The positive predictive value of the fibronectin assay is approximately 25%. Fetal fibronectin testing may be useful in women with symptoms and negative tests, therefore avoiding unnecessary treatment. However, the poor positive predictive value creates clinical ambiguity in patients who test positive.

V MANAGEMENT OF PRETERM LABOR

A Tocolysis.
Treatment with tocolytic medications may not reduce the rate of preterm birth, but it may delay delivery for 48 hours and reduce the associated complications. The time gained allows for transfer to a tertiary center or corticosteroid administration.

1. **Magnesium sulfate**. This agent is currently the most commonly used tocolytic agent in the United States. Randomized controlled clinical trials suggest that it delays delivery by at least 48 hours.

   a. The **mechanism of action** is that magnesium sulfate inhibits uterine contractility. Biochemically, magnesium acts by competitive inhibition of calcium at the motor end plate or the cell membrane, thereby decreasing calcium influx into the cell. It is cleared from the maternal circulation by the kidneys.

   b. **Administration** involves infusing 2 to 4 g/hr to elevate serum levels to above the normal range. The loading dose is 4 to 6 g given over 30 minutes. Once contractions cease, the infusion is reduced to the lowest possible dose to maintain uterine quiescence.

   c. **Precautions**

   (1) Intravenous fluid is limited to 125 mL per hour, and fluid status is observed closely. An indwelling Foley catheter can be used to monitor urine output accurately.

   (2) Deep tendon reflexes and vital signs should be checked hourly.

(3) A pulmonary examination should be performed every 2 to 4 hours.

(4) If signs of magnesium toxicity occur, the infusion should be discontinued and calcium gluconate or calcium carbonate administered as needed.

    d. Complications

      (1) Nausea and vomiting

      (2) Flushing and headache

      (3) Muscle weakness

      (4) Pulmonary edema

      (5) Cardiopulmonary arrest

    e. Contraindications to magnesium therapy include renal failure, myasthenia gravis, and hypocalcemia. In patients with cardiac and pulmonary disease, the effect of this tocolytic on existing pathologic conditions needs to be addressed and the risk/benefit ratio should be considered.

2. β-Mimetics

    a. These agents stimulate β receptors, leading to smooth muscle relaxation and decreased uterine contractions.

    b. Ritodrine is the only agent approved by the Food and Drug Administration for the treatment of preterm labor. Because of its significant maternal side effects, it is not available in the United States.

    c. Terbutaline is the other β-mimetic tocolytic agent, which may be given subcutaneously, parenterally, or orally.

      (1) **Administration** is by three routes. The **subcutaneous dose** is 0.25 mg every 20 minutes three times and then every 4 hours; the **intravenous dose** is 0.125 mg every 4 hours; and the **oral dose** is 5 mg every 6 hours.

      (2) **Side effects** include tachycardia, palpitations, shortness of breath, pulmonary edema, hyperglycemia, hypokalemia, and tachyphylaxis.

      (3) **Contraindications.** Relative contraindications to β-mimetic therapy are diabetes, certain cardiac diseases, and suspected abruption.

3. Indomethacin. This nonsteroidal anti-inflammatory medication inhibits the synthesis of prostaglandins, which are involved in the biochemical process of labor.

    a. Indomethacin, 50 to 100 mg, is initially given rectally. Remaining doses are given orally, 25 to 50 mg every 6 hours. This agent is usually given for no longer than 48 hours.

    b. Maternal side effects include nausea, vomiting, and gastrointestinal bleeding.

    c. A main **neonatal side effect** is **constriction of the ductus arteriosus**.

      (1) Such constriction in a fetus causes tricuspid regurgitation and eventual right heart failure. Ductal constriction is usually transient and responds to discontinuation of the drug. Prior to 32 weeks' gestation, the incidence of ductal constriction is 5% to 10%. **From 32 to 35 weeks' gestation, the incidence of ductal constriction is 50%.**

      (2) Because of this significant side effect, indomethacin is **uncommonly used as a tocolytic after 32 weeks' gestation**.

    d. Other significant neonatal complications include oligohydramnios, pulmonary hypertension, and (possibly) necrotizing enterocolitis.

4. Nifedipine. This calcium channel blocker decreases smooth muscle contractions.

    a. Nifedipine is administered orally, 10 to 20 mg every 8 hours.

    b. Maternal side effects include a decrease in blood pressure and tachycardia.

B Contraindications to tocolytic therapy

1. Absolute

    a. Severe preeclampsia and eclampsia

    b. Nonreassuring fetal heart rate

    c. Significant antepartum bleed

    d. Clinical chorioamnionitis

2. Relative contraindications

    a. Major fetal anomaly

    b. Mild preeclampsia

    c. Maternal cardiac disease

C Refractory preterm labor.   This condition is defined as persistent uterine contractions and cervical change despite maximal tocolytic therapy. Management may include **amniocentesis**, which can be performed to rule out an intra-amniotic infection. However, the prevalence of a positive test is low.

1. A Gram stain is positive for intra-amniotic infection if bacteria are present.

2. A glucose level of less than 14 mg/dL may be a sign of intra-amniotic infection.

3. A positive amniotic fluid culture signals intra-amniotic infection.

D Adjunctive therapy

1. **Corticosteroids**
   a. Corticosteroids are given to women in preterm labor at 24 to 34 weeks' gestation. Repeated courses should not be done outside a research trial.
   b. This medication induces fetal lung maturity, and optimal benefit begins 24 hours after initiation of therapy. Corticosteroids accelerate pulmonary maturity by stimulating the synthesis and release of surfactant from type II pneumocytes.
   c. Corticosteroids decrease mortality, respiratory distress syndrome, and intraventricular hemorrhage.

2. **Antibiotics**. These agents are given as prophylaxis for neonatal group B streptococcal infection.
   a. Antibiotics are started on admission and continued if the group B streptococcus culture is positive. Affected women are treated for 7 days and then retreated during labor and delivery if the latency period is longer than 7 days.
   b. Antibiotics are discontinued if the group B streptococcus culture is negative.
   c. The use of antibiotics to *treat* preterm labor is ineffective and may be harmful.

E Fetal assessment

1. **Ultrasound**
   a. An ultrasound is performed on admission to assess the estimated fetal weight and fetal presentation.
      (1) The estimated fetal weight can indicate whether the fetus has grown appropriately.
      (2) The fetal presentation is important when making a delivery plan. A fetus in breech presentation usually requires a cesarean section.

2. **Fetal well-being**. The fetal heart rate testing should be reassuring before starting tocolytic therapy. If the fetal heart rate is a concern, a biophysical profile should be performed before starting tocolytic therapy.

VI   PRETERM PREMATURE RUPTURE OF MEMBRANES

A Definition.   PPROM is rupture of fetal membranes prior to 37 weeks' gestation.

B Epidemiology

1. PPROM is responsible for 25% to 33% of all of preterm births each year.

2. Between 13% and 60% of patients with PPROM have an intra-amniotic infection.

3. Between 2% and 13% of patients with PPROM have postpartum endometritis.

4. The earlier the gestational age, the greater the potential for pregnancy prolongation; 75% of patients deliver within 1 week.

C Etiology

1. **Intrauterine infection is the major causal factor**.

2. Associated etiologic factors include low socioeconomic status, STDs, prior PPROM and preterm delivery, vaginal bleeding, cervical conization, tobacco smoking, uterine overdistension, and emergency cerclage.

D Evaluation.   A sterile **speculum examination** is performed to evaluate the fetal membrane status and to inspect the cervix.

1. Membrane rupture is confirmed by visualization of amniotic fluid in the posterior fornix or by passing of amniotic fluid from the cervical canal.

2. The vaginal pH is normally 4.5 to 6.0, and the pH of amniotic fluid is 7.1 to 7.3. Nitrazine paper turns blue with a pH above 6.0 to 6.5.

    a. False-positive Nitrazine tests result from semen, alkaline antiseptics, bacterial vaginosis, and blood.

    b. Amniotic fluid from the vaginal pool produces a fernlike pattern on a microscope slide when allowed to dry.

    c. If the patient's history is suggestive of PPROM but the sterile speculum examination is equivocal, an amniocentesis can be performed. Amniotic fluid can be sent for Gram stain and culture. In addition, dilute indigo carmine can be instilled into the amniotic fluid. A tampon is then placed in the patient's vagina. After a few hours it is removed. If the tampon is blue, PPROM has been confirmed. If the tampon is white, the patient does not have PPROM.

3. Once membrane rupture has been confirmed, **digital examination of the cervix should be avoided** until labor or induction of labor.

4. Endocervical samples may be considered for gonorrhea and chlamydia testing if clinically indicated.

5. Group B streptococcus cultures are obtained.

6. May consider sending a urine specimen for culture if clinically indicated.

7. Fetal heart rate and uterine activity monitoring are used to assess fetal well-being and uterine contraction pattern.

8. An ultrasound is performed on admission to assess the estimated fetal weight and fetal presentation.

E Management

1. In the **absence of labor, chorioamnionitis, or nonreassuring fetal heart rate testing**, patients with PPROM can be **expectantly** managed **until 34 to 35 weeks' gestation** with the following medications:

    a. **Corticosteroids**. A complete course is given from 24 to 34 weeks' gestation.

    b. **Broad-spectrum antibiotics**. A 7-day course (2 days intravenous, 5 days oral) is given. Antibiotics prolong the latency period and improve perinatal outcomes in patients with PPROM.

2. Fetal well-being is assessed daily with a nonstress test and a follow-up biophysical profile as needed.

3. Chorioamnionitis, labor, or nonreassuring fetal heart rate testing mandates delivery at any gestational age.

Study Questions for Chapter 15

Directions: *Each of the numbered items or incomplete statements in this section is followed by answers or by completions of the statement. Select the ONE lettered answer or completion that is BEST in each case.*

1. A 25 year-old woman, gravida 3, para 2, comes to labor and delivery at 30 weeks of gestation complaining of regular uterine contractions. Cervical examination reveals 3 cm of dilation and 80% effacement. The patient is administered corticosteroids and tocolytics. The contractions persist despite adding a second tocolytic agent and the obstetrician proceeds with amniocentesis. The amniotic fluid findings reveal presence of bacteria on Gram stain. The next best step is to:

- A Continue tocolytics until 48 hours are completed
- B Discontinue the tocolytic therapy
- C Send the fluid for lecithin-to-sphingomyelin ratio
- D Send a maternal serum specimen for complete blood count
- E Administer the second dose of betamethasone 24 hours after the first dose

2. A 28-year-old woman, gravida 3, para 2, at 28 weeks of gestation, has been admitted to the hospital for several days to treat her preterm labor. Her cervix was dilated to 3 cm and 100% effaced when $MgSO_4$ was started at 2.5 g/hr after a bolus over 30 minutes. An entire workup for preterm labor was done, and she received antibiotics and steroids. Currently, she has three to four contractions per minute that she barely feels on 2 g/hr. Treatment with $MgSO_4$ is most likely to:

- A Reduce rate of preterm birth
- B Reduce morbidity associated with preterm delivery
- C Reduce mortality associated with preterm delivery
- D Stop contractions
- E Delay delivery for 2 days

3. A 22-year-old woman, gravida 1, para 0, at 33 weeks of gestation, presents to labor and delivery and reports cramping and lower back pain. She denies leaking of fluid from the vagina. You perform a speculum examination that shows no pooling, and Nitrazine paper stays yellow after contact with the secretions in the posterior fornix. Cervical cultures are taken. She is placed on fetal heart rate and uterine contraction monitoring, which shows a baseline heart rate of 155 beats per minute and three uterine contractions per a 10-minute period. Her cervix changes from closed and 50% effaced to 2 to 3 cm and 80% effaced. The next best step in management of this patient is:

- A Antibiotics
- B $MgSO_4$
- C Terbutaline
- D Corticosteroids and tocolytic therapy
- E Ultrasound

4. A 29-year-old woman, gravida 3, para 1, spontaneous abortions 1, at 30 weeks of gestation, is in preterm labor. She has received an initial bolus of 6 g of $MgSO_4$ over 30 minutes, and she has been placed on a maintenance rate of 4 g/hr for the last 2 days to reduce her contraction pattern to one every 15 minutes (her contractions are barely noticeable to her). Currently, her vitals are as follows: P = 88, BP = 90/50, R = 9, SaO_2 = 95% on room air. Her deep tendon reflexes are 0 bilaterally. She has crackles on her lung bases on deep inspiration. The next best step in management is:

- A Serum magnesium level
- B Calcium gluconate
- C Switch to terbutaline
- D Discontinue $MgSO_4$
- E Re-evaluate her cervix

Answers and Explanations

1. The answer is B [V C]. When tocolysis requires multiple agents, chorioamnionitis must be considered. The benefit of amniocentesis in this setting is that it tests for the presence of chorioamnionitis. Tests that are available for infection include amniotic fluid glucose concentration (less than 11 to 14 mg/dL), quantitative measure of white blood cell count in the amniotic fluid (values greater than 50/mm³), Gram stain for the presence of bacteria (any organism observed), and amniotic fluid culture. The clinician must evaluate the complete clinical presentation. Laboratory evidence of chorioamnionitis must be considered a contraindication for tocolytics.

2. The answer is E [V A]. Treatment with tocolytic medications may not reduce the rate of preterm birth, but it may delay delivery for 48 hours and reduce the associated complications. The time gained allows for transfer to a tertiary center or corticosteroid administration.

3. The answer is D [V A and D]. The patient is in preterm labor. Tocolytic drugs may prolong pregnancy for 2 to 7 days, which may allow for administration of corticosteroids to improve fetal lung maturity.

4. The answer is D [V A 1]. This patient is probably becoming toxic on $MgSO_4$. Her reflexes are gone, she is lethargic, and her respirations are slow. The magnesium should be turned off and a magnesium level checked. It is also wise to monitor urinary output because magnesium is cleared by the kidneys. Calcium gluconate is given when magnesium levels are too high. (NOTE: Therapeutic serum magnesium levels are 4 to 7 mEq/L. Patellar reflex is lost at 7 to 10 mEq/L. Levels higher than 10 to 15 mEq/L cause pulmonary to cardiac toxicity. Also know this conversion: 1 mEq/L = 2 mM = 1.2 mg/dL.)

chapter 16

Hypertension in Pregnancy

DOMINIC MARCHIANO

I · INTRODUCTION

Hypertensive disease complicates 8% to 11% of all pregnancies. It ranks second only to pulmonary embolism as a cause of maternal mortality in developed countries and accounts for 15% of maternal deaths in the United States.

II · DEFINITIONS

A Chronic hypertension

1. Persistent **blood pressure greater than 140/90 mmHg before the 20th week** of pregnancy
   a. **Mild**: over 140/90 mmHg
   b. **Moderate**: over 150/100 to 170/110 mmHg
   c. **Severe**: over 170/110 mmHg

2. Hypertension initially diagnosed any time during pregnancy that persists for more than 12 weeks postpartum

B Gestational hypertension (pregnancy-induced hypertension [PIH]). Definitions of hypertension based on **incremental increases** in blood pressure over baseline (e.g., diastolic blood pressure at 24 weeks that is 15 mmHg higher than a reading from before 20 weeks) are **no longer used to diagnose PIH.**

1. **Diagnostic criterion**: onset of hypertension after 20 weeks' gestation
   a. Absolute blood pressure of 140/90 mmHg twice over 6 hours, without prior comparison
   b. Absolute mean arterial pressure of 105 mmHg without prior comparison
   c. Blood pressure returns to normal by 12 weeks postpartum

C Preeclampsia: gestational hypertension with proteinuria

1. **Proteinuria** is defined by:
   a. 30 mg/dL on dipstick (1+) on repeated samples **or**
   b. 300 mg on 24-hour urine collection

2. **Preeclampsia** may be **mild or severe** (Table 16-1). Criteria for **severe preeclampsia** suggest end-organ involvement (Table 16-2). After a **grand mal seizure**, preeclampsia is termed **eclampsia.**

3. **HELLP syndrome** (**h**emolysis, **e**levated **l**iver enzymes, **l**ow **p**latelets). This **variant of severe preeclampsia** develops in 10% of women with severe preeclampsia. However, approximately 10% of women with HELLP syndrome are normotensive, which is classified as atypical HELLP syndrome.

4. **Superimposed preeclampsia on chronic hypertension**
   a. New-onset proteinuria after 20 weeks in a woman with chronic hypertension
   b. Sudden increase in proteinuria, edema, or blood pressure or a platelet count less than 100,000/mm^3 in a woman with chronic hypertension and proteinuria before 20 weeks' gestation

TABLE 16-1 Hypertensive Disorders During Pregnancy: Indications of Severity

Abnormality	Mild	Severe
Diastolic blood pressure	<100 mmHg	>110 mmHg
Proteinuria	Trace to +1	Persistent 2+ or more
Headache	Absent	Present
Visual disturbance	Absent	Present
Upper abdominal pain	Absent	Present
Oliguria	Absent	Present
Convulsion	Absent	Present (eclampsia)
Serum creatinine	Normal	Elevated
Thrombocytopenia	Absent	Present
Liver enzyme elevation	Minimal	Marked
Fetal growth restriction	Absent	Obvious
Pulmonary edema	Absent	Present

Reprinted with permission from Cunningham FG, MacDonald PC, Gant NF. Williams Obstetrics. 21st Ed. New York: McGraw-Hill, 2001:570, Table 24-2.

III CHRONIC HYPERTENSION

A Effects on mother

1. Mild chronic hypertension is unlikely to adversely affect pregnancy. Pregnancy is unlikely to hasten the progression of maternal hypertensive end-organ disease.

2. Morbidity is increased over de novo preeclampsia.

B Effects on fetus

1. **Abruptio placentae** is four to eight times more likely in pregnancies complicated by chronic hypertension.

2. When preeclampsia is superimposed on chronic hypertension, preeclampsia occurs earlier and is associated with more pronounced **decreases in uteroplacental perfusion**. Intrauterine growth retardation (IUGR) may result from decreased uteroplacental perfusion.
   a. However, IUGR is not more frequent in cases of mild chronic hypertension.
   b. When preeclampsia is superimposed on chronic hypertension, the incidence of IUGR is 30% to 40%.

3. **Prematurity is more common** with severe chronic hypertension.

4. **Perinatal mortality** approaches 25% in severe chronic hypertension.

TABLE 16-2 Criteria for Severe Preeclampsia

Systolic hypertension >160 mmHg
Diastolic hypertension >110 mmHg
Proteinuria >5 g/24 hr
Oliguria <500 mL/24 hr
Cerebral or visual disturbances
Epigastric pain
Pulmonary edema
Evidence of microangiopathic hemolysis
Hepatocellular dysfunction
Thrombocytopenia
Intrauterine growth restriction
Oligohydramnios

C Antihypertensive management

1. Treatment reduces the risk of maternal morbidity. Whether it reduces perinatal morbidity and mortality remains controversial.

2. Existing antihypertensive therapy should be continued on diagnosis of pregnancy.

3. **Antihypertensive agents**
   a. **α-Methyldopa** is most used frequently and has been studied the most. There is **no evidence of fetal or maternal adverse events**.
   b. **Labetalol** (α- and β-blockade) is associated with a possible increase in growth restriction.
   c. **Nifedipine** has limited data, but it rapidly reduces blood pressure.
   d. **β-Antagonists** have been associated with low birth weight.
   e. **Angiotensin-converting enzyme inhibitors are contraindicated** in pregnancy because of adverse effects on fetal renal function.

D Antepartum management

1. **Baseline evaluation for end-organ disease**
   a. Renal function tests
   b. Ophthalmologic examination
   c. Electrocardiogram

2. Antihypertensive therapy is unlikely to benefit a pregnancy complicated by mild hypertension. It should be reserved for pregnancies complicated by moderate or severe hypertension (diastolic blood pressure more than 100 to 110 mmHg), where it reduces the incidence of cardiovascular and cerebrovascular events.

3. Ultrasound should be used to determine specific gestational age. Serial ultrasound surveillance should be reserved for clinical suspicion of IUGR or superimposed preeclampsia.

4. Nonstress testing and amniotic fluid assessment should be started at 32 to 34 weeks' gestation.

5. Labor induction by 40 weeks' gestation can be considered.

IV PREECLAMPSIA: EPIDEMIOLOGY

A Rate of occurrence: 7% of pregnancies, excluding first-trimester losses

B Risk factors

1. **Pregnancy history**. Primigravidas constitute 65% of cases.
   a. Multiple gestation: 30% incidence
   b. Gestational trophoblastic disease: 70% incidence

2. **Maternal age**. Preeclampsia occurs at extremes of maternal age. However, the association with young age is confounded by the association with primigravidity. However, **maternal age of more than 40 years** is an independent risk factor.

3. **Family history**. Evidence for a genetic contribution includes a 37% incidence in sisters and a 26% incidence in daughters. This pattern is consistent with a dominant gene with reduced penetrance.

4. **Obesity**. Incidence is directly related to degree of obesity.

5. **Chronic hypertension**. Preeclampsia occurs in approximately 25% of women with chronic hypertension.

V PREECLAMPSIA: PATHOPHYSIOLOGY

A Pathophysiologic changes

1. **Cardiovascular system**
   a. Cardiac output remains normal, and increased total peripheral vascular resistance accounts for the hypertension.
   b. Preeclamptic endothelial cells generate less prostacyclin, a vasodilator, than normal endothelial cells. Less prostacyclin allows greater vascular sensitivity to angiotensin II, thus promoting vasospasm and increasing peripheral vascular resistance.

2. Coagulation system
a. Disseminated intravascular coagulation occurs in 10% of patients with preeclampsia.

b. Because of endothelial damage, most of these patients have mild procoagulant consumption and elevated fibrin degradation products.

c. Diffuse intravascular coagulation may arise from vascular damage sustained during vasospasm.

3. Renal function
a. Glomerular changes
(1) Glomerular filtration rate (GFR) is usually decreased in preeclampsia. Deceased renal plasma flow and **glomeruloendotheliosis**, which occludes the capillary lumen, account for the lower GFR.

(2) Protein leaks into urine. The glomerulus, which is normally impermeable to large proteins, becomes more permeable. In part, glomerular damage results from both vasospasm and endothelial damage. This leakage exceeds the tubules' ability to reabsorb proteins.

b. Tubular changes, which affect the clearance of uric acid
(1) Uric acid is normally completely filtered at the glomerulus, secreted, and mostly reabsorbed by the proximal tubules.

(2) Uric acid clearance is 10% of creatinine clearance.

(3) Decreased uric acid clearance is observed prior to a GFR disturbance, suggesting a tubal etiology in which the mechanism remains unknown.

(4) Increased production by hypoxic tissues contributes to increased serum uric acid.

c. Renin-angiotensin-aldosterone system
(1) Levels of the following components are increased:
  (a) Plasma renin activity and plasma renin concentration
  (b) Angiotensinogen
  (c) Angiotensin II
  (d) Aldosterone

(2) The theory that the renin-angiotensin system mediates the pathophysiologic alterations of preeclampsia is suggested by three factors:
  (a) Potent vasoconstrictor effect of angiotensin II
  (b) Stimulation of aldosterone by angiotensin II and consequent sodium retention
  (c) The finding that large doses of angiotensin II can cause proteinuria

(3) It is possible that, despite decreased intravascular volume, preeclamptic vasoconstriction results in a physiologic perception of overfill, which suppresses renin release.

4. Other signs of end-organ disease
a. Visual disturbances result from papilledema and suggest cerebral involvement.

b. Epigastric pain suggests hepatocellular dysfunction and edema and liver capsule distention.

c. Intrauterine growth retardation and oligohydramnios suggest placental vasculopathy and uteroplacental insufficiency.

B Pathologic findings

1. Liver
a. Initially, arteriolar vasodilation results in hemorrhage into the hepatocellular columns. This condition is found on liver biopsy in 66% of patients with eclampsia.

b. Hepatic infarction occurs later and is found on liver biopsy in 40% of patients with eclampsia.

2. Kidney
a. Glomerular endotheliosis is the characteristic renal lesion of preeclampsia.
  (1) Endothelial cells enlarge and may occlude the capillary lumen.
  (2) Podocytes are not altered.
  (3) Changes are completely reversible with resolution of preeclampsia.

b. Nonglomerular changes such as tubular alterations are less common.

3. Placenta and placental site
a. The syncytiotrophoblast is abnormal, containing areas of cell death and degeneration, syncytial knots, and decreased density of microvilli.

   b. Cytotrophoblastic cells proliferate in placental villi.
   c. Placental vascular pathology
      (1) In normal pregnancy, the spiral artery endothelium, elastic lamina, and smooth muscle are replaced by trophoblast. This creates a low-resistance, high-flow system. These changes affect both the decidual and myometrial vessels.
      (2) In preeclampsia, these changes do not uniformly occur or are limited to decidual vessels.
      (3) These observations can be made on first-trimester abortion specimens, suggesting that pathologic change precedes the clinical presentation.

VI   PREECLAMPSIA: CLINICAL MANIFESTATIONS

A Clinical signs

   1. Hypertension is required for diagnosis.

   2. Edema is related to sodium retention, not limited to dependent edema.

   3. Hyperreflexia is common.

B Laboratory findings

   1. Renal function
      a. Proteinuria
      b. Hyperuricemia is likely caused by both altered renal function and increased production of uric acid.
      c. Increased serum creatinine is inversely correlated with creatinine clearance.

   2. Hematology findings
      a. Hemoconcentration as reflected by an increased hematocrit
      b. Thrombocytopenia

   3. Hepatic findings. Increased transaminases, when associated with microangiopathic hemolysis and coagulopathy, suggest HELLP syndrome.

VII   PREECLAMPSIA: MANAGEMENT

A **Delivery** is the only known treatment. At term (37 weeks' gestation), delivery is recommended.

B Route of delivery

   1. Vaginal delivery is preferable to cesarean delivery, which should be reserved for the usual obstetric indications.

   2. Cesarean delivery may be preferred in cases of severe preeclampsia remote from term with an unfavorable cervix.

   3. Some evidence suggests that preeclampsia may expedite cervical ripening and labor induction.

C Antepartum treatment (before 37 weeks)

   1. Mild preeclampsia may be managed expectantly using the following interventions. It is controversial whether in- or outpatient management is preferable.
      a. Bed rest
      b. Blood pressure and urinary protein monitoring
      c. Twice-weekly nonstress tests
      d. Laboratory surveillance

   2. Stable severe preeclampsia
      a. Before 24 weeks. Pregnancy termination should be offered.
      b. Before 32 weeks. Delivery is always a legitimate course of action, but expectant management with blood pressure control is an option.
         (1) Expectant management requires intensive fetal and maternal surveillance.
         (2) Antenatal corticosteroids are recommended.
         (3) Delivery is mandatory if the patient develops thrombocytopenia, abnormal liver function

TABLE 16-3	Effects of Magnesium at Different Serum Levels
Effect	**Level (mEq/L)**
Seizure prophylaxis	4–6
Loss of deep tendon reflexes	10
Respiratory depression	15
General anesthesia	15
Cardiac arrest	25

tests, uncontrollable hypertension, pulmonary edema, oligohydramnios, or abnormal fetal testing.

(4) Presence of proteinuria or controllable hypertension does not require immediate delivery.

c. **After 32 weeks.** Delivery is appropriate after documentation of fetal lung maturity.

(1) If fetal lung maturity is negative, antenatal steroids should be given before 34 weeks.

(2) Alternatively, steroids can be given to all patients between 32 and 34 weeks. Delivery may be effected 48 hours later without documenting fetal lung maturity.

3. **Unstable severe preeclampsia.** Treatment **at any gestational age** involves prompt delivery.

D Intrapartum management

1. **Seizure prophylaxis.** Because there are no signs that accurately predict seizures, **prophylaxis is most effective if all women with preeclampsia are treated.**

a. **Magnesium sulfate** is superior to other antiepileptic medications for preventing eclampsia-related seizures and seizure-related morbidity and mortality.

(1) An intravenous loading dose of 6 g is usually followed by a maintenance infusion of 2 to 4 g/hr.

(2) Patients must be monitored for signs of magnesium toxicity, such as hyporeflexia and respiratory depression.

(3) Magnesium toxicity may be confirmed by testing serum levels (Table 16-3). It can be reversed with 1 g of calcium gluconate.

(4) In instances in which magnesium sulfate cannot be used (e.g., myasthenia gravis, end-stage renal disease [because of impaired magnesium clearance]), phenytoin is safe.

2. **Antihypertensive therapy**

a. **Indications**

(1) Persistent diastolic blood pressure of over 105 mmHg

(2) Isolated diastolic blood pressure of over 110 mmHg

b. **Pharmacologic agents**

(1) **Hydralazine** (preferred agent) reduces afterload but compensates by increasing heart rate; therefore, uterine perfusion is not usually compromised.

(2) **Labetalol** does not reduce afterload.

c. **Invasive cardiac monitoring** should be considered in the presence of oliguria or pulmonary edema.

3. **Type of anesthesia**

a. **Epidural anesthesia** is safe for patients with normal clotting ability and no thrombocytopenia. It can be used for either vaginal or cesarean deliveries.

b. **General anesthesia** should be used with caution because the stimulation of intubation may exacerbate hypertension.

E Postpartum management

1. Magnesium sulfate should be continued for 24 hours but may be discontinued earlier in the presence of pronounced diuresis, because therapeutic levels are not likely attainable.

2. Indications for acute antihypertensive therapy are the same as for the antepartum or intrapartum period.

3. Women who continue to have hypertension but have a persistent diastolic blood pressure of less than 100 mmHg may be discharged on oral therapy.

4. Pregnancy-induced hypertension usually disappears completely by 2 weeks postpartum.

VIII PREECLAMPSIA: PREVENTION

There is no reliable method for preventing preeclampsia. Low-dose aspirin, calcium, antioxidants, low-sodium diet, and fish oil have all been shown to be ineffective.

IX ECLAMPSIA

Eclampsia is preeclampsia complicated by generalized tonic-clonic seizures. Pathophysiology of the convulsions is unknown.

A May occur **before, during, or after labor and delivery**

B May cause maternal death

C Consider cerebral imaging, especially if the seizures occur more than 24 hours postpartum

D **Treatment** includes **magnesium sulfate** to control seizures; **antihypertensive therapy** with hydralazine, labetalol, or nifedipine; **prevention** of aspiration and hypoxia; and **delivery** when the mother is stabilized

X PREECLAMPSIA: PROGNOSIS

With **timely delivery and magnesium sulfate**, the maternal mortality rate should be virtually zero.

A **Recurrence.** The risk is 40% for severe preeclampsia and increases with earlier diagnosis of the index case.

B **Future hypertension.** Preeclampsia does not accelerate hypertension but seems to unmask existing, yet undiagnosed, chronic hypertension.

1. Women with preeclampsia in a first pregnancy are no more likely to develop hypertension than controls.

2. Multiparous women are more likely to develop hypertension, but this is confounded because preeclampsia is unlikely to develop de novo in multiparas. Many of these women had underlying hypertension.

Study Questions for Chapter 16

Directions: *Each of the numbered items or incomplete statements in this section is followed by answers or by completions of the statement. Select the ONE lettered answer or completion that is BEST in each case.*

1. You have been seeing a 23-year-old woman, gravida 1, para 0, at 28 weeks of gestation, throughout her pregnancy. She has no known medical history. She denies blurry vision, epigastric or right upper quadrant pain, severe headache, or trouble breathing. Her blood pressure and urine protein dipstick results for the past three visits are as follows: visit 1, BP = 105/60, U_{dip} = 0; visit 2, BP = 110/65, U_{dip} = 1+; visit 3, BP = 115/68, U_{dip} = 1+. Today her BP = 120/75 and U_{dip} = trace. She reports lots of fetal movement. Her fundus measures 25 cm. Lungs are clear to auscultation bilaterally. Deep tendon reflexes are 2+ symmetric. Results from laboratory studies you sent on visit 3 are the following:

Platelet count = $130 \times 10^3/mm^3$
Leukocytes = 10,400/mL
Peripheral blood smear = no hemolysis
Aspartate aminotransferase = 340 U/L
Alanine aminotransferase = 200 U/L
Blood urea nitrogen = 12 mg/dL
Creatinine = 0.6 mg/dL
Uric acid = 6.0 mg/dL
Glucose = 105 mg/dL

The most accurate diagnosis for this patient is:

- A Chronic hypertension
- B Gestational hypertension
- C Mild preeclampsia
- D Severe preeclampsia
- E Superimposed preeclampsia on chronic hypertension

2. A 20-year-old primigravid woman at 37 weeks of gestation (confirmed by a first-trimester ultrasound) presents to the clinic for routine prenatal care. She reports active fetal movement and abdominal pain. Her blood pressure is 162/103 initially and she has 2+ protein on the urine dipstick. Her physical examination is unremarkable except for diffuse tenderness on the abdomen; however, there is no rebound tenderness. Her fundus measures 36 cm above the symphysis pubis. You send her to labor and delivery where a complete blood cell count, liver enzymes, electrolytes, uric acid, urinalysis, and coagulation profile are drawn. On labor and delivery, her blood pressure is 166/104 and there is 3+ proteinuria on urine dipstick. Her cervix is closed, long, firm, and posterior, and fetal vertex is high. What is the next step in management?

- A Oxytocin
- B Prostaglandin analog and magnesium sulfate
- C Magnesium sulfate
- D Methyldopa
- E Hydralazine

3. A 26-year-old primigravida at 35 weeks' gestation complains of mild headache and facial edema. Her blood pressure is 160/100 and her reflexes are brisk. You suspect that she has preeclampsia. Her urinalysis is likely to show which of the following?

- A Proteinuria
- B Hematuria
- C Glycosuria
- D Ketonuria
- E Leukocytes

4. The diagnosis of preeclampsia would be advanced to eclampsia if the woman in Question 1 developed which of the following?

[A] Severe, unremitting headache
[B] Clonus
[C] Grand mal seizures
[D] Petit mal seizures
[E] Visual scotomata

QUESTIONS 5 AND 6

Directions: The response options for questions 5–6 are the same. For each clinical scenario, select the most appropriate management option.

[A] Immediate cesarean section
[B] Induction of labor
[C] Admission to hospital for observation
[D] Outpatient observation

5. A 38-year-old African-American woman, gravida 1, presents for a routine visit at 39 weeks' gestation. Her blood pressure is persistently 140/90 mm Hg, and her urine protein is +2. Physical examination is otherwise unremarkable, and she is completely asymptomatic. Her cervix is 2 cm dilated and 90% effaced, with the fetal vertex at 0 station.

6. A 25-year-old Asian woman, gravida 2, para 0, presents at 33 weeks' gestation for a routine visit. Her blood pressure is 150/100 mm Hg, and her urine protein is +3. Physical examination is otherwise unremarkable. She reports mild headache, but no right upper quadrant pain or visual scotomata.

7. A 26-year-old nurse, gravida 2, para 1, at 32 weeks of gestation, presents to labor and delivery (L&D) because of elevated blood pressures. She says her systolic blood pressures have been in the high 170s and her diastolic blood pressures have been in the low 110s. She denies abdominal pain, visual disturbances, or severe headache. Her blood pressure at L&D is 150/98 and she has 1+ proteinuria. You send off appropriate labs, admit the patient to the hospital, and keep her on bedrest. Which of the following is an appropriate next step in management?

[A] Induce labor—vaginal delivery
[B] Cesarean section
[C] Phenytoin
[D] Labetalol
[E] Betamethasone

8. A 35-year-old woman, gravida 5, para 1, at 6 weeks of gestation, is seeing you because she just found out she is pregnant. She has a 6-year history of essential hypertension controlled on a diuretic agent. After you perform a routine prenatal examination, you change her blood pressure medication to methyldopa and ask her to use it throughout the entire pregnancy. Which of the following is the best reason for using methyldopa in a patient with chronic hypertension during pregnancy?

[A] It is the best antihypertensive during pregnancy
[B] It decreases the risk of IUGR in the fetus
[C] It decreases the risk of abruptio placentae
[D] It decreases the risk of maternal end-organ damage
[E] It increases uteroplacental perfusion

9. Which of the following is an independent risk factor for pregnancy-induced hypertension?

- A Multiparity
- B Family history of chronic hypertension
- C Age older than 40 years
- D Age younger than 20 years
- E History of seizure disorder

10. Which of the following might be found in a patient with MILD preeclampsia?

- A Oligohydramnios
- B Proteinuria in excess of 3 g per 24 hours
- C Thrombocytopenia
- D Intrauterine growth restriction
- E Elevated transaminases

Answers and Explanations

1. The answer is D [II C and Table 16-1]. Although this patient has normal blood pressures and only mild proteinuria, her blood pressure measurements have been rising steadily over the last few visits. This is the opposite of what happens in normal pregnancy. The most important feature that makes this clinical scenario "severe" is the elevated liver enzymes. Both aspartate aminotransferase (AST) and alanine aminotransferase (ALT) are more than three times normal. [Note: You should have a sense of normal and abnormal laboratory values for common electrolytes, liver enzymes, and cell counts. However, the exact range of normal values will be provided to you in your examination booklet.] This patient has severe preeclampsia, and the clinician should send the patient to the hospital for admission. Gestational hypertension is not a diagnosis and it is an uncommon term. Chronic hypertension is defined as blood pressure greater than 140/90 before week 20 of pregnancy or hypertension that is diagnosed at any time during pregnancy and persists for more than 12 weeks postpartum.

2. The answer is B [VII A and VII E 1]. This clinical scenario is describing severe preeclampsia based on her elevated systolic blood pressure (greater than 160 mmHg) and persistent elevated proteinuria (greater than or equal to 2+). She also has abdominal pain, which is a sign of severe preeclampsia. While awaiting her labs, you should start the delivery process by inducing her with a prostaglandin agent and put her on magnesium sulfate for seizure prophylaxis. It may sound counterintuitive to place someone on magnesium (which is also a tocolytic agent) while attempting to deliver. However, in the management of preeclampsia, magnesium sulfate is used for seizure prophylaxis, and another agent such as a prostaglandin analog or oxytocin (if cervix is favorable; high Bishop score) is used to achieve delivery. Remember, delivery is the only true cure for preeclampsia. Using oxytocin to induce this patient would be unsuccessful because her cervix is unfavorable (low Bishop score). Methyldopa is used for patients with chronic hypertension during pregnancy. Hydralazine is used for persistently high diastolic blood pressure, usually diastolic of over 105 mmHg.

3. The answer is A [II B 2]. Proteinuria is characteristic of the urine of patients with preeclampsia, a form of pregnancy-induced hypertension. Pregnancy-induced hypertension, a multiorgan system disease, commonly involves the cardiovascular, renal, neurologic, and hematologic systems. When renal involvement leads to proteinuria, the disease is called preeclampsia. Blood, glucose, or ketones are not commonly seen in the urine of preeclamptic women, unless other conditions are present.

4. The answer is C [II B 2 b]. Eclampsia is a subset of pregnancy-induced hypertension that is defined by the occurrence of grand mal seizures. Symptoms and signs of impending neurologic instability may include headache, visual changes, hyperreflexia, or clonus, but eclampsia is defined only when a grand mal seizure occurs. Petit mal seizures do not occur with this disease.

5. B [III A 1; VII D 1 b], **6. C** [VII B 2 a–c; V D 1 a (1)–(4)]. The first patient has a diagnosis of mild pregnancy-induced hypertension at term. Because she has proteinuria, her condition may be further classified as preeclampsia. The indicated treatment of PIH of any severity at term is delivery. Because her cervix is favorable, induction of labor is the preferred method of delivery. Induction may be initiated with intravenous oxytocin, and parenteral magnesium sulfate should be used for seizure prophylaxis.

The second patient presents with a more difficult problem because she is preterm. Her hypertension and proteinuria suggest that she has mild preeclampsia, but at this time, she does not satisfy the criteria for severe disease. With mild disease in a preterm patient, observation and evaluation for severe disease are indicated. Because of the serious complications that can occur, the patient is best managed in the hospital until sufficient evaluation to exclude severe PIH is completed. If further evaluation reveals severe disease, delivery is indicated.

7. The answer is E [VII C 1 and C 2 c (1)]. According to criteria discussed in this chapter, this patient represents mild preeclampsia. Management of this case is more complicated because she is preterm (32 weeks). Because definitive management of preeclampsia is delivery, you must weigh the risks of premature delivery for the fetus against the benefits of delivery to the mother. Mild preeclampsia may be managed expectantly (by bedrest, blood pressure and urine protein monitoring, twice-weekly nonstress testing, and lab evaluations) before 37 weeks of gestation. The best course of action (given the above answer choices) is to give antenatal steroids to try to effect fetal lung maturity. Delivery by cesarean section or vaginal birth is not appropriate in someone less than 37 weeks with mild preeclampsia. Anyone who has the diagnosis of preeclampsia needs to be on seizure prophylaxis. The best agent is magnesium sulfate, not phenytoin. Labetalol is used to treat persistently elevated diastolic blood pressure of over 105 mmHg.

8. The answer is D [III C 1]. Treatment of hypertension during pregnancy reduces the risk of **maternal** morbidity probably by preventing end-organ damage. Whether therapy reduces perinatal morbidity and mortality remains controversial. Methyldopa is the most commonly used antihypertensive medication, but it is not necessarily the best. There is evidence that labetalol is as good, if not better, than methyldopa during pregnancy. Methyldopa does not increase uteroplacental perfusion.

9. The answer is C [IV B 2]. While the association of maternal age younger than 20 years with preeclampsia is confounded by primigravity, maternal age greater than 40 years is an independent risk factor for preeclampsia. Personal history of chronic hypertension would be associated with a 25% risk for the development of preeclampsia, but a family history of chronic hypertension does not similarly increase the risk. Seizure disorder and multiparity are not related to preeclampsia.

10. The answer is B [Tables 16-1 and 16-2]. Oligohydramnios, thrombocytopenia, intrauterine growth restriction, and transaminitis are criteria for severe preeclampsia. Proteinuria of 5 gms in a 24-hour specimen is also a criterion for severe preeclampsia. However, proteinuria of only 3 gms would be insufficient for this diagnosis.

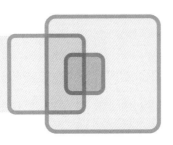

chapter **17**

Medical Complications of Pregnancy

HARISH M. SEHDEV

I   DIABETES

Diabetes affects 2% to 3% of all pregnancies. Of those, approximately 90% are cases of **gestational diabetes**, which is diabetes whose onset occurs during pregnancy.

A Effect of pregnancy on glucose metabolism

1. **Maternal metabolism adjusts** to provide nutrition for both the fetus and the mother.
   a. Increased insulin secretion occurs as a result of β-cell hyperplasia from the increased levels of estrogen and progesterone.
   b. Insulin antagonism results from the increase in human somatomammotropin (produced by syncytiotrophoblasts).
   c. Increased insulin degradation by placental insulinase occurs.

2. A more than 40% **decrease in insulin sensitivity** normally occurs by late in pregnancy, and maintenance of glucose homeostasis results from exaggeration in both the rate and amount of insulin release.

3. Therefore, as pregnancy progresses, women with marginal pancreatic reserve may be unable to meet insulin demands, especially in late pregnancy, and those with preexisting diabetes will need more insulin.

4. **Fetal glucose levels are directly proportional to maternal glucose concentrations**.
   a. Insulin **does not cross** the placenta.
   b. After delivery, insulin requirements for patients with underlying diabetes **decrease** because of the decrease in estrogen, progesterone, placental insulinase, and human somatomammotropin.

B Effects of preexisting diabetes on pregnancy.   Before the use of insulin therapy, complications of diabetes for both the mother and fetus were extremely high. Although insulin therapy has lowered the risk of complications, pregnancies in women with diabetes are still associated with an increased risk of adverse events.

1. **Maternal complications**
   a. Preeclampsia and eclampsia
   b. Diabetic ketoacidosis
   c. Worsening preexisting nephropathy
   d. Worsening preexisting retinopathy
   e. Infection
   f. Polyhydramnios
   g. Cesarean delivery
   h. Postpartum hemorrhage
   i. Mortality

2. **Fetal complications**
   a. Miscarriage
   b. Unexplained stillbirth

    c. Perinatal mortality of approximately 2% to 5% (significantly lower than the risk of approximately 65% before insulin therapy)

    d. Congenital malformations, which account for up to 50% of associated perinatal mortality. Anomalies can affect most organ systems, in particular anencephaly and spina bifida in the **central nervous system**, ventricular septal defects and situs inversus in the **cardiac system**, and a characteristic embryopathy called sacral agenesis or **caudal regression**. These usually occur by **7 weeks' gestation** (see Chapter 7).

    e. Abnormal fetal intrauterine growth (both macrosomia and growth restriction)

    f. Neonatal complications, including respiratory distress syndrome, hypoglycemia, hypocalcemia, polycythemia, and hyperbilirubinemia

C Management of Patients with Diabetes

1. Prior to conception. Appropriate prenatal care for women with **preexisting diabetes** should begin before conception. Such care may decrease the risk of congenital malformations.

    a. Adjust insulin to normalize glucose levels. **Goals** for pregnancy are different than for nonpregnant individuals and are as follows: fasting glucose values **less than 95 mg/dL** and 2-hour postprandial values less than **120 mg/dL**.

    b. Order **hemoglobin A1C** to assess glycemic control.

    c. Provide **folic acid** supplementation.

    d. Provide nutrition counseling.

2. First trimester

    a. Obtain ultrasound between 6 and 8 weeks' gestation if possible for accurate dating.

    b. Order **hemoglobin A1C** to assess glycemic control (the risk for congenital abnormalities increases with higher hemoglobin A1C values).

    c. Assess overall health for effects of background vascular involvement (e.g., renal, ophthalmologic, or cardiac).

    d. Multiple daily injections of insulin (or an insulin pump) may be needed to maintain glucose in the range described above.

3. Second trimester: screening for malformations

    a. Maternal serum α-fetoprotein (AFP) screening at 15 to 20 weeks to assess the risk for fetal neural tube abnormalities

    b. Ultrasound at 16 to 20 weeks to evaluate fetal anatomy

    c. Fetal echocardiography at 20 to 22 weeks to help screen for fetal cardiac abnormalities

4. Third trimester: assessment of fetal well-being

    a. Surveillance of fetal well-being should begin at **28 weeks** with maternal fetal activity assessment (kick counts) because the risk of unexplained stillbirth is increased. **Nonstress testing or biophysical profiles** should begin at 32 weeks or earlier if significant maternal vascular disease exists or there is evidence of fetal growth restriction.

    b. Ultrasound every 4 to 6 weeks to assess fetal growth

5. Timing of delivery. The time at which delivery occurs depends on both maternal glycemic control and the health and maturity of the fetus.

    a. In patients with good glycemic control and reassuring fetal testing, the physician can wait for the onset of labor until 40 weeks' gestation.

    b. If induction of labor is considered before 39 weeks, assessment of fetal lung maturity by amniocentesis should be performed to assess the lecithin-to-sphingomyelin (**L/S**) ratio and the presence of **phosphatidylglycerol** in the amniotic fluid. If testing does not reveal an L/S ratio of at least 2:1 or the presence of phosphatidylglycerol, delivery should be delayed until repeat testing confirms fetal lung maturity, or after 39 weeks as long as fetal testing remains reassuring.

6. Method of delivery. The mode of delivery should be individualized. In patients with diabetes, the fetus can weigh in excess of 4000 g, which increases the risk of **shoulder dystocia** (entrapment of the shoulder after delivery of the head). However, many cases still occur in fetuses that weigh less than 4000 g. Ultrasound assessment of fetal weight is helpful but not completely accurate.

a. If the suspected weight of the fetus does not exceed 4000 g, vaginal delivery (including induction of labor) can be attempted.

b. If the suspected weight of the fetus exceeds 4000 g (macrosomia), elective cesarean delivery can be offered.

c. For all deliveries, euglycemia should be maintained and ketosis avoided.

D **Gestational diabetes** is defined as diabetes whose onset occurs during pregnancy and is attributed to the pregnancy.

1. **Effect of gestational diabetes on pregnancy**
   a. Increased risk of macrosomia
   b. Increased risk of preeclampsia
   c. Increased rate of stillbirth if fasting glucose is elevated
   d. **Fetal anomalies are not increased.**

2. **Screening** for gestational diabetes may be needed based on the following **risk factors**:
   a. Strong family history
   b. Persistent glucosuria
   c. History of unexplained stillbirth or miscarriage
   d. Prior macrosomic fetus
   e. Obesity
   f. Age older than 25 years

3. **Universal screening is recommended** because selective screening may miss up to 50% of cases of gestational diabetes.
   a. The **1-hour glucose tolerance test** consists of a 50-g glucose load. There is no set abnormal value, and the threshold value may be 130, 135, or 140 mg/dL. The lower the threshold, the greater the screen positive rate with a greater sensitivity. An abnormal value requires a standard glucose tolerance test.
   b. The **standard glucose tolerance test is a 3-hour test** consisting of a 100-g glucose load and four serum glucose determinations. Gestational diabetes is diagnosed if there are at least two abnormal values.
   (1) Fasting value: 95 mg/dL
   (2) 1-hour value: 180 mg/dL
   (3) 2-hour value: 155 mg/dL
   (4) 3-hour value: 140 mg/dL

4. **Management**
   a. Provide nutritional counseling and dietary adjustment. If the disease can be controlled by diet alone, patients can be followed similarly to those without diabetes. No evidence supports early delivery.
   b. Monitor fasting and 2-hour postprandial glucose values.
   c. Give insulin if fasting glucose values are greater than 95 mg/dL and 2-hour postprandial values are greater than 120 mg/dL.
   d. Patients who require insulin or are unable to maintain glycemic control should be followed similarly to patients with preexisting diabetes.

5. **Follow-up.** After the postpartum visit, patients with gestational diabetes should be screened routinely for diabetes.

II THYROID DISEASE

Thyroid disease affects up to 1% of all pregnancies.

A **Effects of pregnancy on thyroid function**

1. Plasma inorganic iodine concentration decreases because of increased renal excretion and increased glomerular filtration.

2. Enlargement of the thyroid gland occurs.

3. Serum thyroxine (T_4)-binding globulin is increased.

4. Laboratory assessment of thyroid function is altered.
   a. Increased total T_4
   b. Increased total triiodothyronine (T_3)
   c. Increased radioiodine uptake
   d. Decreased T_3 resin uptake
   e. Unchanged free T_4, free T_3, and thyroid-stimulating hormone (TSH) levels

B **Hyperthyroidism.** This condition occurs in approximately 1 in 200 pregnancies.

1. Effects on pregnancy. The signs and symptoms of normal pregnancy can mimic signs of hyperthyroidism. If hyperthyroidism is untreated, the risk of complications (e.g., preeclampsia, preterm delivery, congestive heart disease, and adverse perinatal outcome) is increased.

2. Causes
   a. Graves disease, an autoimmune process, is the most common cause. This condition is associated with an increase in thyroid-stimulating antibodies that stimulate the TSH receptors. These antibodies can cross the placenta, resulting in fetal thyrotoxicosis.
   b. Gestational trophoblastic disease (see Chapter 18) should be considered, especially if hyperthyroidism occurs early in gestation, and a pelvic ultrasound should be ordered.

3. Diagnosis
   a. Tachycardia
   b. Thyromegaly
   c. Exophthalmos
   d. Poor maternal weight gain
   e. Severe hyperemesis gravidarum
   f. Onycholysis (separation of nail from the nail bed)
   g. Decreased TSH with increased free T_4

4. Management. Therapy can be either medical or surgical with minimal risk to mother and fetus.
   a. Medical therapy
      (1) Propylthiouracil (PTU) prevents both the synthesis of thyroid hormone in the thyroid gland and the peripheral conversion of T_4 to T_3. The drug readily crosses the placenta and may induce **fetal hypothyroidism** and goiter, although this is rare. The goal of treatment is to maintain a maternal high-normal level of free T_4.
      (2) Methimazole prevents only the release of thyroid hormone and has been associated with **aplasia cutis,** a reversible developmental disorder of the fetal scalp.
      (3) Beta-blockers may be used to control tachycardia associated with hyperthyroidism.
      (4) Radioactive iodine is contraindicated in pregnancy because it crosses the placenta and can ablate the fetal thyroid gland.
   b. Surgical therapy. In cases that are refractory to medical therapy, thyroidectomy may be necessary.

5. Thyroid storm is a rare complication of hyperthyroidism that can be associated with heart failure. Treatment includes propylthiouracil, potassium iodide, beta-blockers, hydration, and control of body temperature.

C **Hypothyroidism**

1. Effects on pregnancy
   a. Associated with first trimester miscarriages
   b. Increased risk of preeclampsia, abruptio placentae, stillbirth, and intrauterine growth restriction (IUGR)
   c. Infants of untreated women with significantly increased TSH levels may be at risk for **decreased performance on IQ tests.**

2. Diagnosis. Increased TSH and decreased free T_4 are the basis of diagnosis.

3. Management. Hypothyroidism is treated with supplemental thyroid hormone. Infants of treated mothers are healthy.

III   URINARY TRACT INFECTION

Women are at greater risk for urinary tract infections during pregnancy because of the anatomic and physiologic changes that occur with pregnancy. **A urine culture should be obtained in all women at their first prenatal visit**, and urine dipstick analysis should be performed at all subsequent visits.

A **Asymptomatic bacteriuria.**   This condition is defined as the presence of bacteria within the urinary tract without symptoms.

1. Asymptomatic bacteriuria is present in 5% to 10% of all pregnant women. The incidence is highest in black multiparas with sickle cell trait.

2. **Treatment** requires administration of an antibiotic (e.g., ampicillin or nitrofurantoin) to which the causal organism is sensitive.

3. **Consequences of lack of treatmen**t
   a. Pyelonephritis in up to 40% of affected women
   b. Risk factor for low birth weight

4. A **follow-up culture** is necessary after treatment has been completed.

B **Acute urethritis**

1. Usually, the **etiologic agents** are *Escherichia coli, Chlamydia trachomatis*, and *Neisseria gonorrhoeae.*

2. **Signs and symptoms** include frequency, dysuria, and urgency. Mucopurulent discharge from the urethra may be present.

3. **Urinalysis** reveals white blood cells without bacteria.

4. **Urine culture** and urethral culture for gonorrhea and chlamydia should be performed.

5. **Treatment** is based on the causal agent.

C **Cystitis**

1. **Etiologic agents**
   a. The most common pathogen is *E. coli* (80% to 90% of cases).
   b. Other causal pathogens include *Klebsiella pneumoniae, Proteus* species, and Gram-positive organisms such as enterococci and group B streptococci.

2. **Symptoms** include frequency, urgency, suprapubic pain, dysuria, and hesitancy. Hematuria may be present. Fever is uncommon.

3. **Diagnosis** is made by using a clean catch specimen or one obtained by midstream urine collection or bladder catheterization.

4. **Treatment** involves a short course of antibiotics to which the organism is sensitive. Inadequate treatment may lead to pyelonephritis.

5. A **follow-up culture** is necessary after treatment is complete.

D **Acute pyelonephritis.**   This condition affects 1% to 2% of all pregnancies. It usually results from lower tract infection. Up to 90% of cases are unilateral and usually affect the right side.

1. **Predisposing factors unique to pregnancy**
   a. Ureteral compression at the pelvic brim caused by the enlarging uterus
   b. Decreased tone and peristalsis of the ureters resulting from increased progesterone levels
   c. Decreased bladder sensitivity, which may result in overdistention and the need for catheterization

2. The **most common causative agent** is *E. coli.*

3. **Signs and symptoms** may include:
   a. Fever, chills, and back pain
   b. Nausea or vomiting
   c. Anorexia
   d. Preterm contractions and preterm labor

4. Complications may include:
   a. Bacteremia and septic shock
   b. Pulmonary edema and respiratory distress syndrome
   c. Renal dysfunction
   d. Preterm labor

5. Treatment
   a. Inpatient therapy is preferred.
   b. Hydration is useful.
   c. Intravenous antibiotics are used until the patient is afebrile for 24 to 48 hours; they are followed by oral antibiotics with appropriate sensitivity to complete a 7- to 10-day course of treatment.
   d. Lack of response to treatment should prompt radiologic evaluation for an abscess or renal calculi.
   e. Follow-up therapy includes daily antibiotic suppression for the remainder of the pregnancy.
   f. Up to 30% of patients may develop recurrent urinary tract infections during pregnancy.

IV ANEMIA

Anemia has been defined by the Centers for Disease Control and Prevention as a hemoglobin concentration of less than 11 g/dL in the first and third trimester of pregnancy and less than 10.5 g/dL in the second trimester. Anemia is broadly classified as acquired or hereditary.

A Acquired anemias

1. Iron-deficiency anemia. The most common cause of anemia in pregnancy is **iron deficiency**. The iron requirements of pregnancy are considerable, and most women enter pregnancy with low iron stores.
   a. In pregnancy, a woman needs an additional 1000 mg of elemental iron.
      (1) 300 mg goes to the fetus.
      (2) 500 mg is used to expand the maternal red cell mass.
      (3) 200 mg is shed through the gut and skin.
   b. The level of **hematocrit naturally decreases** during the second trimester of pregnancy, because of the greater expansion of maternal plasma volume compared with the increase in red cell mass and hemoglobin mass.
   c. Late in pregnancy, hemoglobin mass continues to increase while plasma volume remains steady.
   d. Because of the normal transfer of iron from the mother to the fetus, the **fetus does not suffer from iron-deficiency anemia**.
   e. While maternal absorption of iron is increased in pregnancy, treatment involves additional daily elemental iron (200 mg in divided doses) to correct the anemia and maintain adequate stores.

2. Megaloblastic anemia. This condition, which is rare in the United States, is characterized by impaired DNA synthesis. It occurs in pregnant women who consume neither fresh vegetables nor foods with a high content of animal protein.
   a. Folic acid deficiency is the most common form.
   b. Many women also have iron deficiency.
   c. Vitamin B_{12} deficiency is rare but should be checked for in women with a gastrectomy, Crohn's disease, or ileal resection.
   d. Ethanol consumption may be a contributing factor.
   e. Symptoms and signs of megaloblastic anemia during pregnancy include nausea, vomiting, and anorexia.
   f. Treatment includes a well-balanced diet, oral iron, and folic acid (1 mg/day).

B Hereditary anemias, which are characterized by the hemoglobinopathies, result in increases in maternal morbidity and mortality, spontaneous abortion, and perinatal mortality.

1. Sickle cell anemia (hemoglobin SS disease; SS disease). This condition occurs when an individual receives the gene for the production of hemoglobin S, an abnormal variant of hemoglobin, from both parents.

    a. The incidence of sickle cell trait in black adults is 1 in 12; therefore, the theoretical incidence of SS disease is 1 in 576 in the United States. The actual incidence in pregnant women is somewhat lower because of the higher mortality rate in individuals with SS disease. Pregnancy poses an increased risk of adverse outcome for both mother and fetus.

    b. Infectious complications, such as pyelonephritis, cholecystitis, pneumonia, and skin infections, are increased in SS disease.

    c. Complications of pregnancy increase. These include:

        (1) Spontaneous abortion

        (2) Preeclampsia

        (3) Preterm labor and delivery

        (4) IUGR

        (5) Unexplained fetal demise

    d. The number of **vaso-occlusive** crises increases in pregnancy. Treatment includes:

        (1) Hydration

        (2) Analgesics

        (3) Oxygen

        (4) Transfusion

        (5) Screening and therapy for infections

    e. Treatment during pregnancy includes:

        (1) Screening and treatment of asymptomatic bacteriuria

        (2) Urine culture every trimester

        (3) Pneumococcal vaccine (recommended)

        (4) Serial ultrasound to assess fetal growth

        (5) Antepartum fetal surveillance

        (6) Folic acid supplementation

    f. Treatment during labor includes:

        (1) Adequate hydration and oxygen to prevent sickling

        (2) Analgesia

        (3) Packed red blood cell transfusion if a cesarean section is considered and the hemoglobin level is very low.

    g. Although prophylactic transfusions may decrease the number of vaso-occlusive crises, they do not improve perinatal outcome.

2. Sickle cell–hemoglobin C disease (SC disease). Hemoglobin C, like hemoglobin S, results from a change in the sixth position of the β-chain and may be seen in patients of West African or Sicilian descent.

    a. The incidence in the United States is 1 in 823 adult African Americans.

    b. This disease is associated with less morbidity than SS disease but still carries an increased risk of pregnancy loss and pregnancy-induced hypertension.

    c. Affected patients may experience pain crises that are marked by splenic sequestration and that can be associated with thrombocytopenia.

    d. Treatment and follow-up are the same as that for patients with SS disease. The resulting anemia may require transfusion; such treatment is uncommon in the nonpregnant state.

3. Sickle cell–β-thalassemia disease. This condition has a perinatal mortality and morbidity rate similar to that of SC disease, with somewhat less maternal morbidity and mortality.

4. Sickle cell trait is inheritance of the gene for the production of hemoglobin S from one parent and hemoglobin A from the other. This condition occurs in 8.5% of African Americans, and it occurs in individuals of Mediterranean, Caribbean, Latin American, North African, Indian, and Southeast Asian descent.

    a. The anemia in most patients is only mild.

    b. Sickle cell trait does not appear to increase the risk of miscarriage, stillbirth, IUGR, or pregnancy-induced hypertension.

    c. There is an **increased risk for asymptomatic bacteriuria and urinary tract infections**. Therefore, women with the trait should have frequent urine cultures during pregnancy.

    d. Paternal testing may be important because prenatal diagnosis of SS disease is available.

5. **Thalassemias.** The normal adult hemoglobins are A, A$_2$, and F. Ninety-five percent of adult hemoglobin is hemoglobin A (made by two α-chains and two β-chains). Most individuals also have small amounts of hemoglobin A$_2$ (two α-chains and two Δ-chains). The remainder is made up of hemoglobin F (two α-chains and two γ-chains). Patients with thalassemias have a **microcytic anemia** that can be found on their screening complete blood count.

    a. **α-Thalassemia.** The α-thalassemias are characterized by a deletion of one or more of the four genes from the α-chain.

        (1) Deletion of one α-gene does not cause anemia.

        (2) Deletion of two genes causes α-thalassemia trait, characterized by mild anemia.

        (3) Deletion of three genes (hemoglobin H) causes moderate anemia; transfusion or splenectomy is rare.

        (4) Deletion of four genes (Bart hemoglobin) causes severe intrauterine anemia with fetal hydrops and death, as well as maternal preeclampsia and postpartum hemorrhage.

    b. **β-Thalassemia.** The β-thalassemias occur because of point mutations in the genes for β-chain production, leading to a decrease in β-chain formation. This decrease leads to a decrease in hemoglobin A production and a relative increase in the percentage of hemoglobin A$_2$ (more than 4%), which is evident on hemoglobin electrophoresis.

        (1) β-Thalassemia trait occurs when β-globin production is decreased by 50%, causing a mild anemia with hypochromic microcytosis and occasional hepatosplenomegaly.

        (2) β-Thalassemia intermedia occurs when production is decreased by 75%, leading to moderate anemia with occasional need for transfusion, hepatosplenomegaly, and iron overload.

        (3) β-Thalassemia major occurs with no production of the β-chain, causing severe anemia, transfusion dependency, iron overload, bone deformities, and death in early adulthood. (Fetuses and newborns with β-thalassemia are not anemic because of the presence of hemoglobin F.)

    c. Women with the most severe forms of β-thalassemia are transfusion dependent and require close supervision during pregnancy. During pregnancy, women with β-thalassemia intermedia may experience a drop in hemoglobin and hematocrit levels. The red blood cell mass does not expand normally because of deficient hemoglobin production.

        (1) Folic acid supplementation is recommended to keep up with the accelerated red blood cell turnover.

        (2) Iron therapy is indicated only for patients with demonstrable iron deficiency because of the risk of iron overload and hepatotoxicity.

        (3) Pregnancy is well tolerated in patients with α- or β-thalassemia trait.

        (4) Paternal testing may be important because **prenatal diagnosis is available.**

V   HEART DISEASE

A Incidence of heart disease in pregnancy

1. Approximately **1% of pregnancies are complicated by maternal heart disease.** Today, fewer women are seen with heart disease because of the decreased incidence of rheumatic fever and rheumatic heart disease. However, because of advances in corrective heart surgery, more women with congenital cardiac abnormalities reach childbearing age.

2. Women with severe heart disease are **at greater risk for pregnancy complications:**

    a. Miscarriage

    b. IUGR

    c. Preterm delivery

    d. Intrauterine demise

3. **Maternal mortality** with pregnancy depends on the specific lesion. All women with cardiac disease should seek preconceptual counseling with cardiac and perinatal specialists.

    a. The **highest risk** (maternal mortality as high as 50%) is associated with **pulmonary hypertension,** Marfan syndrome with aortic involvement, Turner syndrome with aortic involvement, complicated coarctation of the aorta, and Eisenmenger syndrome.

    b. The **lowest risk** (less than 1%) is associated with corrected tetralogy of Fallot, small atrial and ventricular septal defects, and patent ductus arteriosus.

B Diagnosis of heart disease during pregnancy

1. **Changes associated with normal pregnancy that may place an extra burden on women with heart disease include:**
   a. **Expansion of plasma volume** by as much as 50%
   b. **Increased cardiac output** (30% to 50%)
   c. **Drop in systemic vascular resistance** up to 28 weeks' gestation
   d. **Changes specific to labor**
      (1) Pain, which can increase heart rate and blood pressure
      (2) Shift into the intravascular compartment of as much as 500 mL of plasma with each uterine contraction
      (3) Regional anesthesia, which can decrease cardiac output and blood pressure
      (4) Postpartum increase in blood volume and cardiac output by 10% to 20%. Initially, cardiac output and blood pressure may fall after delivery.

2. **Symptoms of normal pregnancy that can be confused with symptoms of heart disease**
   a. Functional systolic murmurs
   b. Fatigue, dyspnea, and palpitations
   c. Edema, especially in the lower extremities
   d. Enlarged cardiac silhouette on chest radiograph

3. **Signs and symptoms that should lead to suspicion of heart disease**
   a. Progressive limitation of physical activity
   b. Chest pain
   c. Syncope with exertion
   d. Severe dyspnea
   e. Diastolic murmur
   f. Loud systolic murmur
   g. Cyanosis or clubbing
   h. Abnormal heart rhythm on electrocardiography
   i. Abnormal echocardiography

C Management

1. **Preconception**
   a. Counseling about risks
   b. Reviewing current medical regimen

2. **During pregnancy**
   a. Close follow-up with a cardiologist
   b. Frequent maternal echocardiography
   c. Fetal echocardiography at 20 to 22 weeks' gestation (A woman with a congenital cardiac abnormality is at greater risk for having a fetus with a congenital cardiac lesion.)
   d. Careful evaluation of any change in maternal symptoms
   e. Evaluation and treatment for infection and anemia, which could worsen the maternal condition
   f. Anticoagulation, with heparin if appropriate
   g. Hospitalization for signs of deterioration

3. **In labor and postpartum**
   a. Team management, involving cardiology, anesthesiology, and nursing
   b. Invasive monitoring, if necessary
   c. Antibiotic prophylaxis, if necessary
   d. Avoidance of rapid changes in blood pressure and heart rate
   e. **Forceps or vacuum-assisted** delivery in some cases to avoid prolonged second stage of labor
   f. Continued close observation in the postpartum period

VI   PULMONARY DISEASE

A Physiologic changes associated with pregnancy

1. **Mechanical changes of chest cavity**
   a. Upward displacement of diaphragm (as much as 4 cm)

    b. Increase in transverse diameter of chest (2 cm)

    c. Increase in chest circumference (5 to 7 cm)

    d. Increased diaphragmatic excursion

    e. Increase in subcostal angle

2. Changes in pulmonary function

    a. Increased tidal volume (30% to 40%)

    b. Decrease in expiratory reserve

    c. Increase in minute ventilation

    d. Decreased lung volume caused by displacement of diaphragm (Total lung volume decreases 5%, and residual volume decreases 20%.)

    e. No change in forced expiratory volume in 1 second

B **Dyspnea of pregnancy.** As many as 70% of pregnant women report dyspnea, and the etiology is not understood.

C **Asthma.** This condition complicates approximately 1% of all pregnancies and worsens about one-third of cases.

1. Pregnancy complications

    a. If asthma is poorly controlled, it may be associated with increased risk of preterm delivery, IUGR, and perinatal morbidity and mortality.

    b. Use of steroids can be associated with increased risk of gestational diabetes and postpartum hemorrhage.

2. Goals of treatment

    a. Reduce the number of flare-ups.

    b. Prevent severe attacks (status asthmaticus; see VI C 4).

    c. Ensure adequate oxygenation.

3. Treatment

    a. β-Agonists, the primary treatment for acute exacerbations and chronic therapy

        (1) No increase in the incidence of congenital malformations

        (2) Side effects such as tachyphylaxis and arrhythmias

    b. Glucocorticoids

        (1) Inhaled for chronic therapy

        (2) Intravenous and oral therapy for acute exacerbations

        (3) Safe in pregnancy

    c. Aminophylline, which has declined in use

        (1) This drug **crosses the placenta** and has no demonstrable effects on the fetus.

        (2) Levels must be adjusted in pregnancy.

        (3) Side effects are common and include:

            (a) Nausea and vomiting

            (b) Tachycardia

            (c) Arrhythmias

4. Status asthmaticus. Provide immediate treatment using the following interventions:

    a. Oxygenation

    b. Hydration

    c. Subcutaneous catecholamines

    d. Intravenous steroids

    e. Nebulized β-agonists

    f. Intubation, if necessary

D Pneumonia. In addition to being life threatening to the mother when severe, pneumonia is also associated with preterm birth. Chest radiography during pregnancy can be accomplished with little radiation exposure to the fetus using lead shielding to the mother's abdomen.

1. *Streptococcus pneumoniae*: most common bacterial pathogen

    a. Associated with **smoking**

    b. Sudden onset is characteristic. **Signs and symptoms** include:

      (1) Tachypnea
      (2) Fever
      (3) Shaking chills
      (4) Productive cough
      (5) Purulent sputum
   c. Diagnosis
      (1) Lobar consolidation on chest radiograph
      (2) Sputum culture and Gram stain
      (3) Blood culture
   d. Treatment
      (1) Hospitalization
      (2) Intravenous penicillin followed by oral penicillin for 10 to 14 days

2. Other pathogens that cause pneumonia
   a. *Mycoplasma pneumoniae*
      (1) Common in young adults
      (2) Slow onset of symptoms with nonproductive cough
      (3) Clinical diagnosis, with a chest radiograph that reveals patchy infiltrates
      (4) Not responsive to penicillin and should be treated with erythromycin
   b. *Klebsiella pneumoniae* and *Haemophilus influenzae*
      (1) Usually occurs in heavy smokers, alcoholics, and immunocompromised patients
      (2) Requires immediate hospitalization and appropriate antibiotics
   c. Influenza A
      (1) Characterized by sparse sputum production and interstitial infiltrates
      (2) Usually self-limited but can be complicated by secondary bacterial pneumonia
   d. Varicella (chickenpox)
      (1) Has mortality as high as 30%. The risk of pneumonia with primary varicella infection increases in smokers and in pregnant women in the third trimester.
      (2) Requires treatment with intravenous acyclovir. Varicella-zoster immune globulin can be given as prophylaxis to a susceptible woman exposed to the virus.
      (3) The **varicella vaccine** is a live virus and is **contraindicated** in pregnancy. Varicella titers should be checked prior to pregnancy and if the patient is nonimmune, she can be vaccinated.

E **Sarcoidosis.** The etiology of this granulomatous disease is unknown. Sarcoidosis can affect many organ systems.

1. Most commonly, affected individuals are 20 to 40 years of age.

2. The condition is most commonly diagnosed by evidence of **bilateral hilar adenopathy** on routine chest radiography. Definitive diagnosis is made by histology.

3. Most patients are asymptomatic and require no treatment. If therapy is necessary, glucocorticoids are the primary treatment.

4. Pregnancy has no long-term side effects. Sarcoidosis does not appear to affect pregnancy outcome adversely. **Most patients improve** as the pregnancy progresses.

5. In pregnant women, it is necessary to assess renal and hepatic involvement and test pulmonary function.

F **Tuberculosis.** This condition, which is caused by *Mycobacterium tuberculosis,* is unfortunately becoming more common because of HIV infection and increasing immigration from developing countries. Congenital tuberculosis is rare, and most cases of perinatal infection result from horizontal transmission.

1. Symptoms
   a. Lethargy
   b. Cough
   c. Dyspnea
   d. Night sweats

2. **Diagnosis**
   a. Skin testing with subcutaneous dose of intermediate-strength purified protein derivative (PPD)
   b. Chest radiograph
   c. Culture and identification of acid-fast bacilli or fluorescent stain of sputum

3. **Treatment.** The risk of adverse outcome in pregnancy does not appear to increase if treatment is adequate. Therapy has become more complex with the emergence of resistant strains of *M. tuberculosis.*
   a. **Isoniazid** for 9 months: standard therapy
      (1) Side effects: peripheral neuropathy, toxic hepatitis (especially if older than 35 years)
      (2) Prophylactic use in recent PPD converters without active disease
   b. **Ethambutol**: added for resistant strains
      (1) Safe in pregnancy
      (2) Side effect with higher doses: optic neuritis in the mother
   c. **Streptomycin**
      (1) Avoid in pregnancy
      (2) Associated with damage to cranial nerve VIII and renal damage in fetus
   d. **Rifampin**
      (1) Avoid in pregnancy, crosses the placenta
      (2) May increase the risk of congenital malformations

VII THROMBOEMBOLIC DISEASE

A Epidemiology and etiology

1. Thromboembolic disease is **the leading cause of death in pregnant and postpartum women**.

2. Thromboembolic disease occurs in 0.02% to 0.3% of pregnant patients and in 0.1% to 1.0% of postpartum patients.

3. Untreated deep vein thrombosis (DVT) in pregnancy causes pulmonary embolism (PE) in as many as 24% of patients.
   a. The mortality rate is 15%.
   b. If patients are treated adequately, the risk of PE is 4.5%, with a risk of mortality of less than 1%.

4. Most cases of thromboembolic disease in pregnancy are associated with a hereditary thrombotic disorder. These disorders may also be associated with an increased risk for adverse pregnancy outcome in the second and third trimester (early-onset preeclampsia, early-onset intrauterine growth restriction, unexplained stillbirth, and placental abruption). The risk of thromboembolic disease increases significantly with the presence of more than one of the following abnormalities:
   a. Factor V Leiden mutation
   b. Prothrombin mutation
   c. Antiphospholipid antibody
   d. Protein C or protein S deficiency
   e. Antithrombin III deficiency
   f. Homocystinemia

B Pathophysiology

1. Pregnancy is a hypercoagulable state. Increased estrogen production is associated with increases in clotting factors.

2. The gravid uterus may compress the inferior vena cava and pelvic veins, causing venous stasis.

C Diagnosis

1. **Deep vein thrombosis**
   a. **Signs and symptoms**
      (1) Calf pain
      (2) Palpable cord

(3) Tenderness
(4) Unilateral edema of the leg
(5) Homans sign
(6) Dilated superficial veins

b. Real-time ultrasonography with duplex and color Doppler ultrasound is the **procedure of choice** to detect proximal DVT. Although it is highly sensitive and specific for femoral and popliteal thrombosis, real-time ultrasonography **does not detect pelvic vein thrombosis**, which may be responsible for pulmonary embolism.
c. Venography. This procedure is considered the gold standard for diagnosis of DVT.
    (1) Radiation is minimal, and the fetus can be protected by abdominal shielding.
    (2) This procedure is invasive and expensive.
d. ^{125}I radioisotope scanning should **not** be used in pregnancy.
e. Impedance plethysmography is safe, but its sensitivity and specificity have not been well studied in pregnancy.

2. Pulmonary embolism
  a. Clinical findings
    (1) Tachypnea
    (2) Dyspnea
    (3) Pleuritic pain
    (4) Apprehension
    (5) Cough
    (6) Tachycardia
    (7) Hemoptysis
  b. Arterial blood gas analysis
    (1) A PaO_2 of more than 80 mmHg on room air makes the diagnosis unlikely. If signs and symptoms persist, further evaluation is recommended.
    (2) An increased alveolar–arterial gradient may indicate PE.
  c. Ventilation–perfusion scan
    (1) Most patients with a PE have an abnormal ventilation–perfusion scan (sensitivity, 98%).
    (2) Many patients without emboli also have an abnormal scan (specificity, 10%).
    (3) The degree of abnormality is graded low, intermediate, or high probability, with further intervention and therapy guided by clinical suspicion.
  d. Pulmonary angiogram. This technique is the gold standard for diagnosis of PE.
    (1) It is indicated for anticoagulation failures when caval interruption is considered, to distinguish between recurrent embolization and fragmentation of the original clot.
    (2) It is associated with minimal risk to the fetus.
  e. Spiral computed tomography (CT) scan. This is replacing the angiogram as the gold standard, but it may miss small emboli.

D Management

1. Deep vein thrombosis
  a. Bedrest with extremity elevation
  b. Therapeutic anticoagulation with heparin or subcutaneous injections of low-molecular-weight heparin. Both forms of heparin **do not cross the placenta** and are safe when breastfeeding.
  c. Warfarin is a known **teratogen** and should be avoided in pregnancy. It may be used postpartum, even if the mother is nursing.

2. Pulmonary embolism
  a. Oxygen to maintain maternal PaO_2 more than 70 mmHg
  b. Bedrest for 5 to 7 days
  c. Therapeutic anticoagulation with heparin until 3 to 6 months postpartum

E Management of women who have experienced a prior thromboembolic event. The management of women with a prior history of a DVT or PE is controversial. Evaluation for a hereditary thrombotic abnormality should be pursued, and consideration should be made for prophylactic anticoagulation with either heparin or low-molecular-weight heparin.

VIII   SEIZURE DISORDERS

Seizure disorders affect approximately 1% of the population and 1 in 200 pregnancies. Fifteen percent of these cases result from infection, injury, intracranial processes, and metabolic disorders. The remaining 85% are idiopathic (no inciting incident or etiology). Patients with seizure disorders may have reduced fertility.

A **Effects of pregnancy on seizure disorders**

1. Seizure activity may increase. Increased seizure activity can be controlled with appropriate medication and compliance.
2. Pregnancy can affect medication levels.

B **Effects of seizure disorders on pregnancy**

1. **Maternal complications.** No increase in the risk of maternal complications usually results.
2. **Fetal complications**
   a. Increased risk of stillbirth
   b. Decreased birth weight
   c. Increased risk of epilepsy in life
   d. Increased risk of hemorrhagic complications in newborns exposed to anticonvulsants in utero
   e. Increased risk of congenital abnormalities
      (1) Anticonvulsants are associated with increased risk.
         (a) Carbamazepine: neural tube defects, craniofacial defects, and nail hypoplasia
         (b) Phenytoin: microcephaly, dysmorphic facies
         (c) Trimethadione: multiple malformations and mental retardation
         (d) Valproic acid: neural tube defects
      (2) The risk increases with the number of anticonvulsants used in the first trimester.
      (3) It is unclear whether a maternal seizure disorder itself may be a risk factor for fetal anomalies.

C **Management** of pregnant women with a seizure disorder

1. **Preconception**
   a. If the patient is seizure free, consider stopping medications under supervision of a neurologist.
   b. Monotherapy should be used, if possible.
   c. Folic acid supplementation may decrease risk of neural tube abnormalities.
2. **During pregnancy**
   a. Early ultrasound to establish correct gestational age
   b. Monitoring of medication levels
   c. Compliance with medication regimen
   d. Second-trimester screening for congenital abnormalities, including maternal serum AFP, ultrasound, and fetal echocardiography
   e. Serial ultrasound examinations to check for fetal growth restriction
   f. Vitamin K supplementation late in the third trimester (controversial)

IX   Rh ISOIMMUNIZATION

A **Definitions**

1. **Isoimmunization (sensitization)** is caused by maternal antibody production in response to exposure to red blood cell antigens. If these antibodies are directed against fetal red cell antigens, the antibodies can cross the placenta and cause fetal hemolytic disease.
2. **Rh isoimmunization,** a leading cause of hemolytic disease, specifically refers to antibodies against the Rh group, C, c, E, e, and D (the most commonly encountered). Rh antigens are present on fetal cells by the 38th day postconception.

B **Epidemiology**

1. Approximately 1% of all pregnancies are complicated by red blood cell sensitization. The incidence of Rh isoimmunization in the United States has fallen since the 1960s because of anti-D immune globulin.

2. Fifteen percent of Caucasians, 5% to 8% of African Americans, and 1% of Native Americans and Asians are Rh negative (absence of D antigen).

C **Criteria**   (all factors must be present in an Rh-negative pregnant woman)

1. The fetus must be Rh positive.

2. Enough fetal cells must reach the maternal circulation (fetomaternal bleed).

3. The mother must make antibody to D antigen.
   a. Some women are immunogenic nonresponders (as many as 30%).
   b. ABO incompatibility with the fetus can be protective.
   c. The amount of antigen necessary to generate an immune response with anti-D antibody is different for each woman.

D **Prevention of Rh isoimmunization**   (anti-D immunoglobulin)

1. Anti-D immunoglobulin can prevent Rh-negative women from mounting an immune response (producing anti-D antibodies) when exposed to Rh-positive (D-positive) blood.

2. A dose of 300 μg of Rh immune globulin (RhoGAM) can protect (prevent immune response) from an exposure of up to 30 mL of fetal blood.

3. To prevent immunologic response, the patient must:
   a. Not yet be sensitized to the D antigen
   b. Be given enough immune globulin
   c. Be treated in a timely fashion

4. Treatment of Rh-negative women within 72 hours of delivery decreases immunization to less than 1.5%.

5. Treatment of all Rh-negative women at 28 weeks' gestation further decreases risk of sensitization to less than 0.2%.

6. Other indications for use in pregnant Rh-negative, unsensitized women include:
   a. Abortion (spontaneous or elective)
   b. Ectopic pregnancy
   c. Antepartum bleeding, including first and second trimester
   d. Abdominal trauma
   e. After amniocentesis or chorionic villus sampling
   f. After external cephalic version

7. Failure to prevent sensitization may occur in the following conditions:
   a. Inadequate dose (maternal exposure to more than 30 mL of fetal Rh-positive blood)
   b. Treatment delay
   c. Previously sensitized patient

E **Management of the Rh-negative, unsensitized pregnant woman**

1. Type and screen at initial visit.

2. Treat with Rh immune globulin at 28 weeks (it is usual, although not necessary, to confirm that the patient is unsensitized prior to treatment).

3. Treat with Rh immune globulin after delivery (within 72 hours) if the fetus is Rh positive.

4. After delivery, check for "excessive" fetomaternal hemorrhage and treat with additional doses of Rh immune globulin if exposure is greater than 30 mL of fetal Rh-positive blood.

5. The amount of fetal–maternal hemorrhage can be estimated by the **Kleihauer-Betke** test. Treatment of maternal blood with acid elutes the adult hemoglobin from red cells, and only fetal hemoglobin remains. A smear is made and treated with a special stain that detects the red cells with fetal hemoglobin and the **volume of fetal red cells in the maternal circulation can be estimated**.

F **Management of the Rh-negative, sensitized pregnant woman**

1. Accurately assess gestational age with early ultrasound.

2. Determine **paternal blood type**.

  a. If the partner is **Rh negative, there is no need for further evaluation and intervention**.

  b. If the partner is homozygous for D, the fetus is D positive.

  c. If the partner is heterozygous for D, the fetus has a 50% chance of being Rh negative and not at risk for anemia.

  d. With amniocentesis or chorionic villus sampling, DNA analysis can be performed to evaluate whether the fetus is Rh positive.

3. Assess prior obstetric history.

  a. The risk of hemolytic disease tends to be as severe (or more severe) in subsequent pregnancies.

  b. If the mother had a previous hydropic fetus, the risk that the next Rh-positive fetus will become hydropic is 80%.

  c. Hemolysis and hydropic changes usually develop at earlier gestational ages with each successive pregnancy. In general, the risk of severe fetal hemolysis and hydropic changes in the first sensitized pregnancy is low.

4. Assess antibody titer.

  a. In the first sensitized pregnancy, titers should be drawn every 2 to 4 weeks to assess the need for amniocentesis. Amniocentesis should be offered when the "critical titer" is reached. In general, the critical titer is 1:16, and it signifies the titer at which an anemic fetus has been identified. The critical titer is laboratory specific.

  b. In subsequent sensitized pregnancies, antibody titer is not as useful a guide to the timing of amniocentesis. The patient's history should be used to guide the timing of invasive testing and intervention.

5. Use amniocentesis to assess the degree of hemolysis and risk for fetal death. Once invasive testing is initiated, further assessment of antibody titers is not indicated.

  a. Bilirubin in amniotic fluid is a by-product of fetal hemolysis.

  b. Bilirubin enters the amniotic fluid from fetal secretions, and the level of bilirubin in amniotic fluid correlates with fetal hemolysis.

  c. Spectrophotometry is used to assess the level of bilirubin in amniotic fluid.

   (1) Bilirubin causes a shift in optical density away from linearity.

   (2) Shift is greatest at a wavelength of 450 nm.

   (3) Degree of **shift at 450 nm (ΔOD_{450}) is used to estimate the degree of hemolysis**.

  d. In the early 1960s, Liley devised a chart based on the natural history of Rh-sensitized pregnancies from **27 to 41 weeks' gestation**. The chart compares gestational age (x axis) versus assessment of ΔOD_{450} (y axis). Use of the **Liley curve** (Fig. 17-1) is associated with less iatrogenic premature delivery for those pregnancies at low risk of severe fetal anemia.

   (1) The chart is divided into three zones (marked by downsloping lines to reflect increased ability of the fetus to metabolize bilirubin with advancing gestational age).

    (a) Zone I is associated with mild anemia or unaffected fetuses.

    (b) Zone II is associated with mild to severe anemia.

    (c) Zone III is associated with severe fetal anemia and fetal death within 7 to 10 days.

   (2) Management of results in upper zone II or zone III includes cordocentesis to assess fetal hemoglobin, fetal transfusion, or delivery (depending on gestational age).

  e. Prior to 27 weeks, assessment of ΔOD_{450} values is unclear and debatable. Past obstetric history and ultrasound findings may dictate cordocentesis to assess fetal hemoglobin and need for transfusion.

  f. Amniocentesis is associated with an **increased risk of sensitization, infection, rupture of membranes, and fetal loss**.

6. Perform cordocentesis when it is believed that the fetus is at risk for severe anemia.

  a. This technique should be performed with a 22-gauge spinal needle under ultrasound guidance.

  b. This technique may be performed along any portion of the umbilical cord, preferably in the umbilical vein (if transfusion is planned).

  c. The initial sample should assess fetal hemoglobin and hematocrit, platelet count, reticulocyte count, and blood type.

  d. Transfusion should occur if fetal hematocrit is less than 30%.

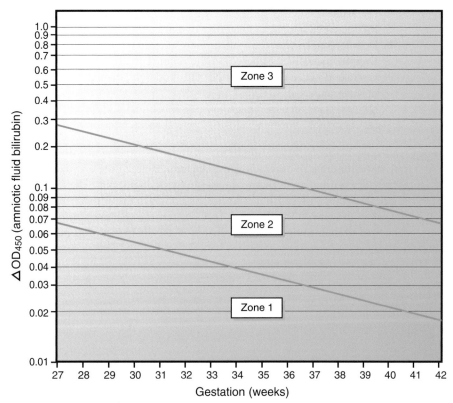

FIGURE 17–1 Liley graph. (From Pritchard JA, MacDonald PC, Gant NF. Williams Obstetrics. 21st Ed. New York: McGraw-Hill, 2001.)

7. If necessary, **perform fetal transfusion** either **intraperitoneally or intravascularly** (through fetal umbilical vein). Intravascular transfusion instantly increases fetal hematocrit, whereas intraperitoneal transfusion requires the fetus to absorb transfused blood through the lymphatic system (severely anemic or hydropic fetuses may do very poorly). The goal is to raise fetal hematocrit.

   a. Donor cells are matched with the mother and fetus (if available from prior cordocentesis).

   b. Donor cells are buffy-coat poor, washed irradiated, filtered, and resuspended in normal saline to a hematocrit of 70% to 75%.

   c. Nomograms exist to determine the amount to be transfused at one time based on donor and fetal hematocrit and on the gestational age of the fetus.

   d. Once transfusion is complete, the final fetal hematocrit is assessed.

   e. The procedure is repeated until the gestational age when the risks of prematurity are minimized. The timing of repeat procedures is based on fetal hematocrit and usually occurs within 2 to 3 weeks. At the time of the first repeat procedure, initial fetal hematocrit can help identify the rate of hemoglobin degradation to help determine the time of future procedures.

   f. Compared with amniocentesis, the **risk** of infection, rupture of membranes, fetal loss, and further sensitization are **increased**.

8. **Consider noninvasive assessment** of the fetus, which can be extremely useful in helping guide initial intervention. Techniques include ultrasound and Doppler velocimetry. Although these modalities are still investigational, they can be extremely useful for guiding timing of initial cordocentesis, especially at gestational ages of less than 27 weeks, when assessment of ΔOD_{450} is not as clear.

   a. Ultrasound. Assessment of fetal anemia includes evidence of:

      (1) Polyhydramnios

      (2) Placental thickening

      (3) Pleural effusions

      (4) Pericardial effusions

        (5) Ascites

        (6) Increased liver size (suggestive of extramedullary hematopoiesis)

    b. Doppler velocimetry. Not all severely anemic fetuses show evidence of hydropic changes. Doppler assessment is based on the premise that fetal anemia is associated with abnormal vascular flow. Fetuses with mild and moderate anemia usually have flow velocities in the normal range.

        (1) Assess for increased peak velocity in the fetal middle cerebellar artery.

        (2) Assess for abnormal velocities in fetal aorta, inferior vena cava, or umbilical vein.

G **Management of maternal sensitization for other antigens.** In addition to the D antigen, red cells have hundreds of other antigens. The frequencies of these antigens depend on the population; fortunately, antibodies to many of these antigens do not place the fetus at risk for severe hemolytic disease. Other antigens that can pose a risk to the fetus by maternal antibody production include the other antigens in the Rh locus (c, C, e, and E), Kell, and Duffy. When a pregnant woman is sensitized to these antigens, the pregnancy is usually managed as outlined above for anti-D.

Study Questions for Chapter 17

Directions: *Each of the numbered items or incomplete statements in this section is followed by answers or by completions of the statement. Select the ONE lettered answer or completion that is BEST in each case.*

1. A 24-year-old primigravida is seeing you for her first prenatal visit. After confirming her pregnancy, you take a complete history and perform a physical examination. She has had type 2 diabetes for 6 years now and has been on oral medications for blood sugar control. Her capillary blood glucose level is 110 mg/dL today. After delivery, her newborn will be at risk for:

- A Elevated blood glucose
- B Low hematocrit
- C Low calcium
- D Elevated potassium
- E Low bilirubin

2. A 22-year-old woman, gravida 2, para 0, at 22 weeks of gestation, presents to you for her routine prenatal visit. She has been seeing you throughout her pregnancy. She had diabetes prior to becoming pregnant and was taking an oral hypoglycemic agent to control her blood sugars. However, since becoming pregnant, she has been self-administering daily regular and NPH (neutral protamine Hagedorn's) insulin. Today, she reports lower back discomfort. Her fundus measures 21 cm and she has 1+ glucose on urine dipstick. Her average fasting blood sugar is 93 mg/dL, and her 2-hour postprandial sugar is 119 mg/dL. What is the next step in management of this patient?

- A Adjust her insulin
- B Measure maternal serum AFP
- C Perform fetal ultrasound
- D Perform fetal echocardiograph
- E Perform magnetic resonance imaging (MRI) of the spine

3. A 28-year-old woman, gravida 2, para 1, at 20 weeks of gestation, presents with increased sweating and palpitations. Her fundus measures 17 cm. T = 98.8, BP = 115/80, P = 132, R = 16. She is found to have elevated total T_4, total T_3, and free T_4, and TSH less than 0.1. What is the initial step in management of this patient?

- A Propranolol
- B Methimazole
- C Propylthiouracil
- D Potassium iodide
- E Fetal ultrasound

4. An 18-year-old woman, gravida 3, para 2, at 28 weeks of gestation, is admitted with right-sided back pain, fever, chills, and severe nausea. She has bilateral costovertebral angle tenderness, with greater discomfort on the right side. T = 102.6°F, with normal complete blood count (CBC), blood urea nitrogen (BUN), and creatinine. Urinalysis revealed more than 100 WBC/hpf. After 3 days of culture-appropriate antibiotics, her temperature is still 103°F. The next step is:

- A Repeat urine culture
- B Repeat CBC
- C Change antibiotics
- D Perform an ultrasound
- E Perform an intravenous pyelogram (IVP)

5. A 20-year-old woman just delivered a viable male neonate at 38 weeks of gestation after being a restrained passenger in a car accident. Upon arriving at the emergency department she was "cleared" by the trauma and orthopedic teams and sent to the labor and delivery floor. There she began having vaginal bleeding and then went into labor spontaneously. The estimated blood loss with delivery was 900 mL, and now she is stable. After obtaining her prenatal information you realize she is Rh negative and antibody D negative. The next step is:

- A Perform a CBC
- B Transfuse packed red blood cells
- C Perform a Kleihauer-Betke test
- D Give additional Rh immune globulin
- E Assess neonatal Rh antigen status

Answers and Explanations

1. The answer is C [I B 2]. A diabetic woman is at higher risk for delivering a baby with respiratory distress, hypoglycemia (low glucose), hypocalcemia (low calcium), polycythemia (high hematocrit), and hyperbilirubinemia (high bilirubin). Potassium levels are usually not affected.

2. The answer is D [I C 3 c]. Women with preexisting diabetes are at higher risk for congenital anomalies, especially cardiac anomalies such as ventricular septal defect and situs inversus. Thus, a fetal echocardiograph should be performed, and the best time to perform one is between 20 and 22 weeks of gestation. Her insulin does not need to be changed because she is below the goals for fasting and 2-hour blood glucose levels. Maternal serum AFP is useful only during weeks 15 through 20. Fetal ultrasound should have already been performed if this is a patient you have been seeing throughout her pregnancy (the optimal time to perform a fetal ultrasound is between 16 and 20 weeks of gestation). The MRI of the maternal spine is unnecessary for her back discomfort, which is a common problem during pregnancy. Further evaluation of her back would be needed if more information in the clinical scenario made you suspicious of a more significant problem.

3. The answer is A [II B 4 a 3]. This patient has hyperthyroidism based on her elevated free T_4 levels and suppressed TSH. Beta-blockers are the initial treatment of choice for her symptoms of tachycardia and palpitations. For this patient, PTU is also necessary to maintain her free T_4 levels near high normal. However, PTU is not the initial treatment to control her significant tachycardia. Methimazole is not used often because it is associated with aplasia cutis and the alternative agent, PTU, is safer. Potassium iodide is one of the agents used to treat a thyroid storm. A fetal ultrasound would be appropriate given the disparity between the gestational age and the fundal height. However, an ultrasound is not the initial step, nor is it a step that will solve this patient's problems.

4. The answer is D [III D 5 d]. The clinical scenario presented is that of pyelonephritis that is not responding to treatment. This finding should always prompt radiologic evaluation to rule out an abscess or renal calculi. The least invasive initial procedure is a renal ultrasound, not an intravenous pyelogram. There is no need to repeat the urine culture or to change her antibiotics since results of her initial urine culture and sensitivity confirm that she is on appropriate antibiotics. Repeating CBC is fine, but it will not tell you why there is lack of response to treatment.

5. The answer is E [IX E 3]. In the management of an Rh-negative, unsensitized (i.e., antibody-negative) patient, you should know the Rh antigen status of the baby. If the baby is Rh negative, then there is no need for Rh immune globulin because the maternal immune system would not form any antibodies directed toward fetal red blood cells. Had the baby been Rh positive, the next step would be to quantitate the amount of fetomaternal blood transfusion by performing a Kleihauer-Betke test. Then, based on those results, you may give additional Rh immune globulin. A CBC or transfusion is not necessary in this scenario because this patient stopped bleeding and is "stable." A CBC or capillary hemoglobin concentration test is appropriate during the first postpartum day for all postpartum patients.

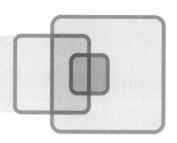

chapter 18

Gestational Trophoblastic Disease

CHRISTINA S. CHU

I INTRODUCTION

Gestational trophoblastic disease (GTD) is the general term for a spectrum of proliferative abnormalities originating from the trophoblast of the placenta.

A Classification (Table 18-1)

1. **Hydatidiform mole. Benign GTD** is also referred to as a hydatidiform mole, or more commonly a "**molar pregnancy.**" It is characterized by abnormal proliferation of the placental trophoblastic cells. These abnormal cells distend the uterus and secrete the polypeptide hormone **human chorionic gonadotropin (hCG)**, mimicking a normal pregnancy. Hydatidiform moles may be **complete (classic)** or **partial (incomplete)**.

2. **Gestational trophoblastic tumor (GTT).** This malignant form of GTD, which arises from the trophoblastic elements of the developing blastocyst, retains the invasive tendencies of the normal placenta and remains able to secrete hCG. GTT can be either **metastatic** or **nonmetastatic**.

B Incidence

1. **Hydatidiform mole.** Benign GTD occurs in 1 of 1500 pregnancies in the United States and in as many as 1 of 125 pregnancies in parts of eastern Asia.
   a. **Complete moles** are the most commonly identified type of molar pregnancy. They are 5 to 10 times more common in pregnancies in women older than 40 years of age. Dietary factors, such as low intake of vitamin A and animal fat intake, are associated with this condition.
   b. **Partial moles** are associated with oral contraceptive use and irregular menses.

2. **GTT.** Malignant GTD is identified in 1 of 20,000 pregnancies in the United States and can occur after any type of pregnancy.
   a. Hydatidiform mole precedes GTT in 50% of cases.
   b. Normal pregnancy precedes GTT in 25% of cases.
   c. Abortion or ectopic pregnancy precedes GTT in 25% of cases.

II HYDATIDIFORM MOLE (Table 18-2)

A Complete mole

1. **Origin.** In 90% of cases, an **"empty" ovum** containing no genomic DNA is fertilized by one **sperm**, which duplicates its DNA, leading to an abnormal 46,XX karyotype, with all DNA paternal in origin. In the remaining 10% of cases, the "empty" ovum is fertilized by two sperm, resulting in an abnormal 46,XX or 46,XY karyotype, again with all DNA of paternal origin. Thus, in a complete mole all the **chromosomes are paternally derived** (Fig. 18-1).

2. **Histologic features**
   a. Marked edema and enlargement of the villi (hydropic villi)
   b. Disappearance of the villous blood vessels
   c. Diffuse proliferation of the trophoblastic lining
   d. Absence of fetal tissue

TABLE 18–1   **Clinical Classification of Gestational Trophoblastic Disease**

Hydatidiform mole (molar pregnancy)
    Complete, or classic
    Incomplete, or partial
 	
Gestational trophoblastic neoplasia
    Nonmetastatic
    Metastatic
        Low risk (good prognosis)
        High risk (poor prognosis)

3. Clinical features

    a. Abnormal uterine bleeding is the most common presenting symptom in the first trimester of pregnancy.

    b. "**Classic symptoms**" occurring later in pregnancy include heavy bleeding (90%), uterine size greater than expected for gestational age (40%), and lack of fetal heart tones. Additional classic symptoms that probably arise from stimulation by excessive hCG are hyperemesis gravidarum (nausea and vomiting; 25% in the past, but about 10% in the modern era), **theca lutein cysts** within the ovaries (50%), preeclampsia (rare in the modern era), and hyperthyroidism. Patients may present with passage of vesicular tissue from the vagina.

    c. A **diagnosis of complete molar pregnancy** rather than miscarriage is suspected when the **hCG level is greater than 100,000 mIU/mL** and when **ultrasound reveals a uterine cavity filled with small vesicles** rather than the expected gestational sac and fetus. Pathologic correlation and cytogenetic analysis for DNA content confirm the diagnosis.

4. Malignant potential

    a. Complete molar pregnancies may result in malignant sequelae in about 2% to 32% of cases.

    b. Up to 25% of cases may eventually display metastatic disease outside of the uterus.

B   **Partial or incomplete mole**

    1. Origin. A partial mole (see Table 18-2) is a normal ovum that is fertilized by two sperm. The resulting karyotype is 69,XXX, 69,XXY, or 69,XYY (Fig. 18-2).

    2. Histologic features

        a. Only focal hydropic villi

        b. Only focal trophoblastic proliferation

        c. Presence of an **umbilical cord, amniotic membrane, and fetus** that is usually not viable and has features of a triploid gestation

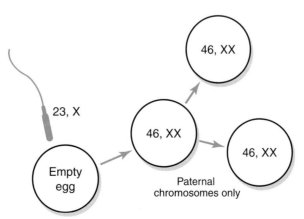

FIGURE 18–1   Chromosomal origin of a diploid complete hydatidiform mole. (Adapted from Kurman RJ. Blaustein's Pathology of the Female Genital Tract. 4th Ed. New York: Springer-Verlag, 1994:1051.)

TABLE 18-2 **Comparison of Complete and Partial Mole**

Feature	Complete Mole	Partial Mole
Age	Greater risk (5–10×) >40 years	Not age related
Karyotype	90% XX, 10% XY	XXX or XXY
	All chromosomes paternally derived	1 chromosome set maternal; 2 chromosome sets paternal
Fetus	Absent	Present
hCG	Often >100,000 mIU/mL	Rarely elevated above normal levels for pregnancy
Primary symptom	Bleeding	Bleeding
Secondary symptoms	Large uterine size for gestational age	Rare
	Hyperemesis	
	Theca lutein cysts	
	Preeclampsia	
	Hyperthyroidism	
Risk of persistence (GTT)	20%	4%

hCG, human chorionic gonadotropin; GTT, gestational trophoblastic tumor.
Adapted from Lu KH, Goldstein DP, Bernstein MR, et al. Managing molar pregnancy. *O G B Manage* 1999;11:67–76.

3. **Clinical features**
   a. **Abnormal uterine bleeding** is the most common presenting symptom in the first trimester of a pregnancy, similar to complete moles.
   b. Excessive vaginal bleeding, hyperemesis, preeclampsia, hyperthyroidism, and ovarian cysts are rare.
   c. **hCG is generally not significantly elevated**, and ultrasound may show a fetus as well as hydropic villi. Pathologic correlation and cytogenetic analysis for DNA content confirm the diagnosis.
   d. Many spontaneous abortions may represent undiagnosed partial moles.
   e. Case reports indicate that normal pregnancies coincident with partial moles have proceeded to term without adverse sequelae.

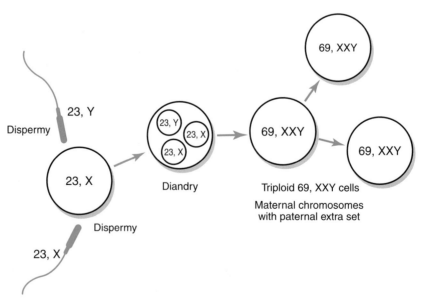

FIGURE 18–2 Chromosomal origin of a triploid partial hydatidiform mole. (Adapted from Kurman RJ. Blaustein's Pathology of the Female Genital Tract. 4th Ed. New York: Springer-Verlag, 1994:1052.)

4. Malignant potential
   a. Less than 5% of partial moles progress to malignant disease.
   b. Only 1% of cases develop extrauterine metastases.

C Management of molar pregnancies (complete and partial)

1. Diagnostic studies
   a. Laboratory tests include a complete blood count with platelets, quantitative hCG, coagulation studies, type and screen, baseline renal function and liver function studies, and thyroid function tests.
   b. Imaging studies include chest radiograph to evaluate for lung metastases and ultrasound.

2. Dilation and suction curettage of the uterus is the primary tool for evacuating a molar pregnancy even when the uterus has enlarged beyond the size expected for a pregnancy of 20 weeks. Simultaneous ultrasound monitoring during the procedure may be helpful.
   a. Intravenous oxytocin should be given to enhance uterine involution after the procedure to minimize blood loss.
   b. Respiratory distress resulting from fluid overload, emboli of trophoblastic tissue, and thyroid storm may occur in as many as 2% of patients in the perioperative period.
   c. Even large **theca lutein cysts** of the ovaries associated with molar gestation resolve as hCG levels drop. These cysts are not an indication for surgical intervention.

3. The **risk of developing GTT** after evacuation is 20% for a complete mole and 4% for a partial mole. **High-risk factors** associated with persistent disease include pretreatment hCG greater than 100,000 mIU/mL, theca lutein cysts greater than 6 cm, age older than 40 years, and previous molar pregnancy.

4. Hysterectomy is a treatment option for patients who do not desire future fertility.

D Follow-up of a complete or partial molar pregnancy.   After evacuation, the expected average time to complete elimination of hCG is 9 to 11 weeks. This period depends on the initial level of hCG, the amount of viable trophoblastic tissue remaining after evacuation, and the half-life of hCG. Follow-up of a molar pregnancy should include:

1. Determinations of hCG made at 48 hours postevacuation, then weekly until the results are negative for 3 consecutive weeks, then every month for 6 months, and then yearly. An increase or plateau in hCG indicates the development of **GTT** and necessitates the initiation of chemotherapy.

2. Physical examination, including a pelvic examination, at regular intervals until remission to ensure adequate involution of pelvic organs.

3. Birth control (recommended for 1 year). Oral contraceptives or medroxyprogesterone (Depo-Provera) injections are recommended. Pregnancy can be attempted after 1 year from the diagnosis.

4. Prophylactic chemotherapy is rarely recommended. Most patients with molar pregnancies are cured with evacuation and do not require any therapy. Serial hCG determinations identify patients who develop GTT (20% of complete moles and 4% of partial moles). The toxicity from prophylactic chemotherapy can be severe, even leading to death.

E Future fertility

1. Normal pregnancy is the most likely result of future gestations.

2. Risk of a second molar pregnancy is 1%; risk of a third molar pregnancy is 33%. Subsequent molar pregnancies may be complete or partial, regardless of the type of initial molar pregnancy.

III **GESTATIONAL TROPHOBLASTIC TUMOR**

A Characteristics.   The occurrence of **GTT** (Table 18-3) after a molar pregnancy may have the **histologic appearance of a mole or choriocarcinoma**. After a normal pregnancy, abortion, or ectopic pregnancy, GTT always has the appearance of **choriocarcinoma**, or occasionally the aggressive **placental site trophoblastic tumor** variant of choriocarcinoma.

TABLE 18-3 Classification of Gestational Trophoblastic Neoplasia

Nonmetastatic: disease confined to the uterus
Metastatic: disease spread outside the uterus

Good prognosis (low risk)	Poor prognosis (high risk)
Short duration: disease present <4 months	Long duration: disease present >4 months
Pretreatment hCG titer: <40,000 mIU/mL	Pretreatment hCG titer: >40,000 mIU/mL
No previous chemotherapy	Brain or liver metastases
	Failure of previous chemotherapy
	Disease after term pregnancy

hCG, human chorionic gonadotropin.

1. **Nonmetastatic GTT (persistent or invasive mole)** is molar tissue that invades the uterine wall, produces persistent hCG elevation, and potentially causes bleeding. It is confined to the uterus and is the most common form of GTT.

2. **Metastatic disease** (disease outside the uterus) may be found most commonly in the lung (80%) and the vagina (30%), but may also affect the liver (10%) and brain (10%). Patients have various symptoms, such as **vaginal bleeding (vaginal metastasis), hemoptysis (pulmonary metastases),** or **neurologic symptoms (brain metastases)**. The disease is often associated with hemorrhage because of the propensity of trophoblastic tissue to invade vessels. Metastases are very friable, and biopsy to confirm diagnosis is not recommended. In the setting of the appropriate clinical history and an elevated hCG, lesions visualized on radiographic studies are treated presumptively.

B Diagnosis

1. **After evacuation of a molar pregnancy**, GTT is diagnosed when there is a documented increase in hCG, the value of hCG reaches a plateau for 3 weeks, or metastatic disease is identified.

2. Weeks or years **after an abortion or ectopic pregnancy**, elevated hCG may indicate GTT or another pregnancy.

C Management

1. **Workup of patients with GTT** should include the following:
   a. Complete history and physical examination
   b. Pretreatment hCG titer, hematologic survey, serum chemistries, and liver function studies
   c. Pelvic ultrasound
   d. Computed tomography (CT) scan of the abdomen and pelvis
   e. Chest radiograph or chest CT
   f. CT or magnetic resonance imaging of the brain in high-risk patients

2. **Nonmetastatic GTT is almost 100% curable.**
   a. **Single-agent chemotherapy** cures more than 90% of patients. Hysterectomy may be offered to decrease the number of treatments required for the patient who does not desire future fertility.
      (1) **Methotrexate** is the most commonly used treatment agent. This **antimetabolite** inhibits purine synthesis by blocking the dihydrofolate reductase enzyme required to process folic acid. This results in arrested synthesis of DNA, RNA, and proteins.
          (a) **Common side effects** include ulcerations of the mouth and gastrointestinal tract mucosa, as well as nausea. **Less common side effects**, seen when multiple or high doses are used, include myelosuppression, hepatotoxicity, nephrotoxicity, alopecia, and pneumonitis.
          (b) **Leucovorin** (folinic acid) is administered 24 hours after each methotrexate dose to rescue normal cells from methotrexate toxicity.
          (c) Folic acid should be avoided during methotrexate treatment as it interferes with the action of the methotrexate.

(2) **Actinomycin D** is an antibiotic that intercalates DNA strands. It is also an effective single-agent treatment for nonmetastatic GTT.

(3) **Failure** of single-agent treatment is rare. Most patients are still curable by switching to another agent or switching to a multidrug regimen.

b. **Follow-up**

(1) hCG titers should be followed carefully: weekly until normal for 3 months, then monthly until normal for 6 months.

(2) Contraception, preferably with oral contraceptives or medroxyprogesterone (Depo-Provera), should be used for 6 to 12 months to allow accurate monitoring of posttreatment hCG levels and to avoid misinterpretation of rising hCG levels due to normal pregnancy.

3. **Metastatic GTT**

a. **Good-prognosis metastatic GTT**

(1) The following factors are associated with a **good prognosis**:

(a) Short duration (less than 4 months)

(b) Low pretreatment hCG titer (less than 40,000 mIU/mL)

(c) No metastatic spread to the brain or liver

(d) No previous chemotherapy

(2) **Single-agent chemotherapy** with methotrexate or actinomycin D can be used to treat good-prognosis metastatic GTT. However, more courses of chemotherapy are usually required, and alternative therapy is needed more frequently.

(3) **Follow-up** is similar to that for nonmetastatic GTT (see III C 2 b).

b. **Poor-prognosis metastatic GTT**

(1) The following factors are **associated with a poor prognosis**:

(a) Long duration (more than 4 months)

(b) High pretreatment hCG titer (more than 40,000 mIU/mL)

(c) Liver or brain metastases

(d) Failure of previous chemotherapy

(e) Disease after a term pregnancy

(2) **Treatment**

(a) Affected patients are treated with **multiagent chemotherapy** such as EMA-CO (**e**toposide, **m**ethotrexate, **a**ctinomycin D, **c**yclophosphamide, and **v**incristine [Oncovin]) and a multiple modality approach (i.e., chemotherapy, surgery, and radiation).

(b) High-risk patients should be treated in centers that have a special interest and expertise in this disease, especially when life-threatening toxicity from therapy is a factor.

(c) The survival rate is approximately 80%.

(d) Hysterectomy usually does not improve the outcome.

(3) **Follow-up**

(a) Three additional courses of chemotherapy after a negative hCG titer

(b) Monitoring of hCG levels (similar to that for nonmetastatic GTT)

(c) Contraception for at least 1 year after negative levels of hCG

D **Recurrence rates**

1. Nonmetastatic GTT: 1%

2. Good-prognosis metastatic GTT: 5%

3. Poor-prognosis metastatic GTT: up to 20%

E **Future fertility.** Fertility after chemotherapy for GTT is usually retained since the chemotherapy agents used do not deplete the oocytes in the ovary. Women who choose to become pregnant should be monitored carefully. A normal intrauterine pregnancy should be documented in the first trimester, the placenta should be histologically evaluated after delivery, and hCG titers should be followed to zero postpartum.

Study Questions for Chapter 18

Directions: *Each of the numbered items or incomplete statements in this section is followed by answers or by completions of the statement. Select the ONE lettered answer or completion that is BEST in each case.*

Questions 1 and 2 are based on the clinical scenario described below.

A 24-year-old woman, gravida 1, para 0, at 24 weeks of gestation by her last menstrual period, presents to the emergency department because of vaginal bleeding. T = 97.8, BP = 135/88, P = 105, R = 16. Her fundus is below the umbilicus and there are no fetal heart tones on Doppler. On speculum examination you see blood emerging from an undilated external os, but no lesions are seen on the cervix or the vaginal walls. Her quantitative hCG level is 85,000 mIU/mL. You are awaiting a formal ultrasound by a radiologist to confirm your suspicion of a molar pregnancy.

1. What is the most likely explanation for this scenario?
   - A. Maternal 0 + Paternal Y (which duplicates)
   - B. Maternal 0 + Paternal X (which duplicates)
   - C. Maternal Y + Paternal X (which duplicates)
   - D. Maternal X + Paternal X + Paternal X
   - E. Maternal Y + Paternal X + Paternal Y

2. Which of the following findings is the most likely on pelvic ultrasound examination?
   - A. A fetus with biparietal diameter consistent with 22 weeks
   - B. Two-vessel umbilical cord
   - C. Two separate placentas
   - D. Left ovary 6 cm and right ovary 3 cm
   - E. Left ovary 6 cm and right ovary 6 cm

3. A 33-year-old woman, gravida 4, para 3, at 16 weeks of gestation by her last menstrual period, presents to labor and delivery complaining of vaginal bleeding. Her vital signs are as follows: T = 98.9, BP = 150/94, P = 103. Fundal height measures 23 cm. A pelvic ultrasound examination reveals a uterus with a diffuse indistinct mass filling the endometrial cavity, and no fetal parts are seen. A dilation and suction curettage is performed and 10 minutes afterwards she is placed on a dilute intravenous oxytocin drip. Complications involving which one of the following organs are most likely to occur at this time?
   - A. Liver
   - B. Kidney
   - C. Vagina
   - D. Lung
   - E. Brain

4. A 27-year-old nulliparous woman presents to the emergency room reporting hemoptysis. She has no medical history other than a pregnancy 3 months ago that resulted in spontaneous abortion. She also has had intermittent vaginal spotting since the miscarriage. Her BP = 110/70 and P = 88. Significant labs are hemoglobin = 9.6 mg/dL and quantitative β-hCG = 35,000 mIU/mL. Her chest radiograph shows several masses in the right middle lobe. Which of the following is the best treatment option for her?
   - A. Dilation and curettage
   - B. Hysterectomy
   - C. Methotrexate and leucovorin
   - D. Actinomycin D
   - E. Methotrexate, actinomycin D, and etoposide

5. A 36-year-old multiparous woman just underwent a hysterectomy because of a molar pregnancy. Other than her treatment for gestational trophoblastic disease, she has no medical problems. She had an appendectomy 3 years ago. She is allergic to penicillin and, although she does not smoke, she admits to drinking at least three to four alcoholic beverages per day. You obtain a β-hCG 2 days after the operation. What is the next best step in management of this patient?

- A β-hCG in 1 week
- B β-hCG in 1 month
- C Methotrexate
- D Levonorgestrel plus ethinyl estradiol
- E Chest radiograph in 1 month

Answers and Explanations

1. D [II B 1], **2.** B [II B 2 c]. The clinical scenario is consistent with a partial or incomplete mole because the uterus is smaller than dates (uterus below umbilicus is less than 20 weeks) and the hCG level is lower than 100,000 mIU/mL. In a partial mole, the ovum is normal and thus contributes only one of its chromosomes. The normal ovum is fertilized by two sperm (each with one sex chromosome). The result is a triploid fetus (69 chromosomes) that usually has the karyotype XXX or XXY. Also, a partial mole will have fetal tissues. The ovaries usually are not enlarged because the hCG levels are not high. Furthermore, even in a complete mole where theca lutein cysts form, the ovaries are usually equally enlarged. Two separate placentas suggest twins.

3. The answer is D [II C 2 b]. After a dilation and suction curettage of the uterus after a molar pregnancy (especially when there is delay in the inception of oxytocin infusion), respiratory distress is a possible complication. The lungs can be injured because of embolic events from trophoblastic tissue at the time of the dilation and curettage, from fluid overload, or as a result of thyroid storm.

4. The answer is C [III C 3 a 2]. This patient has metastatic disease (lung metastasis) with a good prognosis (β-hCG less than 40,000 mIU/mL, no brain or liver metastasis, last pregnancy not normal [spontaneous abortion], disease occurred less than 4 months from the last pregnancy, and no previous chemotherapy). Thus, the best treatment for her is single-agent chemotherapy. Methotrexate is the first-line agent. Note: Leucovorin is not considered multiagent chemotherapy because it is folinic acid added to methotrexate to rescue normal cells from methotrexate toxicity. There is no regimen that consists of only methotrexate, actinomycin D, and etoposide.

5. The answer is A [II D]. The most important step after treatment of a molar pregnancy is to ensure that the patient does not get pregnant within the next year because it would confound follow-up with hCG levels. Had the patient not had a hysterectomy, the next step would be to place her on birth control pills (levonorgestrel plus ethinyl estradiol). Because this patient has had the 48-hour "postevacuation" hCG levels, the next step is to do a weekly hCG until the results are negative three times, then every month for 6 months, and then annually.

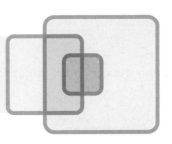

chapter 19

The Menstrual Cycle

THOMAS A. MOLINARO • CLARISA GRACIA

I   INTRODUCTION

The menstrual cycle relies on the cyclic production of estrogen and progesterone that mirrors the regular occurrence of ovulation throughout a woman's reproductive life. The development of predictable, regular cyclic, and spontaneous ovulatory menstrual cycles is regulated by complex interactions of the hypothalamic-pituitary axis, the ovaries, and the genital tract. The menstrual cycle is divided into two phases: the follicular (or proliferative) phase and the luteal (or secretory) phase.

A   Length of the cycle

1. The **mean duration** of the cycle is **28 days**, plus or minus 7 days.
   a. **Polymenorrhea** is defined as menstrual cycles that occur at short intervals (less than 21 days).
   b. **Oligomenorrhea** is defined as menstrual cycles that occur at long intervals (more than 35 days).
2. Menstrual cycles are the most irregular during the 2 years following menarche (i.e., the first menses) and during the 3 years leading up to menopause. At both times, **anovulation** (i.e., absent ovulation) is most common.

B   Follicular or proliferative phase.   This phase lasts from the first day of menses until ovulation, during which time follicles within the ovary grow in response to **follicle-stimulating hormone (FSH)**, and in the uterus **endometrial glands** proliferate under the influence of **estrogen**, primarily **estradiol** produced by the follicle. The follicular phase is characterized by:

1. Variable length, although it averages 14 days
2. Development of ovarian follicles in response to FSH
3. Secretion of estrogen from the ovary
4. Proliferation of the endometrium in response to estrogen
5. Low basal body temperature

C   Ovulation.   Ovulation occurs in response to the **luteinizing hormone (LH)** surge. This phase is characterized by:

1. Release of the oocytes from the follicle in response to FSH induction of collagenases, which enzymatically break down the follicle wall
2. Resumption of meiosis, with oocytes progressing from prophase I through metaphase II
3. Formation of the corpus luteum within the follicle

D   Luteal or secretory phase.   The second part of the cycle extends from ovulation until the onset of menses. The corpus luteum, stimulated by LH, produces progesterone, which causes secretory changes in the endometrium necessary for preparing the endometrium for implantation of the embryo. The luteal phase is characterized by:

1. A fairly constant duration of 12 to 16 days, in contrast to the follicular phase
2. An elevated basal body temperature (higher than 98°F) in response to progesterone production
3. Sustaining of the **corpus luteum** in the ovary, with the secretion of progesterone and estrogen

4. Secretory changes in the endometrium including gland tortuosity and secretion, stromal edema, and a decidual reaction

E Cycle integration. The integration of the menstrual cycle involves the interaction among **gonadotropin-releasing hormone** (GnRH) produced in the hypothalamus, the pituitary **gonadotropins** (FSH and LH), and the ovarian **sex steroids** (i.e., androstenedione, testosterone, estradiol, estrone, and progesterone).

II GONADOTROPIN-RELEASING HORMONE

GnRH is the hypothalamic hormone that controls gonadotropin release.

A Characteristics

1. This hormone, a decapeptide, is produced by hypothalamic neurons, principally from the arcuate nucleus, and is transported along axons that terminate in the median eminence around capillaries of the primary portal plexus.

2. It is secreted into the portal circulation, which carries it to the anterior lobe of the pituitary gland.

B Secretion

1. Gonadotropin-releasing hormone is secreted in a **pulsatile manner**; the amplitude and frequency of the secretions vary throughout the cycle.
  a. One pulse every 60 to 90 minutes is typical of the follicular phase.
  b. One pulse every 2 to 3 hours is typical of the luteal phase.

2. The **amplitude and frequency** are regulated by:
  a. Feedback of estrogen and progesterone
  b. Neurotransmitters within the brain, mainly the catecholamines dopamine (inhibitory) and norepinephrine (facilitatory)

C Action of GnRH on gonadotropin production

1. When GnRH binds to specific receptors on the surface membrane of target cells, it:
  a. Activates a second messenger, **adenyl cyclase**
  b. Changes the concentration of **cyclic adenosine monophosphate (cAMP)**

2. This stimulates the synthesis and storage of both FSH and LH from the same cell.

3. Gonadotropin-releasing hormone activates and moves gonadotropins from the reserve pool to a pool ready for secretion, which leads to their immediate release.

4. High, continuous, or prolonged GnRH exposure saturates the GnRH receptors and inhibits FSH and LH secretion. This is called desensitization or **down-regulation**.

III GONADOTROPINS: FOLLICLE-STIMULATING HORMONE AND LUTEINIZING HORMONE

A FSH is responsible for production of estrogen and growth of the follicle. **Follicle-stimulating hormone receptors** exist primarily on the ovarian **granulosa cell membrane**. FSH stimulates follicular growth by:

1. Increasing the number of FSH and LH receptors on granulosa cells.

2. Increasing the number of granulosa cells by stimulating granulosa cell mitosis in the presence of estrogen

3. Stimulating conversion of androgens to estrogens within the granulosa cell by the enzyme aromatase.

B LH is responsible for the initiation of the luteal phase (ovulation) and maintenance of the luteal phase of the menstrual cycle. **Luteinizing hormone receptors** exist on ovarian **theca cells** at all stages of the cycle and on **granulosa cells** after the follicle matures under the influence of FSH and estradiol.

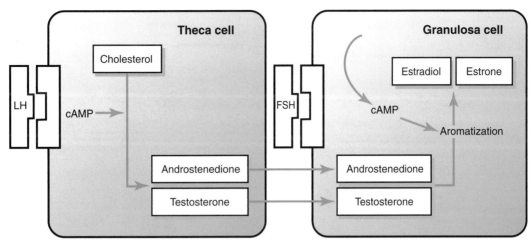

FIGURE 19–1 Two-cell hypothesis of estrogen production. cAMP, cyclic adenosine monophosphate; FSH, follicle-stimulating hormone; LH, luteinizing hormone. (Reprinted with permission from Speroff L, Glass RH, Kase NG. Regulation of the menstrual cycle. In: Speroff L, Glass RH, Kase NG, eds. Clinical Gynecologic Endocrinology and Infertility. 4th Ed. Baltimore: Williams & Wilkins, 1999:207.)

1. Luteinizing hormone stimulates **androgen synthesis** by the theca cells.

2. With a sufficient number of LH receptors on the granulosa cells, LH acts directly on the granulosa cells to cause ovulation.

3. Following ovulation, LH stimulates production of progesterone from the luteinized granulosa cells in the corpus luteum.

C **Two-cell hypothesis of estrogen production** (Fig. 19-1)

1. LH acts on the theca cells to stimulate the conversion of cholesterol to androgens (i.e., androstenedione and testosterone).

2. Androgens are transported from the theca cells to the granulosa cells.

3. Under the influence of FSH, androgens are aromatized to form estrogens (i.e., estradiol and estrone) by the enzyme aromatase in the granulosa cells.

IV OOGENESIS

A **Primordial follicle**

1. The primordial follicle contains an oocyte surrounded by a single layer of granulosa cells (Fig. 19-2).
   a. Each oocyte is arrested in **prophase** of the first meiotic division.

2. A woman is born with a finite number of oocytes, which peak at 6 to 7 million in the 20th week of gestation.
   a. There is a steady decline in the number of follicles from the 20th week of gestation until menopause. This decline is independent of the menstrual cycle and ovulation.
   b. Each month, a cohort of primordial follicles is stimulated to develop into preantral follicles. This process can be independent of gonadotropin stimulation.

B **Preantral follicle**

1. Under the influence of FSH, the number of granulosa cells in the primordial follicle increases.

2. FSH-induced aromatization of androgen results in the production of **estrogen**, which then:
   a. Stimulates preantral follicle growth
   b. Together with FSH, increases FSH receptor content of the follicle
   c. In the presence of FSH, stimulates mitosis of granulosa cells

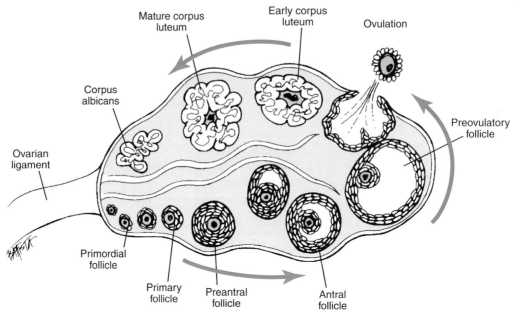

FIGURE 19–2 The process of oogenesis.

C Antral follicle

1. The follicle destined to become dominant secretes the greatest amount of estradiol, which, in turn, increases the density of the FSH receptors on the granulosa cell membrane.

2. Rising estradiol levels result in negative feedback and suppression of FSH release. The dominant follicle is able to respond to the decreasing concentration of FSH due to the greater number of FSH receptors.

3. The other follicles in the cohort become atretic due to fewer FSH receptors, less ability to aromatize androgens to estrogens, and therefore a predominantly androgenic environment.

4. The follicular rise of estradiol exerts a positive feedback on LH secretion.
   a. LH levels rise steadily during the late follicular phase.
   b. LH stimulates androgen production in the theca cells.
   c. The dominant follicle uses the androgen as substrate and further accelerates estrogen output.

5. FSH induces the appearance of LH receptors on granulosa cells.

6. Follicular response to the gonadotropins is modulated by a variety of growth factors.
   a. **Inhibin**, secreted by the granulosa cells in response to FSH
      (1) **Inhibin-A** under the influence of LH suppresses FSH during the luteal phase of the cycle.
      (2) **Inhibin-B** directly suppresses pituitary FSH secretion in the follicular phase of the cycle.
   b. **Activin** augments secretion of FSH and increases pituitary response to GnRH by enhancing GnRH receptor formation on the pituitary.

D Preovulatory follicle

1. Estrogens rise rapidly, reaching a peak approximately 24 to 36 hours before ovulation.

2. Luteinizing hormone increases steadily until midcycle, when there is a surge, which is accompanied by a lesser surge of FSH.

3. Luteinizing hormone initiates luteinization and progesterone production in the granulosa cells within the follicle.

4. The preovulatory rise in progesterone causes a midcycle FSH surge by enhancing pituitary response to GnRH and facilitating the positive feedback action of estrogen.

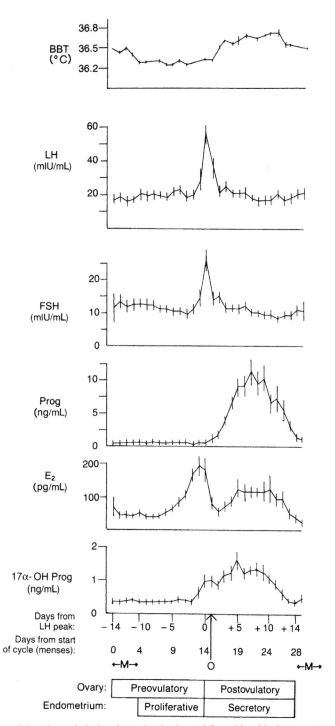

FIGURE 19–3 Hormonal (ovarian and pituitary), uterine (endometrial), and basal body temperature (BBT) correlates of the normal menstrual cycle. Mean plasma concentrations (±SEM) of luteinizing hormone (LH), follicle-stimulating hormone (FSH), progesterone (Prog), estradiol (E_2) [day +1], and 17α-hydroxyprogesterone (17α-OH Prog) are shown as a function of time. Ovulation occurs on day 15 (day +1) after the LH surge, which occurs at midcycle on day 14 (day 0). M, menses; O, ovulation. (Adapted from Thorneycroft IA, Mishell DR Jr, Stone SC, et al. The relation of serum 17-hydroxyprogesterone and estradiol 17-β levels during the human menstrual cycle. Am J Obstet Gynecol 1971;111:947–951.)

E **Ovulation** (Fig. 19-3)

    1. Ovulation occurs approximately 10 to 12 hours after the LH peak and 24 to 36 hours after the estradiol peak. The **onset of the LH surge**, which occurs 34 to 36 hours before ovulation, reliably indicates the timing of ovulation.

2. The **LH surge** stimulates the following:

    a. Resumption of meiosis in the oocyte. The LH surge is responsible for overcoming the oocyte's maturation inhibitor and allowing progression of the oocyte from prophase to metaphase II by the time the oocyte is released from the follicle. An oocyte can only be fertilized if it has progressed through metaphase II.

    b. Luteinization of the granulosa cells. These luteinized granulosa cells are now able to convert cholesterol to progesterone.

    c. Synthesis of progesterone and prostaglandins within the follicle. Prostaglandins and proteolytic enzymes are responsible for the digestion and rupture of the follicle wall leading to release of the oocyte.

F **Corpus luteum**

    1. Peak levels of progesterone are attained 7 to 8 days after ovulation.

    2. Normal luteal function requires optimal preovulatory follicular development.

        a. Suppression of FSH during the follicular phase is associated with:

            (1) Low preovulatory estradiol levels

            (2) Depressed midluteal progesterone production

            (3) Small luteal cell mass

        b. The accumulation of LH receptors during the follicular phase sets the stage for the extent of luteinization and the functional capacity of the corpus luteum.

    3. In the absence of pregnancy, the corpus luteum will undergo apoptosis and cease to produce progesterone by 12 to 14 days after ovulation.

    4. With implantation of an embryo, which occurs approximately 7 days after ovulation, the maternal circulation is exposed to fetal human chorionic gonadotropin (hCG).

    5. In early pregnancy, hCG maintains the secretion of progesterone from the corpus luteum, until placental steroidogenesis (production of progesterone) is established by about the eighth week of gestation.

V   MENSTRUATION

A In the absence of a pregnancy, the demise of the corpus luteum results in decreasing estrogen and progesterone levels, which leads to increased coiling and constriction of the spiral arteries in the endometrium.

    1. The decreased blood flow to the functional portion of the endometrium causes **ischemia** and degradation of endometrial tissue.

    2. The bleeding, or **menses**, is the result of the degraded endometrial tissue, which is desquamated, or shed, into the uterine cavity.

    3. The normal monthly menstrual flow is up to 80 mL of blood. This blood loss can lead to a lower hemoglobin in menstruating women.

B Within 2 days of the onset of menses, the surface epithelium begins to regenerate under the influence of estrogen and continues this process while the endometrium is shedding.

VI   CLINICAL PROBLEMS ASSOCIATED WITH THE MENSTRUAL CYCLE

A **Dysmenorrhea.** Painful menses usually begins with ovulatory menstrual periods and are the most common medical problem in young women. Dysmenorrhea typically does not occur in anovulatory cycles.

    1. Clinical aspects

        a. Dysmenorrhea begins just before or with the onset of menses and lasts 24 to 48 hours.

        b. The pain is suprapubic, sharp, and colicky.

        c. Nausea, diarrhea, and headache may accompany the pain.

        d. Pathologic conditions that cause dysmenorrhea must be considered in those women not responding to therapy. These include endometriosis, müllerian anomalies, and adenomyosis.

2. **Physiology**
   a. Menstrual cramps are the result of **uterine contractions**.
   b. **Prostaglandins** are potent **stimulators** of uterine contractions.
      (1) Endometrial prostaglandins are produced during the luteal phase. If ovulation does not occur, there is no luteal increase in prostaglandins.
      (2) In the first-day menstrual endometrium, the prostaglandin level increases until it is several times higher than its concentration in the luteal phase.

3. **Management**
   a. **Prostaglandin synthetase inhibitors** (e.g., nonsteroidal anti-inflammatory drugs) are first-line therapy because they:
      (1) Decrease levels of endometrial prostaglandin
      (2) Lessen uterine contractions
      (3) Relieve dysmenorrhea best when started prior to or at the first sign of menstrual flow
   b. **Combination** (estrogen plus progestin) **oral contraceptive agents** eliminate ovulation.
      (1) Estrogen followed by progesterone (in ovulatory cycles) is necessary to produce high menstrual levels of prostaglandin in the endometrium.
      (2) Combination oral contraceptives prevent dysmenorrhea by eliminating the natural estrogen-progesterone progression found only in ovulatory cycles.

B Premenstrual syndrome

1. **Definition**. Premenstrual syndrome (PMS) is a group of disorders and symptoms related to the menstrual cycle that include **premenstrual dysphoric disorder (PDD)**. Symptoms must:
   a. Be cyclic
   b. Be sufficiently severe to interfere with some aspects of life
   c. Have a consistent and predictable relationship to the menstrual cycle

2. **Epidemiology**
   a. Eighty percent of women report premenstrual symptoms, and 5% to 10% of women experience PMS that is severe enough to interfere with normal activities, such as work, study, parenting, or relationships.
   b. As many as 50% to 60% of women with severe PMS have an underlying psychiatric disorder.

3. **Etiology**
   a. The causes of PMS are not completely understood but involve fluctuation of ovarian steroids, central nervous system neurotransmitters, genetic predisposition, and psychosocial expectations.
   b. Causal factors include estrogen, progesterone, testosterone, and neurosteroids.
      (1) Symptoms are temporally associated with luteal-phase fluctuations in ovarian hormones. Serum levels of estrogen and progesterone are not diagnostic or predictive of PMS.
      (2) Cyclic ovarian hormone fluctuations are associated with changes in brain neurotransmitters and neurosteroids. Changes in brain chemistry may result in PMS symptoms in biologically susceptible women.

4. **Clinical manifestations**. The most commonly occurring symptoms of PMS are:
   a. Bloating or weight gain
   b. Breast tenderness
   c. Anxiety
   d. Irritability
   e. Food cravings or changes in appetite
   f. Poor concentration
   g. Sleep disturbances
   h. Depressive symptoms or dysphoria
   i. Affective lability
   j. Feeling overwhelmed

5. **Management** (based on the guidelines of the American College of Obstetricians and Gynecologists). Both the physiologic and the psychosocial aspects of PMS must be considered when designing a therapeutic program. Most treatments for PMS are aimed at alleviating symptoms. They include:

a. **Lifestyle changes** (i.e., regular exercise and a balanced diet, avoidance of stressful situations in the premenstrual phase of the cycle)

b. **Calcium supplementation**

c. **Oral contraceptives** (more effective taken continuously) for physical symptoms. These should not be used if mood symptoms are primary.

d. **Long-acting GnRH agonists**. These agents should be limited to short-term use because of long-term effects of hypoestrogenism and the resultant osteoporosis.

e. **Fluoxetine**, a serotonin reuptake inhibitor. This agent can help relieve symptoms of PMS when it is taken continuously throughout the menstrual cycle.

f. **Alprazolam**, a benzodiazepine that acts on the γ-aminobutyric acid receptor complex. This agent has been reported to be beneficial. Because of the addictive potential of alprazolam, it should be reserved for patients who can be monitored reliably and should be restricted to the luteal phase of the menstrual cycle.

Study Questions for Chapter 19

Directions: *Each of the numbered items or incomplete statements in this section is followed by answers or by completions of the statement. Select the ONE lettered answer or completion that is BEST in each case.*

1. A 24-year-old woman, gravida 1, para 1, is seeing you because every month since age 19 she has had severe lower pelvic pain during her periods. She says the pain is similar to "labor pains" and it interferes with her ability to concentrate at work and during leisure activities on the weekends. Her pain has also caused her to become extremely anxious and irritable. She has tried acetaminophen with little relief. She denies having a depressed mood or changes in sleep, energy, or eating patterns. Her past medical history is remarkable for mild asthma controlled with albuterol. She is sexually active, is in a monogamous relationship, and uses condoms for contraception. She has no known drug allergies but admits to drinking a few alcoholic beverages every day. The next step for this woman is:

- [A] Ibuprofen
- [B] Norgestimate plus ethinyl estradiol
- [C] Fluoxetine
- [D] Calcium
- [E] Leuprolide

2. Two female medical students are having a discussion about ovarian reserve. Medical student #1 claims that because women are born with a finite number of follicles and because she has been taking birth control pills since age 16, she has slowed down loss of her follicles every month by inhibiting ovulation. Medical student #2 claims that because she has been pregnant more times than medical student #1, she has a higher ovarian follicle reserve. Which of the following statements is true?

- [A] Medical student #1 has slowed down depletion of her eggs
- [B] Medical student #2 has slowed down depletion of her eggs
- [C] Medical student #1 has higher ovarian reserve than medical student #2
- [D] Both students have slowed down depletion of their eggs
- [E] There is no way to slow down depletion of eggs

3. Hormone X and Y are secreted in the follicular phase and are responsible for suppressing FSH in the late follicular phase prior to ovulation. Hormone Z is responsible for allowing the oocytes to progress through to metaphase II. What are hormones X, Y, and Z respectively?

- [A] Estrogen, progesterone, and LH
- [B] Estrogen, inhibin A, and FSH
- [C] Estrogen, activin, and FSH
- [D] Estrogen, inhibin A, and LH
- [E] Estrogen, inhibin B, and LH

4. Many infertility patients undergo in vitro fertilization (IVF) and embryo transfer (ET) in order to become pregnant. IVF-ET uses many of the principles of the normal menstrual cycle to achieve pregnancy. The patients are given FSH hormone to stimulate multifollicular development, just as occurs in the normal menstrual cycle. Human chorionic gonadotropin is used to "trigger" the ovulation process because it is an analog of LH hormone. Supplemental progesterone is given after the oocytes are retrieved to support the endometrium for implantation. Multiple follicles develop because:

- [A] In an IVF cycle LH hormone is not needed for follicular development
- [B] There is excess FSH available
- [C] hCG is more potent than natural LH
- [D] FSH induces LH release
- [E] Progesterone is not given until after the oocytes are retrieved

Answers and Explanations

1. The answer is A [VI A 3]. The clinical scenario presented here is describing dysmenorrhea (pain only during menses) and not premenstrual syndrome. The best treatment for this woman would be nonsteroidal anti-inflammatory agents (ibuprofen). If the ibuprofen did not relieve her symptoms, then hormonal contraception (norgestimate plus ethinyl estradiol) would be indicated. This medication would not only treat her dysmenorrhea, but would also have contraceptive benefits. Fluoxetine and calcium are useful for premenstrual syndrome, not dysmenorrhea. Leuprolide would suppress menstrual cycles, but is more appropriate for PMS and is associated with significant side effects.

2. The answer is E [IV A 2 a]. Ovarian reserve is primarily a function of age (time). Follicular atresia occurs independent of gonadotropin stimulation. There is continuous growth and atresia of primordial follicles occurring from fetal life through menopause. Pregnancy and oral contraception (i.e., anovulation) do not stop this process. Therefore, women lose a certain number of their follicles every month whether they ovulate or not. Follicular atresia can be increased by chemotherapy and radiation used for treatment of cancer.

3. The answer is D [IV C 2, IV C 5 a, IV E 2 a]. In the follicular phase estrogen and inhibin B both work to suppress FSH directly. This negative feedback leads to less FSH available to stimulate follicular development and as a result only one follicle becomes dominant (sometimes two or more can become dominant, resulting in twins or more). LH is responsible for the three components of ovulation: release of the oocytes from prophase I, together with FSH breakdown of the follicle wall facilitating release of the oocytes, and formation of the corpus luteum with production of progesterone from the luteinized granulosa cells. Inhibin A is important in the luteal phase of the cycle, where it suppresses FSH. Activin stimulates the release of FSH.

4. The answer is B [IV C 2]. During an IVF cycle FSH is given in excess so all the follicles are exposed to adequate stimulation to grow and develop. There is no negative feedback with the pituitary decreasing the FSH concentration leading to only one dominant follicle developing. Endogenous LH hormone is present in high enough concentration to stimulate conversion of cholesterol to androgens in an IVF cycle; additional LH hormone does not need to be given. Although hCG is a more stable compound and therefore preferable for triggering ovulation, both achieve the same result. FSH stimulates LH receptors on granulose cells so that ovulation can occur in response to the LH surge or exogenous hCG administration. Progesterone is not involved in multifollicular development.

chapter 20

Amenorrhea

CLARISA GRACIA • THOMAS A. MOLINARO

I INTRODUCTION

A **Amenorrhea** is the absence of menses for 6 months or longer. In reproductive-aged women, pregnancy should be excluded. The differential diagnosis for amenorrhea is listed in Table 20-1.

1. **Primary amenorrhea** is the absence of menses by 14 years of age in girls without appropriate development of secondary sexual characteristics or by 16 years of age regardless of secondary sex characteristic development.

2. **Secondary amenorrhea** is the cessation of menses for a period of 6 months or a three-cycle interval in women who have been menstruating regularly (most common presentation). Amenorrhea, or anovulatory cycles, is common in pregnancy, during the 2 to 5 years after menarche, and in women approaching menopause.

B **Normal menstrual cycle physiology** requires complex interactions between the hypothalamus, pituitary gland, and end organs (uterus and ovaries).

1. Hypothalamic *pulsatile* release of gonadotropin-releasing hormone (GnRH) secretion stimulates secretion of follicle-stimulating hormone (FSH) and luteinizing hormone (LH) from the anterior pituitary.

2. FSH stimulates a cohort of ovarian follicles to undergo growth and development.

3. Androgens produced in theca cells are converted to estrogens in granulosa cells by the enzyme aromatase.

4. Increasing estradiol levels exert negative feedback on FSH, and the follicle with the most FSH receptors becomes dominant. Other follicles undergo atresia. Estrogen causes endometrial gland proliferation.

5. Increasing levels of estradiol exert positive feedback on LH secretion from the pituitary resulting in the *LH surge*. Shortly after LH levels peak, ovulation occurs.

6. Granulosa cells produce progesterone during the luteal phase, resulting in luteinization of endometrial glands to their secretory form in preparation for a pregnancy. If pregnancy is not established, the corpus luteum regresses and menses ensues as the endometrium experiences progesterone withdrawal.

C Normal menstruation: anatomic requirements

1. Nonobstructed outflow tract

2. Estrogen-primed endometrium

3. Ovaries that are able to respond to FSH and LH, resulting in ovulation

4. Secretion of FSH and LH under the stimulation of GnRH, which is essential to ensure adequate development of a dominant follicle each month

II CLASSIFICATION AND ETIOLOGY OF AMENORRHEA

A **Categories** based on serum gonadotropin levels

1. **Hypergonadotropic**: elevated gonadotropins (typically FSH more than 20 IU/L; LH more than 40 IU/L)

Table 20–1 Differential Diagnosis for Amenorrhea

Hypergonadotropic Amenorrhea	Hypogonadotropic Amenorrhea	Eugonadotropic Amenorrhea
Premature ovarian failure	Anorexia	Androgen excess
45,X		PCOS
45,X/46,XX	Female athlete triad	NCAH
45,X/46,XY		
Deletions of long arm X		
Carriers of fragile X		
Autoimmune causes	Kallmann syndrome	Uterine/outflow disorders
Infectious		Müllerian agenesis
Chemotherapy/radiation	Postpill	Cervical agenesis
	Combined hormonal	Transverse vaginal septum
Turner syndrome 45X	Medroxyprogesterone (Depo-MPA)	Imperforate hymen
Gonadal dysgenesis	Medications	Androgen insensitivity
Swyer syndrome	Phenothiazines	
XY genotype	Reserpine	Asherman syndrome
	Ganglia blockers	
Gonadal agenesis		
	Hypothalamus-pituitary	
Resistant ovary syndrome	Pituitary adenoma	
	Craniopharyngioma	
Galactosemia	Panhypopituitarism	
	Empty sella syndrome	
Enzyme deficiencies		
17α-hydroxylase deficiency	Stress	
Aromatase deficiency		
	Systemic disease	
	β-Thalassemia major	
	Severe renal disease	
	Pubertal delay	

NCAH, nonclassic adrenal hyperplasia; PCOS, polycystic ovary syndrome.

2. **Hypogonadotropic:** low gonadotropin levels (typically FSH and LH less than 5 IU/L)

3. **Eugonadotropic:** normal gonadotropin levels (typically FSH and LH of 5 to 20 IU/L)

B **Hypergonadotropic amenorrhea** commonly, but not always, results from a chromosomal anomaly. The most common genotype is 45,X. Mosaicism (45,X/46,XX) may be seen, and structural aberrations of the X chromosome, including deletions in the long (q) arm, isochromosomes, or ring chromosomes, may occur. For patients with Y-bearing cell lines, gonadectomy should be performed to decrease the risk of future malignancy (e.g., dysgerminoma, gonadoblastoma, and choriocarcinoma). Menopause and premature ovarian failure also manifest as hypergonadotropic amenorrhea.

1. **Turner syndrome**
   a. The most common genotype is 45,X, which is accompanied by nonfunctional streak ovaries. Mosaicism (45,X/46,XX) may occur, and is often accompanied by functional ovarian tissue and leads to secondary amenorrhea.
   b. Phenotypic characteristics include short stature, webbed neck, shield chest, and increased carrying angle at the elbow. It is essential to rule out cardiovascular and renal anomalies in suspected cases.
   c. Other developmental characteristics include spontaneous puberty (10% to 20% of cases) and spontaneous menses (2% to 5% of cases).

2. **Premature ovarian failure**
   a. This condition is defined as secondary amenorrhea with ovarian failure before 40 years of age.
   b. Causes include:
      (1) Genetic (45,X; 45,X/46,XX; deletions in distal segment of the long arm of the X chromosome; fragile X carriers)
      (2) Autoimmune disease. Therefore, it is advisable to assess for the coexistence of other autoimmune diseases such as diabetes, thyroid disease, hyperparathyroidism, pernicious anemia, and hypoadrenalism. **The following laboratory studies may be helpful: fasting glucose, thyroid-stimulating hormone (TSH), thyroid antibodies, calcium, phosphorus, complete blood count, AM cortisol.**
      (3) Infectious (e.g., mumps)
      (4) Chemotherapy or radiation therapy

3. **Gonadal dysgenesis (XY genotype, Swyer syndrome)**
   a. The genotype is XY, and the phenotype is female.
   b. Symptoms and signs include lack of sexual development, a normal female testosterone level, and a palpable müllerian system.

4. **Gonadal agenesis (46,XX karyotype)**: development into prepubertal female

5. **Resistant ovary syndrome**
   a. This condition represents amenorrhea with normal growth and development.
   b. Signs include absent or defective gonadotropin *receptors* or a postreceptor signaling defect and unstimulated ovarian follicles.

6. **Galactosemia**
   a. This condition is an autosomal recessive deficiency in galactose-1-phosphate uridyltransferase activity.
   b. Decreased numbers of oogonia secondary to the toxic effects of galactose metabolites are characteristic.

7. **Enzyme deficiencies**
   a. **17α-Hydroxylase deficiency**
      (1) The ovaries and adrenal glands are affected.
      (2) Presenting signs include absent secondary sex characteristics, hypertension, hypokalemia, and elevated progesterone levels.
   b. **Decreased aromatase enzyme activity** results in lower estrogen levels.

C **Hypogonadotropic amenorrhea** is usually a result of a deficiency in GnRH pulsatile secretion from the hypothalamus. Hypogonadotropic amenorrhea may arise due to a lesion in the central nervous system (CNS) or be secondary to stress, less-than-normal weight, or an eating disorder.

1. **Anorexia**
   a. Anorexia occurs in 1% of all young women. It may identify a dysfunctional family unit.
   b. Signs and symptoms include amenorrhea, bradycardia, dry skin, hypothermia, lanugo hair, constipation, and edema. Bulimia (binging and purging with vomiting, laxatives, or diuretics) may be seen in 50% of patients.
   c. Laboratory markers include decreased FSH, LH, and triiodothyronine (T_3); increased cortisol and reverse T_3 and normal prolactin levels; TSH; and thyroxine (T_4).

2. **Female athlete triad.** This syndrome is defined as a triad of disordered eating, amenorrhea, and osteopenia or osteoporosis.
   a. It is felt to be caused by a mismatch between the energy taken in and the energy expended, leading to hypothalamic suppression.
   b. Body fat is a factor, but does not always explain the symptoms.
      (1) About 17% is necessary for initiating menarche.
      (2) About 22% is necessary for maintaining menstrual regularity.
   c. Associated laboratory results
      (1) Decreased FSH and LH
      (2) Increased prolactin, growth hormone, testosterone, adrenocorticotropic hormone (ACTH), adrenal steroids, and endorphins

3. Kallmann syndrome

a. Deficient secretion of GnRH is associated with anosmia or hyposmia. Kallmann syndrome involves the failure of olfactory axonal and GnRH neuronal migration from the olfactory placode in the nose.

b. Inheritance is either X-linked, autosomal dominant, or autosomal recessive.

c. Symptoms and signs include primary amenorrhea, normal karyotype, infantile sexual development, and the inability to perceive odors.

d. Possible coexisting features include bone and renal anomalies, cleft lip and palate, color blindness, or hearing deficit.

4. Postpill amenorrhea

a. Amenorrhea may occur 6 or more months after patients stop taking oral contraceptive pills or 12 months after they stop taking medroxyprogesterone (Depo-Provera).

5. Medications or drugs

a. Birth control pills may cause amenorrhea.

b. Drugs such as phenothiazine derivatives, reserpine, and ganglia blockers likely interfere with the levels of dopamine and norepinephrine; these agents are also associated with galactorrhea.

6. Pituitary diseases. Evaluation of the sella turcica using magnetic resonance imaging (MRI) with gadolinium or radiography is necessary. Pituitary tumors may be associated with visual changes, galactorrhea, and other hormone deficiencies, including hypothyroidism, amenorrhea, and Addison disease.

a. Craniopharyngioma

(1) Calcifications may be apparent on radiography of the sella turcica.

(2) Frequent manifestations include visual field defects and blurry vision.

b. Adenomas

(1) These tumors vary in size.

(a) Microadenomas (less than 10 mm)

(b) Macroadenomas (more than 10 mm)

(2) The most common are prolactinomas and nonfunctioning tumors.

(a) Elevated prolactin levels cause amenorrhea by suppressing GnRH secretion.

(b) Treatment may involve dopamine agonist therapy (i.e., bromocriptine), surgery, or, in severe cases, radiation therapy.

7. Stress leads to an increased output of corticotropin-releasing hormone, which subsequently results in decreased GnRH pulsatile secretion and thus decreased secretion of FSH and LH.

8. Delayed puberty: idiopathic or constitutional

D Eugonadotropic amenorrhea is a subgroup of amenorrhea that includes disorders of androgen excess and anomalies of the outflow tract or uterus.

1. Disorders of androgen excess: polycystic ovary syndrome

a. The triad of anovulation (or oligo-ovulation), obesity, and hirsutism (androgen excess) is characteristic. Diagnosis is made with inclusion of two of three criteria and exclusion of other causes of amenorrhea.

(1) Menstrual irregularity signifying oligo- or anovulation

(2) The appearance of multiple small ovarian cysts on ultrasound ("**string of pearls**")

(3) Clinical or laboratory evidence of hyperandrogenism

b. Tonically elevated LH and low-normal FSH result in the following events:

(1) Prevention of dominant follicle emergence

(2) Absence of ovulatory cycles

(3) Elevated levels of androgens produced from the theca cells

c. Sex hormone–binding globulin levels are decreased because of elevated levels of androgens.

d. Patients are at increased risk of endometrial hyperplasia secondary to higher levels of free estrogens, primarily estrone (a weakly active estrogen).

e. Evidence suggests that these patients are hyperinsulinemic; as such, they are at increased risk for diabetes mellitus, obesity, and cardiovascular disease.

f. A loss of only 5% to 10% of body weight may help patients re-establish ovulatory cycles.

2. **Disorders of the outflow tract or uterus**
    a. **Müllerian agenesis** (also known as Mayer-Rokitansky-Küster-Hauser syndrome)
        (1) The most common congenital anomaly of the uterus, müllerian agenesis occurs in 1 in 4000 births.
        (2) The underlying mechanism involves unwanted exposure to antimüllerian hormone activity with failed fusion of the müllerian ducts.
        (3) Absence or hypoplasia of the vagina, uterus, and tubes is characteristic. Thirty-three percent of patients may have urinary tract abnormalities, and another 12% may have skeletal anomalies.
        (4) Normal testosterone level differentiates this disorder from androgen insensitivity.
        (5) A renal ultrasound may be obtained to check for associated mesonephric anomalies.
    b. **Other müllerian anomalies**
        (1) **Cervical agenesis or dysgenesis** results in obstruction of flow from the uterus to the vagina and is associated with episodic or cyclic pain, which correlates with menstrual shedding. This is very rare.
        (2) **Transverse vaginal septum**. This anomaly results in occlusion in the upper, middle, or lower segment of the vagina. These patients present with episodic or cyclic pain symptoms.
        (3) **Imperforate hymen**. This anomaly is not technically a müllerian anomaly since the hymen is derived from the urogenital sinus, but it functions and is treated as such. It occurs in 0.1% of female newborns, and may not present until 6 to 12 months after the menstrual lining sheds for first time. The vagina may be distended with more than a liter of old menstrual blood.
    c. **Androgen insensitivity syndrome (AIS)**
        (1) Inheritance is X-linked recessive.
        (2) Patients have male gonads, a normal 46,XY male karyotype with normal male levels of testosterone, and elevated LH.
        (3) The defect is in the androgen receptor. Affected patients have androgen receptors and male levels of testosterone, but the receptors cannot respond to androgen. The affected individuals is phenotypically female, and is usually raised as female.
        (4) Patients have a blind vaginal canal and an absent uterus. Gonadal tissue may be present in the inguinal canal or labia. (The condition should be suspected in a female with bilateral inguinal hernias.)
        (5) Primary amenorrhea, absent uterus, and normal growth and development are evident. The testes are not capable of spermatogenesis.
        (6) **This condition must be differentiated from müllerian agenesis**. Patients with AIS will have absent or sparse pubic and axillary hair, and testosterone levels will be in the male range. Breasts develop normally as significant testosterone is converted to estrogen.
        (7) Gonadectomy must be performed due to the risk of gonadoblastoma, but this condition is one of the only cases in which gonadectomy may be deferred until after puberty.
    d. **Asherman syndrome**
        (1) Intrauterine scarring is usually a result of vigorous curettage during a hypoestrogenic state or in the presence of an intrauterine infection (e.g., postpartum curettage for retained products of conception). However, it may be secondary to other uterine surgical procedures.
        (2) Cyclic pain and bloating, with absent or scant menses, may also occur.
        (3) A high degree of suspicion, with appropriate history, should be maintained.
    e. **Infection**. Tuberculosis and schistosomiasis may cause amenorrhea, usually secondary to intrauterine scarring and adhesions.

III CLINICAL EVALUATION

A **Serum human chorionic gonadotropin (hCG)** to evaluate for pregnancy should be performed in all women with primary or secondary amenorrhea.

B History and physical to evaluate for clues to determine etiology

1. **History**
   a. Review pediatric growth and development charts.
   b. Take a comprehensive menstrual history including age of menarche, duration of menses, and symptoms.
   c. Inquire about childhood or chronic illnesses and medication use.
   d. Ask about sexual history and use of illegal drugs.
   e. Ask about eating habits, exercise patterns, and self-image concerns.
   f. Perform a detailed review of systems, checking for the following conditions:
      (1) Hyperprolactinemia: galactorrhea and amenorrhea
      (2) Hyperthyroidism: nervousness, heart palpitations, weight loss, and heat intolerance
      (3) Hypothyroidism: fatigue, weight gain, and cold intolerance
      (4) Hypothalamic dysfunction or tumor: visual changes or hearing loss
      (5) Outlet obstruction: cyclic pain or bloating
      (6) Ovarian follicle depletion or dysfunction: vasomotor symptoms
      (7) Hyperandrogenic states: hirsutism or signs of virilization (e.g., clitoromegaly, deepening voice, and increased muscle mass)

2. **Physical**
   a. Determine height and weight, calculate the body mass index, assess body habitus, and take vital signs (Cushing disease or steroid use).
   b. Check for cachexia, hypotension, hypothermia, or bradycardia (anorexia).
   c. Palpate thyroid gland.
   d. Assess visual fields and cranial nerves (Kallmann syndrome or pituitary tumor).
   e. Use the Tanner staging of breast and pubic hair development to assess pubertal development, galactorrhea, or androgen excess.
   f. Perform an abdominal examination to check for masses (e.g., pregnancy or ovarian masses).
   g. Examine the genitals and perianal area. (Clitoromegaly may signify androgen excess.)
   h. Check for Turner stigmata (e.g., short stature, webbed neck, or shield chest).
   i. Perform a pelvic examination.
      (1) Check for normal anatomic structures (i.e., presence of vagina and uterus).
      (2) Rule out ovarian masses. If pelvic examination is not sufficient, pelvic ultrasound or a rectoabdominal examination may be necessary.

C **Laboratory evaluation** (Fig. 20-1)

1. **β-hCG to evaluate for pregnancy**

2. **TSH**: treat hypothyroidism with replacement therapy.

3. **Prolactin**: treat hyperprolactinemia with dopamine agonist (cabergoline, pergolide, bromocriptine) after MRI to rule out macroadenoma.

4. **FSH, estradiol**: to determine if patient is hypergonadotropic, hypogonadotropic, or eugonadotropic
   a. In the case of hypergonadotropic amenorrhea, a karyotype should be checked; if normal, then evaluate for other autoimmune disorders.
   b. In hypogonadotropic amenorrhea, an MRI should be obtained to rule out intracranial pathology.
   c. In eugonadotropic amenorrhea, estrogen and progesterone withdrawal may be performed to assess whether an outflow tract abnormality exists; ultrasound MRI of the pelvis may be helpful in these cases as well. In the absence of a structural defect, anovulation is present.

5. Things to consider:
   a. In the case of hypogonadotropic or eugonadotropic amenorrhea, FSH levels may be low or in the normal range, sometimes making diagnosis difficult.
   b. In the patient with pubertal delay, a bone age is helpful to distinguish constitutional delay from true delayed puberty.

IV **MANAGEMENT**

A **Hypergonadotropic amenorrhea**

1. **Hormone replacement therapy**. This treatment aims to prevent bone loss, vasomotor symptoms, urogenital atrophy, and cardiovascular disease due to lack of estrogen.

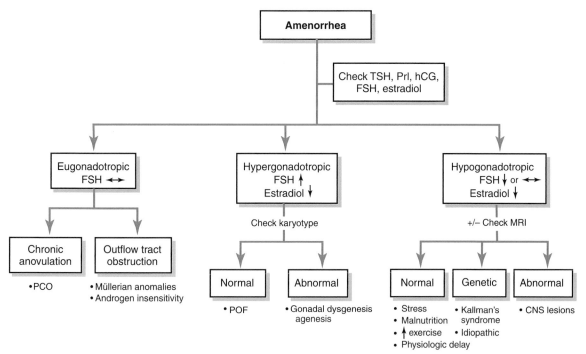

FIGURE 20–1 The laboratory evaluation in amenorrhea. CNS, central nervous system; FSH, follicle-stimulating hormone; hCG, human chorionic gonadotropin; MRI, magnetic resonance imaging; PCO, polycystic ovary syndrome; POF, premature ovarian failure; Prl, prolactin; TSH, thyroid-stimulating hormone.

  a. Estrogen replacement therapy
    (1) Conjugated estrogens or estradiol may be used.
    (2) Estrogen therapy is appropriate for women without a uterus; unopposed estrogen therapy in women with a uterus may lead to endometrial hyperplasia or cancer.
    (3) Administration is daily.
  b. Combined hormone replacement therapy
    (1) Agents
      (a) Conjugated estrogens or estradiol is used in combination with a progestin to protect the endometrium against hyperplasia or cancer.
      (b) Oral contraceptive pills may be used in women who do not desire pregnancy, or in adolescents.

2. **Removal of Y-containing gonads**
  a. In women with a Y-containing karyotype, gonadectomy should be performed to prevent increased transformation into malignant tissue (e.g., gonadoblastoma, dysgerminoma, yolk sac tumor, or choriocarcinoma).
  b. The gonad should be removed as soon as it is detected, except in the case of androgen insensitivity syndrome, where gonadectomy should occur after completion of puberty.

3. **Pregnancy**. Although it is unlikely (but not impossible) that these women will become pregnant with their own oocytes, oocyte donation is an excellent option for these patients. The ultimate success rate depends on the age of the donor (younger age generally means healthier oocytes).

B **Hypogonadotropic amenorrhea.** The mainstay of therapy is treatment of the underlying cause and hormone replacement. In the case of intracranial tumors or adenomas, medical or surgical measures may be necessary.

1. **Hormone replacement therapy** (IV A 1 a–b)
  a. Therapeutic hormones are essential in cases of anorexia or exercise-induced amenorrhea where gonadotropin and estradiol levels are excessively low and if lifestyle changes or therapy has failed to result in menses. Options include conjugated estrogens or estradiol with a progestin to induce menstrual withdrawal bleeding.
  b. Oral contraceptives provide hormonal replacement and contraceptive benefits.

2. **Pregnancy**. Patients who want to become pregnant may be given injectable recombinant gonadotropins. The GnRH pump is also effective, but this option is less popular because it is difficult to use and maintain.

3. **Pituitary tumors**
   a. Asymptomatic nonfunctioning adenoma
      (1) Close surveillance is usually sufficient.
      (2) Treatment with surgery is necessary with symptom occurrence or growth of the adenoma.
   b. Prolactinoma (microadenoma or macroadenoma)
      (1) Medical therapy with a dopamine agonist (bromocriptine, cabergoline) for microadenomas
      (2) For macroadenomas, transsphenoidal resection of the pituitary may be required if medical management fails. In rare cases, surgery may be combined with radiation therapy. Usually, the symptoms can be well controlled.
   c. Craniopharyngiomas and other central nervous system tumors are usually amenable to surgical resection.

4. **Hypothyroidism**. Hypothyroidism is easily treated with T_4 replacement, which re-establishes ovulatory cycles.

C Eugonadotropic amenorrhea. Treatment of disorders of androgen synthesis involves managing the symptoms primarily. The occurrence of a congenital anomaly of the outflow tract usually requires surgery.

1. **Disorders of androgen synthesis (e.g., polycystic ovary syndrome)**
   a. Oral contraceptive pills are useful for anovulatory or oligo-ovulatory patients.
      (1) The progestin component suppresses endogenously elevated LH levels, thereby decreasing androgen overproduction.
      (2) The estrogen component of the pill increases the sex hormone–binding globulin level, thereby decreasing the amounts of free estrogens and androgens.
      (3) The pills also provide contraception.
   b. Cyclic progestins are useful for patients who cannot tolerate or who have contraindications to oral contraceptives.
      (1) Cyclic progestins re-establish monthly bleeding, thereby protecting the endometrium against hyperplasia or cancer.
      (2) Administration is for at least 10 to 12 days each month for maximal endometrial protection.

2. **Treatment of related infertility**
   a. **Clomiphene**. Ovulation induction is used to establish ovulatory cycles.
      (1) The drug may be used with timed intercourse or intrauterine insemination.
      (2) In cases of clomiphene resistance, insulin-sensitizing medications may be used concomitantly, often improving the response to the drug.
      (3) In hyperandrogenic women who respond poorly to clomiphene, some experts advocate the use of dexamethasone at bedtime to decrease the endogenous androgen levels.
      (4) If patients do not respond to clomiphene or dexamethasone, injectable recombinant gonadotropin medications are often used, either in combination with intrauterine insemination or in vitro fertilization.
   b. **Ovarian drilling**. In refractory cases, multiple holes may be drilled into the ovary with electrocautery or laser at laparoscopic surgery to decrease the amount of androgen-producing tissue. However, excessive scar tissue may form after this procedure. Scar tissue may result in blockage of the fallopian tube or pelvic pain.
   c. **Hirsutism**. Several medications can be used to treat hirsutism. These medications serve as androgen receptor blockers or 5α-reductase inhibitors. In these cases, preexisting hair growth is not removed, but new hair growth is inhibited. In the most severe cases, patients may resort to electrolysis, shaving, or depilatory creams.

3. **Asherman syndrome or intrauterine adhesions**
   a. Adhesiolysis may be performed hysteroscopically under direct visualization.
   b. After the adhesiolysis, patients are placed on estrogens postoperatively for 3 to 4 weeks, ending with a course of progestin to promote re-epithelialization of the cavity and subsequent menses.

    c. Other experts advocate intrauterine placement of a Foley balloon to prevent reapposition of the uterine cavity.

4. Congenital anomalies

    a. In the absence of a uterus and vagina, a neovagina may be created with either a surgical procedure or the use of graduated dilators. This requires motivation on the part of the patient.

    b. Patients with no uterus and vagina have ovaries because the ovaries are not part of the müllerian system. Therefore, pregnancy is possible. Patients who are 46, XX can be stimulated to produce multiple follicles, undergo oocyte retrieval, and have the embryos transferred to a gestational carrier.

    c. Patients with androgen insensitivity have no ovaries, and a neovagina may be created; the Y-containing gonads must be removed after pubertal development. These patients should be placed on lifelong estrogen replacement therapy (see IV A 1).

    d. Cervical agenesis is treated by removal of the abnormal cervix and uterus. Trying to preserve fertility by surgically connecting the uterus to the vagina has resulted in infection, multiple surgeries, and death.

    e. Transverse vaginal septum and imperforate hymen are corrected surgically by resecting the septum or hymen to establish vaginal patency. This procedure can be very complicated with a high transverse vaginal septum.

Study Questions for Chapter 20

Directions: *Each of the numbered items or incomplete statements in this section is followed by answers or by completions of the statement. Select the ONE lettered answer or completion that is BEST in each case.*

1. A 24-year-old nulligravid woman presents to your office because of amenorrhea of 4 months' duration. She was started on birth control pills at the age of 18 due to irregular menses. She continued the pills until 4 months ago when she was in a terrible motorcycle accident and had to undergo multiple surgeries on her face to repair fractures. Her past medical and surgical history is unremarkable. Her physical examination is normal. You obtain labs, which reveal the following: hCG less than 5 mIU/mL, prolactin = 12, TSH = 2.2, FSH = 67, estradiol less than 30 pg/mL. Which one of the following is the most likely diagnosis?

- A Stress-induced amenorrhea from the accident
- B Swyer syndrome
- C Turner syndrome
- D Androgen insensitivity syndrome
- E Müllerian anomaly

2. An 18-year-old nulligravid female is seeing you because she has not had a period for the last 8 months. She is a freshman in college majoring in dance. She enjoys hiking to relieve stress. She is sexually active. She began her menses at age 13 and had irregular periods for the first 2 years and then became regular. She is 5 feet 8 inches tall and weighs 90 lb. Her vitals are as follows: T = 96.6, BP = 108/60, P = 52. On examination, she has a normal-appearing vulva and appropriate-sized vagina without any lesions. Her cervix and uterus are unremarkable. You do not appreciate any adnexal masses or tenderness. The rest of her physical examination is unremarkable other than her teeth, on which you see erosion of the upper and lower incisors, especially posteriorly. She also has small scars on the back of her hands. The most likely hormone abnormality in this patient is

- A Increased T_4
- B Decreased FSH
- C Increased TSH
- D Decreased cortisol
- E Increased prolactin

QUESTIONS 3–4

A 25-year-old nulligravid female presents to your office because she has not had a period for the last year. She didn't think too much of it initially due to her hectic schedule, but is concerned now because she recently started a serious relationship. Although she admits she is not yet ready to become pregnant, she wants to have regular periods. She has no significant medical or surgical history. She started her periods at age 12 and they became regular at age 14 until last year. She has never had a major illness. She has no known allergies to medications. She is a major bank executive who travels across the United States and Europe often. She runs 5 miles a day and uses a Jacuzzi often to relax. Her vital signs are as follows: T = 98.9, BP = 135/86, P = 100. Her physical examination reveals a height of 5 feet 6 inches and a weight of 132 lb. The rest of her examination is unremarkable. Labs are as follows: TSH = 1.7, prolactin = 11, FSH = 5.0, estradiol = 45.

3. Abnormality of which structure most likely accounts for her amenorrhea?

- A Hypothalamus
- B Pituitary
- C Ovaries
- D Uterus
- E Vagina

4. The best next step in management of this patient is:

[A] Norgestimate and ethinyl estradiol
[B] Conjugated estrogen and medroxyprogesterone acetate
[C] Clomiphene
[D] GnRH pump
[E] Buspirone

5. A 16-year-old presents to you because she has never had a period. She has no past medical or surgical history. She has never had a major illness. She has no known drug allergies. She is a senior in high school and has been accepted to an Ivy League university. In addition to her excellent academic performance, she is active as a volunteer in the community and enjoys tennis and volleyball. She is 5 feet 7 inches tall and weighs 125 lb. Her vital signs are as follows: T = 98.7, BP = 110/70, P = 70. Her abdomen is unremarkable. She has Tanner stage 4 breast development, axillary hair growth, and pubic hair growth onto her thighs. On sterile speculum examination you discover a short vagina that ends blindly. The diagnosis is:

[A] Androgen insensitivity syndrome
[B] Swyer syndrome
[C] 17α-hydroxylase deficiency
[D] Mayer-Rokitansky-Küster-Hauser syndrome
[E] Kallmann syndrome

Answers and Explanations

1. The answer is C [II B 1]. This patient has hypergonadotropic amenorrhea. The most likely diagnosis is an abnormal karyotype, most common being Turner syndrome 45,X or Turner mosaic 45,X/46,XX. Not all patients with Turner syndrome display the characteristic physical findings. Many patients with Turner syndrome present with secondary amenorrhea. It is important to make sure that there is no Y chromosome present, since this would dictate removal of the gonads. The amenorrhea is unlikely due to stress because that is associated with a low FSH. Androgen insensitivity syndrome is associated with an absent müllerian system, so menstruation would not be possible. Swyer syndrome is associated with primary amenorrhea, which this patient did not have. Her physical examination is normal and her menstrual bleeding is intact; therefore, she cannot have an obstructive müllerian anomaly or absent uterus.

2. The answer is B [II C 1 c]. The clinical scenario described in this question is anorexia nervosa (binging type). She is below the ideal body weight for her height. She has many classic features (amenorrhea, bradycardia, hypothermia, dry skin, erosion of her teeth from stomach acid caused by repetitive induced vomiting, and scars on the back of her hands from inducing vomiting). Patients with anorexia nervosa have decreased gonadotropins (low LH and FSH) and low estrogen, both of which cause amenorrhea. They also have low free T_3 but normal levels of free T_4, TSH, and prolactin. They also have elevated cortisol (because it is a "stress"-related hormone).

3. A [II C 1 and 2], **4. A** [IV B 1 b]. Any type of excessive stress in the form of lifestyle (e.g., busy executive), exercise (e.g., ballet dancer or marathon runner), or major illness (e.g., chronic kidney or lung disease) changes neurotransmitter function within the hypothalamus. Therefore, stress causes hypothalamic dysfunction resulting in changes in the GnRH pulse, which results in low levels of LH and FSH. With hypothalamic amenorrhea, the FSH may be low or normal as in this patient. Before assuming that stress is the cause of her amenorrhea, an MRI of the brain should be performed to evaluate for CNS lesions. The optimal medical treatment of hypogonadotropic amenorrhea is either hormone replacement therapy (e.g., conjugated estrogen or estradiol with progestin) or birth control pills (e.g., norgestimate and ethinyl estradiol). Because this patient is not ready for pregnancy, the latter treatment is more reasonable. Buspirone can be given to a young patient with general anxiety disorder. Clomiphene is used to stimulate follicle development and is therefore not necessary for this patient. A GnRH pump, which is difficult to administer and maintain, is not useful for this patient because she is not trying to become pregnant.

5. The answer is D [II D 2 a] The most common disorder of the outflow tract and the second most common cause of primary amenorrhea is called Mayer-Rokitansky-Küster-Hauser syndrome. Patients with this syndrome have a normal female karyotype with normal ovarian function; therefore, growth and development is normal. The development of the uterus, cervix, and vagina, however, is abnormal. These patients usually have an absent or very short vagina. They lack a uterus and fallopian tubes or can have rudimentary uterine cords that do not connect to the introitus. There is a 33% association with urinary tract abnormalities and only a 12% association with skeletal abnormalities. It is important to distinguish this syndrome from androgen insensitivity syndrome. Individuals with SID have sparse or absent axillary and pubic hair and relatively normal breast size. A testosterone level or karyotype can distinguish between the two. If the individual has AIS, then her gonads need to be removed due to the risk of developing cancer. In Swyer syndrome, a phenotypic female patient with an XY karyotype has a palpable müllerian system, normal female testosterone levels, and lack of sexual development. The syndrome characterized by 17α-hydroxylase deficiency is marked by hypertension, hypokalemia, and elevated progesterone levels in addition to absent sexual development. Kallmann syndrome is amenorrhea caused by hypothalamic dysfunction along with anosmia.

chapter 21

Polycystic Ovary Syndrome

MONICA A. MAINIGI • SAMANTHA M. PFEIFER

I INTRODUCTION

First defined in 1935, Stein and Leventhal described a condition of obesity, amenorrhea, bilateral polycystic ovaries, and "masculinizing changes." More than 70 years later this condition, now known as polycystic ovary syndrome (PCOS), still remains incompletely understood. However, it is now known that polycystic ovary syndrome is the most common cause of menstrual irregularities and infertility in women. The prevalence of PCOS is thought to be between 4% and 10% of reproductive-aged women and varies among race and ethnicity. Using these statistics, there are an estimated 4 to 5 million women of reproductive age affected by PCOS.

II DEFINITION

A **Rotterdam criteria.** In 2003 there was a meeting that took place in Rotterdam to determine a consensus about the diagnostic criteria for PCOS. Up to this point Americans viewed PCOS as primarily an endocrine disorder diagnosed by hormonal testing, while Europeans diagnosed the syndrome primarily by the ultrasound appearance of the ovaries. The following criteria were put forth in an effort to standardize the diagnosis of PCOS. These criteria require two out of three of the following to make a diagnosis in addition to exclusion of other causes of hyperandrogenism and oligomenorrhea (Table 21-1).

1. **Menstrual irregularities.** Most patients with PCOS have menstrual irregularities that begin during adolescence.
   a. **Oligomenorrhea**: less than nine menses per year
   b. **Amenorrhea**: no menses for 6 months or three or more skipped cycles
   c. As a result of irregular ovulation, these women lack adequate progesterone and experience chronic estrogen exposure to the endometrium. This can result in breakthrough or irregular uterine bleeding and can put these patients at increased risk for endometrial hyperplasia and endometrial cancer.

2. **Hyperandrogenism.** Patients may either show signs of clinical hyperandrogenism or have biochemical hyperandrogenism.
   a. **Clinical hyperandrogenism.** Women with PCOS may exhibit hirsutism, acne, or male pattern hair loss.
   (1) Hirsutism is defined as excess pigmented hair in a male pattern, most commonly found on the upper lip, chin, neck, midline on the chest, and lower abdomen. Male pattern baldness is also associated with hyperandrogenism.
   (2) A formal scoring system, known as the Ferriman-Gallwey score, can be used to clinically evaluate hirsutism and a score greater than or equal to 8 is considered abnormal.
   (3) Acne is a very sensitive clinical sign of hyperandrogenism, especially in adolescents and those of Asian descent, who in general have less body hair.
   (4) The rate of hair growth is also clinically important. PCOS is associated with a slow but progressive hair growth. A rapid onset of hirsutism or acne suggests an ovarian or adrenal androgen-producing tumor or drug exposure. In addition, more severe signs of hyperandrogenism such as enlarging of the clitoris or deepening of the voice are rare with PCOS, and are more consistent with tumor or drug exposure.

227

TABLE 21–1 Differential Diagnosis for Polycystic Ovary Syndrome
Nonclassic adrenal hyperplasia
Cushing syndrome
Androgen-producing tumor: adrenal, ovary
Thyroid disease
Hyperprolactinemia
Ovarian failure
Drug exposure

   b. Biochemical hyperandrogenism. Up to 90% of women with PCOS have elevated serum androgen concentration. However, the androgen levels may be normal.
   (1) Typically, testosterone and free testosterone are measured. Extremely high levels of testosterone (greater than 200 ng/dL) suggest an ovarian or adrenal tumor.
   (2) Recently, androstenedione has been suggested as a better marker of androgen excess.
   (3) Dehydroepiandrosterone sulfate (DHEAS) is a marker of adrenal androgen production but is not necessary to measure when considering the diagnosis of PCOS. DHEAS levels greater than 800 ng/dL suggest an adrenal tumor, but this is very rare.

3. **Polycystic ovaries.** A diagnosis of polycystic-appearing ovaries can be made using pelvic ultrasound.
   a. PCOS by ultrasound criteria is defined as 12 or more antral follicles between 2 and 9 mm in size and peripheral in location in at least one ovary (often referred to as the "string of pearls sign").
   b. Transvaginal ultrasound is more sensitive, but may not be appropriate to perform in a young female.
   c. The inclusion of polycystic ovaries in the diagnostic criteria for PCOS remains controversial because of the high incidence of polycystic-appearing ovaries in normal women (12% to 15%) and in women with other causes of hyperandrogenism and oligomenorrhea (up to 100%). However, including this in the diagnostic criteria may encompass more of the spectrum of the disease.

4. **Exclusion of other causes of hyperandrogenism** includes evaluating for:
   a. Nonclassic adrenal hyperplasia
   b. Cushing syndrome
   c. Androgen-producing tumor (both ovarian and adrenal)
   d. Exogenous steroid hormones and drugs with hyperandrogenic effect
   e. Thyroid and prolactin disorders
   f. Premature ovarian failure

III GENETICS AND ETIOLOGY OF PCOS

PCOS is thought to have a multifactorial etiology. Although there is a genetic component, the manifestation of the syndrome is thought to be influenced by nonhereditary factors as well.

A **Genetic studies.** Multiple studies have looked at the inheritance pattern of PCOS.
   1. The prevalence of PCOS among first-degree relatives appears to be between 35% and 40%.
   2. Among siblings of women with PCOS who do not meet the criteria for diagnosis, there appears to be increased rates of either isolated hyperandrogenemia or asymptomatic polycystic ovaries by imaging studies.
   3. The rates of insulin resistance among family members of patients with PCOS also appears to be significantly greater than that of the general population.

B **Candidate genes**
   1. Although PCOS appears to have a genetic origin, at this point no single gene has emerged as a leading candidate in the pathogenesis of PCOS.

2. Candidate genes that have been investigated include genes involved in androgen biosynthesis, secretion, transport, and metabolism, as well as genes involved in the insulin signaling pathway.

IV ▪ PATHOPHYSIOLOGY

The development of the symptoms and signs of PCOS is the result of several abnormalities leading to a state of hyperandrogenism. These include increased gonadotropin-releasing hormone (GnRH) and hyperinsulinism.

A ▪ Increased luteinizing hormone (LH)

1. Women with PCOS have been found to have **increased LH pulse frequency and amplitude** stimulated by GnRH. It is unclear whether this abnormal GnRH secretion is a result of the lack of the feedback mechanism because of the low progesterone levels or an intrinsic defect in GnRH pulse generator.

2. LH stimulates production of **androgens from the theca cells in the ovary** leading to hyperandrogenism. In women without PCOS, much of the androgens are then transported to the granulosa cells and aromatized to estrogens. In patients with PCOS, this stimulation results in hyperandrogenism.

B ▪ Insulin resistance.
Insulin resistance is defined as a decreased ability of insulin to act on peripheral tissues to stimulate glucose metabolism or inhibit hepatic glucose output. This results in hyperinsulinemia. In women with PCOS **insulin resistance is present independent of obesity**. In PCOS selective insulin resistance has been demonstrated: glucose transport and metabolic actions of glucose are affected, but insulin's ability to stimulate ovarian steroidogenesis is preserved. **Insulin has been shown to increase production of androgens in women with PCOS**. Proposed mechanisms include:

1. Direct stimulation of androgens from theca cells. Insulin has been shown to increase production of androgens from theca cells by acting through its own receptor or through insulin-like growth factor (IGF)-I receptor binding.

2. A postreceptor binding defect in the insulin receptor. Normally insulin action is mediated through tyrosine phosphorylation that occurs as a consequence of insulin binding to its receptor. In women with PCOS there appears to be increased serine phosphorylation, which leads to inhibition of glucose action but increased production of androgens.

3. Insulin has been shown to work synergistically with LH to increase theca cell androgen production, possibly through insulin receptors or IGF receptors on the cells. Insulin may also increase androgen production by the adrenal glands.

4. Insulin also decreases the production of sex hormone–binding globulin (SHBG) produced by the liver. This in turn decreases the amount of testosterone bound to SHBG and therefore increases the free metabolically active testosterone.

C ▪ Resulting hyperandrogenism.
Elevated androgen levels in patients with PCOS not only are the result of elevated LH secretion by the pituitary and insulin resistance, but are also due to intrinsic differences between the theca cells of PCOS and control patients.

1. Patients with PCOS at baseline have been found to have elevated 17α-hydroxylase expression in their theca cells and are therefore more efficient at converting androgen precursors to testosterone compared with controls.

2. In addition, the hypertrophy of the theca cells in PCOS may also contribute to increased ovarian androgen production

3. Adrenal androgens have also been noted to be elevated in at least a subset of PCOS patients, suggesting that a defect in the androgen synthesis pathway may be responsible for the phenotype seen.

V HEALTH CONSEQUENCES

PCOS is a metabolic disorder and is associated with the development of other medical conditions. Identifying the patient with PCOS is important so that these conditions can be identified and ideally prevented.

A Diabetes

1. In studies of women with PCOS, the incidence of diabetes has been shown to be as high as 10%.

2. Impaired glucose tolerance diagnosed by a 2-hour glucose tolerance test is seen in approximately 35% of women with PCOS. Impaired glucose tolerance is considered a precursor to diabetes and therefore, if treated, can prevent the development of diabetes.

3. The incidence of diabetes and impaired glucose tolerance in thin women with PCOS has not been determined but may not be as high.

B Obesity

1. Obesity has been reported in between 20% and 80% of all patients with PCOS. The obesity is most often a central obesity with an android appearance and an increased waist-to-hip ratio.

2. Obesity is related to insulin resistance. The incidence of insulin resistance in women with PCOS has been demonstrated to be as high as 60%, but assessing insulin resistance is problematic, and it has been proposed that all women with PCOS are insulin resistant.

3. Women with PCOS find it more difficult to lose weight and appear to gain weight more easily.

C Metabolic syndrome is a constellation of cardiovascular disease risk factors associated with insulin resistance including glucose intolerance, dyslipidemia, hypertension, and central obesity. This syndrome is seen in some but not all women with PCOS.

D Cardiovascular disease. Women with PCOS have many risk factors for cardiovascular disease. These include obesity, hyperlipidemia, high testosterone, and insulin resistance. However, a higher incidence of cardiovascular disease has not been demonstrated in these women. More research is needed to clarify this.

E Endometrial hyperplasia. Menstrual irregularities are primarily on the basis of anovulation. These can range from amenorrhea to continuous bleeding and menorrhagia (excessive flow). The concern in these women is that anovulation places the woman at risk of developing endometrial hyperplasia, which, if left untreated, can progress to endometrial cancer. Therefore, in a woman with PCOS of any age, abnormal bleeding should be evaluated, endometrial biopsy considered, and treatment initiated.

F Infertility. Infertility is associated with PCOS. The cause of the infertility in these women is primarily anovulation. These women may also be at an increased risk for miscarriages, but this has not been confirmed.

VI DIFFERENTIAL DIAGNOSIS

In order to make a diagnosis of PCOS, other causes of ovulatory disorders and hyperandrogenism must be excluded.

A Nonclassic adrenal hyperplasia (NCAH)

1. The enzyme defects in adrenal hyperplasia disrupt the normal pathway converting cholesterol to sex steroids and mineralocorticoids. The most common enzymatic defect in NCAH is 21-hydroxylase deficiency; the lesser two are 3β-hydroxysteroid dehydrogenase deficiency and 11β-hydroxylase deficiency.

2. The defect in 21-hydroxylase leads to accumulation of the precursor 17-hydroxy progesterone (17OHP) in the adrenal gland. This in turn results in elevated production of androstenedione and testosterone.

3. 21-Hydroxylase deficiency is an autosomal recessive disorder. The gene is located on chromosome 6. It is most common in those of Eastern European Jewish, Hispanic, Slavic, and Italian descent.

4. Nonclassic adrenal hyperplasia often presents with premature adrenarche and sometimes premature puberty. The symptoms are very similar to PCOS, the most common being primary amenorrhea, oligomenorrhea, hirsutism, and infertility.

5. The diagnosis is made by checking the 17-hydroxyprogesterone level at 8 AM and in the follicular phase of the menstrual cycle.
   a. 17-Hydroxyprogesterone less than 200 ng/dL: normal
   b. 17-Hydroxyprogesterone greater than 200 ng/dL and less than 400 ng/dL: indeterminate, requires further testing
   c. 17-Hydroxyprogesterone greater than 400 ng/dL: suggestive of NCAH

B Cushing syndrome

1. The findings in Cushing syndrome can resemble those of PCOS and include obesity, hypertension, abdominal striae, hirsutism, acne, and menstrual irregularities.

2. These findings result from excess cortisol production, either from an adrenal neoplasm, excess adrenocorticotropic hormone (ACTH) from a pituitary tumor, or an ectopic source of ACTH.

3. Diagnosis is made by 24-hour urinary collection of free cortisol with the level greater than 100 on two determinations.

C Androgen-producing neoplasm. Early stages of androgen-producing tumors can resemble PCOS and should be considered in cases in which there is a more rapid onset of hirsutism or signs of virilization. The location of the neoplasm could be either the adrenal gland or the ovary. Common ovarian tumors include Sertoli-Leydig cell, granulosa cell, fibroma, thecoma, and luteoma of pregnancy.

D Ovarian hyperthecosis. Ovarian hyperthecosis is a condition of the ovary where nests of luteinized theca cells are present in the ovarian stroma. These patients have elevated serum androgen levels and therefore demonstrate hirsutism, and in fact often show signs of virilization.

E Hyperandrogenic drugs. Drug exposure can lead to a rapid onset of hyperandrogenic symptoms, usually over several months. Implicated drugs include anabolic steroids, methyltestosterone, phenytoin, danazol, cyclosporin, and minoxidil.

F Premature ovarian failure presents with menstrual irregularity. Typical symptoms include hot flushes and night sweats. Diagnosis is made by elevated follicle-stimulating hormone (FSH) and low estradiol in the setting of amenorrhea.

G Severe extremes of hypothyroidism or hyperthyroidism can also lead to menstrual irregularity.

H Hyperprolactinemia results in hypothalamic suppression and amenorrhea. It can also be associated with hirsutism.

VII   EVALUATION

The diagnosis of PCOS can often be suspected by history and physical examination alone. Laboratory evaluation is important to exclude other causes of the symptoms since there is no PCOS test.

A History

1. **Menstrual cycle frequency and duration**
   a. Oligomenorrhea is defined as menses occurring at intervals of greater than 40 days.
   b. Amenorrhea is defined as no menses for 6 months or three menstrual cycles skipped.

2. **Onset and duration of hirsutism and acne**
   a. With PCOS, symptoms start with the onset of puberty and are slowly progressive. The rate and degree of hirsutism is variable among individuals.

   b. An androgen-producing tumor or drug exposure will be associated with a rapid progression of hirsutism, acne, and virilization.

B **Physical findings**

1. **Obesity**
   a. Defined as a body mass index (BMI) greater than or equal to 30 kg/m^2
   b. Incidence of obesity in women with PCOS is 50% to 75%.
   c. Central obesity with an increased waist-to-hip ratio ("apple" versus "pear")

2. **Hirsutism**
   a. Excess male pattern hair growth seen primarily in areas such as the face, jaw, chin, neck, midline on chest and abdomen, and upper thigh
   b. It is important to ask the patient if she has hair growth when seeing her in the office because many women will be meticulous about removing any unwanted hair and it may not be obvious when you see her.
   c. Racial and ethnic differences exist; for example, Asian individuals usually do not have much body hair and therefore may not display significant hirsutism even if high androgen levels are present.
   d. The **Ferriman-Gallwey scoring system** is used to quantify the amount of hair growth. Each area of the body is scored for the amount of hair. A score of greater than or equal to 8 is considered hirsute.

3. **Acne**
   a. May be a more reliable clinical marker of hyperandrogenism than hirsutism in adolescents and ethnic groups without significant hair growth in general (i.e., Asians)
   b. Can involve the face, chest, and back

4. **Acanthosis nigricans**
   a. Raised, velvety, hyperpigmentation of skin, typically seen on the axilla, neck, and intertriginous areas
   b. Marker of insulin resistance
   c. Will go away as insulin resistance improves

C **Laboratory testing**

1. **Making the diagnosis**
   a. Thyroid-stimulating hormone (TSH) and prolactin to exclude these hormonal conditions. Prolactin may be elevated in up to 40% of patients with PCOS, but this is likely secondary to stimulation of the prolactin-producing cells by chronic estrogen and not related to the cause of the disease state.
   b. FSH and estradiol to exclude the possibility of premature ovarian failure in those women with oligomenorrhea or amenorrhea
      (1) FSH should be elevated greater than 40 pg/mL.
      (2) Associated with a suppressed estradiol less than 30 pg/mL
      (3) Measuring LH and FSH to assess the LH-to-FSH ratio is not necessary. Although a ratio of greater than 2 is associated with PCOS, it is only present in approximately 40% of individuals and is not considered diagnostic for PCOS.
   c. 17-Hydroxyprogesterone. It is important to draw this blood sample at a specific time:
      (1) Early in the morning (i.e., 8 AM), due to the diurnal variation of hormone secretion from the adrenal gland. The peak is in the early morning; the lowest production is in the late afternoon.
      (2) In the follicular phase of the menstrual cycle. After ovulation the ovary produces 17-hydroxyprogesterone so the level would reflect secretion from both the ovary and adrenal gland and therefore not reflect just adrenal production.
   d. Increased production of cortisol is associated with Cushing syndrome. Diagnosis is made by:
      (1) 1-mg overnight dexamethasone suppression test
      (2) 24-hour urinary-free cortisol excretion elevated on two separate collections
   e. Total testosterone greater than 200 ng/dL is suggestive of an androgen-producing tumor. Imaging of the ovaries and adrenals is indicated.

(1) Total testosterone levels that are elevated but less than 200 ng/dL associated with anovulation and hirsutism suggest PCOS.

(2) Testosterone may be in the normal range when measured in patients with PCOS.

(3) Free testosterone is often elevated in PCOS. Free testosterone measured by direct immunoassay (most commercial laboratories) is not as accurate as the equilibrium dialysis method.

(4) Measuring SHBG reflects elevated free androgens and is an alternative to measuring free testosterone.

f. DHEAS level greater than 7000 ng/mL is suggestive of an adrenal tumor and warrants imaging of the adrenals.

(1) Moderately elevated DHEAS levels may occur with anovulation, PCOS, or adrenal hyperplasia.

(2) Normal DHEAS levels indicate that adrenal disease is less probable and that ovarian androgen production is more likely.

(3) Measuring DHEAS is not necessary unless an androgen-producing tumor is suspected. A mildly elevated level is nonspecific and does not help in making a diagnosis or determining treatment.

2. Other testing that should be done once the diagnosis of PCOS is determined

a. Insulin resistance. Since most, if not all, women with PCOS have insulin resistance, it may be helpful to assess this.

(1) The most accurate testing is done by the euglycemic clamp technique or the frequently sampled IV glucose tolerance test. However, both of these tests require inpatient monitoring and are therefore best suited for research protocols and not for outpatient screening.

(2) Measuring the glucose-to-insulin ratio is considered to be an alternative with fairly good correlation with the gold standard tests above. The following glucose/insulin ratios have been suggested to diagnose insulin resistance:

(a) Ratio less than 4.5 in obese adult women

(b) Ratio less than 7 in adolescents

b. Diabetes. Since the incidence of diabetes in women with PCOS is 10% and impaired glucose tolerance is seen in up to 35% of women, it is important to screen for these conditions since treatment can prevent significant health problems.

(1) Two-hour glucose tolerance test is the best test to evaluate for these conditions in women with PCOS. This test involves testing fasting level of glucose, then administering a 75-g glucose load, then drawing glucose level at 1- and 2-hour times after (Table 21-2).

(2) A fasting glucose will not detect as many women with impaired glucose tolerance.

c. Lipid levels. Though not involved in the clinical diagnosis of PCOS, abnormal lipid profiles are common in PCOS patients.

(1) Studies have shown that patients with PCOS have elevated total cholesterol, low-density-lipoprotein (LDL), and triglycerides and lower high-density lipoprotein (HDL) concentrations even relative to weight-matched controls, suggesting an inherent defect associated with PCOS.

TABLE 21–2 **Two-Hour Oral Glucose Tolerance Test***	Fasting Serum Glucose (mg/dL)	2-hr Serum Glucose (mg/dL)
Normal	<100	<140
Impaired glucose tolerance	100–126	140–200
Diabetes	>126	>200

*Fasting serum glucose is drawn, then a 75-g oral glucose load is given, and then serum glucose is drawn 2 hours later.

(2) This is thought to lead to a predisposition to vascular and cardiac disease, and therefore measurement and treatment of serum lipid levels may benefit in decreasing the morbidity from cardiovascular risks associated with PCOS.

VIII   TREATMENT

Treatment of PCOS involves treating the various manifestations of the disorder.

A **Obesity** is associated with worsening of PCOS symptoms including menstrual irregularity, insulin resistance, risk of diabetes, and hyperandrogenic symptoms.

1. Weight reduction results in improvement in all symptoms of PCOS. A loss of only 7% to 10% of body weight can result in improved insulin resistance, a significant reduction in testosterone, decreased abdominal fat, and resumption of menses.

2. Dietary composition of the diet has no impact on weight loss, insulin resistance, menstrual cyclicity, and lipids. Although a low-carbohydrate diet may be more effective since it leads to decreased insulin secretion, studies have shown that both low-carbohydrate and low-fat diets are equally effective. Calorie restriction is the most important factor and should be combined with an exercise regimen.

3. Bariatric surgery is becoming more prevalent for treatment of obesity in individuals with BMIs greater than or equal to 40 kg/m^2, or BMIs greater than or equal to 35 kg/m^2 if significant health problems exist. Weight loss of 20 to 40 kg is maintained for up to 10 years.

B **Menstrual irregularity.**   Prolonged unopposed estrogen exposure and amenorrhea can lead to endometrial hyperplasia and endometrial cancer.

1. In patients who have had prolonged anovulation without treatment or have had a history of oligomenorrhea and are older than 35 years, an endometrial biopsy is indicated in order to rule out endometrial hyperplasia and/or cancer.

2. Treatment with progestin is important to prevent hyperplasia and regulate menstrual bleeding.
   a. Combined hormonal contraception: oral contraceptive pills, NuvaRing
   b. Cyclic progestin therapy, administered 12 days a month to induce regular menstrual bleeding

C **Treatment of hirsutism**

1. **Mechanical removal of hair**
   a. Shaving, plucking, bleaching, depilation
   b. Electrolysis achieves permanent hair removal. If done poorly, it may be associated with scarring.
   c. Laser epilation is most effective in women with pale skin and dark hair.
   d. Eflornithine HCl (Vaniqa) inhibits enzyme ornithine decarboxylase, acts directly at the hair follicle, and slows hair growth.

2. **Combined hormonal contraception.** Combined contraception with estrogen and progestin works to treat hyperandrogenism by the following mechanisms:
   a. Decreases androgen production through suppression of LH and therefore suppression of androgen production by the ovarian theca cells
   b. Increases production of SHBG, which in turn decreases free circulating androgens
   c. Decreases androgen secretion by the adrenal gland
   d. Progestins can possess androgen activity in laboratory studies, but clinically there is no difference in the clinical suppression of androgenic symptoms. The best hormonal contraceptive is the one that is best tolerated by the individual.

3. **Antiandrogens** work to suppress hirsutism by competitive inhibition at the level of the testosterone receptor. Several antiandrogens have been used successfully to treat hirsutism. All are equally effective. Improved results are seen when these agents are combined with hormonal contraceptives.
   a. Spironolactone (50 to 100 mg twice daily): may induce hyperkalemia; is important to check potassium after 2 weeks of use

    b. Flutamide (250 to 500 mg/day): rare association with hepatotoxicity in greater than 5% of patients

    c. Finasteride (5 mg/day): 5α-reductase inhibitor

    d. Cyproterone acetate: not available in the United States

D **Metabolic correction.** Since the underlying condition in PCOS is insulin resistance, treating insulin resistance with insulin-sensitizing agents has been shown to result in improvement in PCOS symptoms.

1. **Metformin** is a biguanide that acts by decreasing hepatic glucose production and may also increase peripheral glucose utilization. It is approved for the treatment of diabetes.

    a. Menstrual cyclicity and ovulation rates are improved almost fourfold.

    b. Serum androgens and insulin resistance are improved.

    c. The effect on hirsutism has yet to be determined.

    d. Weight loss occurs only in conjunction with a low-calorie diet and exercise regimen.

    e. The ideal patient who will respond to metformin has yet to be determined.

    f. Side effects are primarily gastrointestinal, including nausea and diarrhea.

2. **Thiazolidinediones.** These insulin sensitizers have been shown to improve androgens and insulin resistance and include rosiglitazone and pioglitazone. These medications have been associated with hepatotoxicity, which has limited their use in PCOS. They are approved for the treatment of diabetes and have limited studies in patients with PCOS.

E **Treatment of infertility.** Women with PCOS often have difficulty conceiving because of the failure to ovulate. The use of ovulation induction agents has been shown to be effective.

1. Clomiphene citrate is an antiestrogen that has been used since the 1960s to induce ovulation. Up to 80% of patients with PCOS will ovulate and 50% will become pregnant.

2. Metformin is associated with a fourfold improvement in ovulation. Recent studies have shown clomiphene to be more successful in achieving ovulation and pregnancy. However, in those who do not respond to clomiphene alone, the addition of metformin may improve ovulation rates in some individuals.

3. Gonadotropins, FSH alone or in combination with LH, are successful in inducing ovulation. However, the risks include high-order multiple gestation.

4. In vitro fertilization is successful in achieving pregnancy and ovulation in women with PCOS.

Study Questions for Chapter 21

Directions: *Each of the numbered items or incomplete statements in this section is followed by answers or by completions of the statement. Select the ONE lettered answer or completion that is BEST in each case.*

1. A 21-year-old nulliparous woman comes to your office reporting several years of irregular menses, occurring only four to five times a year. On physical examination you notice hair on her neck, chin, upper lip, and lower abdomen. Your laboratory workup of this patient should include all of the following EXCEPT:

- A Thyroid-stimulating hormone
- B Serum testosterone
- C 17OH progesterone
- D Leuteinizing hormone/follicle-stimulating hormone
- E Prolactin

2. A 17-year-old woman comes to your office complaining of increased hair growth over the past 6 months, requiring her to wax her upper lip and chin. Her menses have been irregular. Laboratory testing suggests she has PCOS. What is the best recommendation for treating excess hair growth?

- A Combined hormonal contraceptive
- B Combined hormonal contraceptive and electrolysis
- C Antiandrogen and laser or electrolysis
- D Metformin and laser or electrolysis
- E Combined hormonal contraceptive, antiandrogen, and laser or electrolysis

3. An obese 38-year-old woman comes into your office complaining of several episodes of irregular vaginal spotting throughout the past 6 months. She has a long history of irregular periods and was diagnosed with PCOS as a teenager. She is not sexually active and has never been on hormonal contraception. She does not desire fertility at this time. The most important test to perform in this patient is:

- A 2-hour glucose tolerance test
- B Glucose/insulin ratio
- C Serum lipids
- D Endometrial biopsy
- E Pelvic ultrasound

4. A 27-year-old obese nulliparous woman has been on oral contraceptives since age 16 for irregular periods. She comes to your office because she stopped taking her pill 6 months prior but has not had a period since stopping her pill. She and her husband would like to conceive, but she is worried that her weight may be a problem. You counsel her that:

- A Her weight is not a problem
- B If she lost weight, she may start to have periods on her own
- C If she takes metformin, she will lose weight
- D Obesity is a problem and you would recommend gastric bypass
- E A 25% weight reduction is necessary to improve insulin resistance

5. A 32-year-old female, gravida 0, presents with her husband because they want to conceive. She has PCOS diagnosed by you 14 years ago and has been maintained on oral contraceptives and antiandrogens since then. She stopped those medications and started prenatal vitamins as per your instructions 4 months ago and has not had a period since. Her pregnancy test is negative. At this point you would recommend which one of the following approaches to help her achieve a pregnancy?

- A Medroxyprogesterone acetate
- B Clomiphene citrate
- C Metformin
- D Gonadotropins (FSH +/− LH)
- E In vitro fertilization (IVF)

Answers and Explanations

1. The answer is D [IV A–B]. The evaluation of this patient with oligomenorrhea and clinical signs of hyperandrogenism should involve testing for all suspected causes of these symptoms. The most likely etiology is PCOS, but this diagnosis is made by clinical assessment and excluding all other potential causes. In a patient with irregular menses, TSH and prolactin should be checked. The serum testosterone may be elevated in this patient, but levels greater than 200 ng/dL suggest an androgen-producing neoplasm and therefore would require further investigation. Similarly, an elevated 17OH progesterone level will diagnose 21-hydroxylase deficiency, the most common cause of congenital adrenal hyperplasia, which can mimic PCOS. Though the LH-to-FSH ratio may be elevated in up to 40% of individuals with PCOS, this is not necessary for diagnosis. Assessing FSH and estradiol is valuable for diagnosing premature ovarian failure, but this was not offered as one of the answers.

2. The answer is E [VIII C]. The best way to treat hirsutism is by blocking the stimulus to hair growth at as many points as possible while removing existing hair permanently. This would best be accomplished by using a combined hormonal contraceptive (which decreases production of androgens from the ovary and adrenal and increases SHBG, which decreases free [active] androgens) and an antiandrogen (which competitively blocks the action of androgens at the hair follicle) to decrease the new hair growth, while at the same time using laser or electrolysis to remove existing hair. Using a combined hormonal contraceptive and an antiandrogen together is more effective than either alone. Metformin has not been shown to improve hirsutism significantly.

3. The answer is D [II A 1]. This patient, who is over 35 years old and has a long history of irregular menses, is at increased risk for endometrial hyperplasia and endometrial cancer. Therefore, the most important test to perform is an endometrial biopsy. This patient may also be at increased risk for diabetes, insulin resistance, and hyperlipidemia, and therefore tests for these conditions should also be eventually performed, but would not be the most important test. Pelvic ultrasound is helpful to evaluate the abnormal bleeding in this patient, but it is not as important as the endometrial biopsy.

4. The answer is B [VIII A]. Obesity is a problem: it compounds the effects of PCOS, including menstrual irregularity, insulin resistance, and hirsutism, and causes problems during pregnancy for both the mother (higher risk of diabetes, hypertension, and need for cesarean section) and the baby (higher risk of fetal distress). A 7% to 10% decrease in weight is associated with resumption of menses and ovulation and improvement in insulin resistance and androgen levels. Metformin is not a weight loss drug. Weight loss occurs with metformin only in conjunction with a low-calorie diet and exercise regimen. Gastric bypass may be an option for morbidly obese individuals (BMI greater than or equal to 40 kg/m^2), but should be recommended only if less invasive measures, such as diet and exercise and medical management, have failed.

5. The answer is B [VIII E]. In this patient with polycystic ovarian syndrome, the most likely cause for her inability to conceive is anovulation. The majority of these patients (80%) will ovulate on clomiphene citrate, and therefore this is the first-line medication used in these patients to induce ovulation. Metformin is an insulin-sensitizing agent that in some studies has been used to induce resumption of menses and ovulation, but it should not be used as first-line therapy. Metformin has been used with success in patients who fail to ovulate on clomiphene citrate alone. Gonadotropins are effective in inducing ovulation in individuals with PCOS, but have a higher risk of high-order multiple gestation (triplets and higher) in this population and are also associated with hyperstimulation syndrome. IVF is effective, but it is the most aggressive therapy and would not be the first-line treatment at this point.

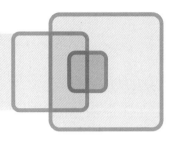

chapter **22**

Hirsutism

SAMANTHA M. PFEIFER

I   **INTRODUCTION**

Increased hair growth in women may be associated with normal or increased levels of **circulating androgens.** It is important to view hirsutism as a potential endocrine abnormality as well as a psychological and cosmetic problem.

A Definitions

1. **Types of hair**
   a. **Lanugo** is soft, short hair covering the fetus that is shed in late gestation and during the neonatal period.
   b. **Vellus** is soft, fine, unpigmented hair that covers apparently hairless areas of the body.
   c. **Terminal** is longer, coarse, pigmented hair that may grow in response to sex hormones (e.g., over the chin and abdomen of men) or may be sex hormone independent (e.g., eyebrows and eyelashes).

2. **Hypertrichosis** is excessive growth of androgen-independent hair in nonsexual areas, such as forearms and legs.

3. **Hirsutism** is the presence of terminal hair in androgen-dependent sites where hair does not normally grow in women. This hair growth is located predominantly on midline portions of the body, including the face, chest, abdomen, and inner thigh.

4. **Virilization** is hirsutism associated with other signs of hyperandrogenism, such as increased muscle mass, clitoromegaly, temporal balding, voice deepening, and increased libido. It can also be associated with signs of defeminization, such as decreased breast size and loss of vaginal lubrication.

B Etiology.   Hair growth, and thus hirsutism, is regulated by:

1. **Number and concentration of hair follicles.** This varies according to racial and ethnic background but not gender. For example, Asian women generally have low concentrations of hair follicles, and hirsutism is rarely seen in these individuals.

2. Degree to which hair follicles are sensitive to androgens and able to convert vellus hairs to terminal hairs

3. **Degree of 5α-reductase activity** in the skin, which determines local androgen activity

4. Ratio of growth to resting phases in affected hair follicles

5. Thickness and degree to which individual hairs are pigmented

II   **ANDROGENS**

These steroids promote the development of male secondary sexual characteristics. In women, androgens are mainly produced by the adrenal gland, the ovary, and peripheral transformation. Testosterone is the most potent androgen; androstenedione, dehydroepiandrosterone (DHEA), and DHEA sulfate (DHEAS) are less potent.

A Testosterone.   Blood testosterone levels are a function of blood production rates and metabolic clearance rates; thus, these levels may not represent the actual state of androgenicity.

1. **Total testosterone** levels in women are usually less than 70 ng/dL.

2. **Sources**:
   a. Ovarian: 25% (in stroma and follicles)
   b. Adrenal origin: 25%
   c. Peripheral transformation of androstenedione to testosterone: 50%

3. **Free testosterone**
   a. Most testosterone in the blood circulates bound to **albumin** (19%) or to **sex hormone–binding globulin** (**SHBG**) (80%). Percentages of free testosterone are as follows:
      (1) Normal women: 1%
      (2) Hirsute women: 2%
      (3) Men: 2% to 3%
   b. Androgenicity depends mainly on the unbound fraction of testosterone because this represents the active form of the hormone.

B **Sex hormone–binding globulin**

1. An inverse relationship exists between SHBG and the percentage of free testosterone. As SHBG decreases, the percentage of free testosterone increases; as SHBG increases, the percentage of free testosterone decreases. However, the total testosterone level may remain normal.
   a. **Factors that decrease plasma SHBG**
      (1) Obesity
      (2) Increased androgen production
      (3) Hyperinsulinemia
      (4) Corticosteroid therapy
      (5) Hypothyroidism
      (6) Acromegaly
   b. **Factors that increase plasma SHBG**
      (1) Estrogen therapy
      (2) Combined hormonal contraceptives
      (3) Pregnancy
      (4) Hyperthyroidism
      (5) Cirrhosis

2. In general, hirsute women have reduced serum concentrations of SHBG and therefore elevated levels of free androgens.

C **5α-Reductase**

1. 5α-Reductase converts testosterone to **dihydrotestosterone (DHT)** in androgen-sensitive tissues such as hair follicles and skin. Levels of this enzyme are significantly elevated in the skin of hirsute women compared with control subjects. The enzyme activity is partly stimulated by elevated circulating testosterone levels.

2. Dihydrotestosterone is responsible for stimulating hair growth and is two to three times as potent as testosterone.

3. **3α-Androstanediol glucuronide (3α-AG)** is the peripheral tissue metabolite of DHT. Although it has been used as a marker of target tissue cellular action, it is not often used clinically.

D **Pathophysiology of androgens in hirsutism.** A combination of the following factors results in hirsutism:

1. Increased concentration of serum androgens, especially free testosterone

2. Decreased levels of SHBG, resulting in increased bioavailable androgen

3. Increased activity of 5α-reductase

III DIAGNOSIS

A **History.** Several factors are important.

1. **Onset of hirsutism**

     a. Gradual onset of hirsutism is associated with acne, oily skin, weight gain, and irregular menstrual cycles. This suggests an underlying endocrine condition, such as polycystic ovary syndrome (PCOS).

     b. Abrupt onset or rapidly worsening hirsutism with signs of virilization should prompt concern for an androgen-producing tumor.

2. Presence or absence of **virilization**

3. **Drug ingestion**. Drugs are usually associated with hypertrichosis, but androgenic drugs (e.g., steroids and phenytoin) may cause hirsutism.

4. **Family history.** A family history of hirsutism may indicate an inherited disorder (i.e., familial hypertrichosis).

5. **Ethnic background**. The pattern of hair growth is genetically predetermined and is associated with differences in 5α-reductase activity at hair follicles.

6. **Local trauma**. Changes in skin and hair growth may occur.

7. **Regularity of menstrual cycles**

     a. Patients with regular menstrual cycles and hirsutism often have idiopathic, ethnic, or familial hirsutism.

     b. Some anovulatory hirsute patients (as many as 40%) appear to have regular menstrual cycles; thus, testing is necessary to determine whether ovulation is occurring.

8. **History of infertility**

B Differential diagnosis

1. **Polycystic ovary syndrome** (see Chapter 21). This heterogeneous endocrine, metabolic, and genetic disorder is seen in 5% to 10% of the general population and is the cause of androgen excess in 65% to 85% of hirsute patients. This syndrome is characterized by hyperandrogenism, oligomenorrhea or amenorrhea (caused by chronic anovulation), and obesity. It is associated with insulin resistance. Patients usually present with hirsutism, menstrual irregularity, and infertility.

     a. The fundamental pathophysiologic defect is not known.

     b. Increased production of androgens may result in:

        (1) Increased secretion of luteinizing hormone (LH) from the anterior pituitary, leading to increased ovarian androgen production

        (2) Insulin resistance and compensatory hyperinsulinemia, stimulating ovarian and adrenal androgen production by direct and indirect mechanisms

     c. Gonadotropin regulation of the menstrual cycle is disrupted, leading to oligo-ovulation or anovulation and menstrual irregularity.

     d. Increased androgen levels inhibit follicular development in the ovary; thus, multiple small atretic follicles are produced. These "polycystic ovaries" are therefore a reflection of the hormonal environment within the ovary rather than the cause of the disorder.

     e. Affected patients are at increased risk for endometrial hyperplasia or cancer, glucose intolerance, type 2 diabetes mellitus, hyperlipidemia, and cardiovascular disease.

2. **Metabolic syndrome** (hyperandrogenism, insulin resistance, hyperlipidosis)

     a. This condition is similar to PCOS, but patients have a greater degree of insulin resistance and hyperinsulinemia.

     b. This disorder is often inherited.

     c. Severe abnormalities of insulin action cause hyperinsulinemia, which stimulates excess ovarian androgen secretion.

3. **Idiopathic hirsutism**. This condition, which accounts for 15% to 30% of hirsute women, is caused by end-organ (skin) hypersensitivity to androgens. Characteristics include:

     a. Regular ovulatory menstrual cycles

     b. Normal circulating androgen levels

     c. Increased peripheral conversion of androgens caused by **increased skin 5α-reductase activity**

4. **Nonclassic adrenal hyperplasia (NCAH)**. This condition is present in approximately 1% of hyperandrogenic women. Patients present at or before puberty. This is a less severe form of congenital

adrenal hyperplasia that is diagnosed in the newborn and is associated with ambiguous genitalia and salt wasting.

  a. Deficiency in activity of adrenal enzymes and thus formation of excess cortisol precursors (e.g., 17-hydroxyprogesterone [17-OHP] and androstenedione) leads to increased production of androgens. The most common enzyme deficiency is 21-hydroxylase.

  b. Inheritance is autosomal recessive, and occurrence is increased in Ashkenazi Jews.

  c. Deficiencies of adrenal enzymes 11β-hydroxylase and 3β-hydroxysteroid dehydrogenase are less common.

5. Cushing syndrome

  a. Adrenocortical hyperfunction leads to excess production of corticosteroids as well as hyperandrogenism, menstrual irregularities, glucose intolerance, and obesity.

  b. Causes are multiple and include adrenal neoplasm, ectopic adrenocorticotropic hormone (ACTH)–producing tumor, and pituitary tumor or Cushing disease.

6. Androgen-producing tumors are associated with sudden-onset hyperandrogenic state, rapid progression, and frank virilization.

  a. Ovarian tumors (e.g., Sertoli-Leydig cell tumor, granulosa-theca cell tumor, thecoma, luteoma of pregnancy)

  b. Adrenal tumors

7. Disorders of pituitary origin

  a. Hyperprolactinemia

  b. Acromegaly

8. Androgenic drug exposure

  a. Without virilization: phenytoin, diazoxide, minoxidil, danazol, corticosteroids, or cyclosporin

  b. With potential virilization: anabolic steroids, androgen therapy, or supplements

9. Y-containing mosaics and **incomplete androgen insensitivity.** These patients show signs of androgen stimulation at puberty.

C Laboratory evaluation

1. Serum testosterone (see II A) is a marker of ovarian and adrenal activity.

  a. Total testosterone levels greater than 200 ng/dL suggest an androgen-producing tumor. However, 10% to 20% of patients with androgen-producing tumors may have low testosterone levels. Imaging is warranted.

    (1) Pelvic ultrasound is best to provide an image of the ovaries.

    (2) Computed tomography or magnetic resonance imaging views the adrenal glands.

  b. Elevated total testosterone levels but less than 200 ng/dL associated with anovulation and hirsutism suggest PCOS.

  c. Testosterone may be in the normal range when measured in patients with PCOS.

2. Serum DHEAS is almost exclusively produced by the adrenal glands and reflects adrenal androgen activity.

  a. Levels greater than 700 μg/dL suggest an adrenal tumor.

  b. Moderately elevated DHEAS levels may occur with anovulation, PCOS, or adrenal hyperplasia.

  c. Normal DHEAS levels indicate that adrenal disease is less probable and that ovarian androgen production is more likely.

3. Elevated levels of **serum androstenedione** suggest ovarian disease, but this test is rarely recommended.

4. Serum 17-OHP

  a. 17-OHP is elevated in 21-hydroxylase deficiency, the most common form of nonclassic adrenal hyperplasia. Normal values should be less than 200 ng/dL.

  b. Circumstances under which 17-OHP must be measured:

    (1) Early in the morning because of diurnal variation of adrenal secretion

    (2) In the follicular phase of the menstrual cycle in ovulatory women to avoid confusion with ovarian production of this hormone in the luteal phase

  c. Baseline values greater than 200 ng/dL are abnormal and should be further evaluated with the ACTH stimulation test to confirm the diagnosis of nonclassic adrenal hyperplasia.

5. Increased production of **cortisol** is associated with Cushing syndrome. Diagnosis is made by:
   a. 1-mg overnight dexamethasone suppression test
   b. 24-hour urinary-free cortisol excretion

6. **Gonadotropins** may be useful. An elevated LH-to-follicle-stimulating hormone (FSH) ratio (2–3:1) suggests PCOS. However, this finding is not present in approximately 40% of patients with PCOS and is not considered diagnostic.

7. **Serum 3α-AG** is rarely measured. Increased levels of 3α-AG indicate an increased activity of 5α-reductase in the periphery and measure peripheral target tissue activity.

8. The evaluation of irregular menstrual cycles and hirsutism also includes **thyroid-stimulating hormone and prolactin**.

IV TREATMENT

A combination of hormonal suppression of hair growth and mechanical hair removal offers the most complete and effective treatment for patients with hirsutism.

A Goals

1. The major goal is **arresting the virilizing process**, not removing hair. Once terminal hair has been established, withdrawal of androgens does not affect the established hair pattern.

2. Amelioration of a specific disease state helps slow the rate of growth by **preventing the establishment of new hair follicles**.

3. Results may not be apparent for 6 to 12 months. Treatment of hirsutism is a **long-term process**.

B Elimination of specific causes

1. **Removal of ovarian or adrenal tumors**

2. **Elimination of drugs** suspected to contribute to the abnormal hair growth

3. Treatment of Cushing syndrome, thyroid disease, or hyperprolactinemia

C Hair removal techniques

1. **Shaving, tweezing, waxing**, and use of **depilatories** are temporary measures, which may need to be repeated daily. These methods neither stimulate hair growth nor increase the rate of hair growth.

2. **Bleaching** is effective for mild hair growth.

3. **Electrolysis** involves the permanent destruction of hair follicles. Multiple treatments are necessary, and scarring may occur. This method should be used after 6 months of hormonal therapy when new hair growth has ceased.

4. **Laser** provides directed damage to hair follicles, which temporarily or permanently removes terminal hair. This method can be used over a larger area than electrolysis, but it is not yet perfected for the treatment of hirsutism. Ideal patients are those with pale skin and very dark hair.

5. **Eflornithine HCl (Vaniqa)**. This topical medication inhibits the enzyme ornithine decarboxylase responsible for hair growth. It acts directly at the hair follicle and slows hair growth.

D Suppression of androgen synthesis

1. In most **idiopathic or ovarian-related hirsutism**, suppression of ovarian steroidogenesis is the goal.

2. **Combination hormonal contraceptives** have a potent negative feedback effect on the pituitary and other effects that ameliorate peripheral androgen stimulation. Low-dose formulations (less than 50 μg estrogen) are effective in treating hirsutism, and a demonstrated benefit has been shown with 20-μg preparations. Although the progestins in the combined hormonal contraceptives are all different and have different levels of androgenicity, there is no proven benefit of one over another in the treatment of hirsutism. The best contraceptive is the one that is best tolerated by the individual patient.
   a. Both **estrogen** and **progestin** in the hormonal contraceptives cause a decrease in gonadotropin secretion with a consequent decrease in ovarian androgen production.

(1) **Estrogen** also stimulates an increase in SHBG, causing increased binding of testosterone and decreased free testosterone levels.

(2) **Progestin** also may displace active androgens at the hair follicle and may inhibit 5α-reductase activity.

    b. Blood testosterone levels are effectively suppressed within 1 to 3 months of therapy. This reduction has been associated with a clinical improvement in the progression of hirsutism.

3. **Medroxyprogesterone acetate** (150 mg intramuscularly every 3 months or 10 to 20 mg orally per day) is effective in suppressing gonadotropin secretion in patients for whom oral contraceptives are contraindicated. It results in:

    a. Decreased production of androgens caused by suppression of LH and FSH

    b. Increased clearance of testosterone from the circulation caused by induction of liver enzymes

4. **Gonadotropin-releasing hormone (GnRH) agonists** suppress the hypothalamic-pituitary-ovarian axis, thereby decreasing ovarian steroidogenesis.

    a. Uses

        (1) In severely androgenized patients refractory to other therapies

        (2) With estrogen and progesterone replacement and with calcium supplements

    b. Side effects include hot flashes, vaginal dryness, and bone loss.

5. **Corticosteroid** suppression of adrenal androgen production is useful in more severe cases of NCAH. For mild cases of NCAH, patients can instead be managed effectively with oral contraceptives and antiandrogen therapy. Long-term side effects or corticosteroids include osteoporosis, diabetes mellitus, and avascular necrosis of the hip, which dictate careful use of this medication.

E **Androgen-receptor blockers.** These medications inhibit binding of DHT to the androgen receptor, thus directly inhibiting hair growth. When combined with oral contraceptives, progestins, or GnRH agonists, further benefit may be obtained.

1. **Spironolactone** is an aldosterone antagonist and diuretic widely used in the United States.

    a. This agent also inhibits 5α-reductase and variably suppresses the ovarian and adrenal synthesis of androgens.

    c. Side effects include initial diuresis and fatigue. Hyperkalemia and hypotension may also occur.

2. **Flutamide** is a nonsteroidal antiandrogen widely used in Europe for treatment of hirsutism.

    a. Side effects include hepatotoxicity; liver enzymes must be monitored.

    b. Contraception must be used with this medication because flutamide may be teratogenic to a male fetus.

3. **Cyproterone acetate** is a potent progestin and antiandrogen.

    a. This agent inhibits gonadotropin secretion (primarily LH), which leads to decreased androgen levels.

    b. It is not currently available in the United States, but is available in Canada and Europe. It is used as a progestin in oral contraceptives.

F **Other medications**

1. **Finasteride** inhibits 5α-reductase activity with negligible side effects.

    a. This agent blocks the conversion of testosterone to DHT.

    b. Contraception must be used with this medication because DHT is necessary in the development of genitalia in a male fetus and is considered a teratogen.

2. **Cimetidine** is a less potent androgen-receptor blocker, rarely used for this indication.

3. **Ketoconazole** blocks ovarian and adrenal androgen synthesis by inhibition of the cytochrome P450 system. This agent has multiple side effects, including the potential for hepatotoxicity and adrenal insufficiency. Therefore, it is rarely used for hirsutism.

4. **Insulin-sensitizing agents**. Metformin and thiazolidinediones are being used in patients with PCOS to improve insulin sensitivity, thus decreasing hyperinsulinemia and androgen levels. Improvement in menstrual cyclicity has been demonstrated, but there is little information regarding the effect on hirsutism. These agents are not approved by the U.S. Food and Drug Administration for treatment of hirsutism.

Study Questions for Chapter 22

Directions: *Match the appropriate hormone(s), substance, or enzyme (which you could measure) with the description that is most likely to account for excessive hair growth in a woman. Each answer may be used once, more than once, or not at all.*

QUESTIONS 1–3

- [A] Testosterone
- [B] 3α-Androstanediol glucuronide
- [C] Androstenedione
- [D] 5α-Reductase
- [E] 17-Hydroxyprogesterone

1. Rapidly progressive hirsutism

2. Hirsutism in a woman with regular menses and no abnormal hormonal measurements

3. Hyperplasia of adrenal gland as source of androgen excess

Directions: *Each of the numbered items or incomplete statements in this section is followed by answers or by completions of the statement. Select the ONE lettered answer or completion that is BEST in each case.*

QUESTIONS 4–6

4. A 33-year-old woman, gravida 2, para 1, spontaneous abortions 1, presents to your office reporting increasing dark hair growth on her chin, upper lip, and lower abdomen. This growth has occurred over many years and has forced her to wax and bleach more often. She denies changes in her voice or size of her clitoris, reduction in breast size, or acne. During her early teen years, she had regular menstrual periods that lasted 4 to 5 days. Now, however, she has to take birth control pills to regulate her cycles. Her past medical history is significant for hepatitis C, which she acquired from a blood transfusion to treat postpartum hemorrhage with her first pregnancy. The next best step in the management of hirsutism in this patient is:

- [A] Depomedroxyprogesterone acetate
- [B] Flutamide
- [C] Spironolactone
- [D] Dexamethasone
- [E] Leuprolide

5. A 23-year-old woman, gravida 1, para 0, abortion 1, has irregular, unpredictable menstrual periods every 30 to 90 days. Physical examination reveals acne on her face and back and several dark, coarse hairs on her chin and lower abdomen. The initial step in diagnosis of androgen excess in this woman is to measure which of the following?

- [A] Androstenedione
- [B] Dehydroepiandrosterone sulfate
- [C] LH and FSH
- [D] 17-Hydroxyprogesterone
- [E] 5α-Reductase

6. A 22-year-old African-American female presents to your office complaining of severe hirsutism on her face. She is currently shaving daily and is very distressed. After you evaluate her you diagnose PCOS. You give her what advice for the best way to manage her hirsutism symptoms?

- A Shaving is bad because it makes the hair grow faster
- B She would be a good candidate for laser epilation
- C Medroxyprogesterone acetate is the best option
- D Combined hormonal contraception with spironolactone is the best option
- E Metformin therapy for PCOS is the best option

Answers and Explanations

1. C [I A 2 and II C 1 and 3], **2.** D [III C 3], **3.** E [III C 4]. Rapid progression of hair growth is suggestive of an androgen-producing tumor. Testosterone is the most likely hormone produced by an ovarian or adrenal tumor. Androstenedione is rarely associated with tumor. Excessive hair growth is caused by the concentration of hair follicles in the skin (which is genetically determined), degree of 5α-reductase activity, and the sensitivity or response of hair follicles to DHT. 3α-Androstanediol glucuronide is the peripheral tissue metabolite of DHT. It is rarely measured for clinical purposes. 21-Hydroxylase deficiency is the cause of the most common form of NCAH. Although moderately elevated DHEAS may occur with adrenal hyperplasia, measurement of 17-OHP is diagnostic for NCAH. The diagnosis can be made by measuring 17-OHP.

4. The answer is C [IV D 1]. The best complement to oral contraceptive pills in the treatment of hirsutism is spironolactone. The mechanism is as follows: it binds to the androgen receptor, preventing the binding of DHT and thus inhibiting hair growth; it also inhibits 5α-reductase and thus the production of DHT. Depomedroxyprogesterone acetate works similarly to oral contraceptive pills (OCPs) in that it suppresses gonadotropins, which decrease ovarian androgen production, but it does not increase SHBG, and therefore does not achieve the same effect. Flutamide, another androgen-receptor blocker, is contraindicated in this woman because of hepatotoxicity. Dexamethasone, a glucocorticoid, suppresses pituitary corticotropin and thus adrenal androgen production, but this drug is used only in patients with elevated adrenal androgen production. GnRH agonists suppress the hypothalamic-pituitary-ovarian axis, which decreases ovarian stimulation and steroidogenesis. This medication is used infrequently for this indication and is not added to OCPs.

5. The answer is D [II A 3]. This patient most likely has PCOS because she has menstrual irregularity and clinical evidence of hyperandrogenism. Therefore, to confirm this diagnosis, all other causes of these symptoms must be excluded. For this reason, a 17-hydroxyprogesterone level must be drawn at 8 AM and just following a menstrual period to evaluate for NCAH. Measuring androstenedione is not going to make a diagnosis. DHEAS is likely to be mildly elevated in several hyperandrogenic syndromes, but the time course of this patient's symptoms does not suggest a tumor, so DHEAS should not be measured. One cannot measure 5α-reductase. 5α-Reductase activity reflects levels of DHT at the skin and can be evaluated by measuring levels of the 3α-androstanediol glucuronide. The LH-to-FSH ratio may be elevated in PCOS, but it is not diagnostic of PCOS and therefore is not necessary.

6. The answer is D [IV A, D, E]. The best treatment option for this young woman is combined hormonal contraceptive with spironolactone. The best results with treating hirsutism are achieved by using more than one modality to stop hair growth, and by using these two medications, androgens are decreased; free androgens are decreased by increasing SHBG and the action of androgens. It would also be good to maximize hair removal procedures to get rid of the hair she already has. Electrolysis would be preferable to laser: since she has dark pigmented skin, laser would not be effective. Shaving can be continued since it does not increase the rate of hair growth. Metformin has not been proven to treat hirsutism in women with PCOS. Medroxyprogesterone acetate would not be as effective as the combined hormonal contraceptive.

chapter 23

Abnormal Uterine Bleeding

SAMANTHA BUTTS

I   DEFINITIONS

A **Abnormal uterine bleeding** is defined as menstrual bleeding that is not regular and cyclic and "normal." The causes of abnormal uterine bleeding can be divided into **structural causes** and **hormonal causes** (see Table 23-1). Structural and dysfunctional causes of abnormal bleeding can be present at the same time.

B **Structural causes** of abnormal uterine bleeding include structural lesions in the uterus that can lead to regular but excessive menstrual flow, intermenstrual bleeding, or prolonged bleeding. These lesions include fibroids, endometrial polyps, adenomyosis, and endometrial or uterine cancer. Bleeding from other sources in the genital tract and systemic illnesses that cause bleeding must also be considered in the differential of abnormal uterine bleeding, since the presentation can be similar. These conditions are covered in detail in other chapters of this text.

C **Dysfunctional uterine bleeding (DUB).** This **abnormal bleeding**, which can be excessive, prolonged, or unpredictable, reflects a disturbance in normal ovulatory function. It is a manifestation of **abnormal hormonal stimulation** of the endometrial lining of the uterus.

1. DUB may be **infrequent or chronic**.

2. DUB results from **abnormalities of endocrine origin** with no demonstrable organic or anatomic cause.

3. DUB is **associated with infrequent or absent ovulation (oligo-ovulation or anovulation, respectively)**. It is often referred to as **estrogen breakthrough bleeding** because it most often results from a hormonal imbalance in which the endometrium receives constant stimulation by estrogen without the influence of progesterone, which checks endometrial growth.

D **Normal menstrual cycle characteristics**   (see Chapter 19)

1. **Purpose of the menstrual cycle**. During the menstrual cycle, multiple organs participate in the orderly and cyclic production of hormones, resulting in:
   a. The recruitment and release of an oocyte and
   b. Proliferation and differentiation of the uterine endometrium in preparation for implantation of an embryo. Menstrual bleeding occurs in cycles where a pregnancy does not occur.

2. **Cycle length**. Most cycles range in length from 24 to 35 days. Fewer than 2% of women have menstrual periods more often than every 21 days or less often than every 35 days.
   a. **Polymenorrhea** is bleeding that occurs more often than every 21 days.
   b. **Oligomenorrhea** is bleeding that occurs less often than every 35 days.
   c. **DUB** may present as **polymenorrhea or oligomenorrhea**.

3. **Cycle regularity**. Although the length of the menstrual cycle may vary from woman to woman, it usually remains the same in a particular individual.
   a. The **follicular phase** represents the first half of the menstrual cycle and is the **source of the person-to-person variation** in cycle length. The follicular phase begins with the onset of menses and culminates in the ovulation of a mature oocyte.
   b. The **luteal phase** is the second half of the cycle and is more consistent in length, lasting **12 to 14 days in most individuals**. If a woman has a 28-day cycle, she tends to ovulate on or about

TABLE 23–1   Differential Diagnosis of Abnormal Uterine Bleeding

Reproductive Tract Pathology	**Endocrine Gland Dysfunction**
Cervicitis	Hypothyroidism
Cervical neoplasia	Hyperthyroidism
Endometritis	Pituitary adenoma
Endometrial polyps	
Endometrial hyperplasia	**Ovulatory Dysfunction**
Endometrial cancer	Anovulation
Uterine leiomyomas	Polycystic ovary syndrome
Uterine sarcomas	Premature ovarian failure
Adenomyosis	Luteal phase defect
Ovarian neoplasms (hormone producing)	Shortened follicular phase
	Prolonged corpus luteum function
Medications	
Estrogen administration	**Pregnancy-related Conditions**
Combined hormonal contraception	Normal pregnancy
Progestin-only contraceptive	Threatened abortion
Contraceptive intrauterine device	Spontaneous/incomplete abortion
Aspirin	Ectopic pregnancy
Anticoagulants	Gestational trophoblastic neoplasm
Psychotropic medications	
	Trauma
Systemic Disease	Laceration
Hematologic disorders	Foreign body
Thrombocytopenia	
Von Willebrand disease	
Hepatic disease	
Renal disease	

day 14 (and has a 14-day follicular phase); if a woman has a 30-day cycle, she tends to ovulate on or about day 16 (with a 16-day follicular phase).

    c. Metrorrhagia refers to bleeding at irregular intervals. When irregular bleeding is excessive, it is termed **menometrorrhagia**.

4. Volume and duration of menstrual bleeding. The normal amount of menstrual blood produced per cycle is 30 to 50 mL. More than 80 mL is considered abnormal. The average duration of menstrual bleeding is 4 to 6 days. **Menorrhagia** is prolonged and excessive bleeding that occurs at regular intervals. Because **DUB** is associated with irregular ovulation, it presents more often as **metrorrhagia** or **menometrorrhagia** than **menorrhagia**. It is important to note, however, that the terms listed here are descriptive and that there is some redundancy in the terminology. It is most important to gather the basic facts about a patient's bleeding and use these terms for documentation and communication with other clinicians.

II   PHYSIOLOGY OF NORMAL MENSTRUAL BLEEDING

A **Postovulatory estrogen-progesterone withdrawal bleeding** describes the hormonal mechanism behind normal menstrual bleeding.

1. During the follicular phase of the cycle, the ovary produces **estrogen**, which results in **endometrial proliferation**. After ovulation, the **corpus luteum** develops from the remnant of the ovulatory follicle. The main function of the corpus luteum is to secrete progesterone (it also produces estrogen), which limits growth of the endometrium and causes it to differentiate. If pregnancy does not occur, the corpus luteum regresses and hormonal support of the endometrium is withdrawn.

2. **Regression of the corpus luteum** and the subsequent **decline in progesterone and estrogen** levels initiate a cascade of events that culminates in menstrual bleeding:

   a. Rhythmic **vasoconstriction** of spiral arterioles leads to ischemia, necrosis, and **sloughing of the surface endometrium**. In addition to playing a key role in the onset of menses, this vasoconstriction helps limit the amount of blood loss during the process. Thrombin and platelet plugging of spiral arterioles also promotes hemostasis.

   b. **Lytic enzymes** are released from intracellular lysosomes, and matrix metalloproteinases are upregulated. This results in **breakdown of endometrial tissue** via degradation of extracellular matrix components and the basement membrane. Endometrial breakdown also leads to the release of significant quantities of prostaglandins (particularly PGF_{2a}), which are potent mediators of myometrial contractions and vasoconstriction.

   c. **Estrogen production** at the beginning of a new menstrual cycle helps control bleeding by healing the raw surface of the endometrium.

III PATHOPHYSIOLOGY OF DYSFUNCTIONAL UTERINE BLEEDING

[A] **Dysfunctional uterine bleeding.** As previously stated, DUB occurs in the absence of the cyclic hormonal changes that regulate the menstrual cycle. In up to 90% of cases it is a manifestation of anovulation leading to **estrogen breakthrough bleeding**.

1. In the absence of ovulation, **estrogen stimulates the endometrium** without the production of progesterone by the corpus luteum. As mentioned previously, progesterone is responsible for endometrial differentiation and also keeps stimulation of the endometrium in check.

2. **Unopposed estrogen stimulation** of the endometrium leads to excessive glandular proliferation with lack of differentiation or development of stromal support. The result is an unstable, fragile, and heterogeneous endometrium that is prone to superficial breakdown and bleeding.

3. As this pattern of unopposed estrogen stimulation continues, the **endometrium sloughs off in isolated locations**. These raw surfaces are restimulated by estrogen just as another part of the endometrium begins to slough off. Prolonged and excessive bleeding results.

4. The **duration and level of unopposed estrogen** stimulation directly affect the amount and duration of bleeding.

5. Estrogen breakthrough bleeding is **unpredictable**. Furthermore, in the absence of estrogen-progesterone withdrawal, there is loss of rhythmic, progressive vasoconstriction of the **spiral arteries**. Without this, there is no periodic, orderly, self-limited shedding of the endometrium.

IV ETIOLOGY OF ABNORMAL UTERINE BLEEDING

[A] **Dysfunctional uterine bleeding**

1. **Common causes of anovulation or oligo-ovulation.** Anovulatory cycles are a symptom of disruption of the normal regulatory mechanisms that control the menstrual cycle. Ovulatory cycles result from a complex interaction of factors involving the hypothalamic-pituitary-ovarian axis. Abnormalities at any of these sites interfere with normal ovulation; a loss of normal ovulatory function occurs because of several causes.

   a. **Polycystic ovary syndrome (PCOS).** This condition involves a complex set of endocrine derangements, including anovulation. It is present in 5% to 10% of women of reproductive age. PCOS is also associated with hyperandrogenism, insulin resistance, and often obesity, each playing a role in the evolution of an oligo-ovulatory state. Signs of hyperandrogenism in PCOS include acne, hirsutism, and elevated serum testosterone. **PCOS is the classic condition that causes DUB due to estrogen breakthrough bleeding.** Women with PCOS are at risk for cardiovascular illness and diabetes mellitus. They are also at increased risk for endometrial hyperplasia and endometrial cancer because of long-term unopposed estrogen stimulation of the endometrium.

   b. **Immaturity of the hypothalamic-pituitary-ovarian axis.** Anovulation and DUB are often seen in postpubertal adolescents shortly after menarche. The onset of the first menstrual period may occur before the hypothalamic control mechanisms of ovulation are fully mature. Gonadotropin-releasing hormone (GnRH) secretion has not yet attained the pulsatile nature characteristic of ovulatory cycles. Estrogen breakthrough is often involved in these instances.

c. **Dysfunction of the hypothalamic-pituitary-ovarian axis.** Any factor that interferes with the normal pulsatile secretion of GnRH leads to anovulation. The following conditions typically cause DUB **not due to estrogen breakthrough bleeding.**

   (1) **Hyperprolactinemia.** Elevation of circulating prolactin may be caused by pituitary adenomas or a side effect of medications, most notably psychotropic drugs. Elevated prolactin inhibits normal GnRH pulsatility and results in anovulation.

   (2) **Stress and anxiety.** Anovulation and menstrual irregularities often occur during times of stress and major life changes. Loss of pulsatile GnRH secretion may occur as a result.

   (3) **Rapid weight loss.** Sudden and rapid weight loss from crash dieting may also interfere with normal GnRH secretion.

   (4) **Borderline anorexia nervosa.** Anovulation occurs early in the course of this disorder. If the anorexia increases in severity, complete loss of ovarian function may occur, resulting in amenorrhea and hypoestrogenism.

   (5) **Hypothyroidism.** This condition may also cause anovulation through dysregulation of a feedback loop that results in increased prolactin levels. Normal GnRH pulsatility is suppressed, as it is in primary hyperprolactinemia.

   (6) **Perimenopause.** This stage describes the years leading up to menopause. Women who are perimenopausal have very few oocytes remaining and as a result, ovulation is infrequent. The intervals between menstrual cycles lengthen as a result.

d. **Abnormalities of normal feedback signals.** Estradiol levels play a critical role in controlling the sequence of events during the normal ovulatory cycle. The rise and fall of estradiol at critical points in the cycle are important feedback mechanisms of cycle control. **Estradiol primarily exerts a negative feedback effect on follicle-stimulating hormone (FSH)** secretion and must decrease appropriately before menses to allow the increase in FSH necessary for initiation of a new cycle. Sustained estradiol levels at this time prevent normal cycling. Elevated estradiol levels can result from persistent secretion, abnormal clearance and metabolism, and production by extragonadal sources. **As in PCOS, estrogen breakthrough is often responsible for DUB in these patients.**

   (1) Certain medical conditions, most notably **hepatic disease or thyroid abnormalities,** may affect the metabolism and clearance of estradiol. The fluctuation in circulating estrogen levels seen in these conditions may cause ovulatory and menstrual dysfunction.

   (2) Conditions that lead to an increase in the production or conversion of estrogen precursors result in extragonadal production of estrogen. **Adipose tissue,** which contains aromatase, is capable of converting peripheral androgens to estrogens. This process increases with increasing body weight.

   (3) Estrogen-producing ovarian tumors such as granulosa cell tumor can cause disruption of the normal feedback mechanism.

B **Hormonally related bleeding.** These types of bleeding are abnormal, but they do not constitute DUB. These patterns are commonly seen and may be confused with DUB.

1. **Estrogen withdrawal bleeding.** This bleeding may occur at **midcycle** when estrogen levels decline briefly just before ovulation. Estrogen withdrawal also causes bleeding that occurs after bilateral oophorectomy.

2. **Progesterone breakthrough bleeding.** In the setting of prolonged progesterone administration, the endometrium receives relatively little estrogenic support. This occurs most often when women use progestin-only contraceptives for extended periods. The antagonistic effect of progesterone on the endometrium combined with inadequate estrogen stimulation results in atrophy. As a result, the endometrial surface bleeds irregularly, varying in amount and duration.

C **Organic causes of abnormal uterine bleeding.** Abnormal uterine bleeding may also be associated with conditions that are not endocrine in nature (Table 23-1). Organic conditions, such as polyps, uterine fibroids, endometritis, endometrial hyperplasia, pregnancy, and blood dyscrasias, must be considered as possible causes of the bleeding. Fibroids, polyps, adenomyosis, and blood dyscrasias usually present with menorrhagia (i.e., excessive cyclic bleeding) since these lesions do not affect ovulatory function. Endometritis, cervicitis, endometrial polyps, and pregnancy-related issues often present with irregular spotting or bleeding usually in addition to regular menstrual function.

V EVALUATION AND DIAGNOSIS OF ABNORMAL UTERINE BLEEDING

A **History.**   In general, structural causes of abnormal bleeding cause a change in the flow pattern of bleeding, but do not affect the menstrual cycle length. Dysfunctional bleeding, however, is defined as a disruption in ovulation and therefore causes a change in the length of the menstrual cycle or leads to an unpredictable and irregular bleeding pattern. A careful history can suggest which is most likely. Women may have structural and hormonal causes of abnormal bleeding present simultaneously, and both need to be diagnosed and addressed.

1. **Contraceptive use/pregnancy**. Pregnancy should always be ruled out in women of reproductive age even if they use contraception. All methods of contraception have small, inherent failure rates when used properly. This rate increases with faulty or erratic use. Moreover, some patients on hormonal contraception experience abnormal bleeding (e.g., progesterone breakthrough bleeding) that either resolves spontaneously or can be remedied with estrogen therapy. Intrauterine devices (IUDs) may also be associated with abnormal bleeding.

2. **Current bleeding history**. It is critical to describe the current pattern of bleeding accurately and to determine to what extent it differs from previous bleeding patterns. Variations from normal cyclic patterns may be a sign of DUB.

3. **Menstrual history**. DUB is most commonly associated with either **oligomenorrhea** or **menometrorrhagia**. Age at menarche, cycle frequency and duration, and presence of cyclically occurring symptoms establish the presence or absence of ovulatory cycles. A history of prolonged DUB identifies women at risk for endometrial hyperplasia and cancer, requiring endometrial sampling. **Menorrhagia** or **intermenstrual bleeding** is often a sign of a structural or an organic cause of bleeding.

4. **Medical history**. The presence of a medical condition associated with abnormal bleeding (e.g., coagulation disorders with or without liver disease) should be considered. Thirty percent of adolescents who present with severe blood loss have an associated coagulopathy, such as **von Willebrand disease**, in which platelets are dysfunctional. In addition, thyroid disease and pituitary adenomas may be the underlying cause of bleeding associated with anovulatory cycles.

5. **Medication history**. Certain medications may be associated with abnormal uterine bleeding (e.g., anticoagulants). Psychotropic medications may secondarily cause DUB through an elevation of prolactin.

B **Physical examination.**   A complete physical examination detects organic causes of abnormal uterine bleeding and signs associated with causes of anovulation and DUB.

1. **General physical examination**. Thyroid enlargement, galactorrhea (prolactinoma), ecchymosis, and purpura may be apparent. Pallor or vital sign instability suggests either brisk bleeding or long-standing bleeding with associated anemia. Such information helps guide the method and acuity of treatment.

2. **Gynecologic examination**. A complete gynecologic examination, including a Papanicolaou smear, detects organic causes of abnormal uterine bleeding. Elimination of anatomic or structural causes of abnormal bleeding is the first step in the diagnosis of DUB.

C **Laboratory studies.**   The history and physical examination determine the need for additional laboratory studies. Not all tests are necessary in all patients.

1. **Pregnancy test**. Modern urine pregnancy tests are highly sensitive, inexpensive, and easy to perform. Such tests should be performed in all premenopausal women with abnormal bleeding.

2. **Complete blood count**. A hemoglobin and hematocrit should be obtained in women with heavy or prolonged bleeding to evaluate for anemia. A white blood cell count may be useful in the diagnosis of endometritis; a platelet count detects thrombocytopenia.

3. **Thyroid-stimulating hormone (TSH) and prolactin.** Levels of these hormones should be obtained whenever bleeding is associated with anovulation.

4. **Coagulation profile.** Prothrombin time, partial thromboplastin time, and a workup for von Willebrand disease should be performed when an associated coagulation disorder is suspected.

5. **Androgen profile.** If there are signs of hyperandrogenism and oligo-ovulation or anovulation, a hyperandrogenic disorder should be considered and tested for appropriately. Total serum testosterone greater than 200 ng/dL suggests a testosterone-producing tumor of the ovary or adrenal. An elevated 17-hydroxyprogesterone level drawn at 8 AM and in the follicular phase of the menstrual cycle can indicate nonclassic adrenal hyperplasia. Polycystic ovary syndrome is diagnosed primarily by clinical signs and ruling out other causes (see Chapter 21).

D **Diagnostic procedures.** The need for additional diagnostic testing is determined on an individual basis.

1. **Ultrasonography and sonohysterography.** Ultrasound evaluation of the uterus can often isolate intrauterine polyps or submucosal fibroids that lead to heavy bleeding. The transvaginal approach is often more sensitive than the transabdominal approach. Sonohysterography, in which saline is instilled into the uterine cavity during transvaginal sonography, can often delineate intracavitary lesions even better than traditional ultrasound. Once the cavity is distended with saline, intracavitary polyps and fibroids can be localized and measured.

2. **Endometrial biopsy. To rule out endometrial hyperplasia or carcinoma**, a sample of the endometrial lining should be obtained in women at risk for endometrial hyperplasia or carcinoma. This includes **any woman over the age of 35 who presents with abnormal bleeding**. Endometrial hyperplasia, especially with atypical histologic features, is believed to be a precursor of endometrial carcinoma and can be treated medically or surgically. Cases of endometrial cancer should be referred to a gynecologic oncologist for further treatment. Endometrial biopsy is performed as an office procedure using a small catheter to obtain the specimen.

3. **Dilation and curettage (D&C).** This procedure is warranted in those women who have DUB and do not respond to medical management with hormonal manipulation. D&C is also required when an endometrial biopsy cannot be performed in the office; this is usually the case if a woman has a stenotic cervical os, making it impossible to pass the biopsy catheter.

4. **Hysteroscopy.** Hysteroscopy involves **direct visualization of the endometrial cavity**. Hysteroscopy and D&C are routinely performed at the same time. Hysteroscopy is particularly useful when a polyp or submucosal fibroid is suspected, because these lesions can be confirmed and resected hysteroscopically. After hysteroscopy, a D&C is performed to rule out coincident endometrial pathology whether a cavitary lesion is visualized or not.

VI **TREATMENT OF ABNORMAL UTERINE BLEEDING**

The cause of the abnormal bleeding should determine the treatment options available to the patient. Hormonal or medical conditions causing the bleeding should be addressed. Structural causes are often addressed surgically (as in the case of fibroids, polyps, or cancers), but conservative therapies may also be appropriate. These treatment options are discussed elsewhere. Patients with structural and hormonal causes of their abnormal bleeding may need multiple or sequential therapies.

A **Hormonal therapy.** The treatment of anovulatory DUB is hormonal therapy with a progestin, an estrogen, or a combination of the two. The choice of therapy is based on the duration of bleeding, age of the patient, and preference of the patient.

1. **Progestins. Progesterone supplementation** is the treatment of choice because most women with DUB are anovulatory. The bleeding represents estrogen breakthrough bleeding that is a manifestation of unopposed estrogen stimulation of the endometrial lining. Addition of progesterone restores the normal controlling influences to the endometrium.
   a. **Progestins act as antiestrogens.** The **antimitotic, antigrowth effect of progestins** supports their use in the treatment of endometrial hyperplasia.

(1) They enhance the conversion of estradiol to estrone, which is then displaced from the cell.

(2) They diminish the effect of estrogen on target cells by inhibiting estrogen receptor replenishment in the cell.

(3) They **support and stabilize the endometrium** so that an organized sloughing of the endometrium occurs after its withdrawal.

a. Progestins may not stop an acute episode of DUB as effectively as estrogen, especially if bleeding has been prolonged. However, **progestin, either alone or in combination with estrogen**, is warranted for long-term control after the acute episode of DUB is controlled.

b. Types of orally administered progestins used to regulate bleeding

(1) Medroxyprogesterone acetate 10 mg daily for 10 to 12 days

(2) Norethindrone acetate 5 mg daily for 10 to 12 days

(3) Oral micronized progesterone 200 mg daily for 10 to 12 days

c. The **levonorgestrel IUD** can reduce menstrual bleeding and is an excellent treatment option for women interested in long-term contraception. It requires replacement every 5 years.

2. **Oral contraceptive therapy**. Frequently, DUB is associated with prolonged endometrial buildup and heavy bleeding in younger women. Combined estrogen-progestin therapy in the form of oral contraceptives is used to treat episodes of acute bleeding. Combined oral contraceptives convert a fragile, overgrown endometrium into a structurally stable lining. Bleeding usually is controlled within 24 hours of initiation of therapy. If no response has occurred by this time, another treatment for the DUB should be pursued.

a. Any low-dose combination oral contraceptive can be used. The pill is administered two or three times a day for 3 to 4 days if excessive and prolonged bleeding is present.

b. A heavy withdrawal bleed is expected after cessation of therapy.

c. After the withdrawal bleed, cyclic therapy with once-a-day administration is continued for 3 months to reduce the endometrial lining to baseline levels. The oral contraceptive can be continued if birth control is desired.

3. **Estrogens**. High-dose estrogen therapy rapidly stops bleeding within 12 to 24 hours. The acute mechanism of action is thought to be **initiation of clotting at the capillary level**. Proliferation of the endometrial surface is a later effect. It is especially useful when bleeding has been **prolonged** or is secondary to **progesterone breakthrough bleeding**.

a. **Conjugated estrogens** (1.25 mg) **or estradiol** (2 mg) are administered daily for 7 to 10 days. If bleeding is moderately heavy, the same doses are administered every 4 hours during the first 24 hours of therapy. Treatment is continued for another 10 days, with the daily dose of estrogen combined with 10 mg medroxyprogesterone. A withdrawal bleed is expected after cessation of therapy.

b. **Intravenous estrogen** is effective in treating **acute profuse DUB**. Estrogen (25 mg) is administered intravenously every 4 hours until the bleeding lessens, or up to 12 hours. A progestin must be started at the same time.

c. After the acute episode is controlled, **chronic therapy** is initiated with the oral contraceptive or periodic progesterone for at least 3 months.

B Medical therapy

1. **Nonsteroidal anti-inflammatory drugs (NSAIDs)**

a. NSAIDs inhibit the synthesis of prostaglandins, which are substances that have important pharmacologic actions on the endometrial vasculature and on endometrial hemostasis. The concentration of endometrial prostaglandins, including thromboxane and prostacyclin, increases progressively during the menstrual cycle.

b. NSAIDs may work by altering the balance between thromboxane and prostacyclin.

c. NSAIDs are primarily effective in limiting menstrual blood loss in women who ovulate, and they reduce excessive blood flow by as much as 50%.

2. **GnRH agonists**. After control of an episode of acute bleeding, GnRH agonists may help achieve amenorrhea in chronically ill patients. Expense and the long-term effects of hypoestrogenism limit therapy. If long-term therapy is chosen, hormone replacement therapy with estrogen and progestin is advised.

3. **Desmopressin**. A synthetic analog of arginine vasopressin, desmopressin is used as a treatment of last resort in patients with coagulation disorders.

C Surgical therapy

1. **D&C** with or without hysteroscopy. This procedure is not the treatment of first choice in DUB. It is undertaken in patients who have bleeding refractory to medical therapy or who are not candidates for hormonal manipulation. It can be a diagnostic and therapeutic modality.

2. **Hysterectomy**. This procedure is a realistic treatment option in the following situations:
   a. For women who have completed childbearing in whom persistent abnormal bleeding is often worrisome or life threatening
   b. For women who do not tolerate medical management
   c. For women diagnosed with atypical endometrial hyperplasia and with an increased risk of endometrial cancer, who may opt for surgical as opposed to medical management

3. **Endometrial ablation**. Ablation of the endometrium is a surgical option for women who have unexplained menorrhagia or who have DUB but are not candidates for hormonal therapy or hysterectomy because of medical conditions or who wish to avoid hysterectomy but choose not to pursue hormonal therapy. It is not indicated in cases where there is endometrial hyperplasia or cancer, or an otherwise structural cause of the bleeding.
   a. Ablation of the endometrium is performed using laser, electrocautery, or thermal destructive techniques.
   b. Fifty percent of women achieve amenorrhea; 90% achieve a decrease in bleeding.
   c. The long-term risk of the occurrence of undetectable endometrial carcinoma in isolated segments of endometrium has yet to be defined.

Study Questions for Chapter 23

Directions: Each of the numbered items or incomplete statements in this section is followed by answers or by completions of the statement. Select the ONE lettered answer or completion that is BEST in each case.

1. A 50-year-old woman, gravida 3, para 2, spontaneous abortions 1, presents to you reporting abnormal vaginal bleeding. Her menstrual cycles used to occur regularly every 30 days and lasted 3 to 4 days. She now has periods every 15 to 22 days and they last for 6 to 7 days for the last 6 months. She denies any past medical or surgical history. Review of systems is negative and she specifically denies light-headedness. Her speculum examination is unremarkable. The bimanual examination reveals a slightly enlarged, regular contour, anteverted uterus that is nontender to palpation. The next best step in management is:

- [A] Low-dose oral contraceptive pills
- [B] Endometrial biopsy
- [C] Dilation and curettage
- [D] Endometrial ablation
- [E] Levonorgestrel IUD

2. A 14-year-old nulligravid girl reports menstrual bleeding every 45 to 50 days and bleeding for 4 days. She experienced menarche at age 13. She is not sexually active. Her physical examination is unremarkable, and her serum pregnancy test is negative. The next best step in management is:

- [A] Low-dose birth control pills
- [B] Reassurance
- [C] NSAIDs
- [D] Hysteroscopy and dilation and curettage
- [E] Coagulation profile

3. A 32-year-old woman, gravida 1, para 1, presents to you reporting bleeding between her periods and lengthening of the time between her periods to more than 40 days. Review of systems is remarkable for a 70-lb weight gain since her pregnancy 2 years ago. She denies any medical problems. She is 5 feet 4 inches tall and weighs 230 lb. Her physical examination is otherwise unremarkable. The most likely explanation for her bleeding is:

- [A] Increased endogenous progesterone
- [B] Increased exogenous progesterone
- [C] Increased endogenous estrogen
- [D] Increased exogenous estrogen
- [E] Increased prolactin

4. An 18-year-old nulligravid girl presents to the emergency department by ambulance because she passed out on the floor of her house and is covered in blood. She is now conscious. She has been bleeding off and on for the past 5 months. Her BP = 98/48, P = 120, RR = 16, and T = 96.2. Her speculum examination reveals blood trickling from the cervical os. There are no lesions in the vagina or cervix. The bimanual examination is unremarkable. Pelvic ultrasound is also unremarkable. Serum human chorionic gonadotropin (hCG) is negative, and her hemoglobin is 7 g/dL. The next best step in management of this patient is:

- [A] Depot-medroxyprogesterone acetate
- [B] Oral conjugated estrogen
- [C] Intravenous estrogen
- [D] Low-dose combination oral contraceptive pills
- [E] GnRH agonist therapy

5. A 38-year-old woman presents complaining of a 2-year history of heavy menstrual flow lasting 9 days, with occasional episodes of soaking her clothes and bedsheets with menstrual blood. Her menses are occurring every 32 days. She denies any bleeding between menses. The rest of her history is notable for hypertension controlled with a diuretic. The next step in evaluation would be:

- [A] Obtain a coagulation profile
- [B] Obtain a pregnancy test
- [C] Perform an endometrial biopsy
- [D] Obtain a pelvic ultrasound
- [E] Obtain a TSH level

Answers and Explanations

1. The answer is B [V D]. The risk of endometrial carcinoma increases with age and should be ruled out in patients with abnormal bleeding who are over age 40 years. In addition, endometrial hyperplasia often develops in women with a history of chronic anovulation and unopposed estrogen stimulation of the endometrium (most likely in this perimenopausal patient). When a woman is diagnosed with endometrial hyperplasia with atypia, she has an increased risk for endometrial carcinoma. Endometrial hyperplasia can be treated with progestin therapy. Many women who are perimenopausal have erratic bleeding because of the transition from regular ovarian folliculogenesis and hormone production to relative ovarian quiescence. An office endometrial biopsy must be performed. Birth control pills will regulate her bleeding but will not tell you about the endometrium. Dilation and curettage is the next step after an endometrial biopsy if the results are not satisfactory (e.g., cervical stenosis and inability to obtain biopsy in the office or no tissue obtained on biopsy) or if the patient is refractory to agents aimed at stopping the bleeding. Endometrial ablation should not be done until you know the endometrium is completely normal. Levonorgestrel IUD is a good treatment option after biopsy of the endometrium.

2. The answer is B [IV A 1 b]. The pattern of bleeding demonstrated by this patient is characteristic of the menstrual pattern seen following menarche. Unless it is prolonged and very heavy (not the case in this patient), it should evolve into a pattern of regular estrogen-progesterone withdrawal bleeding with time (usually by 2 years from menarche). The chance that an anatomic lesion such as a polyp or a fibroid would be the cause of her bleeding is unlikely given her age and pattern of bleeding. Therefore, hysteroscopy with dilation and curettage would not help. Oral contraception and NSAIDs are not indicated at this point unless she desires contraception. Coagulopathy is an unlikely cause of her bleeding because the timing, not the volume, is problematic for this patient.

3. The answer is C [IV A 1 d]. This patient is obese, and therefore likely has increased endogenous production of estrogen from adipose tissue, which can lead to suppression of FSH and anovulation, leading to menstrual irregularity. With estrogen production unopposed by progesterone, the endometrium experiences excessive glandular proliferation without stromal support. As a result, the endometrium sloughs in isolated locations, leading to unpredictable and prolonged bleeding. There is no history of exogenous hormone intake. Progesterone is not being produced. High prolactin typically results in amenorrhea and galactorrhea.

4. The answer is D [VI A 2]. A low-dose oral contraceptive given as three pills a day with taper over 3 to 4 days is an effective way to stop dysfunctional bleeding fairly quickly. Intravenous estrogen is indicated when the bleeding is profuse and the patient unstable. Estrogen (25 mg) is administered intravenously every 4 hours until the bleeding lessens. This patient does not have profuse bleeding, and therefore does not warrant using intravenous estrogen, but she has been bleeding for a long time and is anemic, so a quick method to stop the bleeding would be appropriate. Since this patient has been bleeding for 5 months and is young, she is probably anovulatory. Causes other than normal peripubertal anovulation should be looked for (thyroid disease, bleeding disorder). Just giving estrogen would not help because she is already bleeding due to unopposed estrogen. Depomedroxyprogesterone acetate and a GnRH agonist can both be used to treat anovulation, but they both take a while to work so would not be ideal.

5. The answer is D [IV C]. This woman has a history of regular cyclic menstrual flow, but with menorrhagia. This regular pattern suggests that she does not have an ovulation disorder and that the bleeding is most likely from a structural problem. The next best step would be to obtain a pelvic ultrasound to look for the presence of fibroids, endometrial polyps, or adenomyosis. An endometrial biopsy to look for endometrial hyperplasia or cancer is not warranted since the bleeding is regular and cyclic and there is no bleeding between menses, making this diagnosis unlikely. A coagulation profile is unlikely to be abnormal since this problem is relatively new. A pregnancy test is also not indicated. It is unlikely that hypothyroid abnormalities would cause this regular but heavy menstrual flow. Extreme hypo- or hyperthyroidism can cause irregular menses and anovulation, but not menorrhagia.

chapter 24

Uterine Leiomyomas

MONICA A. MAINIGI · RICHARD W. TURECK

I INTRODUCTION

Uterine leiomyomas, which are also known as myomas, fibroids, or fibromyomas, are proliferative, well-circumscribed, pseudoencapsulated, benign tumors composed of smooth muscle and fibrous connective tissue.

A Leiomyomas are the **most common uterine mass** and the most common neoplasm found in the female pelvis. They are present in 20% to 40% of women 35 years of age or older, and rarely can be present in adolescents.

B They vary in diameter from 1 mm to more than 20 cm.

C Leiomyomas may be single but most often are multiple; 100 or more have been found in a single uterus.

II ETIOLOGY

Leiomyomas are benign neoplasms consisting of a localized proliferation of smooth muscle cells and an accumulation of extracellular matrix. These smooth muscle tumors may be found in organs outside the uterus, including the fallopian tubes, vagina, round ligament, uterosacral ligaments, vulva, and gastrointestinal tract.

A **Cytogenetic studies** suggest that leiomyomas arise from a single neoplastic smooth muscle cell; in other words, they are **monoclonal** tumors resulting from somatic mutations. A variety of chromosomal abnormalities involving chromosomes 6, 7, 12, and 14 have been identified, suggesting a genetic role in the pathogenesis of these tumors. Disruption or dysregulation of the high mobility group genes on chromosome 12 appears to contribute to fibroid development.

B **Hormones** affect growth of leiomyomas but do not appear to be the cause. Evidence that suggests that estrogen is a promoter of leiomyoma growth includes:

1. Leiomyomas are rarely found before puberty and stop growing after menopause.

2. New leiomyomas rarely appear after menopause.

3. Leiomyomas often grow rapidly during pregnancy.

4. Gonadotropin-releasing hormone (GnRH) agonists create a hypoestrogenic environment that results in a reduction of the size of leiomyomas. This effect is reversible on cessation of treatment.

C **Local and paracrine factors**, such as blood supply and proximity to other tumors, may account for variations in tumor volume and rate of growth. In addition, some peptide growth factors may play an etiologic role.

1. Epidermal growth factor (EGF) induces DNA synthesis in leiomyomas and myometrial cells.

2. Estrogen may exert its effect through EGF.

3. Recent studies in animals have shown that pirfenidone, an antifibrotic agent, suppresses leiomyoma growth via its potent inhibition of fibrogenic cytokines, including basic fibroblast growth factor, platelet-derived growth factor, transforming growth factor-β, and EGF.

III CLASSIFICATION AND PATHOLOGY

A **Classification of leiomyomas according to location**   (see Fig. 24-1). Three types of leiomyomas occur based on their location within or on the uterus.

1. **Intramural leiomyomas** are the most common variety, occurring within the myometrium of the uterus as isolated, encapsulated nodules of varying size. As these tumors grow, they can distort the uterine cavity or the external surface of the uterus. These tumors can also cause symmetric enlargement of the uterus when they occur singly.

2. **Submucous leiomyomas** are located beneath the endometrium and can grow into the uterine cavity. They can be **pedunculated** (i.e., attached to the endometrium by a stalk) and may protrude to or through the cervical os into the vagina. These tumors are often associated with abnormal bleeding and menorrhagia severe enough to cause significant anemia.

3. **Subserosal leiomyomas** are located just beneath the serosal surface and grow out toward the peritoneal cavity, causing distortion of the peritoneal surface of the uterus. When leiomyomas extend into the broad ligament, they are known as **intraligamentary leiomyomas**. These tumors may become pedunculated, and reach a large size within the peritoneal cavity without producing symptoms. These potentially mobile tumors may present in such a manner that they need to be differentiated from solid adnexal lesions. Pedunculated leiomyomas may also attach themselves to an adjacent structure such as the omentum, mesentery, or bowel; develop a secondary blood supply; and lose their connection with the uterus and primary blood supply. This situation occurs rarely, and the resulting structures are known as **parasitic leiomyomas**.

B **Pathology**

1. **Gross pathology**. Leiomyomas are **pseudoencapsulated** solid tumors, well demarcated from the surrounding myometrium. The **pseudocapsule** is not a true capsule and results from compression of fibrous and muscular tissue on the surface of the tumor. Because the vasculature is located on the periphery, the central part of the tumor is susceptible to degenerative changes and necrosis. The tumors are smooth, solid, and usually pinkish-white, depending on the degree of vascularity. The surface typically has a trabeculate, fleshy, whorl-like appearance.

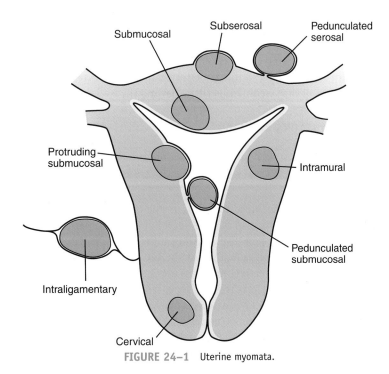

FIGURE 24–1   Uterine myomata.

2. **Microscopic pathology**. Leiomyomas are composed of groups and bundles of smooth muscle fibers in a twisted, whorled fashion. Microscopically, these appear as smooth muscle cells in longitudinal or cross-section intermixed with fibrous connective tissue. Vascular structures are few, and mitoses are rare.

   a. **Cellular leiomyomas** are tumors with mitotic counts of 5 to 10 per 10 consecutive high-power fields that lack cytologic atypia. These are not considered cancerous.

   b. **Leiomyosarcomas** are a distinct clinical entity and are diagnosed based on a **mitotic count** of 10 mitotic figures per 10 high-power fields. Recently, the importance of other factors, such as **cellular atypia** and **coagulative necrosis** of tumor cells, has been recognized. These malignant tumors are found rarely in hysterectomy or myomectomy specimens (incidence 0.2%).

C **Degenerative changes.** A variety of degenerative changes may occur in leiomyomas that alter the gross and microscopic appearance of the tumors. Most of these changes have no clinical significance. Degenerative changes occur secondary to alterations in circulation (either arterial or venous), postmenopausal atrophy, or infection, or they may result from malignant transformation.

1. **Hyaline degeneration**, the most common type of degeneration, is present in almost all leiomyomas. It is caused by an overgrowth of the fibrous elements, which leads to a hyalinization of the fibrous tissue and, eventually, calcification.

2. **Cystic degeneration** may occasionally be a sequel of necrosis, but cystic cavities are usually a result of myxomatous change and liquefaction after hyaline degeneration.

3. **Necrosis** is commonly caused by impairment of the blood supply or severe infection. A specific kind of necrosis is the **red**, or **carneous**, degeneration, which occurs most frequently in pregnancy. The lesion has a dull, reddish hue and is believed to be caused by aseptic degeneration associated with local hemolysis.

4. **Mucoid degeneration** may occur when the arterial input is impaired, particularly in large tumors. Areas of hyalinization may convert to a mucoid or myxomatous type of degeneration; the lesion has a soft, gelatinous consistency. Further degeneration can lead to liquefaction and cystic degeneration.

5. **Infection** of a leiomyoma most commonly occurs with a pedunculated submucous leiomyoma that first becomes necrotic and then becomes infected.

6. **Calcification** of leiomyomas is a common finding in postmenopausal patients.

7. **Sarcomatous degeneration** occurs in less than 1% (0.13% to 0.29%) of leiomyomas. Whether this represents a true degenerative change or a spontaneous neoplasm is a subject of controversy. The presence of a leiomyosarcoma within the core of an apparently benign pseudoencapsulated leiomyoma suggests such a degenerative process. This type of sarcoma is usually of a spindle cell rather than a round cell type. The 5-year survival rate for patients with a leiomyosarcoma arising within a leiomyoma is much better than that for a true leiomyosarcoma of the uterus with extension of the sarcomatous tissue beyond the pseudocapsule of the leiomyoma.

IV ASSOCIATED SYMPTOMS AND SIGNS

A **Symptoms.** These vary greatly, depending on size, number, and location of the leiomyoma or leiomyomas. Most women with leiomyomas are asymptomatic; symptoms occur in 10% to 40% of patients.

1. **Abnormal uterine bleeding**. This is the most common symptom associated with uterine leiomyomas, occurring in as many as 30% of symptomatic women. The typical bleeding pattern is **menorrhagia**, or excessive bleeding at the time of menses (more than 80 mL). The increase in flow usually occurs gradually, but the bleeding may result in a profound anemia. The exact mechanisms of increased blood loss are unclear. Possible factors include necrosis of the surface endometrium overlying the submucous leiomyoma, a disturbance in the hemostatic contraction of normal muscle bundles when extensive intramural myomatous growth occurs, an increase in surface area of the endometrial cavity, or an alteration in endometrial microvasculature. In some cases, abnormal bleeding may be associated with anovulatory states. Leiomyomas can be associated with polyps and endometrial hyperplasia, which may produce an abnormal bleeding pattern. Endometrial sampling is advised if abnormal bleeding is present.

2. **Pain**. Uncomplicated uterine leiomyomas usually do not produce pain. Acute pain associated with fibroids is usually caused by either torsion of a pedunculated leiomyoma or infarction progressing to carneous degeneration within a leiomyoma. Pain is often crampy with a submucous leiomyoma within the endometrial cavity, and severe cramping can occur as the uterus contracts to try to "deliver" the fibroid through the cervical os.

3. **Pressure**. As leiomyomas enlarge, they may cause a feeling of pelvic heaviness or produce pressure symptoms on surrounding structures.
   a. **Urinary frequency** is a common symptom when a growing leiomyoma exerts pressure on the bladder.
   b. **Urinary retention**, a rare occurrence, can result when myomatous growth creates a fixed, retroverted uterus that pushes the cervix anteriorly under the symphysis pubis in the area of the posterior urethrovesicular angle.
   c. **Unilateral uretal obstruction** can be caused by lateral extension or intraligamentous leiomyomas. A markedly enlarged uterus that extends above the pelvic brim may cause ureteral compression, hydroureter, and hydronephrosis.
   d. **Constipation and difficult defecation** can be caused by large posterior leiomyomas.
   e. **Compression of pelvic vasculature** by a markedly enlarged uterus may cause varicosities or edema of the lower extremities. Compression of pelvic vessels can lead to the development of deep venous thrombosis within the pelvis and pulmonary embolus.

4. **Reproductive disorders**. Infertility due to leiomyomas is probably uncommon. Infertility may result when leiomyomas interfere with normal tubal transport or implantation of the fertilized ovum.
   a. **Large intramural leiomyomas located in the cornual regions** may virtually close the interstitial portion of the tube and predispose to ectopic pregnancy.
   b. **Submucous leiomyomas** may impede implantation; the endometrium overlying the leiomyoma may be out of phase with the normal endometrium and thus provide a poor surface for implantation.
   c. **Increased incidences of abortion and premature labor** occur in patients with submucous or intramural leiomyomas.
   d. Less successful results with in vitro fertilization occur in patients who have large submucosal fibroids when compared to controls.

5. **Pregnancy-related disorders**. Uterine leiomyomas, found in 0.3% to 7.2% of pregnancies, are usually present before conception and may increase in size significantly during gestation.
   a. Although women with leiomyomas have a higher **incidence of spontaneous abortion**, the tumors are an uncommon cause of abortion.
   b. **Red degeneration**, or **torsion of a pedunculated fibroid**, may cause gradual or acute symptoms of pain and tenderness. These conditions must be distinguished from other causes of abdominal pain in pregnancy because treatment is conservative with symptomatic relief and observation. Surgical intervention is rarely, if ever, indicated.
   c. **Premature labor** may be increased in women with leiomyomas.
   d. In the third trimester, leiomyomas may be a factor in **malpresentation, mechanical obstruction**, or **uterine dystocia**. Large leiomyomas in the lower uterine segment may prevent descent of the presenting part. Intramural leiomyomas may interfere with effectual uterine contractions and normal labor. Cesarean section may be necessary for delivery.
   e. **Postpartum hemorrhage** is more common with uterine leiomyomas.

B **Signs**

1. **Physical examination**. The diagnosis of uterine leiomyomas can be made with confidence in 95% of cases based on physical examination alone. Uterine size is defined as the equivalent gestational size as determined by abdominal and pelvic examination.
   a. **Abdominal examination**. Uterine leiomyomas may be palpated as irregular, nodular tumors protruding against the anterior abdominal wall. Leiomyomas are usually firm on palpation; softness or tenderness suggests the presence of edema, sarcoma, pregnancy, or degenerative changes.

    b. Pelvic examination. The most common finding is uterine enlargement. The shape of the uterus is usually asymmetric and irregular in outline. The uterus is usually freely movable unless concomitant pelvic disease exists such as endometriosis or pelvic adhesions.

        (1) In the case of **submucous leiomyomas**, the uterine enlargement is usually symmetric.

        (2) Some **subserous leiomyomas** may be distinct from the main body of the uterus and may move freely, which can be confused with adnexal or extrapelvic tumors.

        (3) The **diagnosis of cervical leiomyomas or pedunculated submucous leiomyomas** may be made on examination if the tumor extends through the cervical canal and into the vagina. Occasionally, a submucous leiomyoma may be visible at the introitus.

2. Laboratory evaluation and diagnostic studies. Additional diagnostic studies are based on individual presentation and physical examination. In asymptomatic patients with physical examinations consistent with leiomyomas, it is not necessary to obtain additional studies routinely.

    a. Hemoglobin and hematocrit is obtained in cases of excessive vaginal bleeding to assess the degree of anemia and adequacy of replacement.

    b. Coagulation profile and **bleeding time** are recommended when the history is suggestive of a bleeding diathesis.

    c. Endometrial biopsy is performed in patients with abnormal uterine bleeding who are thought to be anovulatory or at increased risk for endometrial hyperplasia.

    d. Ultrasonography may be used to assess uterine dimension, leiomyoma location, interval growth, and adnexal anatomy.

        (1) Routine ultrasonography does not improve long-term outcome compared with clinical assessment alone. Pelvic ultrasound is appropriate in situations when clinical assessment is difficult or uncertain; when physical examination is suboptimal, as in cases of morbid obesity; or when adnexal pathology cannot be excluded on physical examination alone. Ultrasonography may be used to detect hydroureter and hydronephrosis in the patient with marked uterine enlargement.

        (2) Sonohysterography or intrauterine infusion of sterile saline at the time of ultrasound examination can identify the presence of pedunculated submucous leiomyomas and endometrial polyps.

    e. Hysteroscopy or **hysterosalpingography** may be used to evaluate the endometrial cavity in the evaluation of patients with uterine leiomyomas and infertility or recurrent pregnancy loss.

    f. Magnetic resonance imaging (MRI) is now being used more often in diagnosing and planning treatment for uterine fibroids. MRI has been found to be more effective than ultrasound in demarcating individual myomas, which may affect treatment, and also in assessing risk of malignancy. MRI is also better at discerning other causes of pathology including adenomyosis and adnexal masses.

V   TREATMENT

Therapy for leiomyomas must be individualized and may be nonsurgical or surgical. Treatment decisions are based on symptoms, fertility status, uterine size, and rate of uterine growth.

A Expectant management. In the absence of pain, abnormal bleeding, pressure, or large leiomyomas, observation with periodic examination is appropriate. This is especially true if the patient is nearing menopause, at which time the leiomyomas will atrophy as estrogen levels fall.

1. Bimanual examinations should be performed every 3 to 6 months to determine uterine size and the rate of tumor growth. After slow growth or stable uterine size has been confirmed, annual follow-up may then be appropriate. Rapid growth—a change of 6 pregnancy weeks in size or more in 12 months or less of observation—is suspicious for malignancy and surgical intervention is indicated. Follow-up with pelvic ultrasound or MRI should be performed if physical examination is inadequate because of obesity or if it is necessary to distinguish between a fibroid and an adnexal mass.

2. Endometrial biopsy may be indicated in patients with **abnormal bleeding**.

3. Regular blood counts are warranted; iron deficiency anemia is common with menorrhagia, and iron replacement may be required.

4. **Nonsteroidal anti-inflammatory drugs (NSAIDs)** that inhibit prostaglandin synthesis and are administered on a scheduled rather than as-needed basis can be used to reduce menstrual blood flow. NSAIDs also treat pelvic discomfort or pressure.

5. Low-dose oral contraceptives or progestin therapy may also reduce blood loss.

B **GnRH agonists.** Long-acting GnRH agonists suppress gonadotropin secretion and create a hypoestrogenic state similar to that observed after menopause. They are administered in the form of a subcutaneous implant or an intramuscular depot injection (administered as a monthly or every 3 months injection).

1. Although individual response varies widely, a median reduction in uterine *volume* (not diameter) of 50% has been observed with GnRH agonists. Maximum response is seen after 12 weeks of therapy, with no added advantage to 24 weeks of therapy. Decreased size is secondary to a decrease in blood flow and cell size; cell death and a decrease in cell number are not observed.

2. Leiomyomas rapidly regrow, returning to baseline size within 12 weeks after GnRH therapy is discontinued.

3. Use of GnRH agonist therapy is not recommended for longer than 24 weeks (6 months) because of the long-term effects of a hypoestrogenic state, most notably osteoporosis. Therefore, agonist therapy is often used prior to surgery to achieve a smaller sized fibroid or uterus, which may impact the procedure chosen.

4. Long-term use of GnRH agonists with "add-back" hormone replacement therapy is another alternative, and can be used if the patient is a poor surgical candidate.

5. Because of potential side effects and expense, GnRH agonists are recommended for short-term use in selected cases only. For example:
   a. For large submucous leiomyomas to facilitate hysteroscopic resection
   b. For leiomyomas in symptomatic perimenopausal patients who wish to avoid surgery
   c. As presurgical treatment to decrease bleeding symptoms in patients with anemia who are taking iron in order to increase blood cell count prior to surgery.

C **Surgery**
1. **Indications.** Surgical intervention is indicated when symptoms fail to respond to conservative management.
   a. **Excessive bleeding** that interferes with normal lifestyle or leads to anemia and **chronic pelvic pain or pressure**
   b. **Protrusion** of a pedunculated submucous leiomyoma through the cervix
   c. **Rapid growth** in a leiomyomatous uterus at any age. This finding warrants exploration because it may represent a leiomyosarcoma as opposed to a benign leiomyoma. Most often, leiomyosarcomas represent a distinct clinical entity rather than malignant degeneration within a leiomyoma. Because these malignancies occur primarily in women older than 40 years of age and their incidence increases with advancing age, any increase in uterine size in the postmenopausal woman warrants surgical exploration.
   d. **Repetitive pregnancy loss caused by leiomyomas** after other etiologies have been excluded
   e. **Infertility patients** with leiomyomas after evaluation and treatment of other causes. The location or size of the leiomyoma should indicate that it may be a cause of the infertility.
   f. **Enlarged uterine size** (more than 12 pregnancy weeks) in asymptomatic patients. This criterion has traditionally been cited as an indication for surgery but has recently come under scrutiny. No controlled data indicate that the proposed benefits of surgery outweigh its risks. Expectant management of asymptomatic patients with uterine enlargement of greater than 12 pregnancy weeks' size with stable or slow growth is considered a reasonable treatment option. Surgical intervention is indicated if a patient is concerned about uterine size or is symptomatic.
   g. **Progressive hydronephrosis**, demonstrated by ultrasonography or intravenous pyelography, or **impaired renal function**

2. **Surgical procedures.** The type of surgery to be performed depends on the age of the patient, the nature of the symptoms, the size and the location of the tumor, and the patient's desires about future fertility.

a. **Myomectomy** involves the removal of single or multiple leiomyomas while preserving the uterus. Myomectomy is a reasonable approach in symptomatic women unresponsive to conservative treatment who desire future fertility or uterine conservation. Eighty percent of patients report subjective improvement of symptoms, 15% of patients experience symptom recurrence, and 10% require additional treatment. The **recurrence of leiomyomas after myomectomy** depends on the number of fibroids present prior to myomectomy, race (higher in African Americans), patient age, and the completeness of the original myomectomy. Fifty percent of patients will have evidence of fibroids on ultrasound within 5 years of myomectomy. Fifteen to twenty-five percent of individuals will require further treatment for fibroids in the future.

   (1) **Abdominal myomectomy** is preformed through an incision in the abdomen with gentle dissection of the fibroids out of the uterus followed by careful uterine reconstruction. Risks of this procedure include bleeding, prolonged operative time, and increased postoperative hemorrhage compared to hysterectomy. Experienced surgeons, however, can perform myomectomy with less risk of blood loss than with hysterectomy depending on the technique used. At the time of abdominal myomectomy, it may be necessary to open the uterine cavity to remove intramural or submucous leiomyomas completely. This is considered a risk factor for future uterine rupture and therefore is an indication for cesarean section in future pregnancies.

   (2) **Hysteroscopic resection** can be used in patients with submucous leiomyomas and often leads to an improvement of the menorrhagia associated with these fibroids. A hysteroscope is inserted transcervically into the uterine cavity and the fibroid is resected without having to enter the abdominal cavity. This procedure is associated with significantly less pain and shorter recovery periods compared to an abdominal approach. Up to 20% of women may require additional treatment within 5 to 10 years.

   (3) Indications for **laparoscopic myomectomy** are the same as for abdominal myomectomy. Laparoscopic myomectomy may be associated with shorter recovery times, but uncertainty still exists over whether it is associated with fewer postoperative pelvic adhesions. Large, multiple, deep, and lower posterior wall leiomyomas should be approached with caution; they are technically more challenging and can be associated with a high intraoperative blood loss.

   (4) **MRI-guided focused ultrasound** is a relatively new treatment option that uses ultrasound-generated heat to cause cell death. The fibroids are localized in three-dimension with MRI, and heat from a phased array transducer is able to converge on a focal area and produce protein denaturation. An early study has shown an improvement in symptoms in nearly 60% of patients.

   (5) **Laparoscopic myolysis** (using laser or coagulation current) and **cryomyolysis** (using a $-180°C$ probe) of leiomyomas have resulted in a persistent decrease in the size of fibroids and appear to be another promising therapeutic option.

b. **Hysterectomy** is the definitive treatment for uterine leiomyomas if the indications for surgery are present and **if childbearing is complete and uterine conservation is not important to the individual.**

   (1) With hysterectomy, both the leiomyomas and any associated disease are removed permanently. There is no risk of recurrence.

   (2) In patients with abnormal bleeding, other causes should be evaluated and treated before hysterectomy. Hysterectomy should not be performed on the assumption that the bleeding is caused solely by the leiomyomas. Biopsy of the endometrial cavity is essential before hysterectomy to rule out endometrial neoplasia. The absence of cervical malignancy must also be ascertained before surgery.

   (3) The patient's medical and psychological risks should be evaluated before surgical therapy.

   (4) Ovaries need not be removed in women younger than 40 to 45 years of age. The patient must play an important part in the decision concerning oophorectomy at any age; little evidence supports the contention that the residual ovary after a hysterectomy is at greater risk for development of ovarian cancer. The long-term consequences of estrogen deprivation—osteoporosis and cardiovascular risk—and implications of estrogen replacement therapy should be addressed thoroughly before surgery. Women with a

strong family history of breast or ovarian cancer may benefit from salpingo-oophorectomy and should be counseled appropriately.

c. **Uterine artery embolization (UAE).** Recently, this procedure has emerged as an alternative to traditional surgery. In uterine artery embolization the desired previously mapped artery is injected with embolic material, such as gel-foam pledgets or metal coils. This action occludes the vessel feeding the uterus and leiomyomas, depriving the tumors of their vascular supply and causing shrinking or necrosis and death of the leiomyomas.

(1) Recent studies have shown that uterine artery embolization is relatively safe. It results in a 60% reduction in size of fibroids and controls menorrhagia in more than 90% of cases.

(2) Typical candidates are women with symptomatic fibroids who are approaching menopause, no longer desire fertility, have a large uterus, have multiple health risks for surgery or do not desire surgery, and have uncontrollable menorrhagia.

(3) The most common complication seen in UAE is fibroid expulsion, which can be seen in 3% to 5% of patients and occurs most often in patients with submucosal fibroids. Other complications include vaginal discharge, infection, premature ovarian failure, and persistent pain from fibroid necrosis that may rarely necessitate hysterectomy.

Study Questions for Chapter 24

Directions: *Each of the numbered items or incomplete statements in this section is followed by answers or by completions of the statement. Select the ONE lettered answer or completion that is BEST in each case.*

1. A 25-year-old woman, gravida 4, para 4, with a history of leiomyomas, presents to the emergency department reporting pelvic pressure. She denies cardiac, renal, or hepatic symptoms. A pelvic ultrasound shows a 10-cm left uterine mass that has the echogenicity of a fibroid. Pressure from the fibroid may also cause:

- A Leg ulcers
- B Peau d'orange
- C Superficial thrombophlebitis
- D Deep venous thrombosis of the leg
- E Varicose veins

2. A 30-year-old woman, gravida 2, para 2, presents to you for her annual gynecologic visit. Currently, she has no symptoms. You perform a Pap smear and a pelvic examination that reveals an enlarged, nontender, irregular uterus and no adnexal mass or tenderness. There are no vulvar or vaginal lesions. The most likely type of fibroid is a(n):

- A Anterior intramural fibroid (5-cm size)
- B Submucosal pedunculated fibroid (2-cm size)
- C Subserosal pedunculated fibroid (7-cm size)
- D Posterior intramural fibroid (5-cm size)
- E Intramural fibroid with a submucous component (5-cm size)

3. A 22-year-old woman, gravida 2, para 1, at 20 weeks of gestation, presents to the emergency department reporting acute-onset lower abdominal pain. She has a history of fibroids and an unknown abdominal surgery. Her vital signs are as follows: T = 99.2, BP = 105/68, P = 110, R = 28. There is a linear, 4-cm scar in the right lower quadrant, bowel sounds are present, and the abdomen is nontender except for spot tenderness in the midline, between the umbilicus and the symphysis pubis. There is no rebound tenderness or guarding. There is no costovertebral angle tenderness. Her fundus is 28 cm above the symphysis pubis. Her white blood cells are elevated, urinalysis is normal, and her liver function tests are within normal range. The most likely diagnosis is:

- A Leiomyomatous degeneration
- B Ovarian torsion
- C Cystitis
- D Preeclampsia
- E Appendicitis

4. A 27-year-old woman, gravida 2, para 1, at 30 weeks of gestation, presents to the clinic for a routine prenatal visit. Her pregnancy has been unremarkable thus far. "Serosal fibroids" are listed under her "problem list." Her fundus measures 37 cm from the symphysis pubis. In discussing possible complications of a fibroid uterus during pregnancy, you mention that she is at highest risk for:

- A Preterm premature rupture of membranes (PROM)
- B Placenta previa
- C Pregnancy-induced hypertension (PIH)
- D Breech presentation
- E Placental abruption

5. A 49-year-old woman, gravida 3, para 2, spontaneous abortions 1, who has a known myomatous uterus presents to you because of heavy bleeding during her periods and occasional spotting in between her periods. Her menses occurs every 5 to 6 weeks and lasts 6 to 10 days. It is associated with painful cramps. She has no chronic medical problems. The next best step in management of this patient is:

[A] GnRH agonist for 3 months
[B] GnRH agonist for 6 months and add-back hormones for the last 3 months
[C] Hysterectomy
[D] Endometrial biopsy
[E] Transvaginal ultrasound

Answers and Explanations

1. The answer is E [IV A 3 e]. Compression of pelvic vasculature by a markedly enlarged uterus may cause varicosities or edema (swelling) of the lower extremities. Peau d'orange is a skin edema that occurs in breast cancer. Leg ulcers are common in patients with a history of advanced diabetes or peripheral vascular disease. Superficial thrombophlebitis may result from stasis of blood in this patient, but it is not as common as vein varicosities. Deep venous thrombosis of the leg is not associated with leiomyomas; however, thrombosis of pelvic vessels can occur, which can rarely lead to pulmonary embolus.

2. The answer is C [III A 3]. Subserosal pedunculated fibroids are usually asymptomatic. A larger fibroid does not necessarily cause more symptoms unless it is in a critical location. An anterior large intramural fibroid may cause urinary symptoms because of pressure on the bladder. A large posterior intramural fibroid may cause bowel symptoms (constipation) because of pressure on the rectal area. A submucous fibroid or any intramural fibroid with a submucous component may cause bleeding (because of either local endometrial hyperplasia or a fragile endometrium overlying the fibroid area). The latter can also cause reproductive symptoms by interfering with implantation. A large intracavitary fibroid can even act as an intrauterine device.

3. The answer is A [III C 3]. A patient with a history of fibroids with this question's described physical examination findings during pregnancy most likely has carneous degeneration of her fibroids, which is quite painful. Although ovarian torsion could be an option, in a patient with a history of fibroids, fibroid degeneration would be more likely. The right lower quadrant scar and history of abdominal surgery suggest an appendectomy; therefore, appendicitis is not a possibility. Her blood pressure and urinalysis are normal; therefore, preeclampsia is unlikely. Bladder infection is also unlikely given the lack of urinary symptoms and a normal urinalysis.

4. The answer is D [IV A 5 d]. In the third trimester, leiomyomas may be a factor in malpresentation (breech), mechanical obstruction, and uterine dystocia. PIH and PROM are not related to fibroids (but premature labor is related). Placenta previa and abruption are unlikely with fibroids, especially when they are predominantly in the subserosal location.

5. The answer is D [V A 2 and V B 2]. You cannot assume that abnormal bleeding in a 49-year-old woman is caused by the leiomyomas simply because she has a myomatous uterus. At this age, the risk of endometrial disease, such as polyps, hyperplasia, and carcinoma, is significant and must be ruled out. Endometrial sampling is indicated before considering other therapy. Hysterectomy is the definitive treatment for fibroids and is a therapeutic option for someone who is finished with childbearing and who has inadequate relief with medical management (leuprolide). This option can be contemplated in this case only after endometrial neoplasia is ruled out. A transvaginal ultrasound is unnecessary because you already know that the patient has a fibroid uterus.

chapter 25

Endometriosis

SCOTT E. EDWARDS · RICHARD W. TURECK

I INTRODUCTION

A Definitions

1. Endometriosis is the **presence of functioning endometrial glands and stroma outside their usual location** within the uterine cavity. Significant pelvic adhesions with or without associated inflammatory cells or hemosiderin-laden macrophages often result.

2. Endometriosis is **primarily a pelvic disease** with implants in, or adhesions of, the ovaries, fallopian tubes, uterosacral ligaments, rectosigmoid, bladder, and appendix. Less commonly, endometriosis can be found outside the pelvis, suggesting a metastatic spread.

3. This **generally benign disease** usually affects women in their reproductive years. However, there have been several case reports of endometrioid carcinoma developing within foci of endometriosis.

B Incidence. The estimated incidence of endometriosis is 10% to 15%. Data suggest that 30% to 40% of patients with infertility may have endometriosis. In addition, studies suggest a hereditary tendency of this disease; individuals in certain families tend to develop the more severe and recurrent forms of endometriosis.

II ETIOLOGY

A Causes

1. **Retrograde menstrual flow**. This theory postulates that the retrograde flow of menstrual debris through the fallopian tubes causes the endometrial cells to spread into the pelvis, form implants there, or serve as irritative foci, which stimulate coelomic metaplasia and differentiation of the peritoneal cells into endometrial-type tissue.
   a. **Clinical evidence**. Endometriosis is commonly found in dependent portions of the pelvis, most frequently on the ovaries, cul-de-sac, and uterosacral ligaments. Menstrual efflux from fallopian tubes has been observed during laparoscopy. In addition, patients with outflow obstruction (e.g., müllerian anomalies) have a significantly increased risk of endometriosis.
   b. **Experimental evidence**. Endometrial fragments from menstrual fluid can grow both in tissue culture and after injection beneath the skin of the abdominal wall.

2. **Hematogenous or lymphatic spread**. Endometriosis at sites distant from the pelvis may be caused by vascular or lymphatic transport of endometrial fragments. This could explain the presence of endometriosis at distant sites such as the brain and lungs.

3. **Metaplasia of the coelomic epithelium**. The transformation of coelomic epithelium results from some yet-unspecified stimuli, but it can occur early in puberty after a few menstrual cycles.

4. **Genetic and immunologic influences**. The relative risk of endometriosis is 7% in siblings, compared with 1% in control groups. An altered immunologic response may be involved in the pathogenesis of endometriosis.

B Pain in endometriosis. The commonly suggested mechanisms for pain in endometriosis are the following. One or more of these can exist in an individual.

1. Irritation or direct invasion of pelvic floor nerves by infiltrating endometriotic implants

2. Direct and indirect effects of active bleeding from endometriotic implants

3. Pain may result from growth factors, cytokines, prostaglandins, and histamines in endometriotic tissue and peritoneal fluid of women with endometriosis. In fact, levels of these compounds may be most elevated in patients with the earlier and more atypical forms of the disease.

C **Infertility in endometriosis.** Moderate to severe endometriosis is thought to cause infertility by causing adhesions and scarring of the ovaries and fallopian tubes. Whether minimal endometriosis causes infertility is still under investigation.

1. Patients with endometriosis may have increased concentrations of macrophages in the ampullary portions of the fallopian tubes. Macrophages, chemotactically attracted to areas where endometriosis is present, may interfere with ovulation and corpus luteum formation and with fertilization through gamete phagocytosis. Factors produced by macrophages may interfere with sperm motility.

2. Prostaglandin $F_{2\alpha}$ increases the tone and amplitude of the cervical and uterine musculature and narrows the cervical os. It may increase the venous constriction of the uterus and the intensity of uterine contractions, therefore increasing the degree of dysmenorrhea. Prostaglandins also may interfere with placentation or implantation.

3. Interleukins are also secreted by the activated macrophages. Exposed embryos are less likely to progress to the eight-cell stage at 24 hours. Tumor necrosis factor and other cytokines may stimulate endometrial cell proliferation.

III   SIGNS AND SYMPTOMS

A **Dysmenorrhea.** Secondary dysmenorrhea (menstrual pain secondary to an anatomic pelvic abnormality) is the most common symptom of endometriosis. Typically the pattern with endometriosis is that of increasingly severe menstrual pain over time. With the increased use of laparoscopy, many adolescents with presumed primary dysmenorrhea are being diagnosed with endometriosis.

B Pain with **ovulation** is associated with endometriosis. Unilateral pain can suggest endometriomas within the ovary.

C **Chronic pelvic pain.** Pelvic pain for more then 6 months (diffuse or localized in the pelvis) is considered chronic. However, many women with endometriosis are asymptomatic, and the degree of endometriosis often does not correlate with the existing amount of pain.

D **Dyspareunia.** Painful intercourse may be caused by:

1. Endometrial implants of the uterosacral ligaments

2. Endometriomas of the ovaries

3. Fixed location of uterus and/or ovaries due to endometriosis and adhesions

E **Infertility.** Endometriosis has been demonstrated by laparoscopy in as many as 30% to 40% of women who are infertile. However, it is not clear that endometriosis is the cause of infertility in all those cases; there may just be an association. Endometriosis has also been noted in fertile women undergoing tubal ligation.

F **Associated symptoms**

1. **Urinary**. Urinary symptoms are common in patients with endometriosis; as many as one-third of patients with endometriosis have urinary tract involvement. The highest frequency of such involvement occurs in the bladder, followed in frequency by the lower ureter, upper ureter, and kidney. Symptoms range from intermittent dysuria, frequency, and urgency to complete ureteral obstruction. Gross or microscopic hematuria is present in many patients and frequently follows the menstrual cycle.

2. **Gastrointestinal**. Seven to thirty-five percent of all women with endometriosis have bowel involvement. Symptoms may vary from dyschezia (pain on defecation) and cyclic rectal bleeding form endometrial implants in the large intestine to other symptoms of partial or complete bowel obstruction (e.g., abdominal bloating, intestinal cramps, nausea, and vomiting). Although severe cases of bowel involvement may be diagnosed by magnetic resonance imaging (MRI) or computed tomography (CT), the most practical method of diagnosis remains a radiographic evaluation of the bowel with barium contrast. Because endometriosis induces **severe inflammation** in the serosa, muscularis, and mucosa of the bowel, a "**tethering effect**" is often apparent on a barium enema or upper gastrointestinal series.

G Distant sites for endometriosis

1. **Thoracic**. The thorax is a rare but significant site of endometriosis. The foci of endometriosis can cause cyclic monthly pneumothorax (catamenial pneumothorax), hemoptysis, or hemothorax. The onset of chest pain usually occurs within 2 days of menses. Initial management usually involves hormonal management as outlined below. However, if medical management is unsuccessful, more aggressive measures such as thoracoscopy with pleurodesis may be necessary. Pleurodesis will likely be effective at preventing pneumothorax and hemothorax, but because the implants of endometriosis may still be present, catamenial chest pain may still occur.

2. **Other**. Endometriosis has been documented to occur in other distant sites including nasal passages (monthly nose bleeds), the brain (catamenial seizures), and the umbilicus.

H Differential diagnosis. When considering the diagnosis of endometriosis, one must exclude other diagnoses that can cause the same symptoms. At the same time, it is important to consider these other causes of pain in a patient who is not responding to treatment for endometriosis.

1. **Gynecologic causes**
   a. Ovarian cysts
   b. Müllerian anomalies
   c. Pelvic inflammatory disease (PID) and sexually transmitted diseases
   d. Malignancy

2. **Urinary system**
   a. Interstitial cystitis
   b. Kidney stones

3. **Musculoskeletal system**
   a. Trigger point pain
   b. Pelvic floor dysfunction

4. **Gastrointestinal system**
   a. Irritable bowel disease
   b. Inflammatory bowel disease

IV **DIAGNOSIS**

History and physical examination may be suggestive of endometriosis, but currently the only way to diagnose the condition is by visualization at surgery (usually laparoscopy) or by biopsy of implants.

A History. The patient might have one or more of the characteristic symptoms (see III). A history of endometriosis in the patient's mother or sister is also important.

B Markers for endometriosis

1. **CA-125 is increased** in endometriosis. The CA-125 assay is a test for cell surface antigen found on coelomic epithelium, which includes the endometrium. This test is useful as a marker for response to treatment or recurrence. CA-125 is not a diagnostic test for endometriosis because it **lacks specificity**. It can also be elevated in ovarian cancer, PID, and inflammatory bowel disease.

C Pelvic examination

1. **Nodularity and tenderness of the uterosacral ligaments** are characteristic findings on vaginal and/or rectovaginal examination.

2. **Endometriomas** (ovarian cysts filled with old blood from endometriosis, forming "**chocolate cysts**") are palpated as adnexal masses often fixed to the lateral pelvic walls or to the posterior cul-de-sac.

3. The uterus is often in a **fixed retroverted** position.

4. The pelvic examination in minimal endometriosis is usually normal.

D **Pelvic imaging** is necessary in a woman with pelvic pain in whom endometriosis is suspected in order to look for ovarian endometriomas. Pelvic ultrasound is the best screening tool for visualizing the ovaries and uterus. MRI is better for clarifying the findings on ultrasound. CT scan is not helpful for diagnosing endometriomas. Typical endometriotic lesions are not visualized with pelvic ultrasound or even with MRI. In adolescents with severe dysmenorrhea, pelvic ultrasound should be performed to look for obstructive müllerian anomalies such as a blind noncommunicating uterine horn or a hemi-obstructed vagina with a uterus didelphys.

E **Laparoscopy and the classification of endometriosis.** Laparoscopy is necessary for the diagnosis of endometriosis. A laparoscopy is indicated to look for endometriosis or other causes of pelvic pain if the woman has failed to respond to medical therapy or if there is an abnormality seen on pelvic imaging suggesting endometriosis.

1. **Appearance**
   a. The classic endometriotic implant is characterized as brown or black pigmentation (**powder-burn lesion**) and fibrosis.
   b. Lesions that are **clear vesicular, white opacified, glandular excrescences, polypoid, or red hemorrhagic vesicles** are considered to be "atypical" lesions of endometriosis. Studies also suggest that these implants may be the most metabolically active. These lesions represent the majority of endometriosis seen in adolescents. It is not clear whether these lesions represent a different form of endometriosis or are a precursor to the typical lesions.
   c. White scarring of pelvic peritoneum suggests old burned-out endometriosis.

2. Endometriosis may cause deep tissue damage, resulting in local scarring and reduplication of **peritoneum** and leading to **surface defects** or **Allen-Masters peritoneal defects**. Physicians should strongly suspect the possibility of endometriosis in all patients with demonstrated pelvic peritoneal defects at laparoscopy.

3. **Classification.** The extent of formation of classic lesions, ovarian involvement, and adhesive disease is classified by the American Society of Reproductive Medicine.

V TREATMENT

A **General considerations.** Age of the patient, extent of disease, duration of the infertility, and severity of symptoms are important considerations. The patient's reproductive plans should also be taken into account. Prior to initiating medical treatment for endometriosis, it is important to have made the correct diagnosis by the modalities noted above including laparoscopy.

B **Expectant treatment**

1. Expectant therapy may be appropriate in young women who have pelvic pain with apparent endometriosis on laparoscopy and no immediate interest in pregnancy. Goals are relief of the dysmenorrhea and prevention of further growth of endometriosis.
   a. **Nonsteroidal anti-inflammatory drugs (NSAIDs).** The prostaglandin synthetase inhibitors are effective in controlling endometriosis-related dysmenorrhea. Women with endometriosis show increased concentrations of prostaglandins in the peritoneal fluid. When oral contraceptive pills (OCPs) and NSAIDs are administered simultaneously, they have a synergistic effect.

2. Women with minimal disease and short-term infertility may be managed expectantly, but fertility may be an issue. Recent data have shown that conservative surgery (laparoscopic fulguration of endometriosis) is superior to expectant management in achieving fertility in the next year.

C **Medical therapy.** Ectopic endometrium responds to cyclic hormone secretion in a fashion similar to normal endometrium. It has been well documented that pregnancy tends to alleviate the symptoms of endometriosis. It was this observation that led to the initiation of **hormonal suppression of menses as the basis of medical therapy for endometriosis**. Newer therapies have focused on the specific hormonal triggers for endometriosis. Medical therapy is not indicated for treatment of infertility related to endometriosis.

1. **Oral contraceptive pills**. This is usually the first-line therapy for endometriosis.
   a. **Mode of action**. Continuously administered estrogen–progestin combination OCPs create a "pseudopregnancy" state associated with amenorrhea. The pseudopregnancy causes decidualization, necrobiosis, and resorption of the ectopic endometrium. This treatment is appropriate to control pain associated with menstruation and ovulation with endometriosis.
   b. **Dosage**. The pills are given daily with the placebo pills given every 4 to 12 months to induce withdrawal bleeding. Addition of conjugated estrogens for short periods controls breakthrough bleeding.
   c. **Prognosis**. The recurrence rate is 15% to 25% in the following year, and the pregnancy rate is 25% to 50%.

2. **Gonadotropin-releasing hormone (GnRH) agonists**. These agents are the most commonly used method for medical treatment of endometriosis.
   a. **Mode of action**. GnRH is a decapeptide that controls the release of the anterior pituitary hormones (follicle-stimulating hormone [FSH] and luteinizing hormone [LH]). GnRH has a very short half-life; it is rapidly destroyed by endopeptidases in the hypothalamus and pituitary gland. Normally, the release of GnRH is pulsatile. Chemical alterations of the amino acids at positions 6 and 10 produce synthetic derivatives of GnRH (GnRH analogs, GnRH agonists) that resist cleavage by endopeptidases but retain a high affinity for the pituitary GnRH receptor. The effect is **down-regulation** and **desensitization** of the pituitary with resulting lack of ovarian estrogen production.
   b. **Administration**. GnRH agonists may be administered intranasally, subcutaneously, or intramuscularly daily or as a depot injection every month or every 3 months.
   c. **Adverse effects** are related primarily to the hypoestrogenic state induced by GnRH agonists.
      (1) Menopausal-type symptoms (e.g., hot flashes, decreased libido, vaginal dryness, and headaches) occur because of the hypoestrogenic state.
      (2) Prolonged use (more than 6 months) may result in significant bone loss leading to osteoporosis as a result of the hypoestrogenic state. Using "**add-back therapy**" (low-dose estrogen and progestin) may minimize bone loss while still maintaining pain relief. Oral contraceptives are not used as add-back therapy.
      (3) Flare-ups of endometriotic symptoms may occur in the first few weeks after treatment begins because of the initial temporary rise in estrogen levels after starting GnRH agonists. These symptoms typically abate. GnRH antagonists may have a role in initial suppression in these patients.
   d. **Prognosis**. Amenorrhea and atrophic endometrial changes occur in most patients. Regression of endometriotic lesions occurs in 80% of cases, and symptomatic relief results in more then 50% of cases after 6 months of therapy. However, recurrence rates are 25% to 30% per year after therapy is discontinued.

3. **Danazol**
   a. **Mode of action**. Danazol is an androgenic testosterone derivative that suppresses FSH and LH as well as ovarian estrogen and progesterone production. Danazol also directly acts on endometrial glands to produce an atrophic (thin) endometrium.
   b. **Dosage**. Danazol is administered as 200 mg four times daily for 4 to 9 months. The dose may be lowered to 100 to 600 mg/day after the onset of amenorrhea.
   c. **Prognosis**. Eighty to ninety percent of patients will have clinical improvement on danazol, but significant androgenic side effects such as hirsutism, acne, weight gain, and decreased breast size have limited its use today given the availability of better tolerated therapies.

4. **Aromatase inhibitors**
   a. **Mode of action**. The aromatase enzyme converts androgen precursors such as androstenedione and testosterone to estrone and estradiol. Aromatase inhibitors (AIs) such as letrozole and anastrazole will inhibit the production of estrogen within the endometriotic lesion. AIs will increase FSH and LH by blocking estrogen's negative feedback on the pituitary. These elevated gonadotropins will stimulate ovarian follicular development unless there is concomitant

use of progestins or low-dose OCPs. AIs are currently indicated for the treatment of breast cancer and their use in endometriosis, while promising, should be considered investigational at this point in time.

b. Dosage. Studies have used 2.5 mg of letrozole or 1 mg of anastrazole per day. Therapy continues for 6 to 9 months.

c. Adverse effects. Side effects of AIs are usually benign and include nausea, diarrhea, and headache. Hot flashes are milder and infrequent when compared to GnRH analogs. However, because of the profound reduction in estrogen levels, long-term use carries the risk of bone loss. Concurrent treatment with OCPs or progestins can mitigate this bone loss.

d. Prognosis. Initial small clinical studies have shown approximately 90% pain relief after treatment with anastrazole or letrozole.

D Surgical therapy. Medical therapy does not dissolve adhesions or eliminate endometriomas. Surgery is the treatment of choice in cases that present with considerable anatomic factors (e.g., adhesions and endometriomas). The success of surgery in relieving infertility is directly related to the severity of the endometriosis.

1. **Conservative surgery** involves the excision, fulguration, or laser vaporization of endometriotic lesions; the excision of ovarian endometriomas; and the resection of severely involved viscera, leaving the uterus and at least one ovary and fallopian tube intact. This can usually be accomplished by laparoscopy, but in severe cases laparotomy may be required. Studies have shown that gentle micromanipulation of the tissue, lysis of adhesions, and meticulous hemostasis are important in the patient desiring fertility.

2. **Radical surgery** involves a total hysterectomy and bilateral salpingo-oophorectomy.
   a. This approach is used in patients who do not desire future fertility or in those whose endometriosis is so severe that it precludes any attempt at reconstruction.
   b. The rate of reoperation on women who have a hysterectomy with the ovaries left in place is high and varies from 15% to 40%. This risk may be acceptable for some women who would rather not experience surgical menopause at a young age.
   c. Estrogen replacement therapy is important in patients who undergo radical surgery to prevent osteoporosis and treat hypoestrogenic symptoms such as hot flushes, night sweats, sleeplessness, and vaginal dryness. Estrogen replacement therapy carries only a small risk of inciting growth of residual endometriosis.

Study Questions for Chapter 25

Directions: *Each of the numbered items or incomplete statements in this section is followed by answers or by completions of the statement. Select the ONE lettered answer or completion that is BEST in each case.*

1. A 34-year-old woman, gravida 0, has been trying to get pregnant for the last 3 years and has been unsuccessful. Her history is also significant for pelvic pain for several years and deep dyspareunia. On pelvic examination, you palpate a nodular, tender uterosacral ligament, a retroverted but normal-sized uterus, and a right adnexal mass. A recent pelvic ultrasound reveals a 6-cm right complex ovarian mass. Her CA-125 is elevated. What is the initial next step in management?

- Ⓐ Expectant management
- Ⓑ GnRH agonist
- Ⓒ Diagnostic laparoscopy
- Ⓓ Laparoscopy with cystectomy
- Ⓔ Laparoscopy and right oophorectomy

2. A 23-year-old woman, gravida 1, para 1, reports lower abdominal pain of 1 year's duration. She says that the pain is constant and dull and is worse around the time of her periods. She has no significant medical history and is taking birth control pills for contraception. You perform a laparoscopy and find several deep, typical endometriotic lesions over the bladder and on both uterosacral ligaments and adjacent to both ovaries. All visible lesions are ablated using the laser. What is the next best step in management?

- Ⓐ Oral contraceptive therapy
- Ⓑ GnRH agonist
- Ⓒ Aromatase inhibitor added to oral contraceptive therapy
- Ⓓ Total abdominal hysterectomy and bilateral salpingo-oophorectomy (TAH-BSO)
- Ⓔ Danazol

3. Which of the following patients is unlikely to have endometriosis?

- Ⓐ A 19-year-old with cyclic pelvic pain and bicornuate uterus with a noncommunicating uterine horn
- Ⓑ A 28-year-old patient with cyclic pelvic pain and who has a mother and a sister with endometriosis
- Ⓒ A 25-year-old female with a history of dyspareunia, painful nodular masses in the rectovaginal septum, and a left adnexal mass
- Ⓓ A 28-year-old with menorrhagia and a 4-cm submucosal myoma
- Ⓔ A 32-year-old with infertility and dysmenorrhea and a fixed and retroverted uterus on physical examination

QUESTIONS 4–7

Match the statement below with the best word or words. Each answer choice may be used once, more than once, or not at all.

- Ⓐ Aromatase inhibitor
- Ⓑ Prostaglandins
- Ⓒ Allen-Master lesions
- Ⓓ Pneumothorax
- Ⓔ Powder burn lesions

4. Block production of estrogen within the endometriosis implant

5. Patient with red hemorrhagic vesicles and white lesions who has a pelvic peritoneal defect on laparoscopy

6. Reason why naproxen may alleviate pain symptoms in a patient with endometriosis

7. Complication of extraperitoneal endometriosis

Answers and Explanations

1. The answer is **D** [V D 1]. The most likely diagnosis here is an endometrioma of the right ovary. Because this patient has been attempting to get pregnant, conservative surgery to remove the endometrioma while preserving ovarian tissue and to ablate any endometriotic implants may improve her chances. Expectant management is not appropriate because she is infertile, has a 6-cm ovarian mass, and has significant pelvic pain. Furthermore, other complex ovarian lesions, including ovarian cancers, cannot be ruled out without surgical evaluation. Simple diagnostic laparoscopy without any treatment is also not appropriate. Medical therapy with a GnRH agonist may treat her symptoms, but it will not treat the ovarian cyst or help her get pregnant. It is not necessary to remove what is most likely normal ovarian tissue. CA-125 can be elevated with endometriosis and does not indicate ovarian cancer.

2. The answer is **A** [V C 1-4]. Endometriosis is diagnosed and surgically treated at the time of laparoscopy. Medical management of the endometriosis is indicated at this point to help control the disease. Oral contraceptive pills given continuously would be the best option. The patient had significant pain while on cyclic oral contraceptives prior to the surgery, but the surgery treated the disease and therefore the symptoms may be significantly improved. Also giving the contraceptive on a continuous schedule may improve pain symptoms seen with menses. GnRH agonists would be the next best option if the pain symptoms are not improved with continuous oral contraceptives. GnRH would not be the first medicine tried because of the hypoestrogenic side effects and risk of osteoporosis in this young woman. Danazol is effective for endometriosis, but because of its many androgenic side effects, it is not preferred over leuprolide. Aromatase inhibitors are still considered investigational at this point and would not be recommended. A TAH-BSO is too radical a procedure for this problem and at this point in this patient's life (she is young and still interested in childbearing).

3. The answer is **D** [II A, III A, C, D, H]. Patients with a müllerian anomaly that blocks the egress of menses are at high risk of developing endometriosis. Likewise, patients who have a sibling with endometriosis are at increased risk of the disease (7% versus 1% for controls). The presence of dyspareunia, rectovaginal nodularity, and an adnexal mass in a young woman is highly suggestive of endometriosis and an endometrioma. A complaint of infertility in a patient who has a fixed and retroverted uterus, presumably from scarring, is also very suggestive of endometriosis. Myomas are generally benign proliferations of uterine smooth muscle tissue and are not thought to be associated with endometriosis.

4. A [VC4], **5. C** [IV C d], **6. B** [II C 2], **7. B** [II B 1]. Aromatase inhibitors block the conversion from androgens to estrogens and thereby block the estrogen-dependent proliferation of endometriosis lesions. A patient with endometriosis who has defects in the pelvic peritoneum because of local scarring has Allen-Master defects. Infertility caused by minimal endometriosis may be related to macrophage response and prostaglandin F secretion. Prostaglandins may interfere with placentation and implantation. Naproxen is an NSAID and, as such, is a prostaglandin synthetase or cyclooxygenase enzyme inhibitor. Menstrual cycle–related pneumothorax, or catamenial pneumothorax, is caused by endometriosis present within the pleura. This condition may respond to conservative treatment with continuous oral contraceptives; however, refractory cases may require pleurodesis (scarring to close the pleural space).

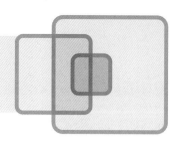

chapter 26

Pelvic Pain

THOMAS A. MOLINARO • RICHARD W. TURECK

I INTRODUCTION

Chronic pelvic pain syndrome is estimated to account for 10% of all visits to gynecologists. Afflicted women report continuous lower abdominal and pelvic pain that markedly hinders their daily activities. Although **acute pelvic pain may be associated with life-threatening illness**, chronic pelvic pain may also have a devastating impact on patients, and physicians should remain compassionate and empathetic. Pain is a subjective experience. The lack of physical findings does not in any way negate the significance of a patient's pain. The **psychological effects** may be considerable.

A The risk of major **depression, sexual dysfunction, and substance abuse** is increased.

B The prevalence of **childhood or adult sexual abuse** is particularly high, and the rate of marital and sexual dysfunction is greater among this cohort of patients.

C Psychological counseling and testing may be necessary to identify patients who require more extensive therapy.

II DEFINITION

Pelvic pain can be acute or chronic, and can be caused by a multitude of conditions in many organ systems. Just because the pain is pelvic in location does not mean that the cause of the condition is gynecologic.

A **Acute pelvic pain** is pain that is located in the anatomic pelvis and is of short duration and sudden onset.

B **Chronic pelvic pain** is noncyclic pain of 6 or more months' duration that localizes to the anatomic pelvis, the anterior abdominal wall at or below the umbilicus, the lumbosacral back, or the buttocks and is of sufficient severity to cause functional disability or lead to medical care.

III ANATOMY AND PHYSIOLOGY OF PELVIC PAIN

Pain perception involves an integration of multiple stimuli through a network of neuronal pathways. Visceral pain is more diffuse than somatic pain, probably because there is no specific identification within the cerebral sensory cortex.

A Neuroanatomy. The pelvic organs receive their innervation from the **autonomic nervous system**, which is composed of both sympathetic and parasympathetic fibers.

1. **Sympathetic nerves** are used to transmit most afferent stimuli through cell bodies that lie in the **thoracolumbar** distribution. Areas that are müllerian in embryonic origin (e.g., uterus, fallopian tubes, and upper vagina) transmit impulses via sympathetic fibers into the spinal cord at the level of T10, T11, T12, and L1. Impulses from the uterus travel through the uterosacral ligaments to the uterine inferior plexus. From the uterus, they join other pelvic afferents to form the hypogastric plexus at the level of the rectum and vagina. The ovaries and distal fallopian tubes derive their nerve supply independently and enter the spinal cord at T9 and T10.

2. **Parasympathetic nerve fibers** are also involved to a lesser extent in the transition of painful stimuli. Impulses from the upper vagina, cervix, and lower uterine segment travel through the parasympathetic system to the sacral roots S2 to S4.

3. **Both sympathetic and parasympathetic fibers** innervate the bladder, rectum, perineum, and anus, which are derived from the urogenital sinus. Fibers from the perineum and anus combine to form branches of the pudendal nerve, eventually terminating in the second and fourth sacral root.

B **Physiology.** Pelvic pain is visceral and may be either **referred** or **splanchnic**.

1. **Splanchnic pain** occurs when an irritable stimulus is appreciated in a specific organ secondary to tension (stretching, distention, or pulling), peritoneal irritation or inflammation, hypoxia or necrosis of viscera, or production of prostanoids.

2. **Referred pain** occurs when autonomic impulses arise from a diseased visceral organ, eliciting an irritable response within the spinal cord. Pain is sensed in the dermatomes corresponding to cells receiving those impulses.

IV EVALUATION

A **Important factors** to assess when determining the clinical significance of pelvic pain include:

1. **Onset** of the pain

2. **Relationship to the menstrual cycle** (Is the pain constant or does it vary?)

3. **Character** of the pain

4. **Location** of the pain

5. **Severity** of the pain (Does it interfere with activities of daily life?)

6. **Presence of associated symptoms** (e.g., dysmenorrhea and deep dyspareunia). Any other symptoms, such as fever, chills, nausea, vomiting, or anorexia, should also be noted.

B **Imaging** studies are useful in determining the etiology of pelvic pain.

1. **Pelvic ultrasound** is particularly useful in identifying abnormalities of gynecologic structures.

2. **Pelvic magnetic resonance imaging (MRI)** may provide additional details when abnormalities are identified.

C **Laparoscopy**, the endoscopic assessment of abdominal and pelvic pathology, is the **gold standard** for the diagnosis of pelvic pain. Laparoscopy is indicated in cases of pelvic pain that are unresponsive to medical therapy or when an organic cause of the pain is suspected. Approximately 40% of laparoscopies are reportedly performed in cases of chronic pelvic pain. This also provides an opportunity to treat as well as diagnose pathology.

V DIFFERENTIAL DIAGNOSIS

A **Acute pelvic pain (Table 26-1)**

1. **Ectopic pregnancy** (see Chapter 27). It is paramount to exclude the possibility of an **ectopic tubal gestation**, a life-threatening condition.
   a. **Pelvic pain** occurs as a result of distention of the fallopian tube caused by the growing pregnancy. The pain is usually **unilateral**. If the pregnancy ruptures through the fallopian tube, rebound tenderness may occur.
   b. **Shoulder pain** may develop as a result of blood in the abdomen causing diaphragmatic irritation and stimulating the phrenic nerves.
   c. A **pregnancy test** is mandated in any woman of childbearing age who presents with acute pelvic pain. If the test is positive, the presence of an ectopic pregnancy must be excluded from the differential diagnosis, particularly in patients with abnormal uterine bleeding.

2. **Ruptured ovarian cyst.** Midcycle pain or **mittelschmerz** is pain in the lower abdomen noticed at or near the time of ovulation. It is believed to be secondary to chemical irritation of the

TABLE 26–1 Causes of Acute Pelvic Pain

Gynecologic	Gastrointestinal	Urologic
Ovarian cyst	Appendicitis	Cystitis
Acute pelvic inflammatory disease	Diverticulosis	Urolithiasis
Adnexal torsion		Pyelonephritis
Ectopic pregnancy		
Endometriosis		
Ruptured ovarian cyst		
Leiomyoma		
Endometritis		

peritoneum from ovarian follicular cyst fluid after ovulation. The pain usually lasts only a few hours and usually no more than 2 days. The use of ultrasonic visualization of the ovaries most often confirms or excludes this diagnosis.

3. **Ovarian torsion**. This involves twisting of the ovary and/or tube and occluding the blood supply. Acute lower abdominal pain may be the primary manifestation.
   a. The clinical presentation depends on the extent of interference with the ovarian blood supply. The more extensive the ischemia, the more severe the pelvic pain is. The pain is usually paroxysmal and unilateral but becomes more constant if infarction occurs. It is associated with peritoneal signs and an elevated white blood cell (WBC) count.
   b. Documentation of ovarian blood flow by **color Doppler ultrasound** is a helpful diagnostic modality in evaluating this medical emergency, but it is not always accurate. Often, **laparoscopy** must be performed to confirm the diagnosis.
   c. If necrotic, the ovary and tube must usually be removed. If the ovary appears viable, it may be untwisted and a cystectomy performed.

4. **Pelvic inflammatory disease (PID)**. Pelvic pain that is acute in onset and associated with cervical motion tenderness and febrile morbidity is characteristic of PID (see Chapter 34). Rebound tenderness and a partial ileus may result from the presence of purulent material within the pelvic and abdominal cavity.

5. **Gastrointestinal disorders**. Gastrointestinal causes of acute lower pelvic and abdominal pain include **appendicitis** and **diverticulitis**; the latter condition is most commonly observed in older women. In appendicitis, the pain is initially not well localized because it results from luminal distention of the appendix by inflammatory exudates. The pain eventually localizes to the right lower quadrant when the parietal peritoneum becomes locally involved in the inflammatory process.

6. **Urologic causes**. Conditions such as cystitis and renal lithiasis may lead to lower abdominal and pelvic pain.

B Chronic or recurrent pelvic pain (Table 26-2).   Chronic pelvic pain may be **cyclic** or **constant**.

1. **Dysmenorrhea** is painful menstruation. It is considered **primary** if it occurs in the absence of identifiable pathology. **Secondary dysmenorrhea** is caused by a defined pelvic abnormality, such as endometriosis or müllerian anomaly.
   a. The **pain** is usually spasmodic or throbbing. It is usually located in the lower abdomen and may radiate to the lower back and legs.
   b. Its onset is concurrent with menses, and the pain lasts for 1 to 3 days.
   c. The etiology of painful uterine contractions involves **prostaglandin $F_{2\alpha}$** produced in the endometrial cells by the action of phospholipase A_2 on lipid cell membranes, forming arachidonic acid.
   d. Associated symptoms include backache, nausea, vomiting, diarrhea, headache, and fatigue.
   e. Therapy is aimed at reducing prostaglandin production. Agents such as **prostaglandin synthetase inhibitors** (nonsteroidal anti-inflammatory drugs [NSAIDs]) or **oral contraceptives** are useful.

TABLE 26–2   Causes of Chronic Pelvic Pain

Gynecologic	Gastrointestinal	Urologic	Musculoskeletal	Psychological
Endometriosis	Constipation	Urinary tract infection	Postural	Depression
Pelvic inflammatory disease/tubo-ovarian abscess	Irritable bowel	Kidney stones	Trigger points	Sexual abuse
Adhesive disease	Gastroenteritis	Interstitial cystitis	Joint pain	Substance abuse
Congenital anomalies	Lactose intolerance	Urethral syndrome	Inflammation	Eating disorder
Ovarian masses	Inflammatory bowel disease		Spinal injury	
Chronic ectopic pregnancy	Appendicitis			
Dysmenorrhea	Hernia			
Leiomyoma				
Endometritis				

2. **Pelvic adhesions**
   a. **Etiology**. Adhesion formation occurs after trauma to the visceral or parietal peritoneum through **operative procedures** (70% of cases), **endometriosis**, or **infection and inflammation**. Foreign body granulomas caused by talc, gauze, or suture material also result in the production of adhesions.
   b. **Pathogenesis**
      (1) In cases that involve ischemic damage to the peritoneum, lysis of fibrin does not occur because of reduced fibrinolytic activity and fibrinous adhesions.
      (2) **Mechanical components** have been proposed as the underlying mechanism of pain sensation caused by adhesions. Patients experience pain via mechanical stimulation of visceral nociceptors because of mechanical stretching of internal organs.
   c. **Diagnosis**
      (1) Patients with adhesions may often have a history of previous pelvic surgery, but many have no past history that may supply a reason for the existence of adhesions. Physical examination of the patient may also be noncontributory. Approximately 25% of patients with adhesions have no preoperative findings on physical examination, which suggests the presence of adhesions.
      (2) **Laparoscopy. Laparoscopic visualization of the abdomen and pelvis is essential**. Detectable pathologic findings are documented in approximately 60% of patients; in 25% of these patients, adhesions are the primary condition. Laparoscopic lysis of adhesions in patients with chronic pelvic pain results in improvement of symptomatology in 65% to 85% of cases. This improvement is maintained in approximately 75% of patients 6 to 12 months after surgery.
3. **Endometriosis** (see Chapter 25). Approximately 25% to 40% of patients who undergo laparoscopy for chronic pelvic pain have evidence of endometriosis.
   a. **Etiology**. Endometriosis is the presence of endometrial glands and stroma at sites other than the uterine cavity. Theories include retrograde menstruation, metastases via vascular and lymphatic channels, altered immune response to ectopic endometrial tissue, and metaplastic transformation of totipotential cells.
   b. **Pain symptoms**
      (1) The amount of disease does not correlate with the degree of pain.
      (2) Pain attributed to endometriosis can be cyclic, acyclic, gastrointestinal, or urologic in nature.
      (3) Deep dyspareunia that is positional is suggestive of endometriosis.
   c. **Diagnosis**
      (1) The definitive diagnostic test is laparoscopy. Visualization of lesions is sufficient for diagnosis. Biopsy of lesions is not essential.

(2) At laparoscopy lesions can be red vesicular, vascular lesions; black "powder burn" lesions; or white largely fibrous lesions.

d. Treatment

(1) Surgical resection of lesions should be accomplished at the time of diagnostic laparoscopy.

(2) Menses can be suppressed using combined hormonal contraceptives in a cyclic or continuous way, or progestin-only depot preparations.

(3) GnRH agonists can be used to suppress menses and create a hypoestrogenic environment. Long-term therapy can be given with add-back therapy with low-dose continuous estrogen and progestin.

(4) Aromatase inhibitors are currently being investigated for use with GnRH agonists or combined hormonal contraceptives for the management of pain associated with endometriosis.

4. Adenomyosis, a condition characterized by the presence of ectopic foci of endometrium within the myometrium, may also cause chronic pelvic pain and severe dysmenorrhea. In the past, adenomyosis was diagnosed in the pathology laboratory after surgical removal of the uterus. Today, magnetic resonance imaging is a useful modality to diagnose adenomyosis and to better plan treatment.

5. Müllerian anomalies

a. Obstructed outflow tract associated with pelvic pain

(1) A partial obstruction of part of the müllerian structures that allows regular menstruation. This category would include conditions such as a noncommunicating obstructed uterine horn, an obstructed hemi-vagina associated with a duplicated cervix and uterine didelphys, and septate or bicornuate uterine fundus.

(2) A complete obstruction associated with amenorrhea. This can lead to chronic pelvic pain if there is functional endometrium in an obstructed uterine remnant, or if an obstruction in the outflow tract has lead to significant endometriosis due to retrograde menstrual flow in the setting of delayed diagnosis.

(3) It is important to consider the diagnosis of obstructed müllerian anomaly when there is increasing dysmenorrhea in a young female who is not responding to medical therapy, and also in the case of müllerian agenesis when pelvic pain is present. Early diagnosis is important.

(4) MRI is the best way to diagnose müllerian anomalies. These are rare and many radiologists are not familiar with the many configurations that can exist. Careful review of the films is important.

(5) Surgical correction is the treatment of choice.

6. Chronic PID and tubo-ovarian abscess

a. Chronic salpingo-oophoritis can lead to pelvic pain. Hydrosalpinges can become reinfected causing significant pain, fever, and occasionally sepsis and death.

b. The organisms are primarily gut flora.

c. Antibiotic therapy is the first line, with surgery reserved for those who do not respond to medical therapy.

7. Adnexal masses. Cysts or tumors on the ovaries or tubes can cause pain. Diagnosis is best made by ultrasound and treatment is usually surgical.

C Nongynecologic causes of chronic pelvic pain

1. Urologic

a. Interstitial cystitis is a chronic inflammatory condition of the bladder wall.

(1) Symptoms include urinary frequency, urgency, and pain.

(2) Other frequently observed symptoms include dyspareunia, premenstrual flare of symptoms, and pelvic pain. These symptoms can be confused with those of endometriosis.

(3) Diagnosis is made by symptoms and cystoscopy to observe typical glomerulations.

(4) Treatment includes avoiding acid-rich foods, antidepressants to treat neurologic pain, and medications including pentosan polysulfate sodium.

b. Other urologic causes include urethral syndromes, bladder malignancy, and chronic urinary tract infections.

2. **Gastrointestinal**: diverticulosis, constipation, carcinoma of the colon, inflammatory bowel disease, and irritable bowel syndrome

3. **Musculoskeletal** pain is most commonly due to chronic repetitive stress and strain, with direct trauma to musculoskeletal structures being less frequent. These conditions are associated with the typical pelvic pain posture, which is increased lumbar lordosis and anterior tilt of pelvis.

   a. **Abdominal trigger points** are defined as a focus of hyperirritability in a muscle or its fascia that is symptomatic with respect to pain. These areas are always tender and prevent full lengthening of the muscle. Typically the pain improves with rest and is exacerbated with activity.

   b. Other musculoskeletal causes include chronic back pain, fibromyalgia, neoplasia of spinal cord, compression of lower vertebrae, and pelvic floor dysfunction.

   c. Physical therapy is the mainstay of therapy for musculoskeletal disorders.

4. **Psychological**

   a. Common causes include depression, history of or current sexual abuse, substance abuse, and eating disorders.

   b. Unless there is good evidence of a psychological reason for chronic pelvic pain, all other organic causes must be investigated and excluded or treated prior to assuming a psychological cause.

[D] Treatments should be aimed at specific etiologies.

1. Oral contraceptives can be useful in patients with dysmenorrhea, endometriosis, and adenomyosis.

2. Analgesics such as NSAIDs and opioids are helpful, although they may become addictive.

3. Local anesthetic injections can be used for nerve blocks and trigger points.

4. Tricyclic antidepressants (i.e., amitriptyline) may help modulate chronic pelvic pain.

5. Physical therapy is often used.

6. Gonadotropin-releasing hormone agonists: Lupron may be useful for endometriosis by inducing chemical menopause.

Study Questions for Chapter 26

Directions: *Each of the numbered items or incomplete statements in this section is followed by answers or by completions of the statement. Select the ONE lettered answer or completion that is BEST in each case.*

1. A 32-year-old woman, gravida 2, para 2, presents to your clinic reporting chronic abdominal and pelvic pain. The pain is intermittent, 6/10 intensity, worse when she lies on her left side, and nonradiating, and occurs at different times throughout her menstrual cycle. Her past medical history is uneventful other than an appendectomy 4 years ago for a ruptured appendicitis. On physical examination of the abdomen in the supine position, you note a small linear scar in the right lower quadrant and active bowel sounds. The abdomen is diffusely tender to palpation, especially in the lower quadrants, and you do not palpate any masses. Her pelvic examination is unremarkable. The most likely diagnosis is:

- [A] Torsion of ovarian cyst
- [B] Mittelschmerz
- [C] Adhesive disease
- [D] Psychogenic cause
- [E] Pelvic inflammatory disease

2. A 19-year-old female, gravida 0, has had increasingly severe menstrual cramps since menarche. Her pain is worse around the time of her menses, but she also complains of dyspareunia, and the pain is worse with movement. She denies any nausea or vomiting, diarrhea, or constipation. She is otherwise healthy and denies any prior surgery. The cause of her pelvic pain is most likely to be:

- [A] Gastrointestinal
- [B] Gynecologic
- [C] Gynecologic or urologic
- [D] Urologic
- [E] Gynecologic, urologic, or musculoskeletal

3. An 18-year-old nulligravid woman presents to your office because she has painful periods. She says she only has pain during the first 2 days of her periods, which are regular. The pain is always midline and 2 cm below the level of the umbilicus. She says Motrin helps ease the pain. She has no other medical or surgical history. Her pain is transmitted via:

- [A] Sympathetic fibers to T10
- [B] Sympathetic fibers to T11
- [C] Parasympathetic fibers to S1
- [D] Parasympathetic fibers to L1
- [E] Pudendal nerve to S2 to S4

4. A 33-year-old woman, gravida 5, para 4, therapeutic abortion (TAB) 1, presents to the clinic with left lower quadrant pain for 2 days. She describes the pain as intermittent initially but now constant, 7/10 intensity, nonradiating, and not associated with any other symptoms. Her last menstrual period was 2 months ago. She had a tubal ligation 3 years ago and a cholecystectomy 7 years ago. Her physical examination is as follows: T = 98.5, BP = 118/76, P = 89, R = 18. Abdominal examination reveals a scar on the right upper quadrant and a small scar within the umbilicus and right lower quadrant, present bowel sounds, slight tenderness to palpation in the left lower quadrant, but no rebound tenderness and no guarding. Her pelvic examination reveals a uterus of normal size, shape, and contour, and no adnexal masses are appreciated. What is the next best step in management?

- [A] Laparoscopy
- [B] Laparotomy
- [C] Antibiotics
- [D] Naproxen
- [E] Serum β-human chorionic gonadotropin (β-hCG)

5. A 25-year-old woman, gravida 4, para 3, spontaneous abortions 1, presents to your clinic for the first time reporting pelvic pain. She has had this pain for the last 10 years and has seen several physicians. She describes the pain as continuous and dull (4/10 intensity) with intermittent exacerbations (10/10). The pain occasionally radiates to her lower back and down her thighs. Nothing she takes or does seems to help her. The pain is not related to her menstrual cycle, which occurs only a few times a year. She has dyspareunia. She has a past medical history significant for asthma, peptic ulcer disease, and major depression. She has had a postpartum bilateral tubal ligation. She has had three hospitalizations within the last 10 years for suicide attempts. She also has a history of sexual abuse by a close family relative that occurred when she was 13 years old. Currently, she is using an albuterol metered dose inhaler, a histamine receptor blocker, and a selective serotonin reuptake inhibitor (SSRI). On pelvic examination, the cervix and uterus are midposition and normal in size and consistency, but there is diffuse pain in all areas of the pelvis, especially the right posterior cul-de-sac. The most likely cause of her pain is:

- [A] Endometriosis
- [B] Uterine fibroids
- [C] Mittelschmerz
- [D] Pelvic adhesions
- [E] Psychogenic cause

Answers and Explanations

1. The answer is C [V B 2]. Due to her previous surgery and the fact that the appendix was ruptured, there is a high likelihood of adhesive disease inside the abdomen and pelvis. The fact that the pain is positional and not related to the menstrual cycle also suggests adhesions. There is no mention or ultrasound report of an ovarian cyst in the clinical scenario. Mittelschmerz is related to the menstrual cycle (occurs around time of ovulation). There is nothing in the scenario that suggests a psychogenic cause, although this should always be in the differential diagnosis. Pelvic inflammatory disease is unlikely given the lack of evidence by pelvic or abdominal examination and lack of other associated findings, such as a fever or high WBC count, or even an elevated erythrocyte sedimentation rate (ESR).

2. The answer is E [Table 26-2]. This patient has pelvic pain that is worse with menses, intercourse, and movement. Therefore, she could have a gynecologic, urologic, or musculoskeletal cause of her symptoms, or a combination of all three. It is important to recognize that chronic pelvic pain can be attributed to gynecologic, urologic, gastrointestinal, musculoskeletal, and psychological causes, or a combination of several. Therefore, if a patient does not respond to therapy, another cause or an additional cause for her symptoms must be considered. In this patient a gastrointestinal cause is unlikely given a lack of gastrointestinal symptoms.

3. The answer is B [III A 1]. Pain from dysmenorrhea is the result of contraction of the upper uterus caused by prostaglandin $F_{2\alpha}$ and can be referred to the dermatome that is equivalent to where the pain signal ends up in the spinal cord. The uterus is innervated by the sympathetic fibers (not parasympathetic), which go to spinal cord segments T10, T11, T12, and L1. Because this patient's pain is slightly below the umbilicus (which is in the T10 dermatome), the pain signal reaches T11 and not T10. The pudendal nerve carries impulses from urogenitally derived structures, such as the bladder, rectum, perineum, and anus.

4. The answer is E [V A 1]. The most important thing is to rule out pregnancy with a serum hCG level, especially because an ectopic pregnancy is a possibility given the patient's history of a tubal ligation. Simply giving an NSAID (naproxen) is not appropriate without ruling out acute causes. A laparoscopy or a laparotomy may be premature at this point given the stable vital signs and lack of other serum studies. Antibiotics are not appropriate because there is no mention of anything that may lead you to suspect pelvic inflammatory disease.

5. The answer is E [I A]. Given the patient's history of major depression, sexual abuse, suicide attempts, and long-standing pelvic pain, the most likely cause may be a manifestation of deep-rooted psychological difficulties. A team approach using a gynecologist, an internist, a psychiatrist, and a social worker would most benefit her. The pain is unrelated to her menses; therefore, you can rule out mittelschmerz and endometriosis. It is unlikely that a postpartum tubal ligation caused any or significant enough adhesions to account for her pelvic pain. There is no evidence of irregular uterine enlargement on pelvic examination.

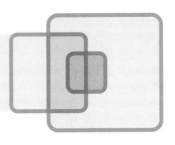

chapter 27

Ectopic Pregnancy

KURT BARNHART

I   INTRODUCTION

An ectopic pregnancy is implantation of an embryo outside the uterus.

A **Location**

1. **Tubal (99%):** anywhere in the fallopian tube
   a. The most common site is the ampulla.
   b. Interstitial (cornual) pregnancies occur in the most proximal tubal segment, which runs through the uterine cornua. This type of ectopic pregnancy can grow to be quite large, and rupture may cause massive hemorrhage.

2. **Ovarian (0.5%):** on the ovary

3. **Abdominal (less than 0.1%):** in the abdomen, with possible adherence to the peritoneum, visceral surfaces, or omentum

4. **Cervical (0.1%):** in the cervix

5. **Heterotopic**
   a. Both intrauterine and ectopic pregnancies may occur concomitantly.
   b. This type of ectopic pregnancy is extremely rare (1 in 4000 in the general population and 1 in 100 in those who conceived with in vitro fertilization [IVF]).

B **Prevalence.**   Ectopic pregnancies constitute 2% of all pregnancies. This proportion has increased over the past few decades, but true prevalence is not known.

C **Significance.**   Ectopic pregnancy may lead to tubal rupture, massive intra-abdominal hemorrhage, and, ultimately, death. It also may result in tubal damage and has been associated with a poor reproductive outcome. It is the leading pregnancy-related cause of death in the first trimester. With reliable serum pregnancy tests and vaginal ultrasound, early detection and treatment of an ectopic pregnancy are possible.

II   ETIOLOGY

A **General considerations.**   The occurrence of ectopic pregnancy has been associated with abnormal function of the fallopian tubes. Normally, the tubes facilitate collection and transport of the oocyte and embryo into the uterus. The integrity of the fimbria, lumen, and ciliated mucosa appears to be important for transport. Conditions thought to prevent or retard migration of the fertilized ovum to the uterus increase the risk for an ectopic pregnancy.

B **Pelvic inflammatory disease (PID).**   The inflammation and scarring of intra- and extraluminal structures resulting from PID impair normal tubal function and foster implantation in the tube. Severe damage may lead to complete tubal blockage and infertility.

C **Tubal surgery.**   Bilateral tubal ligation and tubal reanastomosis may lead to scarring and narrowing of the tube or false passage formation. Other pelvic and abdominal surgeries may also result in peritubal adhesions but have not been directly associated with ectopic pregnancy.

D **Artificial reproductive techniques.** Studies have documented increased risk of ectopic pregnancy with in vitro fertilization, gamete intrafallopian transfer, and superovulation, regardless of previous tubal damage. Retrograde embryo migration may be a possible mechanism.

E **Cigarette smoking.** Studies have shown that cigarette smoking causes tubal ciliary dysfunction. Smoking has been associated with ectopic pregnancy.

F **Intrauterine device (IUD).** Like any contraceptive method, the IUD protects against ectopic pregnancy. However, women who become pregnant with an IUD in place have a higher chance of having a tubal pregnancy than women without an IUD.

III SIGNS AND SYMPTOMS

A **Vaginal bleeding.** Light vaginal bleeding or spotting in the first trimester of pregnancy is the most common symptom of ectopic pregnancy. This bleeding usually begins 7 to 14 days after the missed menstrual period, and patients may interpret the bleeding as a menses.

B **Abdominal pain.** Unilateral pelvic pain is the second most common symptom. The pain may become severe and diffuse and may be associated with shoulder pain (caused by diaphragmatic irritation) if significant intra-abdominal hemorrhage exists.

C **Other symptoms.** Dizziness, fainting spells, and palpitations from hypotension resulting from intra-abdominal hemorrhage may occur.

D **Pregnancy status.** The standard urine pregnancy test is usually positive in the presence of an ectopic pregnancy. However, an ectopic pregnancy may be associated with a lower than expected human chorionic gonadotropin (hCG) level for gestation, and may not be detected in the urine test. The serum pregnancy test, which is more sensitive, should be performed if the urine test is negative and clinical suspicion is high.

IV DIAGNOSIS

Because the symptoms of vaginal bleeding and pain in early pregnancy are not specific for ectopic pregnancy, these findings should not be used in isolation to diagnose this condition.

A **Physical examination.** In the presence of tubal rupture with intra-abdominal hemorrhage, patients may be hypotensive and tachycardic. In these cases, abdominal distention from hemoperitoneum and signs of an acute abdomen may be present with guarding, rebound, and cervical motion tenderness. In the absence of rupture, the physical examination may be completely normal. An unruptured ectopic pregnancy cannot be diagnosed by physical examination alone.

B **Differential diagnosis**

1. Adnexal torsion

2. Appendicitis

3. Spontaneous or threatened abortion

4. PID

5. Hemorrhagic corpus luteum

6. Endometriosis

7. Diverticulitis

8. Ovarian cyst

C **Diagnostic tests.** No single diagnostic test detects all ectopic pregnancies. A diagnostic strategy has been devised involving the use of several diagnostic modalities (Fig. 27-1).

1. **Transvaginal ultrasound.** The first step in the evaluation of a suspected ectopic pregnancy is transvaginal ultrasound.

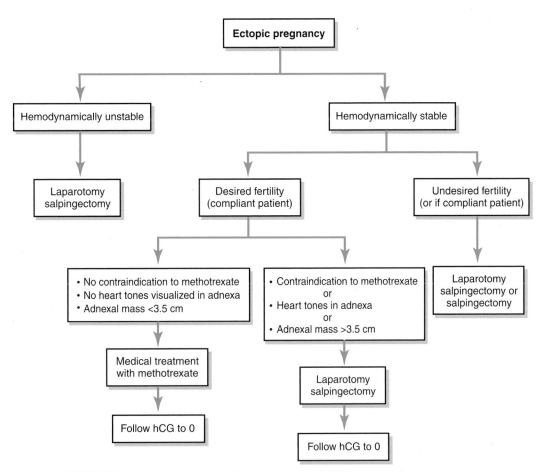

FIGURE 27–1 Treatment algorithm for ectopic pregnancy. hCG, human chorionic gonadotropin.

a. It is difficult to diagnose an ectopic pregnancy by ultrasound alone. However, all viable intrauterine pregnancies can be visualized by transvaginal ultrasound at a gestational age greater than 5.5 to 6 weeks. Therefore, the **best way to diagnose** an ectopic pregnancy is to **rule out the presence of an intrauterine pregnancy** (heterotopic pregnancies are extremely rare).

b. If an intrauterine pregnancy is detected on ultrasound, then ectopic pregnancy has essentially been excluded. If an ectopic pregnancy is visualized, then treatment may be pursued. If the ultrasound is nondiagnostic, then further evaluation is required.

2. **Human chorionic gonadotropin**

a. This hormone, which is produced by trophoblastic tissue, increases linearly in early pregnancy. hCG is used as a surrogate marker for gestational age because the exact gestational age at the time of presentation is often unknown.

b. The **discriminatory zone** is defined as the quantitative hCG level above which all viable intrauterine pregnancies are visible by ultrasound. It is not the lowest hCG at which an intrauterine pregnancy can be visualized. The hCG level for transvaginal ultrasound, which varies by institution, is approximately 2000 mIU/mL. A higher discriminatory zone will decrease the possibility of interrupting a viable gestation.

c. If an intrauterine pregnancy is not identified by transvaginal ultrasound when the quantitative hCG level is higher than the discriminatory zone, then the gestation is, by definition, nonviable (either an abnormal intrauterine pregnancy or an ectopic pregnancy).

3. **Dilation and curettage (D&C).** When an intrauterine pregnancy is not identified by transvaginal ultrasound and the hCG level is greater than the discriminatory zone, a D&C may be performed to determine the location of the gestation. The absence of chorionic villi in the curettage specimen suggests the presence of an extrauterine, or ectopic, pregnancy.

4. Serial hCG testing

a. If the quantitative hCG is below the discriminatory zone and the ultrasound is nondiagnostic, it is necessary to follow serial quantitative hCG levels to distinguish a viable intrauterine pregnancy from a nonviable gestation. Early in viable pregnancies, the **hCG concentration increases in a reproducible fashion** (minimum increase, 50%). If the hCG level increases above the discriminatory zone, a repeat ultrasound should be performed to confirm the presence of an intrauterine pregnancy.

b. hCG levels that fall or stabilize indicate nonviable pregnancies.

(1) When hCG levels decrease, they should be followed until the concentration of hCG is undetectable to confirm the diagnosis of a complete abortion. hCG levels should fall 21% to 35% in 2 days for a woman with a spontaneous abortion (depending on the initial value). Ruptured ectopic pregnancies have occurred at very low hCG concentrations.

(2) When hCG levels fail to rise or decline "normally," a D&C should be performed to distinguish a nonviable intrauterine pregnancy from an ectopic pregnancy.

5. Laparoscopy. If the diagnosis is in doubt, laparoscopy may be performed to directly visualize the tubes and ovaries.

6. Serum progesterone levels. These measurements may be used as an adjunct to ultrasound and hCG. Progesterone levels less than 5 ng/mL are usually associated with nonviable pregnancies, and levels of 25 ng/mL or higher are usually associated with viable intrauterine pregnancies. However, these values are not absolute. Most patients evaluated for ectopic pregnancy have intermediate values, which are not helpful in diagnosis. The usefulness of progesterone is controversial.

V TREATMENT

A Surgical approaches. Surgical treatment of ectopic pregnancy has the advantage of taking care of the ectopic immediately.

1. Salpingectomy, the removal of the fallopian tube containing the ectopic pregnancy, is the treatment of choice in the following situations:

a. Future childbearing is not desired.

b. The tube is severely damaged.

c. Bleeding cannot be controlled.

d. The ectopic is in a fallopian tube where an ectopic occurred previously.

2. Linear salpingotomy, the removal of the gestation through a linear incision in the fallopian tube, may be performed if future fertility is desired.

a. This procedure is associated with a persistent ectopic pregnancy rate of 3% to 20%.

b. Therefore, serial quantitative hCG values must be followed to ensure resolution.

3. Operative laparoscopy may be performed to confirm the diagnosis of ectopic pregnancy and to remove the abnormal gestation via salpingectomy or salpingostomy. This method is typically used in hemodynamically stable patients. Advantages of this technique over laparotomy include:

a. Shorter hospital stay

b. Faster postoperative recovery

c. Better cosmetic result

d. Potentially shorter operative time

4. Laparotomy is typically reserved for hemodynamically unstable patients who require emergent surgery for a ruptured ectopic pregnancy. This method may also be appropriate when laparoscopy is contraindicated or technically challenging because of extensive adhesive disease from prior surgery.

5. Cornual resection may be performed when an interstitial pregnancy occurs. The interstitial portion of the tube is removed via wedge resection into the uterine cornu. Cornual ectopic pregnancies have a higher failure rate with methotrexate and a surgical approach may be more effective.

6. Oophorectomy is indicated only when an ovarian ectopic pregnancy occurs and salvage of the affected ovary is not possible.

B **Medical approach.** Methotrexate, a chemotherapeutic agent, has been used successfully to treat small, unruptured ectopic pregnancies. This approach has the advantage that it avoids surgery, but the patient must be counseled that it may take 3 to 4 weeks for the ectopic to resolve with methotrexate therapy.

1. **Mechanism of action.** Methotrexate is a folic acid antagonist that interferes with DNA synthesis. Its action is principally directed at rapidly dividing cells, such as trophoblastic cells.

2. **Administration.** Methotrexate may be administered in a single intramuscular dose or in multiple doses with folic acid "rescue" (Table 27-1). Serial hCG levels are followed every 2 to 4 days until the hCG level starts to decrease. Once the hCG level is falling, then hCG levels can be checked weekly.

3. **Success rates** (73% to 94%). Decreased success has been noted with ectopic pregnancies of greater than 3.5 cm, with fetal cardiac activity, or with high hCG levels.

4. **Treatment success** using single-dose methotrexate is decreased if the initial hCG value is greater than 5000.

5. **Treatment failures.** Surgical management is usually necessary.

6. **Follow-up.** Serial hCG measurements must be observed after treatment to ensure resolution of the pregnancy.

7. **Complications** (approximately 5% of patients). Mild gastrointestinal symptoms such as nausea, vomiting, diarrhea, and stomatitis are typical. Potential life-threatening complications include pneumonitis, thrombocytopenia, neutropenia, elevated liver function tests, and renal failure.

8. **Contraindications.** Women who are breastfeeding or who have immunodeficiency, liver disease, renal disease, blood disorders, peptic ulcer disease, and active pulmonary disease should not receive methotrexate.

VI PROGNOSIS

A **Fertility.** Reported tubal patency after conservative surgical therapy is approximately 70% to 80%. There appears to be no significant difference in tubal patency after salpingotomy in comparison to methotrexate. As many as 80% of women achieve pregnancy after an ectopic pregnancy, but only 33% deliver live infants. The best chance for future pregnancy in cases of tubal occlusion is in vitro fertilization.

B **Recurrence.** Of those women who achieve pregnancy after an ectopic pregnancy, as many as 27% will have another ectopic pregnancy. All patients should be told about the recurrence risk and should notify a physician as soon as a menses has been missed to determine the location of the pregnancy.

TABLE 27–1 **Methotrexate Treatment in Ectopic Pregnancy**

Treatment Regimen	Single Dose	Two Dose	Multidose
Methotrexate	50 mg/m^2 Day 1	50 mg/m^2 Days 1 and 4	1 mg/kg Day 1 (maybe 3, 5, and 7)
Leucovorin	None	None	0.1 mg/kg alternating with methotrexate
hCG monitoring	Days 1, 4, and 7	Days 1, 4, and 7	Every other day, then weekly until hCG had declined 15%
Repeat dose	Day 7 if hCG did not decline 15% during days 4 through 7	Day 7 if hCG did not decline 15% during days 4 through 7	Administer until hCG declines 15% or up to four doses
Surveillance hCG values	Weekly until level is undetectable	Weekly until level is undetectable	Weekly until level is undetectable

hCG, human chorionic gonadotropin.

Study Questions for Chapter 27

Directions: *Each of the numbered items or incomplete statements in this section is followed by answers or by completions of the statement. Select the ONE lettered answer or completion that is BEST in each case.*

1 A 25-year-old woman, G1, P0, is in the emergency room complaining of lower pelvic pain and spotting for the past week. Her last normal menstrual period was 7 weeks ago. You have obtained a serum β-hCG, which was 4000 IU/L, and a transvaginal ultrasound was performed, which revealed no gestational sac in the endometrial cavity, no adnexal masses, and no free fluid in the cul-de-sac. The next best step in the management of this patient is:

- **A** Repeat β-hCG in 2 days
- **B** Laparoscopy
- **C** Laparotomy
- **D** Methotrexate, single-dose therapy
- **E** Dilation and curettage

2. A 28-year-old woman, gravida 2, para 1, ectopic 1, presents to your clinic for an annual examination. She and her partner would like to try to have another child. Her menstrual cycles are regular, occurring every 28 days. You tell her that it is very important for her to give you a call or to come back to the clinic if she misses her period. The reason for this advice is:

- **A** Given her history, she has a 33% chance of delivering a live infant
- **B** She needs a urine pregnancy test to rule out another ectopic
- **C** Her risk of a recurrent ectopic is approximately 15%
- **D** Her risk of a recurrent ectopic is approximately 30%
- **E** She is at increased risk for pelvic inflammatory disease

3. A 23-year-old woman, gravida 3, para 1, ectopic 1, presents to your office because she missed her last period and has felt a sharp, intermittent pain in her left lower abdomen. She has no past medical history other than a left-sided ectopic pregnancy a few years ago successfully treated with methotrexate, several years after vaginal delivery of her only son. Her serum β-hCG level is 10,500. On physical examination, her BP = 110/74, P = 90, and T = 97.8. She is obese and lacks peritoneal signs, and no masses are appreciated. A transvaginal ultrasound performed in your office reveals no gestational sac in the uterus and a 4.3-cm mass in the left adnexa separate from the ovary. What is the next best step in management of this patient?

- **A** Laparoscopic salpingostomy
- **B** Laparoscopic salpingectomy
- **C** Methotrexate
- **D** Exploratory laparotomy
- **E** Repeat β-hCG in 2 days

4. A 36-year-old nulligravid woman is seeing you for her annual gynecologic care. She has a past medical history significant for pulmonary fibrosis. Within the past 3 years, all of the following are remarkable in her chart: bacterial vaginosis, *Candida*, chronic endometritis, pyelonephritis, history of IUD that was removed 5 years ago, and history of infertility for which she was treated with fertility drugs and in vitro fertilization. She is a nonsmoker but does admit to drinking two to three alcoholic beverages every day. She has a family history significant for colon cancer in her maternal aunt. Which of the following places her at greatest risk for an ectopic pregnancy?

- **A** Age
- **B** Pulmonary fibrosis
- **C** Past IUD use
- **D** Infertility
- **E** Chronic endometritis

5. A 24-year-old woman, gravida 3, para 1, spontaneous abortions 1, presents to the emergency room reporting irregular vaginal bleeding. She is found to be pregnant and her serum hCG is 3500 mIU/mL. She has a past medical history significant for diabetes mellitus and mild asthma. Her BP = 103/68, P = 88, and T = 98.8. Transvaginal ultrasound reveals a uterus with no gestational sac present and a 2-cm right adnexal mass. The least invasive treatment of choice is:

- A Expectant management
- B Methotrexate
- C Laparoscopic salpingostomy
- D Laparoscopic salpingectomy
- E Laparotomy

Answers and Explanations

1. The answer is E [IV C]. When the quantitative hCG level is above the discriminatory zone (usually 2000 mIU/mL, depending on the ultrasound machine) and no pregnancy is visualized by transvaginal ultrasound, the pregnancy either is outside of the uterus or is an abnormal intrauterine pregnancy. To distinguish between the two, a uterine curettage should be performed. The presence of chorionic villi in the uterus indicates that the pregnancy was in the uterus and that the ectopic pregnancy does not exist. Determining the location of the pregnancy is important not only to establish the correct treatment, but also to counsel the patient regarding her risk of having an ectopic in a subsequent pregnancy. Repeating a quantitative hCG is not helpful because the β-hCG level is above the discriminatory level and there is no visualization of a sac in the uterus or adnexa, confirming that the pregnancy is either an ectopic or abnormal intrauterine pregnancy. Methotrexate would not be ideal at this point because it is not clear that the patient has an ectopic pregnancy since there is no pregnancy identified in the uterus and there is no sign of a pregnancy in the tubes by ultrasound. Once the diagnosis has been confirmed by finding no chorionic villi at D&C, then methotrexate would be an option. Neither a laparoscopy nor a laparotomy is necessary yet because no mass has been visualized on ultrasound.

2. The answer is D [VI B]. Of those women who achieve pregnancy after an ectopic pregnancy, as many as 27% will have another ectopic pregnancy. All patients should be counseled about the risk of recurrence. A urine pregnancy test is not as sensitive as a serum hCG and should not be used as the definitive test to determine if a patient is pregnant. Also, a pregnancy test alone cannot differentiate between ectopic and intrauterine pregnancy. This patient is not at increased risk for PID based on the information provided. Although the patient with a history of a prior ectopic does have a 33% chance of delivering a live infant, this would not be the reason to bring her back to the office if she misses a period.

3. The answer is B [V A]. This patient most likely has an ectopic pregnancy in the left fallopian tube, the same tube where she had a prior ectopic pregnancy. The best treatment option is to remove the tube since her rate of another ectopic in the same tube is high. She presumably has another fallopian tube and therefore future pregnancy is possible. Salpingotomy would not be a good idea because leaving the tube in would place the patient at a very high risk for recurrence of another ectopic pregnancy. Methotrexate is contraindicated because the hCG level is too high and the size of the ectopic is too big (greater than 3 cm). Repeating hCG in 2 days is inappropriate because you already know that the hCG level is above the discriminatory level, there is no intrauterine gestation, and there is a mass in the left adnexa, so you have a diagnosis of ectopic pregnancy. Repeating the hCG level would give you no additional information and would just delay the treatment, risking rupture of the ectopic. In a patient who is hemodynamically stable, a laparotomy is not necessary, unless there are medical indications to avoid laparoscopy or the patient has known or suspected intra-abdominal adhesions that would make laparoscopy difficult.

4. The answer is D [II D]. Infertility is a risk factor for ectopic pregnancy. Current IUD use, not past IUD use, places the patient at risk for ectopic pregnancy. Chronic endometritis is not associated with ectopic pregnancy because this inflammation does not involve the fallopian tubes. Age is not a risk factor for ectopic pregnancy. Pulmonary fibrosis is not a risk factor for ectopic pregnancy but would be a contraindication for methotrexate.

5. The answer is B [V B]. This patient has an ectopic pregnancy that is amenable to treatment with methotrexate because she has no contraindications (hCG not high, less than 3-cm adnexal mass, and mild asthma and diabetes mellitus are not contraindications). Although methotrexate and linear salpingostomy have comparable rates of tubal patency and fertility, methotrexate is the least invasive. Expectant management of a growing ectopic pregnancy is not appropriate given possibility of rupture and hemorrhage, which can be catastrophic. Salpingectomy is not preferred to salpingostomy in someone who desires future fertility. Laparotomy is not indicated in this patient, who is hemodynamically stable.

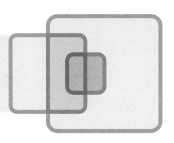

chapter 28

The Infertile Couple

H. IRENE SU • STEVEN J. SONDHEIMER

I INTRODUCTION

A **Infertility** is defined as no conception after 1 year of unprotected intercourse (i.e., without contraception). Predicting fertility prior to attempting pregnancy is difficult and inaccurate.

1. **Fecundability**, or the monthly probability of pregnancy, is about 20% among fertile couples. The cumulative probability of pregnancy after 1 year approaches 85%.

2. **Primary infertility** refers to individuals who have never established a pregnancy.

3. **Secondary infertility** refers to individuals who have conceived previously (including miscarriages) but are currently unable to establish a subsequent pregnancy.

B Incidence.   Approximately 15% of couples are infertile, using the criteria of at least 1 year of unprotected coitus. The longer the period of time that a couple attempts pregnancy without success, the more likely that they will have infertility.

C Causes of infertility

1. The process of achieving pregnancy:
   a. Ovulation
   b. "Competent oocyte"
   c. Fallopian tube patency
   d. Normal uterine cavity and vaginal outflow tract
   e. Spermatogenesis
   f. Coitus

2. Disruptions of these steps necessary in establishing a pregnancy lead to infertility. The following percentages reflect the prevalence of these factors in infertility evaluations. In 20% to 40% of couples, there are multiple causes of infertility. Therefore, the percentages below add up to more than 100.
   a. Ovulatory dysfunction: 25%
   b. Ovarian aging: incidence varies with age
   c. Tubal factor: 35%
   d. Uterine and vaginal outflow tract abnormalities: 3%
   e. Endometriosis: 35%
   f. Male factor: 40%
   g. Coital problems: 5%
   h. Unexplained: 10%

II APPROACH TO TREATMENT

Empathic listening and review of coital technique and frequency is always appropriate. A full infertility evaluation is not usually initiated until 1 year of coitus without contraception. Evaluation should begin sooner in women over age 35 and those with irregular or absent menses; a history of pelvic inflammatory disease, sexually transmitted diseases, or pelvic surgery; or a significant history in the male partner. Early evaluation in a woman without these conditions has the risk of initiating treatment when pregnancy might have occurred spontaneously in a relatively short time. Once the decision to begin evaluation has been made, goals of treatment are as follows:

A Seek out and correct causes of infertility

B Provide accurate information and dispel misinformation

C Provide emotional support, including listening, giving plenty of time for questions, and lending support without blame or criticism

D Provide **preconception counseling**

  1. Smoking cessation and minimal alcohol exposure

  2. Folic acid supplementation to decrease the risk of neural tube defects in the fetus

  3. Genetic counseling
     a. Advanced maternal age carries a higher risk of chromosomal abnormalities and advanced paternal age carries a high risk for new autosomal dominant conditions in the fetus.
     b. Indicated carrier states: certain ethnic populations have a higher risk of genetic problems in the offspring. Examples include Tay-Sachs disease in Ashkenazi Jewish individuals and sickle cell disease in African-American individuals.
     c. A family history of genetic abnormalities in the couple or first-degree relatives, such as congenital cardiac anomalies and mental retardation, could potentially be passed to the fetus.

  4. Maternal–fetal medicine consultation for medical illnesses that could affect the health of the mother or fetus during pregnancy such as diabetes and chronic hypertension

E Provide options for treatment and alternatives when treatment has not been successful or is not possible

III OVULATORY DYSFUNCTION

A Definitions

  1. Inability of the ovaries to release oocytes on a cyclic basis. Normal ovulation requires an **intact hypothalamic-pituitary-ovarian axis.**

  2. **Anovulation** is lack of ovulation.

  3. **Oligo-ovulation** is occasional ovulation.

B Etiology

  1. **Androgen excess**
     a. Polycystic ovarian syndrome
     b. Nonclassic congenital adrenal hyperplasia
     c. Androgen-secreting tumors

  2. **Hypothalamic amenorrhea**
     a. Malnutrition
     b. Weight loss
     c. Excessive exercise

  3. **Hyperprolactinemia**
     a. Medications (many medication classes, including antipsychotics that are dopamine receptor antagonists; a typical example is haloperidol)
     b. Pituitary tumors
     c. Hypothyroidism (Increased thyrotropin-releasing hormone [TRH] secretion stimulates prolactin secretion.)

  4. **Decreased ovarian reserve** (see below)

  5. **Hypothyroidism**

C Diagnosis

  1. **Predictable, regular menses** (every 28 to 35 days) is a very good predictor of ovulation but doesn't confirm that ovulation is occurring.

2. **Basal body temperature monitoring**. The woman takes her temperature upon awakening and before getting out of bed in the morning and graphs the daily temperature. This technique is not helpful in predicting when ovulation will occur, but is helpful in determining that ovulation has occurred.

   a. A **biphasic pattern** is seen with ovulation secondary to the thermogenic effects of progesterone.

   b. Basal temperatures become elevated by 0.5° to 1.0° immediately *after* ovulation in response to progesterone.

   c. At the end of a month-long cycle, the average temperature in the first 10 to 14 days should be lower than in the last 10 to 14 days by approximately 0.3°.

   d. If this pattern is present, it can be assumed that the patient is ovulating.

3. **Urinary luteinizing hormone (LH) kits** may also be used to detect a rise in LH immediately prior to ovulation. Patients begin testing their urine on cycle day 10 and continue testing until they detect a change in color on the indicator stick. It can be assumed that ovulation will occur within the following 12 to 24 hours.

4. A **serum progesterone level** greater than 4 ng/mL suggests ovulation. A progesterone level of 10 ng/mL obtained in the midluteal phase (i.e., 7 days from ovulation) represents an adequate level of progesterone and has largely replaced the endometrial biopsy as an assessment of luteal-phase adequacy.

5. **Luteal-phase endometrial biopsy** is a historic test that was done to confirm ovulation and to determine if the endometrium was in an appropriate stage to allow implantation (i.e., "in phase"). If there is a discrepancy, then a luteal-phase defect, presumably due to lack of progesterone effect, was diagnosed. The idea behind the test is as follows: after ovulation, the corpus luteum produces progesterone, which acts to change the endometrial lining from a proliferative to a secretory appearance. Each day after ovulation the endometrium matures in a characteristic fashion in preparation for embryo implantation approximately 7 days after ovulation (and fertilization). Dating the endometrium by histologic examination on tissue obtained by biopsy and comparing this to the expected appearance based either on the known ovulation date or the onset of the next menses can determine if the endometrium is in phase. However, due to variation in interpretation of the histologic samples and normal variability seen in fertile couples, the test is no longer used.

6. **Thyroid-stimulating hormone (TSH)**, **prolactin**, **total testosterone**, **free testosterone**, **17-hydro-xyprogesterone**, and **follicle-stimulating hormone (FSH)** should be assessed if no evidence of ovulation is detected.

D Treatment

1. **Correction of underlying endocrine disorders**, such as thyroid disease and hyperprolactinemia, leads to spontaneous ovulation in many patients.

2. Induction of ovulation

   a. **Clomiphene citrate** is the **most commonly prescribed fertility drug and is indicated for the treatment of anovulation**. Clomiphene citrate is an estrogen antagonist and works best in women with a functioning hypothalamic-pituitary-ovarian axis (i.e., women with normal estrogen levels and oligo- or anovulation, such as those with polycystic ovarian syndrome). It triggers endogenous release of FSH, which then stimulates follicular development. Clomiphene citrate is well suited for practitioners and patients because of its oral administration, ease of use, and minimal monitoring. The usual starting dose in anovulatory women is 50 mg daily for 5 days early in the follicular phase (usually cycle days 5 to 9). Intercourse can be timed by using a urinary LH predictor kit to predict ovulation or by monitoring follicular development by transvaginal ultrasound. If no measurable response to 50 mg of clomiphene occurs, the dose can be increased by 50 mg in subsequent cycles to a maximum of 150 mg. In **anovulatory women**, each ovulatory cycle induced by clomiphene results in a pregnancy rate of 20%. Cumulatively, the 6-month conception rate in this population is 60% to 75%, mirroring the normal conception rate. The risk of twin pregnancies is 10%, and the risk of higher order multiple pregnancies is less than 1%.

b. Injectable gonadotropins are indicated primarily for women with hypothalamic amenorrhea or for those who have failed to ovulate with clomiphene treatment. Preparations include purified urinary extract of FSH and LH and laboratory-synthesized FSH preparations. Unlike clomiphene, this drug directly stimulates the ovary. Monitoring involves intense serial serum estradiol measurements and transvaginal ultrasounds to assess ovarian response. Ovulation will not occur spontaneously and is triggered by injection of human chorion gonadotropin (hCG; similar structure to LH hormone, which is the natural trigger for ovulation) after both estradiol levels and follicular size suggest follicular maturity. In hypothalamic amenorrheic women, the 6-month conception rate approaches 90%. This rate is lower in women with other causes of anovulation. The risk of twin pregnancies is 10% to 20%, and the risk of higher order multiple pregnancies is less than 5%.

IV "COMPETENT OOCYTE"/DECREASED OVARIAN RESERVE

A A woman's chronologic age and the aging of the ovary correlate with the number and quality of available oocytes and are two independent predictors of fertility.

1. **Age of the woman** is an important predictor of fertility.
   a. Spontaneous loss rates are higher in older women because of higher risk of aneuploidy.
   b. Age-related infertility rates in three age groups are as follows:
      (1) 25 to 29 years: 9%
      (2) 30 to 34 years: 15%
      (3) 35 to 39 years: 22%

2. **Ovarian aging concept.** It is generally accepted that there is a finite number of oocytes in a 46,XX individual. The maximum oocyte number is actually achieved in utero. Throughout a woman's lifetime there is a steady and uninterrupted depletion of oocytes independent of ovulation. Ovarian aging is termed "decreased ovarian reserve" and correlates with a decrease in fertility.

B Diagnosis through **markers of decreased ovarian reserve**

1. **FSH** and **estradiol**
   a. Elevated menstrual **cycle day 3 FSH** is a marker of decreased oocyte number and quality.
      (1) **FSH** level on the third day of the menstrual cycle that is greater than 10 to 12 mIU/mL is considered elevated and correlates with a decrease in fertility. A range is given because these "threshold" levels can vary in value and interpretation in different labs. This FSH level is still considered in the "normal" premenopausal range.
      (2) An elevated **estradiol** level (greater than 80 pg/mL) on the third day can also represent a decrease in ovarian reserve, but it is not as predictive as the FSH level. An elevated estradiol level may suppress the FSH level through negative inhibition and falsely portray a "normal" FSH level.
   b. FSH level greater than 40 mIU/mL associated with amenorrhea is the definition of ovarian failure. If these findings occur in a woman under 40 years old, she has **premature ovarian failure**.

2. An **antral follicle count** is performed by using the ultrasound to visualize the ovaries and to count the total number of follicles between 2 and 5 mm. A low antral follicle count predicts diminished response to fertility treatment.

3. The **clomiphene citrate challenge test** is a **bioassay to FSH response** that reflects ovarian follicular capability. Following administration of clomiphene citrate 100 mg/day on cycle days 5 to 9, an FSH level on menstrual cycle day 10 is compared with a baseline FSH level on menstrual cycle day 3. An FSH value on either day 3 or 10 that is greater than or equal to the threshold level for the laboratory is associated with a decreased likelihood of achieving pregnancy.

C Treatment

Fertility treatment for a patient with decreased ovarian reserve should be approached more aggressively. The chance of success with any treatment option is lower than in an individual with normal ovarian reserve. The decision to proceed should be individualized and must take into account likely success, which depends on the age of the woman and any other factors identified that could affect fertility.

1. **Donor oocytes** through in vitro fertilization can be fertilized with partner sperm, and the embryo(s) can be transferred to and carried by the woman.

2. Adoption

V TUBAL FACTOR

A **Tubal disease.**   The fallopian tube is responsible for efficient transfer of gametes and transport of the dividing embryo to the uterine cavity. It provides an environment in which capacitation of spermatozoa, fertilization, and early development of the embryo take place. Tubal disease or blockage can impair the ability to conceive. Common causes of tubal disease include **pelvic inflammatory disease, tubal ligation**, and **endometriosis**.

B Diagnosis

1. **Hysterosalpingography (HSG)** is a fluoroscopic study that provides visualization of the **uterine cavity** and **internal lumen and patency** of the fallopian tube using a radiopaque dye injected through the cervix. This method neither allows for visualization of the external surface of the tubes nor provides external assessment of pelvic adhesions or anatomic relationships within the pelvis. A hysterosalpingogram is usually obtained before performing a laparoscopy because it is less costly and less invasive.

2. **Laparoscopy** allows direct visualization of the external surface of the fallopian tube to identify abnormalities in structure or location and to detect peritubal or pelvic adhesions. Laparoscopy does not provide any information on tubal patency unless a dye (usually indigo carmine) is injected through the cervix and is allowed to spill into the pelvic cavity under direct visualization.

C Treatment

1. **In vitro fertilization (IVF)** bypasses the fallopian tube and is the most successful.

2. Surgical
   a. **Tubal reanastomosis** for sterilization reversal
   b. Lysis of peritubal adhesions
   c. Neosalpingostomy and fimbrioplasty for occluded fallopian tubes

VI UTERINE AND VAGINAL OUTFLOW TRACT ABNORMALITIES

A **Uterine factor.**   The uterus is responsible for providing an environment suitable for sperm transport, development of the embryo prior to implantation, and carriage of the pregnancy. The following abnormalities are associated more with pregnancy loss than infertility.

1. **Leiomyomas** (fibroids): especially submucosal in location

2. **Uterine polyps**

3. **Synechiae**: scar tissue from prior uterine procedures, also known as Asherman syndrome

4. **Congenital anomalies** such as uterine septum or bicornuate or unicornuate uterus. Recall that **müllerian derivatives do not include ovaries**. Therefore, patients with complete müllerian agenesis (no uterus, fallopian tubes, and upper vagina) should still have normally functioning ovaries.

5. **Cervical factor:** current infertility diagnosis and treatment do not approach the cervix separately from the uterus. While cervical changes such as prior cone biopsy or loop electrosurgical excision procedures (LEEPs) for cervical dysplasia may affect fertility (through miscarriages), they are rarely the cause of infertility.

B **Vaginal outflow tract** abnormalities such as congenital transverse vaginal septum and vaginal adhesions (a rare consequence of graft versus host disease in bone marrow transplant patients)

C Diagnosis

1. **HSG** allows visualization of the internal contour of the uterine cavity by injection of a radiopaque dye under fluoroscopic radiography through the cervix. Aside from detecting tubal

pathology, this **technique detects synechiae, congenital anatomic anomalies**, and **polyps** and **fibroids** if they distort the uterine cavity.

2. If an abnormality is detected on HSG, a **hysteroscopy** can be performed to confirm the abnormality. Hysteroscopy allows for direct visualization of the uterine cavity.

3. If a congenital uterine anomaly is suspected after hysterosalpingography, a **pelvic magnetic resonance image (MRI)** may be helpful to noninvasively assess the external and internal contours of the uterus. This technique also allows inspection of the urinary tract given a high rate of associated anomalies. **Laparoscopy** is a more invasive method of obtaining information about the external contour of the uterus.

4. **Sonohysterography** is performed by placing a small balloon-tipped cannula into the uterus via the cervix and infusing the cavity with sterile saline. A vaginal ultrasound is performed simultaneously to visualize the internal uterine contour. Small polyps and fibroids impinging on the uterine cavity can be detected by this method. However, this method **does not allow assessment of the external surface of the uterus**.

D Treatment

1. **Surgical correction**. Many abnormalities, including synechiae, fibroids, polyps, and uterine septae, can be surgically corrected at the time of hysteroscopy.

2. **IVF** can be performed in patients without an intact uterus, and embryos can be transferred to and carried in a **gestational carrier**.

VII ENDOMETRIOSIS

A **Endometriosis** (see Chapter 25) is a common gynecologic disorder estimated to affect 71% of women with pelvic pain alone and nearly 85% of women with both infertility and pelvic pain. Endometriosis is postulated to affect fertility through:

1. **Anatomic distortion** of the pelvis secondary to endometriotic lesions or adhesions

2. Other *hypothesized* mechanisms, including:
   a. Interference in oocyte pick-up by the fimbriae and inhibition of fertilization due to increased concentration of macrophages, prostaglandins, interleukin-1, and tumor necrosis factor in the peritoneal fluid of patients with endometriosis
   b. Altered endometrial receptivity

3. Though the exact mechanism for endometriosis affecting fertility has not been elucidated, it is suggested by the following:
   a. Laparoscopic correction of minimal or mild endometriosis results in a small but significant improvement in fertility.
   b. IVF outcomes are worse in patients with endometriosis.

B Diagnosis

1. **Laparoscopy with visual confirmation of endometriotic lesions or biopsy-confirmed histology** is the only way to confirm the diagnosis.

2. History of worsening or severe dysmenorrhea and/or pre- or postmenstrual bleeding is suggestive of endometriosis.

3. A **pelvic ultrasound**, especially if done by the vaginal route, can often diagnose echogenic ovarian masses that correspond to **endometriomas** ("chocolate cysts"). The presence of endometriomas suggests the possibility of moderate to severe endometriosis.

C Treatment

1. **Surgical ablation and adhesiolysis** typically by laparoscopy is the treatment of choice in those with moderate to severe disease.

2. **Empiric fertility treatment** without laparoscopic confirmation of endometriosis can be undertaken, especially if mild or minimal endometriosis is suspected.

3. **Gonadotropin-releasing hormone (GnRH)** agonist therapy is not indicated for treatment of endometriosis in those who are trying to conceive.

VIII MALE FACTOR INFERTILITY

A Male factor infertility occurs when abnormalities in semen volume, sperm count, or motility significantly affect a couple's ability to conceive. **Paternal age** greater than 40 years is associated with a 20% greater chance of birth defects in the offspring. The capacity to fertilize is maintained.

B Diagnosis

1. **Semen analysis** should be the initial test obtained on all males in couples seeking evaluation. The sample is generally collected by masturbation after 2 to 5 days of abstinence. Ideally two samples should be analyzed. The World Health Organization standards are as follows:
   a. **Volume**: 1.5 to 5.0 mL
   b. **Concentration**: greater than 20 million sperm/mL
   c. **Total sperm number**: greater than 40 million per ejaculate
   d. **Percent motility**: greater than 50%
   e. **Progression**: greater than 2 (scale 0 to 4)
   f. **Morphology**: more than 30% with normal, oval heads and a single tail
   g. **White blood cells**: less than 1 million/mL

2. Differential diagnosis
   a. **Azoospermia** is the absence of sperm in the ejaculate.
      (1) Obstructive azoospermia: vasectomy, congenital bilateral absence of vas deferens (CBAVD), postsurgical obstruction
      (2) Nonobstructive azoospermia: hypogonadotropic hypogonadism: Kallmann syndrome, pituitary tumors; testicular failure: chemotherapy/radiation, trauma, mumps, idiopathic; chromosome abnormalities: Klinefelter syndrome (47,XXY), translocations/deletions, Y chromosome microdeletions

3. Evaluation of the male with azoospermia or severe oligospermia (in absence of prior vasectomy or vasectomy reversal)
   a. Review of medications, medical history, surgical history
   b. FSH and **testosterone levels** to evaluate for hypo- or hypergonadotropic disorders
   c. **Karyotype**: 10% to 15% of azoospermic men will have an abnormal karyotype. Klinefelter syndrome is the most common and accounts for two-thirds of chromosomal abnormalities in infertile men.
   d. **Y chromosome microdeletion** is found in 10% to 15% of men with azoospermia or severe oligospermia. These deletions are not seen on a karyotype. This test is performed by polymerase chain reaction (PCR), followed by gel electrophoresis.
   e. Prolactin and thyroid-stimulating hormone if indicated
   f. Testicular ultrasound
   g. **Cystic fibrosis screening** in CBVAD. Approximately two-thirds of men with CBAVD will have a mutation in the cystic fibrosis transmembrane conductance regulator (CFTR) gene.
   h. Referral to a urologist for examination

4. Historic tests: no longer recommended
   a. **Postcoital test (PK test)** is no longer used since the results of the test do not predict success of any particular treatment. The purpose of the PK test is to check receptivity of the cervical mucus and the ability of sperm to reach and survive in the mucus. Cervical mucus is examined microscopically between 2 and 12 hours after coitus at midcycle for the number of sperm per high-power field and percentage and quality of motility.
   b. Tests of **fertilizing capacity of spermatozoa** have been devised to assess the ability of sperm to fertilize an ovum, but are also not used clinically because of **unclear prognostic value** and **lack of standardization**.
      (1) **Zona-free hamster ovum penetration test** evaluates the ability of sperm to penetrate a hamster ovum without a zona present. The patient's sperm is compared with a known, fertile sperm sample.
      (2) **Human zona binding assay** tests the ability of sperm to attach to the zona. The ratio of the number of patient sperm attached to the zona is compared with the number of a known, fertile control.

C Treatment. In deciding how to proceed with the treatment of the male, the factors identified in the female must be considered.

1. **Medical therapies** include:
   a. Correction of underlying hormonal disorders (e.g., thyroid disorders, prolactin excess, and dietary disturbances)
   b. Use of hCG to stimulate sperm production in cases of hypothalamic dysfunction

2. **Surgical therapies**
   a. Varicocele repair
   b. Vasectomy reversal: may not be advised if the female partner is older due to the length of time needed for sperm to be seen in the ejaculate after reversal

3. **Intrauterine insemination** with sperm. This technique involves washing the semen specimen to concentrate the actively motile sperm and placing the specimen high in the reproductive tract, closer to the fallopian tubes, at the time of ovulation. This technique is performed in conjunction with administering a fertility drug to the female. This procedure is well suited to mild male factor infertility as well as unexplained infertility.

4. **IVF.** This technique is indicated as primary treatment in those with severe oligospermia or in cases of obstructive and nonobstructive azoospermia with surgical collection of sperm. It is combined with intracytoplasmic injection of sperm (ICSI) to achieve fertilization. Surgical techniques to acquire sperm for IVF/ICSI include:
   a. Percutaneous epididymal sperm aspiration
   b. Testicular sperm aspiration/extraction (biopsy)
   c. Microsurgical testicular sperm extraction

5. Insemination with **donor sperm** can be performed in a woman's natural ovulatory cycle or in combination with fertility drugs or IVF.

IX   COITAL PROBLEMS

A The **most fertile days** are up to 4 days prior to ovulation and on the day of ovulation. Coitus should occur during this period.

B Diagnosis by **history**. Are vaginal penetration and ejaculation occurring? Is successful intercourse occurring during the most fertile days? In some ethnic groups, ideal timing of coitus is difficult due to a mandatory waiting period between the end of menses and when intercourse is allowed.

C Treatment. **Regular coitus** (on average every other day) without long intervals of abstinence is the best way to ensure that the fertile window is included.

X   UNEXPLAINED INFERTILITY

A **Unexplained infertility** refers to couples in whom **no identifiable causes or mild abnormalities** are present, such as mild male factor or minimal to mild endometriosis.

B Diagnosis. Diagnosis of exclusion. A laparoscopy is not necessary to make the diagnosis.

C Treatment. **Empiric superovulation with either clomiphene citrate or injectable gonadotropins, along with timed intrauterine insemination, is usually attempted before considering assisted reproductive technology**. During superovulation the follicular growth and number is monitored by ultrasound and serum estradiol levels; hCG injection is used to induce ovulation, and timed intrauterine insemination of washed concentrated sperm, resuspended in a balanced salt solution free of semen proteins and prostaglandins, is also used. Unlike with ovulatory infertility, where unifollicular development is desired, development of three to five follicles is the goal. The problem with this treatment, however, is the risk of high-order multiple gestation because there is no control over how many oocytes fertilize or implant.

XI   **ASSISTED REPRODUCTIVE TECHNOLOGY**

A **IVF** involves ovarian follicular stimulation followed by **ultrasound-guided oocyte retrieval**. The oocytes are then fertilized with sperm in the laboratory, and resultant embryos are transferred back into the uterus.

1. **Injectable gonadotropins** are used to stimulate ovaries to produce multiple follicles.

2. Endogenous ovulation/LH surge is suppressed through **pituitary suppression** with GnRH agonists and antagonists.

3. Ovulation is triggered by hCG because it is more stable than LH and has an almost identical structure (hCG shares the same α subunit as LH, and the β subunit differs by only 30 amino acids).

4. Approximately 36 hours after exogenous stimulation of ovulation, oocytes are usually retrieved transvaginally under ultrasound guidance. In rare circumstances, oocytes can be retrieved transabdominally, transvesically, and laparoscopically.

5. Oocytes are incubated with sperm in a dish to allow for fertilization overnight. Fertilized eggs are then monitored for division.

6. **Embryo transfers** back into the uterus through the cervix typically occur on **day 3** (8- to 10-cell stage) or **day 5** (blastocyst stage) after retrieval.

7. **The number of embryos transferred depends on age, embryo morphology, and prior patient history**. In the United States, there are guidelines from the American Society of Reproductive Medicine to help direct the number of embryos transferred. In multiple European countries, there are guidelines for single embryo transfers. The goal is to ensure successful pregnancies and deliveries while minimizing the number of multiple pregnancies.

B In **ICSI**, a micromanipulation technique, a sperm is injected directly into the cytoplasm of the oocyte to enhance fertilization. This method is often used for **male factor infertility**. Pregnancy rates are independent of any semen analysis parameter because sperm are directly injected into ova by an embryologist.

C In **preimplantation genetic diagnosis (PGD)**, a single cell or polar body is biopsied from the embryo prior to embryo transfer during an IVF cycle and subjected to genetic testing. Currently, this technique is most often used in identifying affected embryos of single gene disorders such as Gaucher disease and cystic fibrosis. With the results from testing, an unaffected embryo is transferred back into the uterus. PGD serves as an alternative to chorionic villus sampling or amniocentesis for diagnosis and possible abortion of affected fetuses.

D In **gamete intrafallopian transfer (GIFT)**, oocytes are retrieved from ovaries as previously mentioned. The oocyte and spermatozoa are not placed into a dish for fertilization but are placed together within the distal fallopian tube, allowing for natural fertilization. However, the fertilization rate and embryo development are unknown. This procedure normally requires a **laparoscopic approach**.

E Another procedure that involves the same principles as GIFT is **zygote intrafallopian transfer (ZIFT)**, except that a zygote (present after fertilization in vitro) is placed into the fallopian tube for further development. This also requires a **laparoscopic approach**. Both GIFT and ZIFT are seldom used since they require laparoscopy and success is just as likely if not better with conventional IVF.

Study Questions for Chapter 28

Directions: *Match each clinical scenario with the most likely cause of infertility. Each answer may be used once, more than once, or not at all.*

QUESTIONS 1–6

- A. Ovulation
- B. Oocyte quality
- C. Tubal factor
- D. Uterine factor
- E. Male factor
- F. Unexplained

1. A 25-year-old woman, gravida 2, para 2, has been trying to get pregnant for the last 2 years. She has no medical problems. She had surgery for a ruptured appendix 5 years ago. Her periods are regular and last 3 to 4 days. She denies smoking, drinking alcohol, or using drugs. Her husband is 28 years old, is healthy, and has a normal sperm count.

2. A 29-year-old woman, gravida 5, para 1, spontaneous abortions 4, presents to you because she has not been able to carry a pregnancy successfully since the birth of her son 8 years ago. Although she becomes pregnant easily, she miscarries the pregnancy at 10 to 14 weeks. Her bimanual examination reveals an irregularly enlarged uterus (14-week size). Her husband is 34 years old and is healthy.

3. A 30-year-old nulligravid woman presents to you because she and her husband have been trying to get pregnant for the past 2 years. She has no prior medical history. She has regular, 30-day menstrual cycles and denies dysmenorrhea. Her pelvic examination is normal. Laboratory testing on cycle day 3 is normal. Ovulation is confirmed by a midluteal-phase progesterone level. You perform a hysterosalpingogram that shows a normal uterine cavity and patent bilateral fallopian tubes. Her husband is 31 years old and has a normal semen analysis.

4. A 39-year-old woman, gravida 1, para 0 (spontaneous abortion 2 years ago), presents with 2 years of secondary infertility. She has no other medical history and has regular 30-day menstrual cycles. On her pelvic ultrasound, you noted an antral follicle count of four from the two ovaries. The hysterosalpingogram that you performed showed a normal uterine cavity and bilateral tubal patency. Her husband's semen analysis is normal.

5. A 27-year-old woman, gravida 2, para 2, presents to you because she has not been able to get pregnant after reversal of her husband's vasectomy. She has no medical problems.

6. A 22-year-old nulligravid woman and her husband have been trying to get pregnant for the last 18 months. She has no known medical problems and has never had any surgery. She says her periods are irregular. She gets about four to five periods per year. She is 5 feet 2 inches tall and weighs 210 lb. On review of systems, she reports hair growth on her abdomen and chin.

Directions: *Each of the numbered items or incomplete statements in this section is followed by answers or by completions of the statement. Select the ONE lettered answer or completion that is BEST in each case.*

7. Among 100 healthy, fertile couples, approximately how many will become pregnant within 1 month if they have regular intercourse?

- [A] 15
- [B] 20
- [C] 35
- [D] 45
- [E] 85

8. A 26-year-old nulligravid and her 26-year-old husband are seeing you because they have not been able to get pregnant for the last 3 years. The woman has regular periods every 30 days that last 4 days. Both of them have no medical problems or past surgical history. Both deny smoking, caffeine use, herbal remedy use, alcohol abuse, or drug use. The husband's sperm analysis reveals a volume of 2.5 mL, total count less than 0.1×10^6 sperm/mL, 10% forward progression, and 30% normal morphology. The next best step in management of this couple is:

- [A] Semen wash, intrauterine insemination (IUI) with clomiphene citrate
- [B] IVF with ICSI and embryo transfer (ET)
- [C] Conventional IVF and ET (IVF-ET)
- [D] Karyotype, FSH, testosterone, Y microdeletion testing

Answers and Explanations

1. C [V A], **2.** D [V A 1], **3.** F [X A], **4.** B [IV A], **5.** E [VIII B 2], **6.** A [III B 1]. In question 1, the woman has had surgery for a ruptured appendix. When an intra-abdominal infection is present (from either a ruptured viscus or pelvic inflammatory disease), there is a risk of adhesion formation, including adhesion of the fallopian tubes to other structures. This prevents proper egg retrieval and transport by the tube, which can lead to ectopic pregnancy. This diagnosis can be confirmed by hysterosalpingography or laparoscopy. In question 2, this patient most likely has submucosal fibroids in her uterus that are contributing to her miscarriages. Other things to consider would be uterine anomalies such as uterine septum or bicornuate or unicornuate uterus. It would be important to know if she had trouble carrying her first child and if she delivered at term. A fibroid may have developed since the birth of her child so that it was not present when she was pregnant earlier. The first step would be a pelvic ultrasound followed by a hysterosalpingogram or hysteroscopy and MRI if uterine abnormality is suspected. In question 3, the couple has a normal infertility workup, rendering the diagnosis of exclusion: unexplained infertility. A laparoscopy is not necessary to make this diagnosis. In question 4, this older patient has a low antral follicle count and an otherwise normal workup. Her infertility is likely due to decreased ovarian reserve. A cycle day 3 FSH and estradiol level would be helpful in confirming the diagnosis. In question 5, reversal of vasectomy may not work. A semen analysis would show azoospermia. The next step would be to use donor sperm versus percutaneous epididymal sperm aspiration performed in conjunction with IVF. In question 6, this patient's signs and symptoms suggest polycystic ovarian syndrome. These patients are oligo-ovulatory.

7. The answer is B [I A 1]. The fecundability, or monthly probability of pregnancy, is 20% among fertile couples.

8. The answer is D [VIII B 3]. In this clinical scenario, it appears that the wife is ovulatory and has no reason for having tubal or uterine abnormalities. The husband, however, has abnormal sperm parameters, namely severe oligospermia. The workup of severe oligospermia includes a karyotype to evaluate for Klinefelter syndrome and Y chromosome microdeletion testing. These abnormalities have implications not only for this couple's fertility, but also for possible transmission to their offspring and therefore should be performed prior to treatment. ICSI is a micromanipulation technique in which sperm is injected directly into the cytoplasm of the oocyte to enhance fertilization. This method is often used for severe male factor infertility (as in this case). Should this couple proceed with fertility treatment after workup of severe oligospermia, they will most likely undergo IVF with ICSI. In cases of severe male factor, IVF with ICSI has better success than conventional IVF (without ICSI). Sperm washing with IUI combined with fertility drug treatment in the woman is a treatment for mild oligospermia, but in this situation, the sperm count is so low that IUI is not likely to be successful.

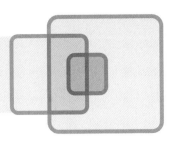

chapter 29

Recurrent Pregnancy Loss

KAT LIN • SAMANTHA BUTTS

Recurrent pregnancy loss (RPL) is one of the most devastating conditions for couples wishing to conceive. The grief experienced by couples affected with this disorder is often compounded by frustration due to the fact that many will have an evaluation that reveals no identifiable cause of their pregnancy losses. Couples affected with RPL require genuine empathy and specialized care focusing on complete evaluation, adequate explanation, and sound guidance in their pursuit of subsequent pregnancies.

I DEFINITION

A **Classically, RPL is defined as two to three or more *consecutive* spontaneous abortions of clinically recognized pregnancies prior to 15 weeks of gestation.** However, the requirement for consecutive miscarriages as opposed to cumulative miscarriages (i.e., three in a row vs. three total) has been challenged by some authorities.

1. Spontaneous abortion, pregnancy loss, and miscarriage are interchangeable terms.

2. Excluded from the definition of recurrent pregnancy loss are abnormal pregnancies such as ectopic and molar pregnancies.

3. If a miscarriage occurs after ultrasound identification of a viable pregnancy with a demonstrable fetal heartbeat (approximately 7 weeks gestational age), the miscarriage may be characterized in one of two ways:
   a. Early spontaneous miscarriage: before 12 weeks' gestation
   b. Late spontaneous miscarriage: after 12 weeks' gestation

4. These designations are important because certain causes of RPL are more or less common depending on the gestational age of the pregnancy at the time of the loss. For instance, genetic causes are less common than other etiologies after 10 weeks' gestation.

5. Recurrent fetal loss at or beyond 14 weeks of gestation is infrequent.

II INCIDENCE

A The risk of early miscarriage in any pregnancy is 30% to 50% of all conceptions and 15% of pregnancies greater than or equal to 6 weeks of gestation.

B RPL affects 5% of couples who are trying to establish a family.

C The risk of recurrent pregnancy loss increases with maternal age, and this trend parallels the general increase in odds of miscarriage in older women.

III ETIOLOGY OF MISCARRIAGES IN THE GENERAL REPRODUCTIVE POPULATION

In each pregnancy there is a risk of miscarriage.

A Advanced age
1. Risk of clinical pregnancy loss in women younger than 35 years of age: 9% to 12%
2. Risk of clinical pregnancy loss in women older than 40 years of age: up to 45%

B Chromosome anomaly accounts for 50% of miscarriages and risk increases with age of the mother.

1. Trisomy: 50%

2. Polypoid: 20%

3. Monosomy for chromosome X: 18%

4. Unbalanced translocations: 4%

C Congenital anomalies. These may not be associated with gross chromosome anomalies.

D Structural anomalies of the uterus

1. Uterine fibroids

2. Uterine septum

3. Endometrial polyp

E Hormonal conditions

1. Hypothyroidism

2. Luteal-phase deficiency

IV ETIOLOGY OF RECURRENT PREGNANCY LOSS

A In 50% or more of cases, the etiology of RPL is not known and couples have a completely normal evaluation.

B **Genetic/parental chromosomal abnormality.** An occult chromosomal abnormality in either the male or female partner is the cause of RPL in 3% to 5% of all cases. These chromosomal abnormalities are termed "occult" because the individuals who carry them have a normal amount of DNA and appear normal (they are often described as abnormal but balanced). However, portions of their chromosomes are rearranged in a way that makes them less capable of producing cytogenetically normal gametes and predisposes to RPL.

1. **Parental balanced translocations are most common.** Segregation of homologous chromosomes during meiosis in gametes of the affected parent often results in duplication or deficiency of chromosome segments. If an unbalanced gamete from the carrier of the translocation joins with a balanced gamete from the partner, embryonic aneuploidy (abnormal chromosome number) and early pregnancy loss can ensue.

2. **Reciprocal translocation accounts for 60% of translocations seen with RPL.** This occurs when the distal portion of one chromosomal arm (e.g., A* from parent chromosome A) is exchanged for the distal portion of a second chromosome (e.g., B* from parent chromosome B) during meiosis.
   a. Two new chromosomes emerge from this exchange.
      (1) A with a distal portion of B (B*).
      (2) B with a distal portion of A (A*).
   b. As no DNA is lost during this translocation, the affected individual is "balanced" and shows no outward evidence of the rearrangement.
   c. In many cases, adults with balanced translocations are initially diagnosed during an evaluation for RPL.

3. **Robertsonian translocation** occurs when genetic information is exchanged between two acrocentric chromosomes. **Acrocentric chromosomes** are unique because their centromeres are near the end of the chromosome and their short arms encode redundant genes (chromosomes 13, 14, 15, 21, and 22).
   a. During a robertsonian translocation, the long arms of two acrocentric chromosomes fuse at the centromere and the two short arms are completely lost.
   b. A person carrying a robertsonian translocation appears completely normal because the loss of nonessential, redundant DNA on the short arms of the involved chromosomes is well tolerated.
   c. As is the case with those who have reciprocal translocations, gametes of the affected individual may become unbalanced.

4. **Chromosomal inversions** involve the rearrangement of a segment of the chromosome such that it is reversed within itself. DNA is rarely lost and the affected individual appears normal. While some inversions have been associated with production of unbalanced gametes and RPL, in general, they account for a very small percentage of abnormal parental chromosomes in RPL.

C **Antiphospholipid syndrome (APS)** is an autoimmune condition characterized by poor obstetric outcomes (recurrent or late pregnancy loss, stillbirth) and thrombophilia in the setting of autoantibodies that cause hypercoagulation in vivo. It accounts for approximately 15% of RPL.

1. These autoantibodies promote placental thrombosis and inflammation and may impair normal invasion of fetal trophoblastic tissue into maternal blood vessels/uterine endometrium. The end result is increased risk of pregnancy loss.

2. To ensure the accuracy of this diagnosis, at least one of the following clinical criteria and one laboratory criterion must be fulfilled.
   a. **Clinical criteria (one of two)**
      (1) **Thrombosis**: one or more episodes of venous or arterial vascular thrombosis, which should be confirmed by radiologic imaging, such as Doppler studies
      (2) **Pregnancy morbidity (one of three)**:
         (a) One or more unexplained fetal deaths of a morphologically normal fetus beyond 10 weeks' gestation
         (b) One or more premature births of a morphologically normal neonate less than or equal to 34 weeks' gestation, due to either eclampsia/preeclampsia or placental insufficiency as evidenced by fetal testing suggestive of fetal hypoxia, oligohydramnios, or postnatal birth weight less than the 10th percentile for gestational age
         (c) Three or more *consecutive* spontaneous abortions before the 10th week of gestation, with other causes excluded
   b. **Laboratory criteria (at least one of the following)**
      (1) Anticardiolipin antibodies, IgM or IgG, in medium or high titers (while these are rarely standardized across laboratories, they are commonly reported as greater than 40 GPL (IgG) or MPL (IgM) units, or greater than the 99th percentile of anticardiolipin antibodies within a normal population). The same antibody must be elevated on at least two occasions, 6 to 12 weeks apart.
      (2) Lupus anticoagulant antibodies, detected by the following steps, on two occasions, 6 weeks apart:
         (a) Prolonged phospholipid-dependent coagulation on a screening test, such as activated partial thromboplastin time (aPTT), kaolin clotting time, dilute Russell viper venom time, dilute prothrombin time, or Textarin time
         (b) Failure to correct the prolonged clotting time by mixing with normal platelet-poor plasma
         (c) Shortening or correcting of the prolonged coagulation time by the addition of excess phospholipids
         (d) Exclusion of other coagulopathies
         (e) It is important to emphasize that although the **antiphospholipid syndrome** causes abnormal clotting clinically, lupus anticoagulants cause prolonged bleeding in vitro.
         (f) Other antiphospholipid antibodies, including anticardiolipin IgA antibody, antiphosphatidylserine, and anti-β_2-glycoprotein I antibodies, are not significantly associated with RPL.

D **Anatomic causes** account for 15% of RPL. Congenital abnormalities of the uterus have been strongly associated with early recurrent pregnancy loss and second-trimester loss.

1. **Müllerian anomalies**. The uterine abnormalities associated with recurrent and late miscarriage arise from failure of the embryologic precursors of the reproductive tract to develop.
   a. During embryologic development of a normal female fetus, paired müllerian ducts arise, which are destined to develop into the fallopian tubes and fuse to form the uterus, cervix, and upper third of the vagina.

b. If this process does not occur properly, müllerian anomalies can arise. It is thought that pregnancy failure in the setting of müllerian anomalies is the result of poor uterine vascularization and/or limited uterine volume.

    (1) Uterine septum results when fusion of the paired müllerian ducts has occurred normally but the medial septum between the ducts has not been completely resorbed. Septums are the most common uterine abnormality diagnosed in women with recurrent pregnancy loss.

    (2) Unicornuate uterus occurs when one of the paired müllerian ducts fails to develop; a uterus with a limited cavity size results.

    (3) Bicornuate uterus arises due to the incomplete fusion of the müllerian ducts resulting in two separate uterine cavities joined at a common cervix.

    (4) Uterine didelphys is the result of complete failure of the müllerian ducts to fuse, but normal differentiation of each duct system. The final outcome is two separate uteri and cervices, with each uterine horn smaller than a normal uterus.

2. Other structural abnormalities in the uterus

    a. Uterine fibroids are benign, fibromuscular tumors that arise in the uterus. Fibroids in a submucosal location are believed to cause miscarriages because of inadequate blood supply if the placenta implants on the fibroid. Tumors greater than 5 cm are usually implicated.

    b. Constricted uterine cavity may result from drug exposure in utero (diethylstilbestrol) or from uterine surgery (myomectomy, Asherman syndrome).

3. Diagnosis of uterine abnormalities. Several imaging modalities exist to evaluate the uterus for abnormalities during the workup for recurrent pregnancy loss. Each modality has benefits and drawbacks. Selection of a particular imaging modality depends on accessibility, pretest suspicion, and patient characteristics.

    a. Hysterosalpingogram (HSG). Radiographs of the pelvis are performed while radio-opaque dye is instilled into the uterine cavity. This is usually the first-line test for patients suspected of having uterine anomalies as a cause for RPL.

    b. Ultrasound. Real-time images of the pelvis are acquired using sound waves. This modality is less accurate for septums than it is for diagnosing other müllerian anomalies.

    c. Saline sonohysterography. Saline is instilled into the uterine cavity while ultrasound is performed. This test highlights the shape of the uterine cavity.

    d. Magnetic resonance imaging (MRI). Multiplanar images of the pelvis are generated with the use of magnets rather than x-rays. MRI is superior to HSG for distinguishing a bicornuate uterus from a uterine septum.

    e. Hysteroscopy. This minor surgical procedure involves direct visualization of the uterine cavity with a camera attached to a small telescope. This is the gold standard for evaluating the cavity for müllerian anomalies and can also be used for correcting uterine septums and removing submucosal fibroids, polyps, and adhesions.

E Endocrinologic factors

1. Untreated hypothyroidism may increase the risk of miscarriage.

2. Luteal-phase deficiency has been implicated in the cause of RPL. Progesterone is responsible for the progressive changes of the endometrium following ovulation. A lack in progesterone or progesterone activity has been associated with a short luteal phase and RPL.

    a. This is diagnosed by a midluteal-phase progesterone level of less than 10 ng/mL.

3. Elevated prolactin levels have been associated with RPL. High levels of prolactin cause hypothalamic dysfunction and lack of progesterone, leading to miscarriage.

4. Polycystic ovarian syndrome (PCOS) involves a constellation of features including oligo-ovulation/amenorrhea, hyperandrogenemism (either clinically as hirsutism or acne, or elevated serum androgens), and/or polycystic-appearing ovaries on ultrasound. It is the most common endocrinopathy in reproductive-aged women, with a prevalence of 5% to 10%.

    a. It has been suggested by observational studies that women with PCOS have a spontaneous miscarriage rate (20% to 40%) that is twofold higher than that in the general population. However, emerging clinical trail data suggest that these data might be overestimates of the true risk of miscarriage associated with PCOS. **PCOS as a cause for pregnancy loss has yet to be confirmed.**

    b. The potential mechanism of miscarriage in PCOS is controversial and not well understood. It has been postulated, for example, that high circulating androgen levels and insulin resistance seen in this condition may adversely affect endometrial receptivity and implantation of an early embryo.

    c. No strong data exist supporting a role for treatment of PCOS and improved pregnancy outcomes.

5. Poorly controlled insulin-dependent diabetes mellitus, particularly with hemoglobin A1C (a measure of disease control) values above 8%, increases the risk of miscarriage and the risk of major congenital malformations in the fetus.

    a. This is most likely due to hyperglycemia and maternal vascular disease.

    b. No increased risk of miscarriage is seen with well-controlled diabetes mellitus.

6. Thrombophilias other than antiphospholipid syndrome can predispose to microvascular thrombosis, which then impairs placental development and growth leading to spontaneous abortion. Usually, this affects late fetal loss with intrauterine growth restriction, placental abruption, and preeclampsia.

    a. A relationship with early pregnancy loss has not been clearly established.

    b. Therefore, inherited coagulopathies (e.g., factor V Leiden, prothrombin gene mutation, and deficiencies in protein S, protein C, and antithrombin) and other thrombophilic factors (e.g., factor VIII, factor XIII) should **not** be considered definitive etiologies of RPL.

V RPL EVALUATION OVERVIEW

In a couple with RPL, initial evaluation should focus on a thorough history and record review.

A Gestational ages of all miscarriages should be ascertained as well as any workup or treatment performed previously.

B In the initial evaluation, lab work including APS evaluation and thyroid-stimulating hormone (TSH) should be obtained; other labs should be measured in accordance with the couple's individual medical history.

C Imaging of the uterus should be scheduled to evaluate the possibility of a müllerian anomaly.

D A karyotype is usually performed last because a translocation is far less common than other causes of RPL. However, a karyotype may be ordered at any point in the evaluation.

E It should be noted that even if one abnormality is discovered, a complete evaluation is still recommended given the possibility of a multifactorial etiology for the RPL.

VI TREATMENTS FOR WOMEN WITH RECURRENT PREGNANCY LOSS

A Overview

    1. Many women with RPL have a normal evaluation and therefore are classified as idiopathic.

    2. Some treatments that have been targeted at this population have unsubstantiated efficacy and possible harm. This section will focus on treatments with proven benefit for patients falling into specific etiologies of RPL.

    3. For those women with idiopathic RPL, counseling about the odds of a future successful pregnancy without treatment and supportive care should be emphasized.

B Treatments for parental genetic abnormalities. If it is determined that a member of the couple has a balanced chromosomal translocation, several options exist. Reproductive or medical genetic counseling can be extremely useful in managing these patients.

    1. The couple could continue to try to conceive on their own. If one person is affected with a balanced translocation, there still exists the possibility of a spontaneous normal conception (approximately 25% if the woman carries the translocation and 40% if the male is the carrier).

    2. In vitro fertilization (IVF) and preimplantation genetic diagnosis (PGD) in an attempt to select normal embryos for conception

    a. Oocytes are harvested from the female partner and combined with sperm outside the body.

    b. Embryos that are generated from this process can be biopsied (usually a single cell from a six- to eight-cell embryo) and evaluated for chromosomal abnormalities using fluorescence in situ hybridization (FISH).

    c. Embryos with a normal karyotype can be selected and transferred to the uterus of the patient.

    d. At present, limited data and experience exist with respect to IVF and PGD for the treatment of RPL and parental translocations. However, there may be a more significant role for **IVF/PGD** in this area in the future.

  3. Donor gametes can be used (egg donation if the female carries the translocation or sperm donation if the male is affected) in combination with fertility treatments.

C **Treatment of antiphospholipid antibody syndrome.** Prior to treatment of antiphospholipid antibody syndrome, the diagnosis (criteria described above) must be confirmed.

  1. Adequate treatment of antiphospholipid antibody syndrome requires that the affected individual receive subcutaneous heparin injections and low-dose aspirin throughout her pregnancy.

  2. Long-term treatment with heparin can be unpleasant for patients and has potential risks (bleeding, osteoporosis, and heparin-induced thrombocytopenia).

  3. Despite these drawbacks, the combination significantly improves the odds of a live birth in those treated (up to twofold increase in clinical trials).

  4. The benefit of this regimen is in its prevention of placental microthrombi and possible treatment of inflammation. Aspirin is usually given at a dose of 80 mg/day. Heparin can be administered as unfractionated or low-molecular-weight heparin (neither form of heparin crosses the placenta).

D **Treatments for müllerian anomalies**

  1. **Uterine septums** are the most common and most strongly associated defect with RPL and can be surgically removed. This is best accomplished by use of a **hysteroscope**, which allows the surgeon to visualize the septum while hysteroscopic scissors are introduced to resect the septum from its distal aspect to its proximal aspect.

  2. For women with a **bicornuate uterus** or **uterine didelphys**, careful obstetric management is the preferred approach. A **metroplasty** is a surgical procedure to unify the cavities and reconstruct the uterus and can be performed when pregnancy outcomes have been particularly poor despite excellent and aggressive prenatal care in previous pregnancies. Unlike the septum resection, which is often a minor surgical procedure, metroplasty is a major abdominal surgery.

  3. For women with a **unicornuate uterus**, surgical options to prevent first-trimester miscarriage are limited. Metroplasty is not an option because these patients have only one developed uterine horn. In some patients, a stitch or **cerclage** can be placed in the cervix early in the second trimester to prevent premature cervical dilation and a late miscarriage.

  4. Patients should be counseled extensively before going forward with any surgical procedure for recurrent pregnancy loss. Surgical risks and potential benefits should be reviewed. A patient who has a metroplasty, for example, must have a cesarean section for all deliveries because the nature of the surgery makes labor and vaginal delivery extremely risky. For patients with particularly poor obstetric histories who decline surgery, are not surgical candidates, or have failed surgical treatment, the use of a gestational carrier who carries the pregnancy as a surrogate may be a consideration.

E **Treatment controversies.** As mentioned previously, several approaches (listed below) have been explored for women with unexplained recurrent pregnancy loss. None of these treatments has demonstrated efficacy in the treatment of RPL, and paternal leukocyte immunization may increase the odds of miscarriage. Its use for the treatment of RPL has been restricted by the Food and Drug Administration.

  1. Low-dose **aspirin**

  2. **Progesterone** supplementation after ovulation

3. Immunomodulation of the female partner using **intravenous immunoglobulin (IVIG)**. It has been postulated that an abnormal maternal immune response to the early conceptus may play a role in RPL and that IVIG could suppress this response.

4. Immunomodulation of the female partner through vaccination **with paternal leukocytes** (before reattempting conception) to sensitize the mother to the paternal components of the fetus

F Natural history/observation. Many couples with unexplained RPL can be reassured that their odds of having a successful future pregnancy are reasonable even if no treatment is utilized. This is especially true if the couple has ever experienced a live birth. For instance, a woman with a history of three unexplained miscarriages and one prior liveborn infant has a 32% chance of the next pregnancy being a miscarriage—in other words, a 68% chance that the pregnancy will develop normally. Education and reassurance is an extremely important facet of the care provided to these couples.

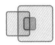

Study Questions for Chapter 29

Directions: *Each of the numbered items or incomplete statements in this section is followed by answers or by completions of the statement. Select the ONE lettered answer or completion that is BEST in each case.*

1. A patient with a history of three miscarriages presents to your office. The only workup she has had done so far was a lab evaluation that showed the following results: lupus anticoagulant screen negative, anticardiolipin IgA high positive, IgG low positive, and IgM normal. What would you offer the patient next?

- A Discuss with her that she has antiphospholipid syndrome and devise a treatment plan based on this diagnosis
- B Repeat antiphospholipid screen in 6 to 8 weeks
- C Start heparin and baby aspirin treatments immediately
- D Start baby aspirin with next pregnancy
- E None of the above

2. A couple with RPL gets karyotype analysis and the male partner is found to have a robertsonian translocation involving chromosomes 14 and 21. The female partner is normal. The next most appropriate step in the treatment of this couple is:

- A Offer IVF as an option for treatment
- B Discuss the role of donor gametes in treatment
- C Offer the couple in vitro fertilization with preimplantation genetic diagnosis (PGD)
- D Close observation with next pregnancy
- E Send the couple for a consult with a genetic counselor

3. A patient with a history of three miscarriages presents to your office. The only workup she has had done so far was a lab evaluation that showed the following results: lupus anticoagulant screen negative, anticardiolipin IgG high positive, and IgM normal. What would you offer the patient next?

- A Discuss with her that she has antiphospholipid syndrome and devise a treatment plan based on this diagnosis
- B Repeat antiphospholipid screen in 6 to 8 weeks
- C Order a hysterosalpingogram
- D B and C
- E None of the above

Answers and Explanations

1. The answer is E [IV C]. The patient does not have antiphospholipid syndrome based on these lab results. Anticardiolipin IgA being positive is not part of the diagnostic criteria, and the low-positive IgG is also not positive. There is no need to repeat these tests again. Since the patient does not have the syndrome, there is no need to initiate anticoagulant therapy, but alternative causes of her RPL should be sought.

2. The answer is E [IV A, B, VI B]. The couple should hear from an experienced geneticist or genetic counselor what the implications of their translocation are for their offspring (e.g., if the pregnancy survives and the fetus is affected with a trisomy) and the exact statistics with respect to odds of a normal pregnancy with no intervention. A discussion of donor egg, donor sperm, or IVF with preimplantation genetic diagnosis should occur with a reproductive endocrinologist who can explain and offer these treatments. Ideally these treatment possibilities should be discussed after the patient has been seen by a genetic counselor.

3. The answer is D [IV C, D]. In order to confirm the diagnosis of antiphospholipid syndrome, either anticardiolipin antibodies or lupus anticoagulant screen must be significantly positive twice, with at least 6 to 8 weeks between positive tests. Of note, the same lab abnormality must be present each time. For instance, if this patient had a positive lupus anticoagulant screen and a normalized anticardiolipin IgG, this would not represent a positive result. In addition, if the full panel of labs for the antiphospholipid screen were negative, other etiologies for RPL must be sought. It is reasonable to schedule the patient for uterine imaging while waiting for the repeat antiphospholipid screen to rule in or out an anatomic cause of RPL.

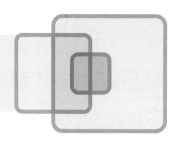

chapter **30**

Pediatric and Adolescent Gynecology

SAMANTHA BUTTS • SAMANTHA M. PFEIFER • MICHELLE VICHNIN

I   **INTRODUCTION**

An awareness of the problems that are unique to pediatric and adolescent gynecology is invaluable for proper management of the young patient. Particular care is essential in addressing gynecologic concerns in this age group because both physical and emotional trauma may be inadvertently inflicted. It is important to establish rapport and reassurance in a young patient who may be uncomfortable with pelvic or genital examinations. A female adolescent does not need a pelvic examination unless she is experiencing abnormal symptoms. Even then, noninvasive imaging (e.g., pelvic ultrasound and magnetic resonance imaging [MRI]) can be performed instead of a pelvic examination. Once an adolescent is sexually active, a regular pelvic examination is indicated.

A   **Normal findings in a pediatric patient** include the following:

1. A mucoid vaginal discharge and even vaginal bleeding in an infant for up to 2 weeks after birth; caused by maternal estrogens

2. An introitus that is located more anteriorly than normal and a clitoris that is more prominent than normal (1 to 2 cm)

3. A redundant hymen that may protrude on straining and that remains essentially the same size until 10 years of age

4. A vaginal epithelium that is uncornified and erythematous with an alkaline pH

5. A small uterus (2.5 to 3 cm in length), with the cervix comprising two-thirds of the organ (the reverse of adult proportions)

6. A cervical os that is covered with glandular epithelium and normally appears red (ectropion)

B   **Normal findings in an adolescent patient**

1. Intact hymen in those not sexually active

2. Postpubertal gynecologic examination in an adolescent is similar to an adult female.

C   **Visualization of the vagina.**   Instruments for visualizing the vagina include the vaginoscope, the urethroscope, and the pediatric speculum. Stirrups are usually not necessary for the preadolescent; a simple "frog-leg" position is usually sufficient. Occasionally, intravenous sedation may be necessary to accomplish a thorough genital examination. To determine the presence or absence of internal genitalia, ultrasound and MRI are helpful.

D   **Rectal examination** is often more informative than a vaginal examination because the short posterior vaginal fornix cannot be distended and a cul-de-sac does not exist.

II   **VULVOVAGINAL LESIONS**

A   **Lichen sclerosus et atrophicus**

1. **Clinical picture**. The child can present with vulvar itching. A white, papular lesion resembling leukoplakia may cover the vulva and perianal regions. As the disease progresses, there

may be loss of normal architecture, including loss of demarcation of the labia and scarring of the clitoral hood.

2. **Etiology**. Causes are unknown, though hypoestrogenic state is thought to play a role.

3. **Diagnosis**. Biopsy, which shows superficial hyperkeratosis with basal atrophic and sclerotic changes, should be performed to clarify the diagnosis.

4. **Management**. This condition is benign and can be self-limiting. Improved hygiene is the first line of therapy. Low-potency topical steroid cream is not usually effective, and high-potency topical steroids may be necessary in cases with severe itching. Progesterone cream has been used with variable success. Testosterone, used in the past for treatment of adults with this condition, should be avoided. The condition may resolve at puberty but is usually chronic.

B Trauma

1. **Clinical picture**
   a. **Tears, abrasions, ecchymoses, and hematomas** are common in preadolescent girls. The incidence is highest in children between 4 and 12 years of age. The most common mechanisms of injury are sexual abuse, straddle injuries, accidental penetration, sudden abduction of the extremities, and pelvic fractures. Most genital trauma results from straddle injuries, such as a child landing on the center bar of a boy's bicycle. The injury may appear as a small ecchymotic area or a large vulvar hematoma. The clinician must always suspect sexual abuse when a child presents with genital trauma.
   b. **Sexual abuse** necessitates immediate medical attention, including a complete physical examination, cervical and rectal smears, serologic tests, and psychological evaluation and follow-up. Genital findings, when present, should be recorded very carefully because of their importance in supporting allegations of abuse in court proceedings. The colposcope is used to document specific normal and abnormal findings, and photographs can be placed in the patient's chart. However, in cases of sexual abuse, 96% of patient abnormalities are detected with the unaided eye.

2. **Management**
   a. When vaginal bleeding occurs because of pelvic trauma, **a complete and thorough examination is mandatory**. This includes evaluation of the urinary system and rectum. A vaginoscope is used to visualize the vagina to locate sources of bleeding. A large vaginal laceration may result in an expanding hematoma in the retroperitoneal space. Superficial abrasions and lacerations of the vulva, if not actively bleeding, can be cleaned and left alone. If adequate visualization cannot be performed, examination under anesthesia is required.
   b. **Conservative therapy** for most traumas consists of rest, ice, and analgesics.
   c. In sexual abuse, **antibiotic therapy** is advised as prophylaxis against sexually transmitted diseases. Current Centers for Disease Control and Prevention (CDC) recommendations from 2006 are ceftriaxone, metronidazole, and azithromycin as well as hepatitis B vaccination if the patient has not been previously vaccinated.

C Labial agglutination

1. **Clinical picture**. Adhesion of the labia minora in the midline is the usual presentation. This vertical line of fusion distinguishes labial agglutination from imperforate hymen or vaginal atresia. The agglutination encourages retention of urine and vaginal secretions and can lead to vulvovaginitis or a urinary tract infection. Labial agglutination is believed to result from vulvar inflammation or skin disease, and the hypoestrogenic state.

2. **Management**
   a. If asymptomatic, **improved hygiene** may be all that is necessary. Treatment is indicated if there is a chronic vulvovaginitis or difficulty urinating.
   b. **Lubrication of the labia** with a bland ointment and **gentle manual separation** over several weeks may be effective.
   c. **Topical estrogen**, applied twice daily, induces cornification of the epithelium and promotes spontaneous separation. The use of estrogen in the prepubertal female, if prolonged, may stimulate breast growth and vaginal bleeding. Therapy must be limited to 2 weeks.

d. Surgical separation is rarely necessary, but when necessary should be performed bluntly and not with a scalpel.

e. Once separation of the labia has occurred, continuation of nightly emollient application such as petroleum jelly can be useful to avoid recurrences.

D Prolapsed urethra

1. **Clinical picture.** A small, hemorrhagic, friable mass surrounding the urethra is the most common presentation. The average age at diagnosis is 5 years. The bleeding is usually painless. The prolapse is thought to result from increased intra-abdominal pressure. The lesion can easily be confused with a condyloma but can be distinguished by applying a dilute acetic acid solution: a condyloma turns white, whereas a prolapsed urethra remains pink and fleshy.

2. **Management**
   a. If voiding is uninhibited, **local therapy** may be all that is needed. Topical estrogen and sitz baths are the mainstays of therapy. The prolapse usually resolves after 4 weeks of therapy.
   b. If urinary retention or necrosis is present, **surgical repair** and catheterization are necessary.

E Vaginal discharge

1. **Clinical picture**
   a. A **mucoid discharge** is common in infants for up to 2 weeks after birth; it results from maternal estrogen. It is also a common finding in prepubertal and postpubertal girls, who experience increased estrogen production by maturing ovaries.
   b. **Pathologic discharge** may result from any of the following conditions:
      (1) **Infections with organisms,** such as *Escherichia coli*, *Proteus*, *Pseudomonas*, yeast, *Gardnerella*, *Neisseria gonorrhoeae*, *Chlamydia*, and *Trichomonas*
      (2) **Hemolytic streptococcal vaginitis**, which results in a bloody or serosanguineous discharge, usually after a streptococcal infection elsewhere (e.g., skin or throat)
      (3) **Monilial vaginitis**, which is common in children with diabetes or after antibiotic therapy
      (4) **A foreign body**, which can cause persistent vaginal discharge, sometimes with pain and bleeding
      (5) **Nonspecific vaginitis** from local irritation, scratching, manipulation, or poor hygiene

2. **Management.** Conservative management is advisable, as follows:
   a. **Culture** to identify causative organisms. Preliminary search for *Monilia*, nonspecific bacteria, and *Trichomonas* can be accomplished by examining the discharge on a laboratory slide with saline and sodium hydroxide (20%) preparations added.
   b. **Urinalysis** to rule out cystitis
   c. **Review proper hygiene.** Instruct the child's caretaker to avoid placing the child in tight clothing or using perfume soaps, bubble bath, and powders. The child should avoid prolonged periods in moist clothing.
   d. **Perianal examination** with transparent tape to test for pinworms
   e. **In cases of persistent discharge, examination under anesthesia is indicated to rule out foreign body.**

III **NEOPLASMS**

A **Tumors of the vagina,** although uncommon, are most often malignant. **Sarcoma botryoides** is the most common malignant vaginal tumor.

1. **Clinical picture**
   a. Sarcoma botryoides arises from mesenchymal tissue of the cervix or vagina, usually on the anterior wall of the upper vagina. It grows rapidly, fills the vagina, and then protrudes through the introitus.
   b. It appears as an edematous, grape-like mass that bleeds readily on touch. It is usually multicentric and extension is usually local, with rare instances of distant metastases.

2. **Management.** A combination of surgery and chemotherapy is most commonly used.

B Ovarian tumors

1. **Clinical picture**. Although uncommon in children, ovarian tumors may present as torsion (twisting) of the ovaries. Among ovarian neoplasms, 40% are of non–germ cell origin (coelomic epithelium), and 60% are of germ cell origin. Most ovarian neoplasms in adolescents are also endocrine secreting regardless of origin.
   a. **Non–germ cell origin**
      (1) Lipoid cell tumors (estrogen producing)
      (2) Granulosa-theca cell tumors (estrogen producing), of which approximately 20% are malignant
   b. **Germ cell origin**
      (1) Benign cystic teratomas
      (2) Benign cysts
      (3) Arrhenoblastomas (androgen producing)
      (4) Dysgerminomas and gonadoblastomas (tumors of dysgenetic gonads)
      (5) Endodermal sinus tumors
      (6) Embryonal carcinomas (human chorionic gonadotropin [hCG]-secreting tumors)
      (7) Immature teratomas, which account for 20% of malignant germ cell tumors

2. **Therapy**. **Treatment is surgical**, alone or in combination with chemotherapy, depending on the tumor. Radiation is sometimes used to treat dysgerminomas.

IV **CONGENITAL ANOMALIES IN THE PEDIATRIC PATIENT**

A Müllerian agenesis (Mayer-von Rokitansky-Kuster-Hauser [MRKH] syndrome). Vaginal and uterine agenesis (atresia). Represents a failure of the caudal müllerian duct to fuse with the urogenital sinus

1. **Clinical picture**
   a. This condition most often is diagnosed at the time of puberty because of the resulting amenorrhea. **Ovarian development is normal**, but there is only a vaginal dimple at the introitus and the **uterus is usually absent or fails to develop** beyond a rudimentary structure.
   b. Vaginal agenesis (normal 46,XX karyotype) must be distinguished from androgen insensitivity syndrome (male 46,XY karyotype), which is also associated with an absent vagina (see V E).

2. **Management**. Surgical creation of a neovagina and nonsurgical dilation techniques both successfully create a vagina. However, treatment should be deferred until after puberty, when the patient has a good understanding of the condition and is emotionally ready to consider treatment.

B Ectopic ureter with vaginal terminus

1. **Clinical picture**
   a. Ectopic ureter, the most common cause of vaginal cysts in infants, presents as a **ureterocele**, which appears as a cystic mass protruding from the vagina. If the ureter is patent, constant irritation and vaginitis may be presenting signs.
   b. The ectopic ureter is usually one of a pair to a single kidney, and it usually drains the rudimentary upper renal pole of the kidney.
   c. **Hydroureter** and **hydronephrosis** may develop.

2. **Diagnosis**. The existence of an ectopic ureter is made using **intravenous pyelography**, which allows visualization of the entire urinary tract.

3. **Management**. It is preferable to **resect the lowest portion of the ureter** and **implant it into the bladder** rather than remove the ureter and the associated portion of the kidney.

C Vaginal ectopic anus

1. **Clinical picture**. Vaginal ectopic anus is an **imperforate anus associated with rectovaginal communication**. Only a skin dimple is found at the normal anal site.

2. **Management**. **Surgical correction** is indicated.

V DEVELOPMENTAL DEFECTS OF THE EXTERNAL GENITALIA (AMBIGUOUS GENITALIA)

Ambiguous genitalia results when hormones with androgenic activity are present during development of a female fetus, or androgens or androgen activity are absent during development of a male fetus. The resulting appearance of the genitalia can be incomplete, or a mixture of male and female features, making identification of sex difficult at birth. Early diagnosis is important to guarantee proper assignment of sex during the neonatal period. The management plan should be established at that time to minimize psychological problems and to help establish the gender role.

A **Congenital adrenal hyperplasia (CAH).** This condition results when enzymatic regulation of the biosynthesis of cortisol and aldosterone is impaired at various steps in the pathway. Adrenocorticotropic hormone (ACTH) secretion by the pituitary is increased because of low levels of blood cortisol. Both the precursors immediately preceding the impaired step and the by-products have biologic activity, predominantly androgenic, that can lead to the clinical and biochemical features observed. **The 21-hydroxylase defect is the most common cause of distinct virilization of the female newborn**. Its incidence is 1 in 5000 births, and it accounts for 95% of all cases of congenital adrenal hyperplasia, which is inherited as an **autosomal recessive trait**.

1. **Clinical picture**. The chromosomes, gonads, and internal genitalia are female, but the external genitalia are virilized to varying degrees. The degree of closure of the urogenital orifice varies, and clitoral enlargement and accentuation of labial folds are characteristic. The disorder is progressive if untreated.

2. **Diagnosis**. Serum 17-hydroxyprogesterone and dehydroepiandrosterone (DHEA) obtained after 24 hours of life are both elevated. A blood karyotype should be obtained. **Serum electrolytes should be followed because salt wasting, which may be life threatening, may occur**.

3. **Management**. Hydrocortisone is administered indefinitely to all patients.

B **Adrenal tumors.** These tumors, which may cause virilization of the external genitalia after infancy, should be suspected in children with high levels of dehydroepiandrosterone sulfate (DHEAS).

C **Maternal ingestion of androgenic substances.** This condition can result in **masculinization of the female fetus**. Causal agents identified include androgens, danazol, and synthetic progestins (in doses much higher than in oral contraceptive pills).

1. **Clinical picture**. Masculinization is limited to the external genitalia. The clitoris is enlarged and the labia may be fused, but the vagina, tubes, and uterus are normal. Growth and development are normal, and progressive virilization does not occur.

2. **Diagnosis**. The condition can be diagnosed based on a positive history and on exclusion.

3. **Management**. Clitoral reduction and surgical correction of the fused labia may be necessary.

D **Childhood ingestion of androgens.** This condition usually involves preparations that have androgenic activity.

1. **Clinical picture**. Clinical manifestations are the same as those resulting from maternal ingestion of androgenic substances (i.e., masculinization; see V C 1).

2. **Management**. Therapy involves clitoral reduction and surgical correction of the fused labia, if necessary.

E **Androgen insensitivity syndrome (testicular feminization)**

1. **Clinical picture**. A 46,XY genotype is present, but a female phenotype develops.
   a. Androgens are produced by the testes (which develop in the presence of a Y chromosome) and by the adrenal glands. A defect in the androgen receptor prevents tissue from responding to androgen stimulation.
   b. External genitalia are feminized because normal (male) development of these structures is prevented by lack of response to the androgen dihydrotestosterone. These babies are thought to be normal females at birth, and are ultimately reared as girls. In incomplete forms of the syndrome, there is some response to the circulating androgens, and ambiguous genitalia occur.

    c. The testes produce müllerian inhibitory substance; as a result, there is no uterine, cervical, upper vaginal, or fallopian tube development. A short vagina that ends in a blind pouch and labia, which often contain testes, develops in these patients.

    d. Lack of responsiveness to testosterone during embryonic sexual differentiation affects development of internal genitalia. Normal male internal genitalia do not develop because testosterone is required for that process to occur.

    e. An incomplete form (Reifenstein syndrome) occurs in which external genitalia appear virilized.

  2. Diagnosis. Patients with complete androgen insensitivity syndrome are usually diagnosed at puberty with primary amenorrhea and a blind or absent vagina. Because of the inability to respond to androgens, there is lack of pubic and axillary hair development. **Breast development does occur because estrogen concentration is high due to conversion of testosterone produced after puberty.** This syndrome is distinguished from MRKH by absent axillary and pubic hair development and a high testosterone level. A karyotype can be performed for confirmation.

  3. Management. The gonads should be removed because of an increased risk of malignancy (3% to 4% before 25 years of age). However, removal should be performed **after** puberty.

  F **True hermaphroditism**

    1. Clinical picture. The genotype of most true hermaphrodites is 46,XX. The external genitalia may appear male, female, or ambiguous. Both male and female internal genitalia may be present. Sex assignment and rearing should be consistent with the dominant appearance of the external genitalia and with surgical correctability.

    2. Management. The genitalia that are inconsistent with sex assignment should be surgically removed or modified.

  G **Maternal virilizing tumor during pregnancy** (luteoma of pregnancy). This condition may result in masculinization of the female fetus. The clinical picture and therapy are similar to those for the maternal ingestion of androgenic substances (see V C). Psychological development and mental capacity are consistent with chronologic age. Reproductive potential is not adversely affected, and the patient can become pregnant.

VI   NORMAL AND ABNORMAL PUBERTAL DEVELOPMENT

  A **Normal puberty.** Puberty encompasses the psychological, physical, and endocrinologic changes beginning in late childhood that ultimately allow for reproductive capacity. In North America, the average age of onset of puberty in girls is 9 years. Once initiated, it proceeds over an average of 4 to 5 years and culminates in the onset of menses. Increased production of luteinizing hormone and follicle-stimulating hormone, as well as other factors (such as leptin), is responsible for the initiation of the pubertal process.

  B The normal physical changes associated with puberty were studied and outlined in detail by two British physicians in the late 1960s, Marshall and Tanner. Their work resulted in the Tanner stages of breast and pubic hair development. Tanner stages are currently used to evaluate pubertal development in children (Table 30-1). Components of the normal puberty include the following:

    1. Growth spurt. The growth spurt begins before the onset of other signs of puberty. The peak growth velocity occurs at an average age of 11 to 12 years, usually 1 year before menarche.

    2. Thelarche. The onset of breast development usually begins between 9 and 11 years of age. It is a sign of ovarian estrogen production and is completed over approximately 3 years. Tanner stages describe the normal changes in the transition from the prepubertal to the mature breast contour (Fig. 30-1).

    3. Adrenarche and pubarche. Adrenarche refers to the production of androgens from the adrenal gland, and pubarche is the development of axillary and pubic hair that results from the adrenal and gonadal androgens. Adrenarche is not regulated by the same hypothalamic-pituitary process that governs the rest of puberty. Pubarche usually follows thelarche in the pubertal

TABLE 30–1   Tanner Staging

	Breast	Pubic Hair
Stage 1 (prepubertal)	Elevation of papilla only	No pubic hair
Stage 2	Elevation of breast and papilla as small mound; areola diameter enlarged; median age: 9.8 years	Sparse, long, pigmented hair chiefly along labia majora; median age: 10.5 years
Stage 3	Further enlargement without separation of breast and areola; median age: 11.2 years	Dark, coarse, curled hair sparsely spread over mons; median age: 11.4 years
Stage 4	Secondary mound of areola and papilla above the breast; age: 12.1 years	Adult-type hair, abundant but limited to mons; median age: 12 years
Stage 5	Recession of areola to contour of breast; median age: 14.6 years	Adult-type spread in quantity and distribution; median age: 13.7 years

Adapted with permission from Speroff L, Glass RH, Kase NG. Clinical Gynecologic Endocrinology and Infertility. 6th Ed. Philadelphia: Lippincott Williams & Wilkins, 1999:397.

sequence but can be the first sign of puberty in up to 20% of girls. Again, Tanner stages are used to describe normal pubic hair development (Fig. 30-2).

4. **Menarche**. In menarche, vaginal bleeding occurs in response to hormonal changes, specifically production of estrogen by the ovary, for the first time. The average age of the first menses is 12 to 13 years. For the first 2 years following menarche, menses are often irregular because of anovulation or sporadic ovulation.

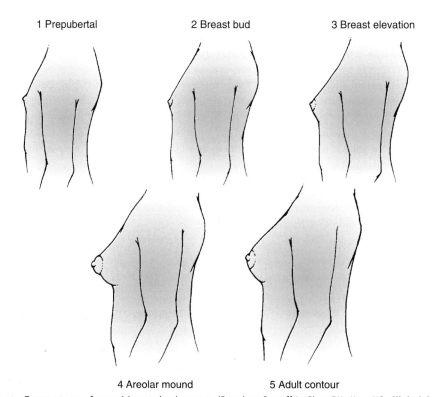

FIGURE 30–1   Tanner stages of normal breast development. (Based on Speroff L, Glass RH, Kase NG. Clinical Gynecologic Endocrinology and Infertility. 6th Ed. Philadelphia: Lippincott Williams & Wilkins, 1999:398.)

1 Prepubertal   2 Presexual hair   3 Sexual hair

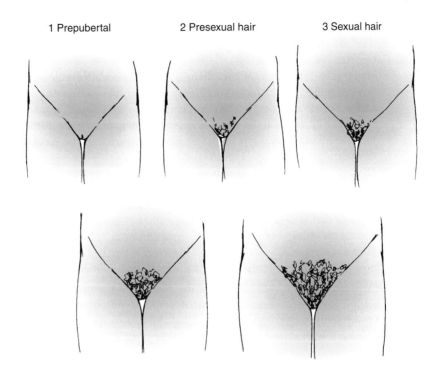

4 Mid-escutcheon   5 Female escutcheon

FIGURE 30–2   Tanner stages of normal pubic hair development. (Based on Speroff L, Glass RH, Kase NG. Clinical Gynecologic Endocrinology and Infertility. 6th Ed. Philadelphia: Lippincott Williams & Wilkins, 1999:399.)

C Precocious puberty.   This condition is characterized by the onset of secondary sexual characteristics before 8 years of age in Caucasian girls and before 7 years of age in African-American girls. Besides the psychological ramifications inherent in this syndrome, there exists the risk of short stature from early epiphyseal closure. Most cases of precocious puberty are idiopathic.

1. **Forms of precocious puberty**
   a. **Central precocious puberty**. This type of precocious puberty is caused by early activation of the hypothalamic-pituitary-gonadal axis, leading to the onset of hormonal secretion from the ovaries. The most common cause is idiopathic (74%). Other causes are rare and include central nervous system lesions such as infection, craniopharyngioma, astrocytoma, neurofibroma, hemangioma of the hypothalamus, hydrocephalus, and neoplasm of the floor of the third ventricle.
   b. **Peripheral precocious puberty**. This type of precocious puberty is caused by secretion of sex steroids from the ovary or exogenous hormone ingestion. These include hormone-producing ovarian or adrenal tumors, McCune-Albright syndrome, ectopic gonadotropin production, and primary hypothyroidism.

2. **Diagnosis**. Physical and radiologic signs are the basis of diagnosis. Assessment of bone age is critical, usually with a plain film of the wrist of the nondominant hand. An endocrine profile including gonadotropin levels and thyroid function tests must be evaluated. In addition, imaging of the brain with computed tomography (CT) or MRI is essential to rule out an intracranial mass.

3. **Management**. Therapy is aimed at slowing down accelerated growth; reducing pituitary, ovarian, and adrenal function; and inducing regression of secondary sex characteristics. **For idiopathic precocious puberty, the treatment of choice is gonadotropin-releasing hormone (GnRH) agonists, which suppress the pituitary and halt the progression through puberty.** The treatment is continued until an appropriate age has been reached for resumption of pubertal development. In cases of known etiology, recommended therapy is with surgery, chemotherapy, or radiation therapy as indicated.

D **Delayed puberty.** Delayed puberty is characterized by the absence of breast development by age 13 years or the absence of menses by age 16 years (see Chapter 20).

1. **Categories**
   a. **Hypergonadotropic hypogonadism.** This condition affects almost 50% of all patients with delayed puberty. It includes conditions in which the ovaries or gonads are not functioning and are unable to respond to gonadotropins; as a result, gonadotropin levels are high. Examples include Turner syndrome (45,X), idiopathic premature ovarian failure, autoimmune ovarian failure, gonadal dysgenesis, and ovarian failure secondary to radiation therapy or chemotherapy.
   b. **Hypogonadotropic hypogonadism.** This condition accounts for 10% to 15% of patients with pubertal delay. The ovary is normal; however, there is a lack of production of hormonal stimulation from the hypothalamus. Hypogonadotropic hypogonadism includes Kallmann syndrome (isolated GnRH deficiency); hypothalamic suppression by stress, severe disease, or malnutrition; and tumor invasion of the pituitary (prolactinoma or craniopharyngioma).
   c. **Eugonadotropic.** Constitutional delay accounts for 10% to 20% of cases. These patients have normal progression of the stages of puberty; the initiation of the process is simply delayed.

2. **Management.** Treatment is based on the etiology of the delay. In cases of gonadal dysgenesis when a Y chromosome or fragment of a Y chromosome is present, the gonads should be removed at diagnosis because of the risk of neoplastic degeneration. Otherwise, hormone replacement with estrogen, and subsequently both estrogen and progesterone, is required to promote sexual development and menarche.

VII SPECIAL PROBLEMS OF THE ADOLESCENT

A **Dysmenorrhea** is defined as cramp-like pain in the lower abdomen associated with menstrual flow.

1. **Etiology**
   a. **Primary dysmenorrhea** accounts for most cases and is attributed to increased prostaglandin production with menses in the presence of normal anatomy.
   b. **Secondary dysmenorrhea** results from conditions such as endometriosis and müllerian anomalies with an obstruction in a portion of the outflow tract, which leads to pain in the obstructed segment, but menstrual flow is not affected. Examples include obstructed hemiuterus and uterus didelphys with obstructed hemivagina.

2. **Clinical picture.** Severe, cyclic, cramp-like pain located in the lower abdomen and pelvis is associated with menses. Pain may radiate to the thighs and back and be accompanied by nausea, vomiting, and diarrhea.

3. **Management.** First-line therapy is prostaglandin inhibitors (nonsteroidal anti-inflammatory drugs [NSAIDs]). If the symptoms are not adequately controlled, then the next step is to empirically start oral contraceptives or obtain a pelvic ultrasound to evaluate for abnormal anatomy depending on the location, progression, and severity of the symptoms. If the pain symptoms do not respond to NSAIDs and combined hormonal contraception, then a pelvic ultrasound is indicated. If medical management fails to control the symptoms and the pelvic ultrasound is normal, then laparoscopy is recommended for definitive diagnosis.

B **Dysfunctional uterine bleeding (DUB)** (see Chapter 21). DUB is defined as excessive, prolonged, or irregular bleeding not associated with an anatomic lesion. Most adolescent girls have anovulatory menstrual periods for the first 2 to 3 years following menarche. Approximately 2% of adolescents ovulate regularly in the first 6 months after menarche and 18% by the end of the first year, making DUB common in this age group.

1. **Etiology.** The cause of DUB in 75% of cases is an immature hypothalamic-pituitary axis, resulting in anovulation. Other causes include psychogenic factors, juvenile hypothyroidism, and coagulation disorders (von Willebrand disease).

2. **Clinical picture**
   a. **Menometrorrhagia** (irregular, heavy bleeding) is the most characteristic symptom.

b. Bleeding can be prolonged and heavy, in some cases leading to severe anemia.

c. The condition is usually self-limited.

3. Management. Therapy involves the use of cyclic hormonal manipulation with progestins or combined oral contraceptive pills. Bleeding disorders must be ruled out in patients with heavy bleeding as up to 20% of teens with menorrhagia have some sort of bleeding problem.

C **Amenorrhea** (see Chapter 20). Primary amenorrhea is defined as no menstrual flow by 16 years of age, or within 2 years of breast development. Chromosomal abnormalities account for approximately 30% to 40% of all cases of primary amenorrhea. Secondary amenorrhea is menstruation that ceases for more than 6 months.

1. Müllerian anomalies and **vaginal agenesis** cause amenorrhea in 20% of cases. The incidence of renal or urinary tract anomalies in patients with müllerian anomalies is approximately 45%. Treatment is usually surgical.

a. Mayer-von Rokitansky-Küster-Hauser syndrome involves vaginal agenesis with or without uterine agenesis. Adolescents may present with cyclic abdominal pain and amenorrhea when endometrial tissue is present within one or both of the uterine remnants (see Chapter 20).

b. Imperforate hymen results in obstructed outflow of menstrual blood. Affected patients present with amenorrhea and cyclic abdominal pain. A bulging introitus and pelvic mass are present on examination. An imperforate hymen is not a true müllerian anomaly because the hymen is derived from the urogenital sinus. However, it is treated as a müllerian anomaly.

2. Hypogonadotropic hypogonadism. This condition is characterized by a deficiency of hypothalamic hormone secretion. It accounts for 40% to 50% of all cases of amenorrhea.

a. Kallmann syndrome is a rare autosomal dominant disorder that involves a deficiency of GnRH. It is associated with anosmia.

b. Central nervous system lesions, including craniopharyngioma and pituitary adenoma, may cause hypogonadotropic amenorrhea.

c. Anorexia nervosa, a condition characterized by extreme weight loss with no known organic cause, can affect adolescent development and result in amenorrhea. Psychiatric symptoms may be present, and occasionally the outcome is fatal.

d. Female athlete triad is a syndrome defined by amenorrhea, disordered eating, and osteoporosis. Typically, this condition is seen in athletes whose performance is enhanced by a lean physique, such as ballet dancers, ice skaters, and long-distance runners. The etiology most likely involves an inadequate caloric intake for the level of energy expended, which leads to hypoestrogenism and amenorrhea.

3. Gonadal dysgenesis (hypergonadotropic hypogonadism). This condition is characterized by absence of secondary sex characteristics, infantile but normal genitalia, and streak-like gonads that are devoid of germ cells and appear as fibrous white streaks. The presence of a Y chromosome dictates early removal of the gonads because of their propensity for malignancy (25% of cases occur by the age of 15 years). The different forms of gonadal dysgenesis are as follows:

a. Turner syndrome (45,X) is characterized at birth by low weight, short stature, edema of the hands and feet, and loose skin folds on the neck. Adolescent patients have short stature, lack of sexual maturation, a low posterior hairline, prominent ears, a broad chest, widely spaced nipples, and epicanthal folds. Cardiac anomalies are common in these patients.

b. Swyer syndrome (46,XY) is characterized by a female phenotype with amenorrhea and lack of secondary sex characteristics. Growth is usually normal, and some virilization may occur after puberty, especially when gonadal tumors are present. Swyer syndrome is inherited as an X-linked recessive trait. The clinical picture without virilization and tumor propensity may also occur in 46,XX individuals. This condition is termed pure gonadal dysgenesis and is an autosomal recessive inheritance.

c. Mixed gonadal dysgenesis (45,X/46,XY mosaicism) is characterized by sexual ambiguity in newborns. Internal structures include müllerian and wolffian derivatives. Asymmetric development of the gonads is expressed as a testis or gonadal tumor on one side with a streak-like, rudimentary gonad or no gonad on the other side.

d. **Abnormalities of the X chromosome** (e.g., mosaicism, isochromosome, short-arm X deletion, long-arm X deletion, and translocation) result in amenorrhea and varying degrees of Turner syndrome.

4. **Ovarian failure.** This condition, which is rare in adolescents, is usually attributed to genetic defects (e.g., Turner mosaic [45X/46XX], or deletion a portion of the long arm of the X chromosome), autoimmune conditions, radiation or chemotherapy for cancers, or galactosemia. Treatment involves estrogen and progesterone replacement.

5. **Polycystic ovary syndrome.** This condition is the **most common cause of anovulation** and secondary amenorrhea in the adolescent age group. This syndrome is characterized by oligomenorrhea, hirsutism, acne, and polycystic-appearing ovaries on ultrasound. The syndrome is associated with obesity (50% to 70%), insulin resistance, and the development of diabetes. Combined hormonal contraceptives are the mainstay of therapy for menstrual cycle regulation and control of hirsutism and acne. Antiandrogen agents are also beneficial, especially in combination with combined hormonal contraceptives. In addition, weight loss effectively improves symptoms in obese individuals (see Chapter 21).

6. **Systemic illnesses.** Renal failure, diabetes mellitus, cystic fibrosis, and hemoglobinopathies (sickle cell anemia and thalassemia) may cause hypothalamic amenorrhea.

7. **Other endocrine gland disorders.** Thyroid disease, late-onset congenital adrenal hyperplasia, Cushing syndrome, and pituitary adenomas may all cause amenorrhea.

D Contraception. Most sexually active adolescents do not use contraception, especially at the time of the first sexual act. Because younger patients probably do not mention contraception, a discussion about the use of contraceptives and preventing the transmission of sexually transmitted diseases should follow a physical examination, regardless of whether the patient is sexually active.

E Sexual abuse. Defined as sexual touch by someone at least **5 years older than the adolescent**, sexual abuse incorporates a wide range of behavior, from coerced seduction to violent assault. Rape is a form of sexual abuse. Seven percent of American men and women between 18 and 22 years of age have experienced at least one episode of nonvoluntary sexual intercourse.

1. Lack of findings on examination does not mean that abuse did not occur. A thorough history, assessment of family and environment, and laboratory studies should accompany the examination to establish the diagnosis.

2. Follow-up studies suggest that many people, particularly adolescents, may remain psychologically impaired and even suffer from posttraumatic stress disorder long after the abuse has ended.

Study Questions for Chapter 30

Directions: *Each of the numbered items or incomplete statements in this section is followed by answers or by completions of the statement. Select the ONE lettered answer or completion that is BEST in each case.*

1. A 15-year-old female is brought to your office complaining of severe dysmenorrhea that has become progressively worse since the onset of menses. Menarche occurred at age 13. The pain is located predominantly on the right side, lasts for the duration of the menstrual flow, and at its worst is associated with nausea and vomiting. She has had to miss school with every menstrual period for the past year. She has tried nonsteroidal medications, which initially helped but no longer relieve the pain significantly. The next step in management is:

- A Take the maximal dose of nonsteroidal medications and see if pain is improved
- B Refer her to psychiatry since this may just be a ploy to get out of school
- C Start combined oral contraceptive hormone pills
- D Obtain a pelvic ultrasound
- E Perform a laparoscopy to evaluate for endometriosis

2. An 8-year-old girl is brought to your office by her mother because of occasionally bloody vaginal discharge. Her mother suspects sexual abuse because she doesn't "know of any other reason why a little girl should be bleeding from her vagina." She has no other medical history except for a throat infection a few weeks ago, which was treated with penicillin. On physical examination, she has enlargement of both breasts and enlarged areolae. There is no axillary hair growth. No pubic hair is apparent. The external genitalia have an age-appropriate clitoris and normal labia minora. There are no bruises, hematomas, or lacerations. You take a culture of the vaginal discharge, which is pink to red colored and not foul smelling. You are not able to perform a more through examination. The most likely cause of her vaginal bleeding is:

- A Precocious puberty
- B Sexual abuse
- C Foreign body
- D Bacterial infection
- E Pinworm

3. A 6-year-old girl is brought to your office because she has had four urinary tract infections within the last 3 months. While the mother is holding her, you examine her genitalia. There is lack of pubic hair. The labia minora are in apposition but are easily separable with gentle traction. You note a 1-cm sized clitoris. There is a 0.3-cm cystic structure in the inferior aspect of the urethra, which is nontender to cotton swab palpation; however, it has left a red hue on your cotton swab. You order a urinalysis and a urine culture and sensitivity. The safest and next best step in management is:

- A Estrogen cream
- B Sitz baths
- C Intravenous pyelography
- D Low-potency steroid cream
- E Surgical repair

4. A 24-year-old woman, gravida 1, para 1, just delivered a live female infant by natural birth. The infant weighed 3990 g and had APGARs of 8 and 9 at 1 and 5 minutes, respectively. Upon inspection of the neonate, the pediatricians are unable to assign a gender because there is clitoral hypertrophy and the labia majora are partially fused. You do not palpate any masses within them. The most important next step in management of this condition is:

- A 17-OH-progesterone level
- B Dehydroepiandrosterone level
- C Serum sodium level
- D Tell the parents they have a baby girl
- E Karyotype

5. You are a world-renowned reproductive endocrinologist and are asked to make a diagnosis for a patient who has ambiguous genitalia. Here are the data:

Karyotype	XY
Spermatogenesis	Absent
Müllerian structures	Absent
Wolffian structures	Present
External genitalia	Male hypospadias
Breast	Gynecomastia

The diagnosis is:

- [A] True hermaphroditism
- [B] Mixed gonadal dysgenesis
- [C] Swyer syndrome
- [D] Complete androgen insensitivity
- [E] Reifenstein syndrome

Answers and Explanations

1. The answer is D [VII, A, 1–3]. The significant factors in this patient's history are the progression of her symptoms, the severity, and the localized nature of the pain. Primary dysmenorrhea may be severe, but is usually diffuse throughout the pelvis and does not become progressively worse over time. The history in this patient suggests secondary dysmenorrhea, possibly an obstructive müllerian anomaly. For this reason the next step should be a pelvic ultrasound. Combined hormonal contraceptives would be the next step if the pain didn't localize and there was no significant progression of pain symptoms with each menses. She is already on NSAIDs, so increasing the amount would not be beneficial given the severity of the symptoms. A laparoscopy would not be appropriate at this point without first performing an ultrasound and maximizing medical therapy. Though sometimes pelvic pain can be attributed to psychiatric causes, it is rare, and the patient should have all structural abnormalities investigated and optimal medical therapy tried first.

2. The answer is D [II E 1 b 2]. Given the clinical scenario, the only cause that is consistent is hemolytic streptococcal throat infection that has translated into vaginitis weeks later. Although sexual abuse should always be suspected with bloody vaginal discharge, the evidence is lacking, and the mother has no good reason to believe that her daughter has been sexually abused. Precocious puberty is unlikely in an 8-year-old girl with isolated development of the breast (thelarche) without pubarche. Pinworm would present with intense vaginal and perianal itching, especially at night. Given her older age and lack of information in the clinical scenario (especially because the discharge is not foul smelling), foreign body is less likely.

3. The answer is B [II D 2 a]. The diagnosis is prolapsed urethra, characterized by a small, hemorrhagic, friable (blood on cotton swab), painless mass surrounding the urethra. The safest and least expensive initial therapy is sitz baths. The bathtub is filled with lukewarm water with or without Epsom salt, and the patient sits in the bathtub a few times each day. Estrogen cream would be the next step in treatment. Intravenous pyelography would be useful if the diagnosis were ectopic ureter. Low-potency steroid creams are useful for lichen sclerosus. Surgical repair of prolapsed urethra is not necessary unless the patient has urinary retention or necrosis is present.

4. The answer is C [V A 2]. Because congenital adrenal hyperplasia, especially 21-hydroxylase deficiency, is the most common cause of distinct virilization of the female newborn, efforts should be made to obtain serum electrolytes immediately because the salt-wasting type of CAH can be life threatening. Diagnosis of CAH is best accomplished by finding elevated levels of 17-OH-progesterone. A karyotype can be obtained later to rule out other causes of ambiguous genitalia, such as hermaphroditism and mixed gonadal dysgenesis. You should not assign a gender until you have all of the information.

5. The answer is E [V E 1 e]. The two most important syndromes that have an XY karyotype are the androgen insensitivity syndromes (AIS) (complete, Reifenstein [incomplete], 5-α-reductase) and Swyer syndrome. Complete androgen insensitivity syndrome (CAIS) has the following features: XY, no spermatogenesis, absent müllerian structures, absent wolffian structures, *female external genitalia*, and female breast development. Reifenstein syndrome is exactly the same as CAIS except for more "male influence": wolffian structures are present, external genitalia are male (male hypospadias), and breasts are not as well developed (gynecomastia). Swyer syndrome is different from AIS in that there is more of a "female influence." This syndrome is characterized by the *presence of müllerian structures, absence of wolffian structures*, infantile female external genitalia, and lack of breast development. Mixed gonadal dysgenesis is characterized by mosaicism for 45,X/46,XY. There is usually a streak gonad on one side and a functioning testis on the other side. Both wolffian and müllerian structures are present and the external genitalia are ambiguous (although a wide range of phenotypes is possible). A true hermaprodite has both testicular tissue (XY genotype plus testicular tissue histology) and ovarian tissue (XX genotype plus ovarian tissue histology). One gonad can be a testis and the other an ovary, or one gonad can have both tissue types ("ovotestis"). True hermaphrodites have ambiguous external genitalia, which are most often more in the male spectrum than in the female. They also have gynecomastia.

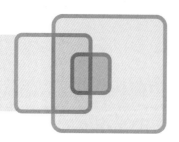

chapter 31

Menopause

ANN L. STEINER

I   DEFINITIONS

A Menopause

1. **Menopause** is a natural biologic process, and is not defined as a disease of estrogen deficiency. It is the **permanent cessation of menses occurring as a result of loss of ovarian activity**. Menopause is retrospectively defined as the absence of menses after the **final menstrual period (FMP)**. The FMP can only be determined when it is followed by amenorrhea for 1 year. The cessation of menses reflects the reduction of ovarian estrogen production to **levels insufficient to produce proliferation of the endometrial lining**.

2. Menses usually cease spontaneously between **40 and 58 years of age**; the median age of menopause is 51.4 years, with 90% becoming menopausal between the ages of 45 to 55 years of age. Chronologic age is a poor indicator of the menopause transition because of the wide range of age for spontaneous menopause. The average age of menopause has been stable worldwide for centuries, in spite of increasing longevity. However, age of menopause can be affected by current cigarette smoking and genetic predisposition.

3. **Premature menopause** is defined as the permanent cessation of menses occurring before 40 years of age.

4. **Menopause** can be spontaneous or induced by surgery, chemotherapy, radiation, or other exogenous influences.

B Perimenopause

1. The **perimenopause** or **menopause transition** refers to the period just before menopause. It ends with the FMP.

2. This period is marked by variation in menstrual cycle length and flow, reflecting a rise in levels of **follicle-stimulating hormone** (FSH).

3. The median age of onset of menstrual irregularity is 47.5 years; the transition lasts an average of 4 years. Nevertheless, 10% of women abruptly stop menstruating without having cycle irregularity.

C **Postmenopause** begins with the FMP and continues for the duration of the woman's life.

II   PHYSIOLOGY OF PERIMENOPAUSE

A Ovarian function.   A period of waxing and waning ovarian function occurs before menopause. It is a time of fluctuation in hormone production and reduced fecundability. It may be difficult to differentiate changes due to menopause from those related to aging.

1. The **number of remaining ovarian follicles is reduced** and those remaining are less sensitive to gonadotropin stimulation. Aging of the female reproductive system begins at birth, and consists of the steady loss of oocytes from atresia or ovulation. Follicular function varies not only from one individual to another, but also from cycle to cycle within the same individual. As follicular maturation declines, ovulation becomes less frequent in perimenopause.

2. Although fertility rates are markedly reduced, **conception** can occur during this time of fluctuating ovarian activity.

B Endocrinology

1. **Inhibin** production by the ovary depends on the number of existing ovarian oocytes and therefore is reduced. Inhibin B exerts a negative feedback on the secretion of FSH by the pituitary.

2. An **increase in FSH** levels results from the decreased circulating levels of inhibin and the loss of negative feedback. This is the earliest evidence of a change in ovarian function. Elevated FSH levels can be seen with both normal and abnormal cycles. The hallmark of reproductive aging is the elevation of FSH to greater than 10 mIU/mL in the early follicular phase (between day 2 and 5 of the menstrual cycle).

3. **Luteinizing hormone (LH)** secretion escapes the negative feedback of inhibin, and LH levels are not affected by the loss of inhibin production. LH levels rise much later in the transition than FSH levels; sustained elevations may not be seen until after menopause.

4. **Estradiol** levels fluctuate but remain within the wide range of normal until follicular development ceases altogether. Estradiol levels may actually rise in perimenopause due to an increase in the number of recruited remaining follicles from the increase in FSH levels. Estradiol also has a negative feedback effect on FSH levels.

5. **Progesterone** levels fluctuate depending on the presence and adequacy of ovulation and are frequently low during perimenopause.

6. **Androgen** levels are unchanged or slightly decreased in perimenopause. Levels are more affected by aging than by failing ovarian function.

C Menstrual cycles.
Changes in the menstrual cycle reflect changes in ovarian function and circulating levels of ovarian steroids and pituitary gonadotropins.

1. **Changes in menstrual cycle regularity** occur as a woman progresses through her 40s. Cycle length is determined by the length of the follicular phase. The secretory phase should be a constant 12 to 14 days. The length of time between menses, or cycle length, is variable and may be normal length, shortened, or prolonged. Bleeding may be heavier or lighter than previous menses and last for longer or shorter duration of time than was previously usual.

2. **Shortening of cycle length** often occurs early in perimenopause and is associated with ovulatory cycles, a shortened follicular phase, and elevated FSH levels.

3. **Anovulatory cycles** and **prolonged cycles** become more frequent as menopause approaches, resulting in **dysfunctional uterine bleeding (DUB)** and oligomenorrhea. DUB is defined as abnormal bleeding not caused by pelvic pathology, medications, systemic disease, or pregnancy. It is a diagnosis of exclusion.

III PHYSIOLOGY OF MENOPAUSE

A Ovarian function.
Follicular reserve is depleted and is finally manifested by a permanent cessation in menses.

1. **Few follicular units remain in the postmenopausal ovary**, and those present are no longer capable of a normal response despite stimulation by markedly elevated gonadotropins.
   a. **FSH receptors** are absent on a cellular level.
   b. **Estradiol** production by the ovary depends on FSH stimulation of follicles, and is negligible in the postmenopausal ovary. The greatest decline in estradiol levels are in the first year after the FMP and decrease more gradually in subsequent years.
   c. **Estrone,** a less potent estrogen than estradiol, is produced in negligible amounts by the postmenopausal ovary. It is derived from metabolism of estradiol and from peripheral aromatization of androstenedione in adipose and muscle tissue. Estrone becomes the predominant estrogen in menopause.

2. **Ovarian stromal tissue** continues to produce androgenic steroid hormones for several years after menopause.
   a. Although there is a lack of FSH receptors, ovarian stromal cells possess LH receptors and respond with the production of **ovarian androgens** (e.g., androstenedione, testosterone, and dehydroepiandrosterone [DHEA]).

    b. Androstenedione and **DHEA** production continues but at a decreased rate. **Testosterone** production remains stable or may be slightly increased.

    3. When menses have been absent for 1 year and FSH levels are persistently greater than 30 mIU/mL, conception is no longer an issue.

B Endocrinology

1. **FSH levels** are elevated 10 to 20 times above premenopausal levels, reaching a plateau 1 to 3 years after menopause, after which there is a gradual decline. This reflects loss of the negative feedback effects of both inhibin and estradiol. FSH levels never return to the premenopausal range, even with estrogen replacement therapy, reflecting the influence of inhibin.

2. **LH levels** rise two- to threefold after menopause, reaching a plateau in 1 to 3 years, after which there is a gradual decline. This reflects the loss of the negative feedback effect of estradiol. LH levels never reach those of FSH because of the shorter circulating half-life of LH (30 minutes as opposed to 4 hours).

3. Although **ovarian estrogen production** is negligible after menopause, there is individual variation in circulating estrogen levels because of peripheral conversion of androgenic precursors to estrone.
   a. **Androgens**, which serve as precursors for estrone, continue to be produced by the postmenopausal ovary and the adrenal gland.
   b. **Aromatase enzymes** that convert androgens to estrone primarily (and estradiol to a lesser degree) are present in peripheral tissues but are **predominantly present in adipose tissue**.
   c. Estrogen levels vary with the degree of adiposity. **Obesity** can lead to a state of relative estrogen excess.

4. **Peripheral testosterone levels** are decreased despite sustained or increased production rates by the ovary. Circulating testosterone levels are the net result of androstenedione and testosterone production by the adrenal gland and the ovary.
   a. Testosterone and androstenedione production by the adrenal gland continue to fall with progressive age.
   b. Testosterone production by the ovaries does not decrease for several years after menopause.
   c. Androstenedione production by the ovary is markedly reduced after menopause and accounts for the fall in circulating testosterone levels.

5. **DHEA levels** are reduced after menopause. However, DHEA sulfate levels, which reflect adrenal gland activity, are unchanged.

6. **Sex hormone–binding globulin (SHBG)** is decreased by 40% in association with the decrease of estradiol. As a result of the decrease in SHBG, the ratio of free androgen to SHBG is increased, allowing more circulating unbound testosterone.

C **Premature menopause** or **premature ovarian failure** is the cessation of menses in a woman **younger than 40 years of age**. Premature ovarian failure can be transient. When it is permanent, it is equivalent to premature menopause.

1. The frequency of premature ovarian failure is 0.3%. This is the diagnosis in 5% to 10% of women with secondary amenorrhea.

2. Most women with premature menopause undergo premature oocyte atresia and follicular depletion. This results from one of three mechanisms:
   a. Decreased initial germ cell number at birth
   b. Accelerated oocyte atresia after birth
   c. Postnatal germ cell destruction

3. A small number of affected women have abundant remaining follicles and elevated gonadotropins, suggesting a resistance to gonadotropin stimulation or the presence of biologically inactive gonadotropins.

4. Etiologies of premature ovarian failure and hypergonadotropic amenorrhea are diverse and fall under one of the following categories (See Chapter 20):
   a. Genetic and cytogenetic abnormalities
   b. Enzymatic defects
   c. Metabolic defects

    d. Physical insults and iatrogenic causes

    e. Autoimmune disturbances

    f. Abnormal gonadotropin structure or function

    g. Idiopathic

IV CLINICAL MANIFESTATIONS OF PERIMENOPAUSE

A **Manifestations of estrogen excess.** During perimenopause, some women present with evidence of estrogen excess rather than deficiency, due to a transient increase from increased FSH levels.

1. **Abnormal uterine bleeding (AUB)** is bleeding that is excessive in amount, duration, and frequency. It can occur due to prolonged exposure of the uterine lining to estrogen stimulation unopposed by progesterone. It may also be due to structural or systemic abnormalities. AUB without known structural or endocrine causes is called **dysfunctional uterine bleeding (DUB)**.

   a. Anovulatory cycles, common to the perimenopausal transition, lead to unopposed estrogen stimulation of the endometrial lining. This in turn can cause **AUB**, due to dyssynchronous shedding of the endometrium, which occurs with increased frequency in perimenopausal women. The type of AUB seen most commonly in the perimenopause transition is due to anovulatory cycles.

   b. Increased endogenous estrogen can also be caused by **increased peripheral conversion of androgen** precursors to **estrone** and estradiol. This is most frequently seen in obese perimenopausal women.

   c. Less commonly, pathologic conditions are associated with increased estrogen production (ovarian tumors) or decreased metabolic clearance of estrogen (hepatic or renal disease), leading to elevated circulating estrogen levels.

   d. There are many other **causes of AUB not related to sex hormone fluctuation**. Examples are endometrial polyps, fibroids, pregnancy, infection, coagulopathy, disorders of thyroid or prolactin regulation, chronic illness, and exogenous medications.

   e. Uterine leiomyoma, previously present, may grow during menopause transition due to estrogen excess. This may result in AUB and pelvic symptoms such as pain or pressure.

2. **Endometrial neoplasia**

   a. Prolonged unopposed estrogen stimulation of the endometrial lining may lead to excessive endometrial proliferation and subsequent endometrial pathology.

   b. Abnormal uterine bleeding that occurs either in a woman older than 40 years of age or in a younger woman with risk factors (history of chronic anovulation or unopposed estrogen, prolonged bleeding, obesity) must be evaluated with pelvic examination, pregnancy test, lab work as indicated by history, and endometrial sampling to rule out disease. Office **endometrial biopsy, with or without pelvic ultrasonography**, is usually sufficient. **Dilation and curettage (D&C) with hysteroscopy** and **sonohysterography** are alternatives for diagnostic testing.

   c. Simple endometrial hyperplasia has low risk of progression to endometrial carcinoma and can be treated medically.

   d. Complex endometrial hyperplasia without atypia is a more advanced type of hyperplasia, with a 3% risk of progressing to endometrial carcinoma. Complex hyperplasia may also be treated medically, followed up with posttreatment tissue sampling.

   e. Complex endometrial hyperplasia with atypia is associated with an increased risk of an associated endometrial carcinoma. Because of an approximately 25% risk of progression to endometrial carcinoma, hysterectomy is the treatment of choice for this condition. However, if medical management is elected, hysteroscopy with D&C is necessary first to rule out the coexistence of endometrial cancer.

   f. Endometrial cancer should be suspected in all perimenopausal women who present with abnormal bleeding. As much as 10% of postmenopausal bleeding is secondary to a carcinoma. Treatment is surgical.

B **Manifestations of hormonal fluctuation**

1. **Menstrual cycle changes.** Some change in the character of established menstrual cycles is the most common manifestation of perimenopause. Ninety percent of women may experience menstrual changes in perimenopause.

a. **Menorrhagia** is defined as increased blood flow (**more than 80 mL**) during menses, or bleeding that lasts longer than 7 days. Cycles are **regular** and ovulatory. Increased flow may result from a relative reduction in progesterone levels. Increased bleeding at regular intervals is also called **hypermenorrhea**.

b. **Metrorrhagia** is bleeding at **irregular intervals or between menses**. Shortening of cycle length is a common change reported early in the menopausal transition. Cycle length remains longer than 21 days but is typically shorter than cycles experienced during the reproductive years. Cycles are ovulatory with a shortened follicular phase.

c. **Oligomenorrhea is the decreased frequency of menstruation.** As menopause approaches, missed periods are common, and cycle length increases until a permanent cessation of menses occurs.

d. **Amenorrhea** is the absence of menses.

2. **Other symptoms**. Many women who are still menstruating experience a variety of symptoms traditionally attributed to menopause.

a. **Hot flashes** are symptoms of vasomotor instability. This is the second most common perimenopausal symptom, reported by 75% of perimenopausal women. Hot flashes can come and go over time and are not consistent from cycle to cycle. They typically are present for up to 2 years after the FMP, but may persist for up to 10 years. When they occur with sleep and are associated with perspiration, they are called **night sweats**. Peripheral vasodilation is associated with a rise in skin temperature, resulting in a hot flash. There may also be a modest increase in heart rate at the same time. Although there is no objective link between alcohol, caffeine, and hot flashes, there are anecdotal reports supporting an association.

b. **Headaches** may worsen during perimenopause, and then improve again after menopause. There may be a hormonal link, but this has not been well studied.

c. **Sleep disturbance.** Interrupted sleep, with or without hot flashes, is reported by one-third to one-half of U.S. women in this age group.

d. **Mood disturbance** is reported by 10% of perimenopausal women. This includes symptoms of irritability, depression, insomnia, fatigue, and difficulty with memory or concentrating. Sleep deprivation and midlife stresses may be strong contributing factors. There is no evidence that cognitive function actually deteriorates with perimenopause or menopause.

e. **Sexual function** such as libido, arousal, and vaginal lubrication and elasticity can be affected by the onset of perimenopause. These changes can be due to many causes, including hormonal fluctuation, medications, sleep disturbance, loss of partner, and life stresses.

f. **Weight gain** occurs for many women during the menopause transition, possibly due to aging and lifestyle. Obesity increases a woman's risk for other health problems, such as cardiovascular disease and diabetes. A theory that weight gain during this time may also be due to a decrease in metabolically active tissue and less overall time spent in the secretory phase of the cycle as menses become farther apart needs further study.

C Treatment

1. **Progestogen (natural progesterone or synthetic progestin) supplementation.** Periodic administration of a progestogen is used to treat conditions associated with estrogen excess.

a. **DUB** can be treated with intermittent progestogen in 12- to 14-day monthly cycles, which provides estrogen antagonism and allows for the orderly sloughing of the endometrium. Therapy may also be administered continuously, preventing withdrawal bleeding. These therapies decrease the incidence of anovulatory uterine bleeding and the development of endometrial neoplasia.

(1) **Medroxyprogesterone acetate (MPA)** is the most commonly used progestogen for DUB. Therapy may be used for only one cycle, continued cyclically until there is absence of withdrawal bleeding, or used continuously to suppress bleeding altogether. Absence of withdrawal bleeding signifies a reduction of estrogen levels to the menopausal range.

(2) **Norethindrone acetate**, also a progestin, can be used as an alternative to MPA.

(3) **Oral micronized progesterone**, derived from plant sources, is also an alternative.

(4) **The progestin-containing intrauterine system** delivers continuous low-dose progestin (levonorgestrel) directly to the endometrium. Ninety percent of women who use it have a reduction in blood flow and 20% have complete absence of any bleeding.

    b. Simple and complex hyperplasia may be treated effectively with progestogen supplementation. Treatment with progestin or progesterone as described for DUB is prescribed. Follow-up biopsy is performed after 3 months of treatment to verify resolution of the hyperplasia.

    c. Complex hyperplasia with atypia may be treated with high-dose progestogen if surgical therapy is not an option, once the presence of carcinoma has been excluded by such methods as ultrasonography, hysteroscopy, and D&C. Follow-up biopsy after 3 months of treatment is mandatory to verify resolution.

        (1) Progestogen is given daily for 3–6 months.

        (2) Megestrol (a strong progestin) is given daily for 3–6 months.

2. Combination (estrogen–progestin) hormonal contraceptives are useful for both contraception and treating symptoms in perimenopausal women who are normotensive nonsmokers without other risk factors. Choices include oral contraceptive pills, vaginal ring, and contraceptive patch.

    a. Low-dose combination hormonal contraceptives (35 μg ethinyl estradiol or less) can be an effective treatment for abnormal bleeding and hot flashes associated with perimenopause.

    b. These medications are obviously also an effective method of contraception for women in whom this is still a concern. There is no increased risk using combination hormonal contraceptives in perimenopausal-aged women **without risk factors** compared to younger women.

    c. Because **combination hormonal contraceptives** contain **five to seven times the estrogen equivalent of postmenopausal hormone therapy**, it is desirable to change therapy with the onset of menopause. FSH levels fluctuate rapidly and are not consistent in perimenopause. Therefore, FSH is not a reliable test for evaluating or predicting menopause status and the need for contraception. One suggested option is to continue combination hormonal contraception in women who tolerate it and have no risk factors until the age of 50 to 55.

    d. Other methods of contraception may be considered as well, as long as pregnancy is an issue.

3. Hormone therapy (HT) refers to the combined use of estrogen and progestogen in subcontraceptive doses. **Estrogen therapy (ET)** refers to the use of estrogen without a progestogen, usually only given in women who have undergone hysterectomy.

    a. HT and ET may be used to treat perimenopausal symptoms in women with oligomenorrhea before permanent cessation of menses. There are many variations in dose, drug types, and delivery systems for HT and ET.

    b. Progestogen is added to estrogen in women who have their uterus. Otherwise, **unopposed estrogen** increases the risk of **endometrial neoplasia** in these women. The risk is related to duration of use and dose. The absolute risk of endometrial cancer is 1 per 1000 in postmenopausal women. In general, the risk increases to 1 per 100 in women on unopposed estrogen.

4. Scheduled **nonsteroidal anti-inflammatory drugs (NSAIDs)** effectively reduce menstrual blood flow in 40% to 60% in women with ovulatory cycles. NSAIDs block prostaglandin synthetase activity and should be initiated at the onset of menses and given on a regular schedule until past the risk of heavy flow. NSAIDs may be useful in the treatment of menstrual migraines.

5. Alternative therapies such as herbal remedies, acupuncture, and non–Food and Drug Administration (FDA)-approved hormones require further study.

V CLINICAL MANIFESTATIONS OF MENOPAUSE

A **Target organ response to decreased estrogen.** Estrogen-responsive tissues are present throughout the body. Chronic reduction of estrogen may result in any of the following manifestations:

1. Urogenital atrophy. The vagina, urethra, bladder, and pelvic floor are estrogen-responsive tissues. Decreased estrogen levels after menopause result in a generalized atrophy of these structures. About 25% of women seek medical help for associated symptoms. These symptoms often improve with the use of topical or systemic estrogen.

    a. There is a reduction in the thickness of **vaginal epithelium** and vaginal vascular flow and increased vaginal pH. The vaginal epithelium shows a loss of rugation and elasticity. Maturation of the vaginal epithelium is estrogen dependent. After menopause, there is a shift in the maturation index, with a preponderance of immature cell types (basal and parabasal) over mature cell types (intermediate and superficial).

    b. The vaginal walls lose elasticity and compliance; the **vagina becomes smaller**, and the size of the upper vagina diminishes. This results in increased likelihood of trauma, infection, **dyspareunia** (painful intercourse), and painful pelvic examination.

    c. The **labia minora** have a pale, dry, thin appearance, and there is a reduction of the fat content of the **labia majora**.

    d. The **pelvic tissues and ligaments** that support the uterus and the vagina may **lose their tone**, predisposing to disorders of pelvic relaxation.

    e. The **epithelium of the urethra and bladder** mucosa becomes atrophic; there is a loss of urethral and bladder wall elasticity and compliance.

    f. **Urinary tract symptoms** resulting from changes in the mucosal lining of the urethra and bladder may lead to increased symptoms of dysuria, nocturia, urinary frequency, urgency, and urge incontinence.

    g. Urinary conditions such as **urinary stress incontinence** may progressively worsen after menopause because of urethral changes and a loss of pelvic support. There is an increased incidence of **asymptomatic bacteriuria** and urinary tract infection in the postmenopausal woman.

2. Uterine changes

    a. The **endometrial tissue becomes thin**, with atrophic histologic changes.

    b. The **myometrium atrophies**, and the **uterine corpus decreases in size**. There is a reversal of the corpus:cervical length ratio compared with the reproductive years.

    c. The **squamocolumnar junction** of the cervix migrates higher in the endocervical canal; the cervical os frequently becomes stenotic.

    d. **Fibroids**, if present, may reduce in size but do not disappear.

3. Breast changes

    a. Progressive fatty replacement of breast tissue with atrophy of active glandular units occurs, with regression of fibrocystic changes.

    b. After menopause, the mammographic appearance of the breast becomes progressively more radiolucent in response to decreasing sex hormone levels.

    c. HT increases breast density and reduces the sensitivity of mammograms.

4. Skin changes

    a. Skin collagen content and skin thickness decrease proportionately with time after menopause.

    b. Sunlight and cigarette smoke exposure accelerate skin aging.

5. Hair changes. As estrogen decreases, circulating androgens increase and the chance of developing increased facial hair and androgenic alopecia increases.

6. Central nervous system (CNS) changes

    a. Estrogen receptors are located throughout the brain. Cognitive function, as measured by some parameters, may decline with advancing age.

    b. Reduced estrogen levels may affect cognitive function and moods after menopause, although the precise contribution has not been fully defined. It is unclear to what extent giving hormone therapy affects cognitive function. Giving HT in menopause does not appear to have a beneficial effect on the prevention of Alzheimer disease.

7. Cardiovascular disease

    a. The incidence of cardiovascular disease increases after the age of 50 years in women, coincident with the age of menopause.

    b. Cardiovascular disease is the cause of the largest number of deaths of menopausal women. The mortality rate from cardiovascular disease among American women is greater than the next 14 causes of death combined.

    c. Endogenous estrogen appears to protect against cardiovascular disease in premenopausal women. Nevertheless, taking HT in menopause may not protect against and may increase the risk of some vascular disease. This is especially true in women with a prior history of cardiovascular disease.

8. Vasomotor symptoms (VMSs) or hot flashes

    a. **Hot flashes** are the second most common perimenopausal/menopausal symptom after abnormal bleeding. There are differences in incidence depending on the ethnic background of the woman. African-American women report hot flashes the most frequently, followed by Hispanic, Caucasian, Chinese, and Japanese Americans. Differences in body mass index may be a more important predictor of hot flashes than ethnic background.

(1) These symptoms have a circadian rhythm and are more frequent in the early evening. No clinical trials have confirmed that hot flashes are precipitated by caffeine, alcohol, or stress. They do appear to be exacerbated by cigarette smoking, sedentary lifestyle, and induced menopause.

(2) Hot flashes last for **1 to 2 years** in most women but may last for as long as 10 years.

b. Symptoms are the result of **inappropriate stimulation of the body's heat-releasing mechanisms** by the thermoregulatory centers in the hypothalamus. Although the core body temperature is normal, the body is stimulated to lose heat. The role of estrogen in causing VMSs is unclear. Estrogen administration diminishes the frequency and severity of symptoms in a dose-dependent manner.

c. VMSs are characterized by **progressive vasodilation of the skin over the head, neck, and chest**, causing a skin temperature rise. They are accompanied by reddening of the skin, a feeling of intense body heat, and perspiration. Palpitations or tachycardia may accompany the flush. The flush may last 1 to 5 minutes and recur with variable frequency. Flashes may vary from being annoying to totally disruptive to normal life function.

d. **Treatment**

(1) **Lifestyle changes,** such a regular exercise, avoiding smoking, wearing cool clothes, and lowering room air temperature, may help to minimize symptoms.

(2) **HT and ET** consistently reduce or eliminate hot flashes, as do combined hormonal contraceptives such as birth control pill. Results are dose related, and optimal results may be achieved over several weeks.

(3) **Progestogen, clonidine, gabapentin, and herbal remedies** are used to treat hot flashes in women in whom estrogen is contraindicated. Relief is not as complete as that seen with estrogen therapy.

(4) **Venlafaxine and selective serotonin reuptake inhibitors (SSRIs),** given in low doses, have been effective in reducing or eliminating vasomotor instability in up to 60% of symptomatic women.

9. **Altered menstrual function.** Oligomenorrhea is followed by amenorrhea. If irregular vaginal bleeding or bleeding after 6 months of amenorrhea occurs, endometrial disease (e.g., polyps, hyperplasia, or neoplasia) must be ruled out.

10. **Osteoporosis** is a disorder characterized by **compromised bone strength** predisposing to an **increased risk of fracture.** Bone strength reflects the integration of two main features: bone density and bone quality. Osteoporosis may be a primary disease state, resulting from estrogen deficiency or aging, or may be secondary to other diseases, conditions, or medications that affect calcium and bone metabolism. It is a "silent" disease, becoming symptomatic only when fractures have occurred.

a. Epidemiology and etiology

(1) Peak trabecular bone mass is reached in the late 20s and peak cortical bone mass in the early 30s. Thereafter, there is a gradual loss of bone with aging. **Bone loss is accelerated for the first 5 to 10 years after menopause** as a direct result of declining estrogen levels. Osteoporosis is more common in women than in men because of lower peak bone mass and higher rates of bone loss. Trabecular bone loss is more rapid in early postmenopause, resulting in an increase in distal forearm fractures after age 45 and vertebral fractures beginning at age 55. Cortical bone loss is more gradual, resulting in an increased incidence of hip fractures in women after age 65.

(2) **Major risk factors for fracture** are advanced age, Caucasian or Asian race, and female gender as well as a personal history of fracture after age 50 or a family history of osteoporosis or related fractures in a first-degree relative. Other risk factors include, but are not limited to, current low bone mass, low body mass index, inadequate calcium and vitamin D intake, sedentary lifestyle, cigarette smoking, hypothalamic amenorrhea, premature menopause, use of certain medications such as glucocorticoids or gonadotropin-releasing hormone agonists, medical conditions such hyperthyroidism and hyperparathyroidism, and excessive use of alcohol.

(3) Osteoporosis has reached epidemic proportions in the United States, causing an estimated 1.5 million fractures annually. Four out of five Americans with osteoporosis are women. In 2002, an estimated $18 billion was spent in direct care expenditures for osteoporotic fractures.

   (a) Approximately 25% of white American women older than 60 years of age who are not treated have **vertebral compression fractures**. These are the most common fractures. There are about 700,000 osteoporosis-related vertebral fractures a year.

   (b) Approximately 32% of untreated white American women older than 75 years of age suffer **hip fractures**; 24% over the age of 50 will die in the first year after fracture. Of those who survive, 20% no longer live independently. There are over 300,000 hip fractures a year. Fractures also can occur at the distal forearm and other sites.

(4) Osteoporosis results when **bone resorption outweighs bone formation**. Trabecular bone is at greater risk than cortical bone because it is more metabolically active and structurally more porous.

b. Diagnosis. Osteoporosis is a silent disease, becoming symptomatic only when a fracture occurs. Most common fractures are vertebral compression fractures (which can be symptomatic or asymptomatic), a Colles fracture of the forearm, or a hip fracture, although all bones are at risk.

c. Imaging modalities can be used to detect bone loss and bones at risk for fracture at an earlier stage. However, not all osteoporotic fractures are associated with measured low bone mass.

   (1) Peripheral densitometry devices such as quantitative ultrasound (QUS) can be used on the wrist, finger, or heel. Precision is poorer than with x-ray–based studies. QUS should not be used for monitoring therapy.

   (2) Dual-energy x-ray absorptiometry (DEXA) is the most popular technique used today to measure bone mass. It is the gold standard to which all other methods are compared, having excellent precision and low radiation dose. Independent measurements can be made at the hip, spine, and, if indicated, distal forearm.

   (3) Quantitative computed tomography gives the most precise measurement of bone mass at specific sites. However, its use has been limited by expense and higher radiation dose.

d. The definition of osteoporosis is based on DEXA T scores. A T score is based on the mean peak bone mass of a normal young adult population and is expressed in standard deviations from the mean in this reference group. A T score equal to 0 is average, greater than 0 is above average, and less than 0 is below average. The lower the T score, the higher the risk of having a fracture is. **Osteopenia** (decreased bone density) is defined as a T score between −1 and −2.5. **Osteoporosis** is defined as a T score less than −2.5.

e. Prevention and treatment of osteoporosis is important. The higher a woman's bone mass at the onset of menopause, the more bone she will have to lose to be at risk for osteoporotic fractures. Although no one can alter her genetic predisposition, many lifestyle factors can affect fracture risk.

   (1) Adequate calcium intake can be obtained through diet or supplementation; 1500 mg of elemental calcium daily is recommended after the age of 50. This can be obtained through diet or supplements.

   (2) Vitamin D is essential for the absorption of calcium and reduces fracture risk as well as the risk of falling: 600 to 800 IU/day is recommended, although up to 2000 IU/day is safe. Vitamin D can be obtained through diet, supplementation, and sun exposure to the unprotected skin.

   (3) Weight-bearing **exercise** has a positive effect on the skeleton and may reduce fracture risk and decrease the risk of falling.

   (4) Reducing the risk of falling is essential for the prevention of fractures. This includes safety factors such as optimizing medications that may affect balance, removing dangerous obstacles, providing aids for ambulation and lighting, and using hip protectors.

   (5) Cigarette smoking and excessive alcohol consumption increase the risk of fractures and are associated with lower bone mass.

f. There are many medications used to prevent bone loss and/or treat low bone density. With the exception of Teriparatide, these work by slowing bone breakdown during bone remodeling. They are called antireabsorptive agents.

(1) **Bisphosphonates** are very effective at preventing bone loss and decreasing the risk of fractures in people with low bone mass. Some are also approved for treating glucocorticoid-induced osteoporosis. Dosing is variable, ranging from once a week to once a year, depending on the type of bisphosphonate. They can be administered orally or intravenously.

(2) **Selective estrogen receptor modulators (SERMs)** such as Raloxifene are taken orally daily and are related to tamoxifen. Raloxifene is approved for prevention of osteoporosis and is effective in reducing the vertebral fracture rate.

(3) **Calcitonin** nasal spray in limited studies has been shown to increase vertebral bone mass and decrease vertebral fracture risk.

(4) **HT and ET** are effective in preventing osteoporosis and reducing hip and vertebral fractures. However, due to other medication-associated risk factors, it is not recommended that they be used primarily for this indication unless other medications are not appropriate.

(5) **Teriparatide (rhPTH 1-34)** is given as a daily injection for up to 18 to 24 months. It has an anabolic bone effect and decreases vertebral and nonvertebral fractures. Effect on hip is not proven.

VI HORMONE THERAPY

A Benefits and indications. The goals of HT are to (1) reduce symptoms resulting from estrogen depletion such as hot flushes, sleeplessness, and mood disorders; (2) treat vaginal dryness and atrophy; and (3) minimize the risk of disorders that may be more frequent during hormone therapy. Randomized controlled trials and observational studies published since 1998 highlighted the benefits of hormone therapy. However, studies published after 2002 suggested a small but significant increase in the rate of cardiovascular disease, stroke, venous thrombotic embolism, and breast cancer associated with use of HT. As a result of this information, the percentage of women aged 50 to 74 taking HT increased between 1995 and 2001 from 33% to 42%. By mid-2003, however, the number had decreased to 28%. Hormone or estrogen replacement therapy is the most effective treatment for the relief of menopause-related symptoms and menopausal osteoporosis. However, each woman has a unique risk profile that may lead to more or less overall benefit from HT. It is important to consider the relative risks and benefits of HT for each patient before recommending these medications. If the decision is made to use HT, it should be given in the lowest doses for the duration of time needed to achieve the desired effect.

B Recent studies. Table 31-1 lists recent large studies published on the use of HT in menopause. Data from these studies show that HT:

1. Is the most effective treatment for hot flushes. Some, but not all, studies showed a benefit in sense of well-being.

2. Significantly improves vaginal atrophy and dyspareunia.

TABLE 31–1

Title	Acronym	Year
Randomized controlled trials		
Postmenopausal Estrogen/Progestin Interventions trial	PEPI	1998
Heart and Estrogen/Progestin Replacement Study	HERS	1998
Women's Health Initiative Hormone Trials	WHI-HT	2002, 2004
Observational studies		
The Nurses Health Study	NHS	2000
The Million Women Study	MWS	2003
Women's Health Initiative Observational Study	WHI-OS	2005

3. Has been shown to prevent and treat osteopenia and osteoporosis and decrease incidence of bone fractures.

4. Does not seem to prevent cognitive impairment or dementia in menopausal women.

5. Does not protect against cardiovascular disease in menopause, though lipid profiles are improved. The Women's Health Initiative (WHI) study showed a slight increase in non-fatal cardiovascular events primarily in the first year of therapy. Death due to cardiac disease was not increased with HT in that study.

6. Increases the risk of stroke in users. The absolute risk is approximately from 20 to 25 cases per year among 10,000 otherwise healthy postmenopausal women.

7. Increases the risk of venous thromboembolism (VTE). The incidence of VTE in healthy post-menopausal women is 16 to 22 cases per 10,000 women per year. HT increases this risk twofold.

8. With combined estrogen and progestogen does not increase the risk of endometrial cancer. Estrogen alone is associated with an increased risk of developing endometrial cancer and should therefore not be used in women with a uterus.

9. Increases the incidence of breast cancer in users, but the risk returns to normal within 5 years after discontinuation. The effect of hormones on breast cancer risk is similar to that of alcohol consumption, obesity, and parity. The risk is slightly higher in those women using both estrogen and progestogen compared to estrogen alone. The risk of breast cancer in healthy post-menopausal women is approximately 30 cases per 10,000 women per year. The use of HT adds approximately 8 to 17 cases per 10,000 women per year to this baseline risk.

C Current studies to watch

1. **Kronos Early Estrogen Prevention Study (KEEPS)** is an ongoing study evaluating estrogen given either orally or transdermally to recently postmenopausal women to see if starting HT earlier modifies the effect on atherosclerotic disease. Progesterone is given to women who have their uterus.

2. The **Early versus Late Intervention Trial with Estradiol (ELITE)** study is currently evaluating women less than 6 years postmenopausal versus women greater than 10 years postmenopausal and the effect of estradiol on the development of atherosclerotic changes. Progesterone is given to women with their uterus.

3. The **Study of Women Across the Nation (SWAN)** is observing midlife transition and normal aging in women of five different American ethnic groups.

D Risks and contraindications

1. **Absolute contraindications** include:
   a. Undiagnosed abnormal genital bleeding
   b. Known or suspected breast cancer or estrogen-dependent neoplasia
   c. Active or history of thrombosis
   d. History of stroke or myocardial infarction in the previous year
   e. Active liver dysfunction or disease
   f. Known or suspected pregnancy
   g. Known hypersensitivity to HT/ET

2. **Endometrial cancer**. Estrogen therapy increases the risk of endometrial hyperplasia and carcinoma when used without progestogen in a woman with her uterus.
   a. **Addition of a progestogen** for at least 12 days per month reduces that risk of endometrial cancer to less than 1% to 2%. There is a decreased relative risk of endometrial cancer in women who are on combined estrogen and progestin replacement therapy compared to women who take no HT.
   b. In some cases hormone therapy may be considered in women who have been successfully treated for stage I endometrial carcinoma and are asymptomatic.

3. **Commonly used schedules of HT**
   a. The mainstay of HT is estrogen, which is usually given in a daily or continuous fashion. **Progestogen** is added to **estrogen** therapy to prevent endometrial hyperplasia and carcinoma in women who have their uterus.

(1) **Cyclic therapy.** Continuous estrogen therapy is given, and progestogen is added for 12 to 14 days each month. This results in a predictable withdrawal bleed following monthly cessation of progestogen in 80% of women. The duration and flow may decrease with time and cease altogether. Oral micronized progesterone, medroxyprogesterone acetate, or norethindrone acetate for 12 to 14 days a month can be used.

(2) **Continuous combined therapy.** Progestogen given continuously with daily estrogen does not induce cyclic bleeding but is associated with unpredictable irregular bleeding in up to 40% of women in the first 6 months of therapy. By 1 year this is reduced to 10% to 25% of users. Oral micronized progesterone, medroxyprogesterone acetate, or norethindrone acetate is taken daily with estrogen.

b. **Abnormal bleeding** that occurs with HT must be evaluated with **endometrial sampling** and possibly ultrasound to rule out endometrial disease. Bleeding that continues after sampling and appropriate management should be evaluated with **hysteroscopy** or **sonohysterography.**

c. **Side effects** of progestogens may be associated with their mineralocorticoid antagonist activity. Premenstrual tension syndrome–like symptoms such as fluid retention and swelling, mood disturbance and depression, mastalgia, and headache are reported. Adjustment in dose, schedule, and route of administration may help relieve symptoms. Concerns about the possible effect of **progestogen with estrogen and increased risk of breast cancer have been raised by results of the WHI study.**

4. **Route of administration of systemic hormones** affects first pass through the liver, metabolism, and resulting serum levels of hormones. HT and ET may be administered through the following routes with FDA-approved products.

a. **Transdermal patches** contain either estrogen alone or estrogen plus progestogen and are changed once or twice a week, depending on the product.

b. **Percutaneous gel or emulsion** dispenses estrogen in metered doses and is used daily.

c. The **vaginal ring** contains estrogen only and is changed every 3 months.

d. **Oral estrogen or oral estrogen plus progestogen** is the most common route of administration. When administering HT, a single pill containing both estrogen and progestin may be given or they may be given in separate pills, on a daily basis.

5. **Local applications**

a. **Topical estrogen** is used intravaginally to treat symptoms of **urogenital atrophy** and **dyspareunia.** Estrogen-containing creams, tablets, and synthetic rings are available for this use. Peak systemic absorption is in the first few days of initial use. Once the vaginal mucosa becomes cornified, there is minimal systemic absorption of estrogen.

b. **A progestin-containing intrauterine device** may provide endometrial protection and avoid the side effects of systemic progestogen.

VII RECOMMENDATIONS FOR CARE OF THE MENOPAUSAL WOMAN

A Health risk assessment and physical examination

1. Identification of risk factors in medical, surgical, social, family, and lifestyle history

2. Assessment for problems including abnormal bleeding, sexual function issues, sleep disturbance, urinary dysfunction, and hot flashes

3. Annual determination of height, weight, and blood pressure

4. Annual physical examination, including breast and pelvic examination

B Age–risk-appropriate screenings. Evidence-based testing is performed to detect early disease in low-risk, asymptomatic patients.

1. Lipid profile assessment every 5 years beginning at age 45

2. Fasting blood sugar screening every 3 years beginning at age 45

3. Thyroid-stimulating hormone testing every 5 years beginning at age 50

4. Mammography every 1 to 2 years from 40 to 50 years of age, annually after 50 years of age

5. Cervical cytology every 1 to 3 years depending on age, risk, high-risk human papilloma virus DNA testing, and previous Pap history

6. Osteoporosis screening beginning at age 65 years, and earlier in women with risk factors for fractures or in women whose decision to begin treatment would be influenced by screening results

7. Routine screening for colon cancer beginning in low-risk women at age 50 years. Options include yearly fecal occult blood testing and/or flexible sigmoidoscopy every 5 years, colonoscopy every 10 years, or double-contrast barium enema every 5 years.

C Promotion of a healthy lifestyle

1. Discuss smoking cessation and alcohol limitation as needed.

2. Make nutritional assessment and recommendations about weight control, dietary fat, cholesterol, calcium, vitamin D, and caloric intake.

3. Assess contraceptive needs and risk for sexually transmitted diseases.

4. Make exercise assessment and recommendations.

5. Identify physical, emotional, and substance abuse risk and history, as well as high risk behaviors.

6. Screen for symptoms of depression.

7. Counsel about prevention of falls in appropriate women.

8. Encourage home and occupational safety, as well as seat belt and safe firearm use.

9. Provide individually appropriate patient education.

10. Assess vaccination update status.

BIBLIOGRAPHY

Spearoff, Fritz. Clinical Gynecologic Endocrinology and Infertility. 7th Ed. Philadelphia: Lippincott Williams and Wilkins, 2005.

Management of osteoporosis in postmenopausal women: 2006 position statement of the North American Menopause Society. Menopause 2006;13(3):340–367.

Primary and preventive care: periodic assessment. ACOG Committee Opinion #292, November 2003.

Study Questions for Chapter 31

Directions: *Each of the numbered items or incomplete statements in this section is followed by answers or by completions of the statement. Select the ONE lettered answer or completion that is BEST in each case.*

1. A 50-year-old woman has menses every 2 to 3 months and hot flashes that wake her. She falls asleep in the afternoon at work because she doesn't sleep well at night. She is otherwise healthy and has no medical risk factors. She asks you if she is at risk for becoming pregnant with unprotected intercourse and wants your advice regarding managing her symptoms. You should:

[A] Check FSH levels
[B] Advise her that she is too old to possibly conceive
[C] Advise her to use natural family planning for reliable protection against becoming pregnant
[D] Discuss using a low-dose combination hormonal contraceptive with her
[E] Recommend she have a tubal ligation

2. A healthy 35-year-old woman, G2P2, presents with a history of regular menses since age 14, until her last period 1 year ago. Her human chorionic gonadotropin (hCG) is negative, serum estradiol less than 20 pg/mL, FSH and LH greater than 100 mIU/mL, and prolactin less than 20 ng/mL. She has hot flashes and dyspareunia that disrupt her life. Which of the following is NOT true?

[A] The patient is at an increased risk of bone loss and fracture compared to menstruating women her age
[B] The patient has premature ovarian failure and should be offered HT both for her symptoms and to protect her from bone loss
[C] This is a typical menopausal woman
[D] This patient should receive progestogen in addition to estrogen if she chooses to take systemic hormones
[E] Vaginal estrogens will relieve her genitourinary symptoms

3. Current studies regarding the risks and benefits of HT/ET put perimenopausal and menopausal women in a treatment dilemma. Which of the following is true?

[A] Women using HT have twice the risk of developing breast cancer compared to healthy menopausal women
[B] HT prevents all-cause dementia in women who begin medication after the age of 65 years
[C] HT/ET should be given in the lowest doses for the shortest duration of time needed to achieve the desired effect
[D] If a woman with breast cancer has symptoms due to chemotherapy-induced menopause, she has no available pharmacologic agents available to her
[E] HT/ET is indicated for prevention of skin changes due to estrogen deficiency and for prevention of cardiovascular disease

4. A frail 70-year-old woman with her FMP at age 51 complains of back pain and a 4-inch loss in height. Spine films confirm the presence of multiple osteoporosis-related vertebral compression fractures. Her DEXA hip T score = –2.7. Your concerns for management include all but which of the following?

[A] Potential risk of future hip fracture
[B] Assessment of risk of falling
[C] Concern that the patient's positive smoking history will exclude her from therapy to prevent future fractures
[D] Concern that a SERM may not be as effective as a bisphosphonate in treating this patient
[E] Concern that the patient's immobility may limit her ability to perform weight-bearing exercise or go outside for sun exposure to increase endogenous vitamin D

5. A 55-year-old woman with her FMP at age 50 presents with a history of 3 days of light vaginal bleeding. You should:

- A Give her vaginal estrogen for atrophic vaginitis and tell her to come back if the bleeding doesn't get better
- B Perform a hysterectomy and bilateral salpingo-oophorectomy to rule out endometrial cancer
- C Take a history, perform a physical examination, perform endometrial tissue sampling, and order a pelvic ultrasound or perform hysteroscopy
- D Recommend she go on a diet, since there is increased production of estrone in obese women
- E Start ET instead of HT, since adding a progestogen may make her bleed

Answers and Explanations

1. The answer is **D** [IV B, C]. If the patient qualifies medically for low-dose combination contraception such as oral contraceptive pills or the vaginal ring, it will provide both adequate contraception and relief of vasomotor symptoms. FSH is not a reliable marker for menopause in this patient and should not be used to determine potential to conceive if she is still having periods. Gonadotropins are released in a pulsatile fashion during perimenopause. Age is a poor predictor of menopause status or fertility during perimenopause, although fecundity decreases with advancing age. Natural family planning becomes less reliable in a woman with irregular menses. While tubal ligation is an excellent method of contraception, it does not provide any relief of this woman's VMSs. If she desires, a short-term solution for both of her issues, without the risks of anesthesia or surgery, is optimal.

2. The answer is **C** [III C]. This is not a typical menopausal woman because she is so young. She has premature ovarian failure, defined as menopause prior to age 40. Early menopause is a risk factor for increased fracture risk because of long-term low estrogen levels. HT will provide relief of VMSs and genitourinary symptoms, as well as providing protection against loss of bone mass in this very young woman. Unopposed estrogen should not be used in a woman with her uterus intact, due to an increased risk of endometrial neoplasia with unopposed estrogen. Vaginal estrogen will relieve her vaginal dryness and dyspareunia if she declines systemic HT.

3. The answer is **C** [VI B]. Because there is an increased risk of blood clots and stroke in women on HT/ET, and in women on ET an increased risk of breast cancer, women who desire treatment should take the lowest dose for the shortest duration necessary to achieve treatment goals. HT is associated with a small increase in risk of breast cancer. HT does not prevent decline of cognitive function or dementia and increases the risk of all-cause dementia in new starters after age 65. In a woman in whom hormone therapy is contraindicated, there are several off-label alternatives for sleep disturbance and VMSs. These include SSRIs, gabapentin, and clonidine. HT/ET is indicated for relief of moderate to severe VMSs and vaginal dryness. Due to potential serious risks, it is not indicated for what are considered minor symptoms such as estrogen deficiency–related skin changes. HT is associated with an increased risk of CHD events, primarily in the first year of use, and is not considered protective against cardiovascular disease based on current studies. Newer studies are ongoing to evaluate whether HT, if started early in the menopause process, can prevent cardiovascular changes associated with menopause.

4. The answer is **C** [V A 10]. Smoking is a major risk factor for osteoporosis and fracture. Current smoking is not exclusionary from any of the approved osteoporosis medications. A history of vertebral fracture is the greatest risk factor for future fractures. Therefore, this patient's history of vertebral compression fractures increases her risk of future hip fracture. The risk of falling and sustaining fractures can be modified by assessment and intervention of the patient's living and activity environment. There are no SERMs currently approved for prevention of hip fracture, although there are such bisphosphonates available. This patient is likely to have limited weight-bearing activity due to her vertebral compression fractures. She is likely to be vitamin D deficient because of limited mobility and access to sun exposure, increasing the risk of fracture and falling.

5. The answer is **C** [IV 1–2]. Although postmenopausal bleeding is common, it is not normal. This patient needs to be evaluated for endometrial neoplasia. She requires a workup and close follow-up. A tissue diagnosis is indicated before definitive surgical treatment (i.e., hysterectomy) for presumed endometrial neoplasia. Although obesity is a risk factor for endometrial neoplasia, a definitive diagnosis is required. ET/HT is contraindicated in patients with vaginal bleeding of unknown etiology.

chapter 32

Family Planning: Contraception and Complications

COURTNEY A. SCHREIBER

I CONTRACEPTIVE EFFICACY

The number of pregnancies per 100 woman-years is the number of pregnancies in 100 sexually active, fertile women who use a given method of contraception for 1 year. The expected pregnancy rate in women using no method of contraception is 85 pregnancies per 100 woman-years.

II BARRIER METHODS

A Condoms. One of the oldest surviving forms of birth control, condoms are effective, safe, and relatively inexpensive. Moreover, their effects are reversible. Condoms are effective if used consistently.

1. **Mode of action**. Both female and male condoms act as physical barriers to semen.

2. **Advantages**
   a. **Protection from sexually transmitted diseases (STDs)**
      (1) **Latex condoms protect against STDs** caused by herpes simplex virus, *Neisseria gonorrhoeae*, *Chlamydia trachomatis*, *Ureaplasma urealyticum*, *Mycoplasma hominis*, *Trichomonas vaginalis*, *Treponema pallidum*, and HIV, but not human papilloma virus.
      (2) **Natural, or nonlatex, condoms do not protect against most STDs** because they contain small pores that allow passage of microbes.
   b. Easy accessibility
   c. Few side effects

3. **Disadvantages**
   a. Must be used in each act of intercourse
   b. Requires cooperation of both partners

4. **Types of condoms**
   a. **Female condoms** line the entire surface of the vagina and partially shield the perineum. They can be inserted up to 8 hours in advance but should be removed immediately after each act of intercourse. Female condoms should not be used in conjunction with male condoms.
   b. **Male condoms** cover the glans and the shaft of the penis and must be used from the beginning to the end of each act of intercourse to be effective. Some condoms contain spermicidal agents. **Condoms impregnated with spermicide are no more effective than condoms alone**.

5. **Efficacy. Pregnancy rate** is 3 to 21 per 100 woman-years of use.

B Spermicides. Creams, jellies, aerosol foams, nonfoaming and foaming suppositories, and vaginal films are commonly used with other forms of contraception, such as diaphragms, sponges, and condoms. Only about 3% of women use spermicides alone.

1. **Mode of action**. Spermicides serve as a **chemical barrier** to sperm. The **active agents** in spermicides (e.g., nonoxynol 9) disrupt the outer lipoprotein surface layer of spermatozoa, killing the sperm, decreasing their motility, or inactivating the enzymes needed to penetrate the ova.

2. **Advantages**
   a. Increase the efficacy of vaginal sponges, diaphragms, and cervical caps
   b. Available over the counter

        c. No need for medical consultation

        d. Few side effects

    3. Disadvantages

        a. Need for insertion with each act of intercourse

        b. Limited duration of effectiveness

        c. Possible increase in the risk of HIV transmission caused by disruption of vaginal epithelium. This increased risk appears to be dose dependent: people who use these products multiple times per day should be wary of this effect.

    4. Efficacy. **Pregnancy rate** is as much as 26 in 100 woman-years of use. As with mechanical barrier methods, efficacy depends on the couple's motivation to use spermicides correctly with every act of intercourse.

C **Vaginal sponges**

    1. Mode of action. Vaginal sponges release spermicide during coitus, absorb ejaculate, and physically block the entrance to the cervical canal.

    2. Advantages

        a. Use for as long as 24 hours regardless of frequency of sexual intercourse

        b. Few systemic side effects

    3. Efficacy. **Pregnancy rate** is 40 in 100 woman-years of use in parous women and 20 in 100 woman-years of use in nulliparous women.

D **Diaphragms.** These dome-shaped contraceptives are 50 to 105 mm in diameter and are made of latex rubber. They rest between the posterior aspect of the symphysis pubis and the posterior fornix of the vagina, thus covering the anterior vaginal wall and the cervix.

    1. Mode of action. Diaphragms act as physical barriers to sperm and are effective vehicles for holding spermicide over the cervix.

    2. Advantages

        a. Contraception for up to 6 hours after placement

        b. Few side effects

    3. Disadvantages

        a. Need to keep in place for at least 6 hours after intercourse to ensure that no motile sperm are left in the vagina

        b. Requirement for use with a spermicidal agent

        c. Need to replace spermicide with each act of intercourse

        d. Associated with an increased risk of urinary tract infections

        e. Need to be fit by a clinician

    4. Efficacy. **Pregnancy rate** is reported to be 5 to 10 in 100 woman-years of use.

E **Cervical caps.** These contraceptives are as effective as diaphragms but are more difficult to fit.

    1. Mode of action. The cervical cap has the same mode of action as the diaphragm.

    2. Advantages

        a. Ability to leave in place up to 48 hours (compared to 6 hours with the diaphragm), regardless of number of acts of intercourse

        b. Effectiveness without the addition of a spermicidal agent

    3. Disadvantages

        a. Need to keep in place for at least 6 hours after intercourse (same as the diaphragm)

        b. Few physicians are trained in the placement and use of the cervical cap.

    4. Efficacy. **Pregnancy rate** is reported to be about 5 to 10 in 100 woman-years of use.

III INTRAUTERINE DEVICES

These reversible methods of contraception are one of the most widely used throughout the world. Intrauterine devices (IUDs) are extremely effective in reducing the risk of pregnancy. The copper IUD

(ParaGard) and the progestin-only IUD (Mirena) are currently available in the United States. Both IUDs have multiple mechanisms of action but primarily act by preventing sperm mobility and oocyte fertilization. Evidence does not support the claim that IUDs are abortifacients.

A Types

1. The **copper-impregnated IUD** is approved for 10 continuous years of use. Evidence demonstrates that it is effective for 12 years.

2. The **progestin-impregnated IUD**, with levonorgestrel 20, is approved for 5 years and then must be replaced.

B Mode of action

1. **Copper-impregnated IUD**
   a. **Copper itself acts as a spermicide**.
   b. The IUD causes a local, sterile inflammatory reaction in the uterus, and the intrauterine environment becomes spermicidal.
   c. The copper intensifies the inflammation in the uterine cavity, producing a lining that is unfavorable for implantation.

2. **Progestin-only IUD**
   a. This IUD exerts its contraceptive effect locally on the endometrium and the cervix. Progestin alters the endometrium, rendering it unfavorable for implantation.
   b. In addition, both uterine and tubal motility are impaired, thereby impairing sperm–egg interaction. Thickening of the cervical mucus makes the passage of sperm difficult.

C Advantages. These IUDs do not interfere with lactation and are not coitally dependent. IUDs and implants are the most effective reversible methods of contraception currently on the market.

1. **Copper-impregnated IUD**
   a. As many as 12 years of continuous contraceptive efficacy from one IUD
   b. Can be inserted at any time during the menstrual cycle
   c. Resumption of fertility on removal

2. **Progestin-only IUD**
   a. As many as 5 years of continuous contraceptive efficacy from one IUD
   b. Useful for treatment of menorrhagia (heavy menstrual bleeding) and dysmenorrhea (painful menses)
   c. Resumption of fertility on removal of the IUD

D Disadvantages

1. **Insertion**. Although the copper-impregnated IUD may be inserted at any time during the menstrual cycle, the progestin-only IUD should be inserted within the first 7 days.

2. **Uterine perforation**. This complication occurs in about 1 in 1000 insertions and should be suspected if the patient can no longer feel the string.

3. **Infection**. Risk is highest in the first 2 weeks after insertion because of possible introduction of bacteria into uterine cavity at the time of insertion. The risk of infection increases in women with a history of recent pelvic infection.

E Efficacy. **Pregnancy rate** among users of either type of IUD is less than 2 to 3 in 100 woman-years of use.

F Contraindications

1. **Known pregnancy**

2. Recent (less than 3 month) history of endometritis or purulent cervicitis

3. Distorted uterine cavity (increases expulsion rate)

G Pregnancy-related issues. If a woman becomes pregnant with an IUD in place, it should be removed immediately because the IUD increases the risk of pregnancy loss and preterm labor. In addition, the risk of increased infection necessitates the removal of the IUD early in pregnancy.

1. The **spontaneous abortion rate** is about 50% if an IUD remains in place. The risk of miscarriage after removal in early pregnancy is about 20% to 30%. This is compared to the risk of first-trimester miscarriage in the general population of 20% to 25%.

2. In general, **ectopic pregnancy** is prevented by both the progestin-only and copper-impregnated IUDs. If a pregnancy does occur with an IUD in place, about 5% of women have an ectopic pregnancy.

3. The chance of a **premature birth** is 12% to 15% in pregnancies when an IUD is left in place. This is compared to the baseline risk of preterm labor of about 10% in the United States.

IV PROGESTIN-ONLY METHODS

A Mode of action

1. Diminishing and thickening cervical mucus, thereby preventing sperm penetration

2. Producing a thin, atrophic endometrium, precluding implantation

3. Reducing the ciliary action of the fallopian tube, preventing sperm and egg transport

4. Diminishing the function of the corpus luteum

5. Occasional inhibition of ovulation by suppressing the midcycle peaks of luteinizing hormone (LH) and follicle-stimulating hormone (FSH)

B "Minipill" (Micronor, others). Less than 1% of oral contraceptive prescriptions in the United States are for this progestin-only oral contraceptive; however, typical use failure rates approximate the typical use failure rates of combined oral contraceptive pills.

1. **Advantages**
   a. No alteration of milk production and nearly 100% effectiveness in breastfeeding women
   b. Tolerance in women who are unable to take estrogen
   c. Independent of sexual intercourse

2. **Disadvantages**
   a. Irregular vaginal bleeding
   b. No protection against STDs
   c. Need for daily administration
      (1) Progestin-only pills are taken continuously for 28 days without a pill-free interval. Because these pills have a dose of progestin that is very close to the threshold of contraceptive efficacy, they must be taken at approximately the same time each day.
      (2) Suppressed ovulation occurs in only a proportion, and contraceptive efficacy depends on the other progestin-related mechanisms previously listed (see IV A).

3. **Efficacy. Pregnancy rate** is 5 in 100 woman-years of use. Consistent administration is necessary. A difference of a few hours may contribute to reduced contraceptive protection.

C Injectable progestin. Medroxyprogesterone (Depo-Provera), the most commonly used injectable form of contraception, is given as a deep intramuscular injection every 12 weeks. Menstrual patterns may be irregular during the first year of use; this is a common reason for discontinuation. Fifty percent of women develop amenorrhea within 1 year of use.

1. **Advantages**
   a. Effective for 12 weeks
   b. Independent of sexual intercourse
   c. Safe for use during breastfeeding
   d. Women on antiepileptic medications may have fewer seizures, and those with sickle cell disease may have fewer sickle cell crises.

2. **Disadvantages**
   a. No protection against STDs
   b. Irregular bleeding and spotting
   c. Weight gain in certain populations (year 1, 5 lb; year 2, 16 lb)
   d. Prolonged return of fertility (median time from discontinuation to return of fertility, 8.5 months)

3. **Efficacy. Pregnancy rate** is less than 1 in 100 woman-years of use.

D Implantable progestin.   Implantable progestin-containing rods release hormones at a low but constant rate.

1. **Advantages**
   a. Effectiveness for up to 3 to 5 years
   b. Independent of sexual intercourse
   c. Almost immediate return of fertility after removal

2. **Disadvantages**
   a. Menstrual irregularity
   b. No protection against STDs
   c. Weight gain
   d. Higher rate of failure with high body mass index (BMI)
   e. Need for surgical placement and removal
   f. Less effective in women who take antiseizure medications or rifampin

3. **Efficacy. Pregnancy rate** is less than 1 in 100 woman-years of use.

4. **Specific types of implants**
   a. **Original form (Norplant)** is no longer manufactured. It consists of six implants each containing levonorgestrel, and is effective for up to 5 years. It is no longer available in the United States.
   b. **Implanon**
      (1) This single implantable rod contains 3-keto-desogestrel, a progestin that is more potent than levonorgestrel. Studies have shown that serum hormone concentrations remain adequate for at least 3 years. Implanon users have a lower incidence of prolonged or irregular menstrual bleeding compared with users of Norplant; however, the incidence of oligomenorrhea (infrequent menses) and amenorrhea is higher.
      (2) Implanon has just been approved by the Food and Drug Administration (FDA) and is now available in the United States.

E Progestin-only IUD   (see III B)

V   COMBINATION ORAL CONTRACEPTIVE PILLS

A Composition.   Combination oral contraceptive pills (OCPs) contain various amounts of estrogen (ethinyl estradiol) and one of a variety of progestins. The current preparations contain low doses of estrogen (usually 20 to 35 µg per pill). Most are taken for 21 days, with 1 week between pill packs, in either monophasic or triphasic combinations. Continuous use with intermittent menstrual withdraw (four menses a year) is becoming more widespread.

B Mode of action.   The primary mechanism is inhibition of the LH surge.

1. Suppression of ovulation

2. Thickening of the cervical mucus, resulting in ineffective sperm migration

3. Alteration of tubal motility

4. Alteration of endometrium to make it thin and inactive, thus hampering implantation

C Efficacy.   **Pregnancy rate** is 5 in 100 woman-years.

D Current controversies regarding complications

1. **Venous thromboembolism**
   a. Estrogen causes an increase in serum levels of several clotting factors, especially factor VII. Antithrombin III levels fall within 10 days of starting OCPs.
   b. The incidence of both superficial and deep vein thromboses is increased in OCP users. Risk increases as estrogen dose increases.
   c. Despite these risks, it is still safer for a woman to use OCPs than to become pregnant. The **attributable risk**, or the number of venous thromboembolic events attributable to estrogen in OCPs, is approximately 6 in 100,000 woman-years. The estimated risk in pregnant women is 20 in 100,000 woman-years.

    d. Initial epidemiologic studies reported that women using **third-generation** (those that contain gestodene or desogestrel) OCPs have increased rates of venous thromboembolism compared with those using **second-generation** (containing norethindrone and levonorgestrel) OCPs. Additional studies demonstrated an inconsistent and weak association between OCPs and venous thromboembolism (strength of association, 0.7 to 2.3).

    e. Women with **inherited thrombophilias** who take OCPs have an increased risk of thromboembolism. The risk of thrombosis with OCP use is six times higher in **carriers of antithrombin and protein C and protein S defects**. The odds of having a venous thromboembolism event are 10 times higher in OCP users than in nonusers in carriers of the **factor V Leiden** mutation and seven times higher in carriers of the **prothrombin G20210A mutation**. Patients with a personal or family history of deep venous thrombosis or pulmonary embolus should be screened for these thrombophilias prior to starting OCPs. It is not necessary to screen all potential users of OCPs.

2. Cardiovascular disease

    a. There is no evidence to support an increased or decreased risk of **myocardial infarction** resulting from past or current use of OCPs. The strength of association between OCP use and **stroke** is weak, with an odds ratio of 1.1:1.8 (most 95% confidence intervals cross 1.0).

    b. However, a **synergistic effect** exists **between OCPs and smoking** as causes of cardiovascular events. **Heavy smoking, hypertension, severe diabetes mellitus with vascular complications**, and **obesity** (more than 50% above ideal body weight) are independent risk factors for cardiovascular disease. Women older than 35 years of age are at the highest risk for a cardiovascular event. However, women older than 35 years with no risk factors can safely use OCPs.

3. Hypertension. Plasma renin activity, angiotensin levels, aldosterone section, and renal retention of sodium are all increased in OCP users. The resulting hypertension in a small number of OCP users may represent the failed suppression of plasma renin activity that occurs with elevated levels of angiotensin. The length of OCP use appears to relate to the development of hypertension, which develops in approximately 5% of users after 5 years of use. Normotensive levels return in almost all women who developed hypertension while taking OCPs when the contraception is discontinued.

4. Liver tumor. An association between the use of OCPs and the subsequent development of a rare liver tumor, **hepatocellular adenoma**, has been reported. The associated risk increases when OCPs have been used for 5 years or more. Tumor development occurs at a rate of 3 in 100,000 woman-years of use.

5. Neoplasia

    a. Breast cancer

        (1) Progestins antagonize the stimulating effect of estrogen on breast tissue. The incidence of breast cancer has remained fairly constant during the past 15 to 20 years despite widespread use of OCPs.

        (2) A **small but statistically significant increase in risk of breast carcinoma exists in current (relative risk, 1.24)** and recent users (relative risk, 1.16) of OCPs, but not in past users.

            (a) This increased risk equates to a small increase in the actual number of new cases of breast cancer, and it disappears after 10 years of use.

            (b) **Cancers diagnosed** in recent or current OCP users **are not advanced and tend to be localized** compared with OCP nonusers.

        (3) Patients with a **family history of breast cancer have no additional risk**.

    b. Cervical cancer. Although this finding is controversial, there may be a small increased risk of cancer of the cervix. This may be especially true with use of more than 5 years and in women who test positive for human papillomavirus. Cervical hypertrophy and eversion are seen in OCP users.

    c. Endometrial cancer. Progestins reduce the stimulating effect of estrogen and prevent the normal proliferative endometrium from progressing to hyperplasia, thus **decreasing the risk of endometrial cancer by 50%** (see V E 2).

    d. Ovarian cancer (see V E 1)

  E **Noncontraceptive benefits**

1. Ovarian cancer. OCPs suppress ovarian activity and inhibit ovulation; the interruption of a significant number of ovulatory cycles in oral contraceptive users may lead to a decreased incidence of ovarian cancer.

a. Users of OCPs are less likely to develop ovarian cancer than those who have never used OCPs. An average decrease of 40% in the likelihood of ovarian cancer is seen in women who have taken OCPs at some time. Protection is provided after as little as 3 to 6 months of use and persists for at least 15 years after discontinuation. Recent data also suggest that OCPs serve as primary prevention for women at risk for hereditary ovarian cancer.

b. In particular, the risk of ovarian cancer is **significantly reduced in current and past users** of OCPs. This risk reduction increases as the period of OCP use increases. Women at increased risk for epithelial ovarian cancer may benefit from OCP use.

2. **Endometrial cancer.** Users of OCPs have a 50% reduction in endometrial cancer compared with those who have never used OCPs. Risk is reduced with longer use of pills. The actual duration of protection is unknown but lasts for a minimum of 15 years.

3. **Benign breast disease.** Fibrocystic change and fibroadenoma development are significantly reduced with OCP use. Larger amounts of progestin and longer periods of use decrease the risk of benign breast disease. The risk is lowest in current OCP users.

4. **Ectopic pregnancy.** The contraceptive effect of OCPs prevents ectopic pregnancy. The protection rate is 90% in current OCP users.

5. **Iron deficiency anemia.** OCPs decrease menstrual blood loss and regulate menstrual bleeding, thus decreasing likelihood of iron deficiency anemia. This action benefits both past and current OCP users.

6. **Pelvic inflammatory disease (PID).** OCPs protect against only those patients with PID who require hospitalization. At least 12 months of OCP use is necessary, and protection is limited to current users. No protection against lower genital tract infections (e.g., cervicitis) and tubal infertility is evident.

7. **Dysmenorrhea.** OCPs improve primary dysmenorrhea. OCPs have also been shown to improve dysmenorrhea caused by endometriosis.

8. **Hirsutism and acne.** OCPs improve hirsutism and acne caused by hyperandrogenism by decreasing production of androgens by the ovary and adrenal and increasing sex hormone–binding globulin production by the liver.

F New combination OCP preparations

1. Packaging to allow continuous use with menstrual withdrawl every 3 months instead of monthly

2. An OCP containing ethinyl estradiol with a new progestin, drospirenone, which is an analog of spironolactone

VI   OTHER COMBINATION HORMONAL METHODS

A Contraceptive vaginal ring (NuvaRing). This contraceptive device consists of a 5.4-cm flexible ring made of ethylene vinyl acetate copolymer containing ethinyl estradiol and etonogestrel. The ring is inserted into the vagina and the hormones are absorbed into the systemic circulation.

1. **Use.** The vaginal ring is worn continuously for 3 weeks and then discarded; a new ring is inserted into the vagina 1 week later. If the ring is left in place for more than 4 weeks, its contraceptive efficacy may be reduced.

2. **Mode of action** is similar to that of combined OCPs (see V B).

3. **Advantages**
   a. Beginning of contraceptive effect within the first day of use
   b. Inserted by the user, does not need to be fitted
   c. Does not need to be removed for sexual intercourse
   d. Rapid resumption of fertility on discontinuation
   e. Fewer side effects (e.g., weight gain, acne, bleeding irregularities, and breast tenderness) than combined OCPs
   f. Does not require daily attention

4. **Disadvantages** include no protection against STDs.

5. **Efficacy** is similar to that of combined OCPs.

B Transdermal patch (Ortho Evra). The once-weekly contraceptive patch releases norelgestromin, the active metabolite of norgestimate, and ethinyl estradiol daily to the systemic circulation.

1. **Use.** Typical use includes placement of the patch on the same day of each week for 3 consecutive weeks followed by a patch-free week.

2. **Mode of action** is similar to that of combined OCPs (see V B).

3. **Advantages**
   a. Maintenance of normal activity, including bathing, swimming, and heavy exercise while using the patch
   b. Noncontraceptive benefits. The noncontraceptive effects of transdermal administration have not yet been studied but are expected to be similar to those of combined OCPs.
   c. Independent of sexual intercourse
   d. Rapidly reversible on discontinuation
   e. Does not require daily or coital attention

4. **Disadvantages** include no protection from STDs.

5. **Efficacy** is similar to that of combined OCPs.

6. **Controversies. The FDA recently issued a warning that the Ortho Evra patch may be associated with a greater risk of VTE than is found with combination OCPs.** One published study reported no significant difference in risk of VTE with the two methods of contraception. A second study, not yet published, reported a significantly higher risk with the patch compared with the oral contraceptive. In response to the second study, the FDA mandated a labeling change warning of increased risk of VTE with the patch. The attributable risk remains low.

VII EMERGENCY CONTRACEPTION

The primary **advantage** of this type of contraception is that it has no medical contraindications except previously established pregnancy. Its primary **disadvantage** is lack of protection against STDs. Methods of emergency contraception include the combined and progestin-only contraceptive pills, copper-impregnated IUD, and mifepristone (RU486).

A Overall mode of action. A single mechanism of action has not yet been established. Emergency contraception probably prevents pregnancy by causing anovulation or delaying ovulation. An effect on the endometrium preventing implantation has also been suggested.

B Overall efficacy. The efficacy declines with increasing delay between episode of unprotected intercourse and initiation of treatment. Among the oral contraceptives, the progestin-only method is more effective in preventing pregnancy than the combination-pill, or Yuzpe, method (85% effective versus 57%). The copper-impregnated IUD is significantly more effective than the use of hormonal emergency contraception, which has a failure rate of 0.1%.

C "Morning-after pill"

1. **Combination method.** The most common regimen involves four tablets that are a combination of ethinyl estradiol and norgestrel, given as two tablets twice over 12 hours. The necessary **minimum effective dose** of ethinyl estradiol and norgestrel is 100 μg and 1.0 mg, respectively (**Yuzpe method**).

2. **Progestin-only method.** The most common regimen is levonorgestrel, 0.75 mg, taken 12 hours apart. The necessary **minimum dose** of levonorgestrel is 1 mg. A single dose of 1.5 mg has been shown to be even more effective than the two doses of 0.75 mg.

3. Prepackaged, commercially available emergency hormonal contraception
   a. **Plan B** is a **progestin-only method** that consists of two tablets, each containing 0.75 mg of levonorgestrel, and detailed instructions for both physicians and patients.
   b. This preparation is available over the counter in the United States for women over the age of 18 years.

4. **Use.** The "morning-after pill" is best taken within 120 hours of unprotected coitus; use within 24 hours increases efficacy: the sooner the better.

5. **Side effects**. Most common side effects include nausea (about 50% of women) and vomiting (about 20% of women). An antiemetic is often needed with combination pills but *not* with progestin-only pills.

[D] The **copper-impregnated IUD** can be used as an alternative method. It should be inserted up to 5 to 7 days after ovulation to prevent pregnancy. The copper IUD is significantly more effective than the use of hormonal emergency contraception; the failure rate is 0.1%.

[E] Mifepristone (RU486) is a progestational antagonist that binds to the progesterone receptor and prevents or interrupts progestational action. A single oral dose (600 mg) is associated with an efficacy rate of nearly 100%.

VIII NATURAL FAMILY PLANNING

This contraceptive method entails avoiding pregnancies by abstaining from sexual intercourse during the fertile phase of the menstrual cycle. Drugs, devices, and surgical procedures are not used. Coitus is limited to before and after the fertile period each month.

[A] Fertility awareness. Women are most fertile several days around the time of ovulation.

1. Fertility status can be determined by charting basal body temperature, maintaining a menstrual calendar, and monitoring changes in cervical mucus.

2. Fertility determination depends on a couple's ability to identify and interpret signs of fertility.

[B] **Basal body temperature** is the temperature of the body at complete rest after a period of sleep and before normal activity, including eating.

1. The basal body temperature exhibits a biphasic pattern during an ovulatory cycle (i.e., it is lower in the first half of the cycle, increases at the time of ovulation, and remains higher for the rest of the cycle).

2. The basal body temperature **increases 0.4 to 1.0°F during the postovulatory phase** of the cycle because the secretion of progesterone has a thermogenic effect.

3. **As an indicator of fertility**, the basal body temperature can detect only the end of the fertile phase because the temperature elevation is detected after ovulation

4. **To avoid pregnancy**, a couple must restrict sexual intercourse from the end of menses to 1 to 2 days after the temperature elevation.

[C] Menstrual calendar calculations

1. Calculations are based on the following assumptions:
   a. Ovulation occurs on day 14 (plus or minus 2 days) before the onset of menses.
   b. Sperm remain viable for about 5 days.
   c. The ovum survives for about 1 day.

2. Lengths of previous cycles give an estimate of when to avoid intercourse during a current cycle.

[D] Cervical secretions

1. Varying concentrations of estrogen and progesterone affect the quantity and quality of cervical mucus.

2. Secretions **during the fertile period are abundant, clear or white, slippery, and stretchy**. Ovulation occurs within 1 day before to 1 day after the appearance of this discharge.

3. **After ovulation**, as progesterone levels increase, cervical secretions become **thick, cloudy, and sticky**.

4. It is presumed that the **fertile period** begins when cervical secretions are first noted until 4 days past the peak of the slippery discharge. **To avoid pregnancy, couples should abstain from intercourse during the fertile period.**

[E] Advantages

1. Acceptance by some religions that disapprove of other methods of contraception

2. Involvement of both partners

3. Minimal cost

4. No medical consultation needed

F Disadvantages

1. No protection against STDs

2. Difficulty of use with irregular menses

3. Ovulation can occur unpredictably even in women with generally regular cycles.

G Efficacy. **Pregnancy rate** among women using natural family planning is 10 to 23 in 100 woman-years of use.

IX   SURGICAL STERILIZATION

These procedures have become one of the most widely used methods of contraception. Both tubal ligation and vasectomy are designed to be permanent. Depending on the technique used, tubal sterilization has a failure rate during the first year of 0.7% to 5.4%. Counseling is essential; nearly 6% of women regret their decision, but this is much more common in women under 30. Vasectomy has a failure rate during the first year of 0.1%.

Study Questions for Chapter 32

Directions: *Match the description below with the best method of contraception. Each answer may be used once, more than once, or not at all.*

QUESTIONS 1–4

A Depot-medroxyprogesterone acetate
B Progestin-only pill (minipill)
C Combination birth control pill
D Progesterone IUD
E Vaginal contraceptive ring

1. A 24-year-old woman, gravida 3, para 3, who just delivered a healthy boy and is breastfeeding him. She is a successful model and cannot tolerate excessive weight gain. She has never been able to remember to take a pill daily.

2. A 29-year-nulliparous woman who has factor V Leiden deficiency and a bicornuate uterus. She is a librarian who exercises 6 days a week in order to maintain her physique. She has had several tumultuous relationships this year. She tries to use condoms in addition to this contraceptive method to prevent STDs.

3. A 28-year-old nulliparous physician who has a history of major depression. She is on call in the hospital every 4 days and sometimes forgets to take her antidepressant medication. She has been in a new relationship for the past 2 months. She always uses condoms in addition to this contraceptive method to prevent STDs.

4. A 26-year-old woman, gravida 4, para 4, is happily married . She has regular periods that last 9 to 10 days, are extremely heavy, and are associated with severe cramping. She is fairly sure she has completed childbearing.

Directions: *Each of the numbered items or incomplete statements in this section is followed by answers or by completions of the statement. Select the ONE lettered answer or completion that is BEST in each case.*

5. Your 24-year-old multiparous patient is interested in long-term contraception, but is concerned that the copper IUD acts as an abortifacient. The best guidance you could give her is:
A She should not use the copper IUD because its main mechanism of action is as an abortifacient
B The main way in which the copper IUD prevents pregnancy is by acting as a spermicide
C Tubal ligation is a more effective long-term contraceptive than an IUD, so she should consider that instead
D IUD is associated with a high rate of infection (pelvic inflammatory disease)

6. A 25-year-old woman, gravida 1, para 0, therapeutic abortions (TAB) 1, presents to the emergency department and is being evaluated for date rape, which occurred 12 hours ago. She says that the rapist forced himself onto her and had time to ejaculate inside her. She has no past medical history. In addition to prophylactic treatment for STDs, complete rape evaluation, and counseling, the most effective and widely available management to prevent pregnancy is:
A Ethinyl estradiol and norgestrel, two tablets now and two in 12 hours
B Ethinyl estradiol and norgestrel, two tablets now and two in 12 hours, and prochlorperazine
C Plan B 150 mg now
D Levonorgestrel, 0.75 mg now and another in 12 hours
E Mifepristone (RU-486)

Answers and Explanations

1. D [IV B], **2.** B [IV B], **3.** E [VI B], **4.** D [III C 2]. Women who are breastfeeding should use progestin-only contraceptive methods so as to not affect their quantity and quality of breast milk. This first patient cannot tolerate depot-medroxyprogesterone acetate because it is associated with 5-lb-per-year weight gain in a subpopulation of women. The progestin-only pill may not be ideal since she cannot remember to take pills daily and the efficacy of this pill is dependent on taking the pill at the same time each day. Therefore, the IUD would be the best option. The second patient would benefit from the progestin-only pill because (1) she should avoid estrogen-containing contraceptive methods (combination pills or patch) because of her inherited thrombophilia; (2) she should avoid depot-medroxyprogesterone acetate because she is concerned with weight loss; and (3) she is not a candidate for an IUD because she has an abnormal uterine cavity. The third patient has depression, and depot-medroxyprogesterone acetate has been associated with major depression. She may forget to take any form of daily (pill) contraceptive because of her busy schedule. The IUD is not contraindicated in nulliparous women, but does require insertion, which may be uncomfortable for this patient. Therefore, the vaginal contraceptive ring is the best option. The fourth patient would benefit from the progestin-releasing IUD because her dysmenorrhea and menorrhagia would improve. She is also in a monogamous relationship, which makes her the perfect candidate for this form of contraception.

5. The answer is B [III B]. The copper IUD predominantly gets its efficacy from the spermicidal action of the copper. The IUD is as effective as a tubal ligation, does not have to be removed for 12 years, and is reversible. It is not associated with a high rate of PID.

6. The answer is C [VII B and VII C 3 a]. The progestin method is more effective in preventing pregnancy than the combination pill method. Taking both pills at once increases the efficacy; therefore, taking Plan B 150 mg at once is a better choice. The combination method is associated with severe nausea and should be used with antinausea medication. The copper IUD is even more effective than the progestin method, but it is not in the answer choices. Although RU-486 has a nearly 100% efficacy rate, it is not widely available in the United States.

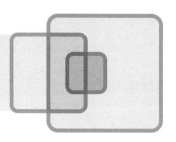

chapter 33

Sexually Transmitted Diseases

ANN HONEBRINK

I INTRODUCTION

A **Sexually transmitted diseases (STDs)** are among the oldest described conditions in medical history. References to gonorrhea can be found in the Bible. The number of protozoan, bacterial, viral, and ectoparasitic infections that have been identified as sexually transmitted has continued to increase since biblical times.

B **Control of STDs** is currently a major public health concern, especially because there is a growing appreciation that individuals infected with other STDs are more susceptible to infection with HIV. In the developed world, the United States has the highest incidence of STDs, with an estimated cost of more than $17 billion per year.

C **Evidence-based treatment and cure** is available for the majority of STDs. Currently accepted treatment regimens in the United States are based on recommended regimens published and regularly updated by the Centers for Disease Control and Prevention (CDC). Primary prevention of STDs focuses on counseling at-risk individuals in an attempt to control this major health problem. Because incidence rates of many STDs are highest among adolescents, it is essential that prevention counseling, screening, and treatment strategies include the special needs of this age group.

II BACTERIAL SEXUALLY TRANSMITTED DISEASES

A **Gonorrhea.** The cause of this STD is the Gram-negative diplococcus *Neisseria gonorrhoeae*. Humans are the only natural host of this bacterium, which has a predilection for **columnar and transitional epithelium**. In **women**, who often have mild or no symptoms, gonorrhea may cause cervicitis, urethritis, pelvic inflammatory disease (PID), and acute pharyngitis. In **men**, who are usually symptomatic, infection causes urethritis, prostatitis, and epididymitis. Systemic sequelae (see II A 2 f, g) later develop in both men and women. In **newborns**, exposure at birth may cause blindness, infection of the joints, or even serious sepsis.

1. **Epidemiology**
   a. In 2005, 339,593 cases of gonorrhea were reported to the CDC; this figure is believed to represent about half of the total infections in the United States. Infection rates have fallen since the mid-1970s but seem to have plateaued since the mid-1990s. In 2005, the rate of gonorrhea detection was 115.6 cases per 100,000 population in the United States. **Approximately 75% of reported cases occur among 15- to 29-year-old individuals**. In 2005, rates of infection were 18 times greater for African Americans than for whites.
   b. **Transmission** from men to women by sexual contact is likely to result in infection after a **single exposure. Risk factors** include:
      (1) Young age
      (2) Multiple sexual partners
      (3) Failure to use barrier contraception
      (4) Early sexual activity
2. **Clinical presentation.** In both sexes, when symptoms occur, they usually appear 2 to 5 days after exposure but may not be evident for 30 days. Although women may often be initially

asymptomatic, symptoms of gonococcal PID often occur after a menstrual period. Symptoms include:

a. Mucopurulent discharge, as occurs in acute cervicitis in women and urethritis in men

b. Lower abdominal pain, anorexia, and fever, as is characteristic of acute PID; perihepatitis can also occur because of peritoneal spread of infection.

c. Dysuria (men and women)

d. Pharyngitis (in men and women after oral contact with an infected penis)

e. Proctitis in male or female recipients of anal intercourse

f. Disseminated gonococcal infection occurs in 1% to 3% of infected patients and is more common in men than in women.

    (1) Arthritis (both tenosynovitis and purulent, mono- or polyarticular)

    (2) Pustular or vesicopustular skin lesions may accompany arthritis.

    (3) Septicemia

    (4) Endocarditis, meningitis and osteopyelitis (all rare)

g. Other sequelae

    (1) Women: increased risk of infertility, chronic pelvic pain, ectopic pregnancy

    (2) Men: risk of epididymitis with subsequent infertility and urethral scarring, chronic prostatitis

    (3) Both sexes: three to five times increased risk of acquisition of HIV infection with HIV exposure

3. Diagnosis. Exact diagnosis depends on identification of *N. gonorrhoeae* by one of several methods:

a. Thayer-Martin culture medium. This technique is selective for *N. gonorrhoeae*. Culture specimens must be incubated at 35 to 36°C in a 5% CO_2 atmosphere. This culture technique is highly sensitive and specific, inexpensive, and suitable for use for specimens taken from a variety of body sites (e.g., rectum, pharynx, cervix, and urethra). In addition, it can test for antimicrobial sensitivity. Culture is preferred for children or other individuals in which the diagnosis may have legal implications.

b. Gram stain, looking for Gram-negative diplococci in polymorphonuclear leukocytes. This test is actually useful only in male intraurethral specimens because samples from other sites may yield results that can be confused with normal flora, decreasing both sensitivity and specificity.

c. Nucleic acid amplification test (NAAT). This test, which uses nucleic acid sequences unique to a specific organism for identification, does not require viable organisms to produce a positive result. The NAAT has a sensitivity of 96.7% in endocervical specimens using culture as a standard. The NAAT can also be used on male urethral specimens and male and female urine specimens but is not reliable on pharyngeal or rectal specimens.

4. Treatment. Because coinfection with *Chlamydia trachomatis* occurs often in patients infected with *N. gonorrhoeae*, consideration should be given to treatment plans that cover both organisms, especially in populations at high risk for STDs.

a. For **uncomplicated gonococcal infection of the urethra, cervix, and rectum,** all recommended regimens involve a **single treatment**, which is important in increasing compliance. CDC-recommended regimens include:

    (1) Cephalosporins, such as cefixime 400 mg by mouth or ceftriaxone 125 mg intramuscularly. Ceftriaxone is also a recommended option for treating pharyngeal gonorrheal infection.

    (2) Quinolones, such as ciprofloxacin 500 mg orally (also recommended for pharyngeal infections), ofloxacin 400 mg orally, or levofloxacin 500 mg. Quinolones should not be used in children under 18 years of age who weigh less than 45 kg and should not be used in pregnant women. In the United States, 9.1% of gonorrhea isolates were quinolone resistant in 2005, up from 4.1% in 2003. Twenty-nine percent of isolates found as the result of homosexual male contact were resistant and resistance is higher in certain areas of the country, including Hawaii and California. This has caused the CDC to recommend that quinolones NOT be used in infected homosexual men or in infected individuals from areas where a high rate of quinolone resistance has been found.

    (3) Alternative regimen: spectinomycin 2 g intramuscularly (may be difficult to obtain)

       (4) Azithromycin 2 g orally (single dose) is also effective, but expense and gastrointestinal side effects at this dose limit use.

   b. When treating for presumed or proven coinfection with *C. trachomatis*, it is necessary to add either azithromycin 1 g orally (single dose) or doxycycline 100 mg orally twice daily for 7 days. (Doxycycline should not be used in pregnant women or in children.)

   c. More complex, inpatient treatment is required for patients with PID (see Chapter 28); infected infants; and individuals with disseminated gonorrhea, gonorrheal meningitis, or endocarditis.

5. Follow-up. As with any STD, patients with gonorrhea should be tested for other STDs, including HIV and hepatitis B. All sexual partners should also be evaluated and treated. Although tests of cure are no longer necessary when patients are treated successfully with the previously described regimens (see II A 4), tests for reinfection should be considered in individuals at high risk. When using **nucleic acid tests**, remember that the test **can remain positive for up to 3 weeks after treatment**; live organisms need not be present for a positive test. Repeat testing is also warranted in individuals with persistent symptoms.

B **Chlamydia.** *Chlamydia*, a genus of obligatory Gram-negative intracellular bacteria, is the pathogen in a broad spectrum of infections. *C. trachomatis* (serotypes B, D, E, F, G, H, I, J, and K) is the obligate intracellular bacterium that causes sexually transmitted chlamydial genital infection.

1. Epidemiology. Chlamydia is the **most commonly reported STD** in the United States; 976,445 cases were reported in 2005. Infection rates have increased from 35 per 100,000 to 332 per 100,000 from 1986 through 2005. Chlamydia is most commonly diagnosed in adolescents and young adults up to 25 years of age but can also occur in older, at-risk individuals. Detection rates in women are three times that in men, probably reflecting more aggressive screening in women. Coinfection with *N. gonorrhoeae* is common, and susceptibility to HIV infection in individuals with chlamydia is estimated to be increased three- to fivefold. Routine screening of asymptomatic, at-risk individuals has been shown to decrease occurrence of PID by up to 60%.

2. Clinical presentation

   a. Women are asymptomatic 75% of the time.

   b. In symptomatic women, **mucopurulent cervicitis** can be demonstrated.

   c. Symptoms of **urethritis** and **pyuria** and a **negative urine culture** in sexually active women suggest a chlamydial infection.

   d. Fever and **lower abdominal pain** suggest PID, which occurs in as many as 40% of women with untreated chlamydia (see Chapter 34). These infections may be more insidious and protracted in duration than those associated with gonococcal PID.

   e. Although 50% of chlamydial infections in men are asymptomatic, urethritis may occur.

   f. In exposed infants, *C. trachomatis* may cause conjunctivitis and pneumonia.

3. Diagnosis

   a. Culture. Testing should be done from the endocervix in women and urethra in men. This highly specific technique has been the gold standard for diagnosis of chlamydia and should be used in children and in other cases that have potential legal implications. Antimicrobial susceptibility testing can be performed on isolates. However, culture techniques involving tissue culture are expensive and technically challenging, and the results are difficult to standardize. All of these factors limit culture sensitivity.

   b. Nucleic acid amplification test. This sensitive test amplifies organism-specific nucleic acid sequences, most commonly using either polymerase chain reaction (PCR) or ligase chain reaction (LCR). Urine testing is possible to detect genital infection in both men and women; however, endocervical sampling in women may be more sensitive. With a sensitivity of 85% and a specificity of 99%, NAATs have become the most utilized tests for chlamydia testing. However, it should be noted that when the prevalence in a population is less than 2%, a positive test only has a positive predictive value of 63% and therefore should be interpreted with care.

4. Treatment. The therapy for PID is discussed in detail in Chapter 34. Treatment for uncomplicated cases of urethritis and cervicitis includes:

   a. Doxycycline 100 mg orally twice daily for 7 days (contraindicated in pregnancy)

   b. Azithromycin 1 g orally

   c. Ofloxacin 400 mg orally twice daily for 7 days (contraindicated in pregnancy)

    d. Erythromycin base 500 mg orally four times daily for 7 days

    e. Levofloxacin 500 mg orally for 7 days (contraindicated in pregnancy)

5. Follow-up

    a. Retesting for cure may not be necessary after treatment with single-dose azithromycin or a complete course of doxycycline. In fact, retesting using nucleic acid technology less than 3 to 6 weeks after treatment may yield false-positive results in adequately treated individuals because nucleic acid technology does not rely on live organisms to produce a positive test.

    b. However, retesting is advisable when reinfection is suspected and compliance with medication is not certain, especially in cases in which symptoms persist. Because reinfection with chlamydia is common in studies of previously infected women, the CDC recommends that rescreening be considered 3 to 4 months after treatment. In addition, test of cure at 3 or more weeks after treatment is recommended when erythromycin (commonly used in pregnancy) is used for treatment.

6. Sequelae. Complications may include PID, ectopic pregnancy, and infertility.

C Chancroid. The Gram-negative coccobacillus *Haemophilus ducreyi* causes this genital ulcerative disease.

    1. Epidemiology

        a. Chancroid is rare in the United States but common worldwide. In 1999, only 143 cases were reported in the United States, where this STD is seen most frequently in discrete outbreaks. However, it is probably underdiagnosed and underreported. Trauma facilitates entry into mucosal vulvar tissues in women. The incubation time is 3 to 5 days.

        b. Chancroid is a known cofactor in HIV transmission, and there is a high incidence of coexisting HIV infection among individuals with chancroid worldwide. Ten percent of patients in the United States with chancroid may also be infected with syphilis or herpes. Coinfection is more likely when chancroid is acquired outside the United States. Testing for HIV should be done on all persons diagnosed with chancroid.

    2. Clinical presentation. Lesions begin as small papules and progress to painful genital ulcers in 2 to 3 days. If the lesions are left untreated, buboes and inguinal ulcers may develop, accompanied by regional lymphadenopathy.

    3. Diagnosis. Culture is not widely available and is only 80% sensitive. PCR tests are being developed, but none in the United States has yet been approved by the Food and Drug Administration. Probable diagnosis is made when painful genital ulcers are present without evidence of herpes (culture) or syphilis (darkfield examination and serologic testing). Diagnosis is supported by coexisting painful inguinal adenopathy, which occurs in up to one-third of cases.

    4. Treatment. Sexual partners should receive treatment as well. Ulcers should start to improve by 3 days posttreatment and resolve by 7 days; larger ulcers may take longer to heal. Lack of response to treatment should cause reconsideration of the diagnosis. Therapeutic regimens include:

        a. Azithromycin 1 g orally

        b. Ceftriaxone 250 mg intramuscularly

        c. Ciprofloxacin 500 mg orally twice daily for 3 days

        d. Erythromycin base 500 mg orally three times daily for 7 days

D Granuloma inguinale. This genital ulcerative disease, which is also known as donovanosis, is caused by *Klebsiella granulomatis*, a Gram-negative intracellular bacterium.

    1. Epidemiology. This STD is rare in the United States, but it is endemic in some tropical areas including some parts of India, Africa, and Australia. Ulcers appear after an 8- to 80-day incubation period. Coinfection of ulcers with other STDs may occur.

    2. Clinical presentation. Affected individuals present with a painless, beefy red, friable ulcerative lesion without regional lymphadenopathy but with accompanying inguinal groin swelling caused by subcutaneous spread of granuloma. This condition may lead to lymphedema and elephantiasis of the external genitalia.

    3. Diagnosis. Culture of *C. granulomatis* is difficult. When the diagnosis is expected based on appearance of lesions, scrapings of ulcers show pathognomonic cells—mononuclear cells with inclusion cysts containing Gram-negative pleomorphic rod-like organisms, known as Donovan bodies.

4. **Treatment**. Repeat courses of treatment may be necessary. Treatment should be continued until all ulcers have completely healed. Treatment of asymptomatic sex partners is controversial. One of the following therapeutic regimens may be used:

a. **Doxycycline** 100 mg orally twice daily for at least 3 weeks
b. **Trimethoprim–sulfamethoxazole** 160 mg/800 mg orally twice daily for at least 3 weeks
c. **Ciprofloxacin** 750 mg orally twice daily for at least 3 weeks
d. **Erythromycin base** 500 mg orally four times daily for at least 3 weeks
e. **Azithromycin** 1 g orally once a week for at least 3 weeks

E **Bacterial vaginosis (BV).** This vaginal infection results from the replacement of the normal H_2O_2-producing *Lactobacillus* with high concentrations of other bacteria, such as *Gardnerella vaginalis*, *Mobiluncus*, *Bacteroides*, and *Mycoplasma*. BV is included in this chapter, but it is not considered to be a STD. BV is associated with new or multiple sexual partners but is thought to result from alteration in balance in normal flora as opposed to sexual transmission of an infectious agent.

1. **Epidemiology**. BV is the most common cause of vaginal discharge and odor, but 50% of women who meet criteria for diagnosis (see I D 2) are asymptomatic. In addition, BV has also become increasingly associated with pregnancy complications, PID, and postprocedure endometritis and cuff cellulitis.

2. **Diagnosis**. BV may be diagnosed by the use of clinical or Gram stain evidence. Clinical diagnosis requires three of the following criteria:

a. Homogenous, grayish, noninflammatory discharge that adheres to vaginal walls
b. Saline preparation of vaginal secretions that reveals squamous cells whose borders are obscured by coccobacillary forms, known as **clue cells**
c. **pH** of secretions greater than 4.5
d. Fishy odor after addition of **10% potassium hydroxide ("whiff" test)**
e. Newer DNA probe tests for *G. vaginalis* as well as card tests for elevation of pH, trimethylamine, and proline aminopeptidase may be useful for diagnosis.
f. Vaginal culture for *G. vaginalis* and Pap smears are not useful because of low sensitivity and specificity.

3. **Treatment**. Women with symptomatic disease who are not pregnant require treatment. Whether treatment in pregnant women reduces pregnancy-related complications, most notably preterm labor, remains controversial. Studies have shown a reduction in postoperative infections in women who received preoperative treatment. **Effective treatments** include the following:

a. **Metronidazole** 500 mg orally twice daily for 7 days
b. **Metronidazole gel** (0.75%) one applicator intravaginally once daily for 5 days
c. **Clindamycin** cream (2%) one applicator intravaginally at bedtime for 7 days

F **Lymphogranuloma venereum (LGV).** *C. trachomatis,* serotypes L_1, L_2, and L_3, causes LGV, producing a wide variety of local and regional ulcerations and destruction of genital tissues.

1. **Epidemiology**. LGV rarely occurs in the United States and is more frequently seen in tropical countries. It is endemic in some parts of Africa, India, Southeast Asia, and the Caribbean.

2. **Clinical presentation**. Between 34 and 21 days after exposure, primary genital ulcers appear at the site of inoculation. The lesions resolve spontaneously. Two to six weeks after this, tender, secondary unilateral inguinal or femoral adenopathy develops, which can develop into buboes and rupture. When the rectum is infected, both men and women experience proctitis with accompanying perianal inflammation and lymphatic involvement, which can lead to tertiary fistula formation and strictures. Genital elephantiasis and infertility can also occur in tertiary disease.

3. **Diagnosis**. Usually, diagnosis is made serologically or by exclusion of other causes of inguinal lymphadenopathy. **Complement fixation** is the test of choice. Titers greater than 1:64 indicate active infection. The CDC also has recently developed an accurate polymerase chain reaction assay. Culture is a difficult and therefore unreliable diagnostic tool.

4. **Treatment**
   a. **Doxycycline** 100 mg orally twice daily for 21 days
   b. **Erythromycin** 500 mg orally four times daily for 21 days
   c. **Surgical reconstruction** may be required for patients with considerable tissue destruction in the tertiary stage. Buboes may need to be incised and drained
   d. **Sexual partners** of patients diagnosed with LGV should be treated as well. If asymptomatic, partners can be treated with 1 mg azithromax or doxycycline 100 mg bid for 7 days.

III SYPHILIS

The cause of this systemic STD is the spirochete *Treponema pallidum*. It can be transmitted by direct sexual contact with an infected lesion, by contact with the infected blood, or by intrauterine transmission from mother to fetus (congenital syphilis). Syphilis has been called the "great imitator" because of its association with a variety of signs and symptoms.

A Epidemiology. With the introduction of penicillin treatment and public health programs in the 1940s, syphilis was nearly eliminated in the United States by 1957. Since then, national epidemics have occurred in a cyclic fashion every 7 to 10 years. Since reporting was initiated in 1941, the lowest rate of primary and secondary syphilis was reported in 2000. Cases have increased recently, with 8,724 new cases of primary and secondary syphilis being reported to the CDC in 2005. In 2005, the rate of congenital syphilis was 8 per 100,000 live births. The presence of syphilis increases the risk of acquiring HIV by a factor of two to five.

B Clinical presentation

1. The **initial lesion** of primary syphilis is a painless, ulcerated, hard **chancre**, usually on the external genitalia, although vaginal and cervical lesions may also be detected. Incubation time from exposure to first symptom is 10 to 90 days. The primary lesions resolve in 2 to 6 weeks.

2. In **untreated patients**, this chancre is followed in 6 weeks to 6 months by a **secondary or bacteremic stage** in which the skin and mucous membranes are affected. A **maculopapular rash** of the palms, soles, and mucous membranes occurs. **Condyloma latum** and **generalized lymphadenopathy** are seen as well. These lesions usually resolve within 2 to 6 weeks.

3. Approximately 33% of untreated patients progress to **tertiary syphilis** with **multiple organ involvement**. Endarteritis leads to aortic aneurysm and aortic insufficiency, tabes dorsalis, optic atrophy, and meningovascular syphilis, as well as gummatous lesions.

4. **Latent infection** occurs in infected individuals with no clinical manifestations of the disease. Latent infection is detected serologically and classified as **early latent** (infection of less than 1 year's duration) or **late latent** (infection of more than 1 year's duration) or latent syphilis of unknown duration.

5. Identification and treatment of pregnant women with diagnosed syphilis is the mainstay of prevention of **congenital syphilis**. Untreated congenital syphilis may cause stillbirth, nonimmune hydrops, jaundice, infant hepatosplenomegaly, and skin rash and pseudoparalysis of an arm or leg.

C Diagnosis. **Darkfield examination** of fresh specimens detects spirochetes in the primary and secondary stages of the disease. **Serologic tests** are helpful in diagnosing syphilis in patients who have progressed beyond primary disease. In the primary stage, infected individuals have not had sufficient time to mount an immune response that can be serologically detected. There are **two types of serologic tests**.

1. **Nontreponemal tests**, which are measured quantitatively in titers and usually correlate with disease activity. These tests usually become negative after treatment, but a low-level positive titer can persist for many years. A fourfold increase or decrease in titer using the same test is believed to be clinically significant. There are two nontreponemal tests:
   a. Rapid plasma reagin (**RPR**)
   b. Venereal Disease Research Laboratory (**VDRL**)

2. **Treponemal antibody tests**, which can remain positive for life. Early treatment of primary syphilis makes it more likely that treponemal antibody tests will become negative. Treponemal

antibody titers are not used to assess treatment response because they correlate poorly with disease activity. There are two treponemal antibody tests:

    a. Fluorescent treponemal antibody absorption (**FTA-ABS**)

    b. *T. pallidum* particle agglutination (**TP-PA**)

3. Both types of serologic tests should be used to diagnose syphilis because various medical conditions can cause a false-positive RPR or VDRL. When treponemal antibody testing confirms true infection, serial nontreponemal test titers are utilized to guide management.

D Treatment

1. General considerations

    a. Need for treatment. Individuals with a history of sexual contact with a person with documented syphilis, a positive darkfield examination, or a positive FTA-ABS test should be treated. Sexual contacts of patients receiving therapy should also be treated. Possible reinfection should also prompt treatment; a fourfold increase in a quantitative antitreponemal test implies reinfection.

    b. Safety of therapeutic regimens. Treatment regimens are based on duration and severity of syphilis. Alternative treatments are listed for penicillin-allergic patients, but much less objective evidence exists for optimum dosing and duration of these alternative regimens. The **Jarisch-Herxheimer reaction**, an acute febrile reaction that may be accompanied by myalgias, headache, and other systemic symptoms, can occur within 24 hours after treatment of syphilis at any stage, especially early disease.

2. Specific regimens

    a. Early disease: primary, secondary, early latent, and asymptomatic recent sexual contacts:

        (1) Benzathine penicillin G 2.4 million units intramuscularly in a single dose

        (2) Doxycycline 100 mg orally twice daily or **tetracycline** 500 mg orally four times daily for 2 weeks in nonpregnant patients with penicillin allergy

    b. Late disease: late latent or latent syphilis of unknown duration as well as tertiary syphilis (not including neurosyphilis):

        (1) Benzathine penicillin G 2.4 million units intramuscularly every week for 3 weeks

        (2) Doxycycline 100 mg orally twice daily or **tetracycline** 500 mg orally four times daily for 4 weeks in nonpregnant patients with penicillin allergy

    c. Neurosyphilis

        (1) This form of syphilis may occur at any stage of infection with *T. pallidum*. It should be suspected in patients who are HIV positive, fail initial treatment, have an initial titer in excess of 1:32, have neurologic or ophthalmic signs or symptoms, or are diagnosed with aortitis or gummas. Diagnosis is made by testing the cerebrospinal fluid (CSF).

        (2) Recommended treatment is aqueous crystalline **penicillin G** 18 to 24 million units per day, given 3 to 4 million units intravenously every 3 to 4 hours or by continuous infusion for 10 to 14 days. Alternatively, **procaine penicillin** 2.4 million units can be given once daily with **probenecid** 500 mg orally four times daily, both for 10 to 14 days. For penicillin-allergic patients, **ceftriaxone** 2 g/day, either intramuscularly or intravenously, for 10 to 14 days may be used. The use of ceftriaxone in penicillin-allergic patients is limited by the possibility of cross-allergy to cephalosporins. However, other treatment regimens have not been tested adequately for patients with neurosyphilis.

    d. Penicillin-allergic pregnant patients. These patients should undergo **skin testing** followed by **penicillin desensitization** for two reasons: tetracycline and doxycycline are contraindicated in pregnancy, and only penicillin has been proven to prevent fetal infection.

    e. Congenital syphilis

        (1) Treatment is recommended for infants who are strongly suspected of being born with syphilis because of specific abnormalities on physical examination, serum nontreponemal serologic titer four times greater than the maternal titer, positive darkfield examination of infant body fluid, or history of inadequately treated maternal syphilis.

        (2) The recommended regimen is aqueous crystalline **penicillin G** 100,000 to 150,000 units/kg/day, administered in divided doses of 50,000 units/kg intravenously every 12 hours for the first 7 days of life and every 8 hours after this for a total of 10 days. Alternatively,

procaine penicillin G 50,000 units/kg/dose, intramuscularly once daily, can be given for the first 10 days of life.

E **Follow-up**

1. Patients should be tested by VDRL or RPR at 3, 6, and 12 months. Patients with early syphilis should have a fourfold decline in titer by 3 months posttreatment. Retreatment should be considered for a fourfold increase in titer, for failure of an initial titer greater than 1:32 to decrease fourfold 12 to 14 months after treatment, or if symptoms or signs of disease occur after treatment. Close serologic follow-up is warranted in patients treated with alternative regimens.

2. All patients diagnosed with syphilis should be tested for HIV. When neurosyphilis has been diagnosed and treated, follow-up CSF examination should be performed every 6 months until the cell count is normal.

IV **VIRAL SEXUALLY TRANSMITTED DISEASES**

A **HIV.** Originally identified in 1981, this unique retrovirus is believed to be responsible for severe deficiencies in cell-mediated immunity, leading to unusual opportunistic infections, malignancy, and, eventually, death. The disease caused by HIV is known as **AIDS**. If left untreated, AIDS develops in almost all HIV-infected individuals; 87% develop AIDS within 17 years of HIV infection.

1. **Epidemiology.** In 2001, 40 million individuals were estimated to be infected with HIV worldwide, including 950,000 individuals in the United States.
   a. Exhaustive epidemiologic studies have demonstrated that male homosexuals and bisexuals, intravenous drug users, female heterosexual consorts of infected men, recipients of tainted blood or concentrated blood products, and neonates born to infected women are the predominant populations at risk. In addition, African Americans and Hispanics are more likely than Caucasians to become infected with HIV. Recent studies show that the most rapidly increasing subset of AIDS cases in the United States results from heterosexual transmission of HIV.
   b. Transmission is both horizontal and vertical. **Incubation or latency time** is between 2 months and 17 years. The **prevalence in the general population** is estimated to be 22 in 100,000. Men are affected more frequently than women, but the prevalence in women is increasing.
   c. Other STDs increase susceptibility to HIV infection in two ways.
      (1) Genital ulcers cause breaks in the mucosa and skin in areas exposed to HIV through sexual contact, facilitating entry of HIV.
      (2) Nonulcerative STDs, such as chlamydia and gonorrhea, increase the local concentration of immune system–mediated HIV target cells, such as CD4+ cells. In addition, when HIV-infected individuals have other STDs, HIV is more likely to be present in their genital secretions. These observations support the value of HIV testing whenever another STD is diagnosed, as well as contact tracing and treatment of sexual partners if STDs are diagnosed.
   d. Most HIV infections in the United States are caused by HIV type 1 (HIV-1). However, rare cases of HIV type 2 (HIV-2) have been documented in the United States. Epidemiologic risk factors for HIV-2 are a sex partner from western Africa, where HIV-2 is endemic, or a history of nonsterile injection or blood transfusion in West Africa.

2. **Clinical presentation.** Approximately 80% to 90% of infected individuals are asymptomatic carriers. The median time between infection with HIV and the development of AIDS in adults is 10 years; this period ranges from a few months to more than 17 years.
   a. **Initial exposure to HIV** results in a retroviral syndrome in about 70% of patients.
      (1) The **usual incubation period is 2 to 4 weeks**.
      (2) **Symptoms** include febrile pharyngitis, fever, sweats, myalgia, arthralgia, headache, and photophobia.
      (3) **Lymphadenopathy** is usually generalized and begins in the second week.
   b. Later, a **more severe form of the disease** may occur.
      (1) **Symptoms** are generalized lymphadenopathy, night sweats, fever, diarrhea, weight loss, and fatigue.

(2) Infections such as **herpes zoster virus** and **oral candidiasis** may occur.

(3) Within 4 to 5 years, 30% of cases progress to AIDS.

c. AIDS is the final stage in HIV infection

(1) It is manifested by **severe alterations of cell-mediated immunity** (reversal of the CD4 [helper T cell]–to–CD8 [suppressor T cell] ratio).

(2) Lymphadenopathy, Kaposi sarcoma, opportunistic infections, malaise, diarrhea, weight loss, and death result.

3. Diagnosis

a. Serologic screening with **enzyme-linked immunosorbent assay (ELISA)** for individuals at risk detects more than 95% of patients within 3 months of infection.

b. A positive ELISA is confirmed by a repeat ELISA and then a **Western blot analysis**, which is more specific.

c. Many states require pretest and posttest counseling and written informed consent for HIV testing.

d. If acute retroviral syndrome is suspected, viral load testing for HIV plasma RNA should be performed. If HIV is detected, another test should be performed for confirmation purposes. Current research suggests that early treatment at this time may be beneficial.

e. HIV screening should be offered to all people at risk, especially those seeking treatment for other STDs as well as pregnant women.

4. Treatment. Care of HIV-positive patients involves:

a. A thorough history and physical examination, including gynecologic examination and Pap smear

b. Evaluation for associated diseases, such as STDs and tuberculosis (TB)

c. Identification of patients in need of immediate medical care and antiretroviral therapy or prophylaxis for opportunistic infections

d. Determination of need for referral

e. Administration of recommended vaccines

(1) Pneumococcal

(2) Influenza

(3) Hepatitis B if susceptible

(4) Measles if needed

(5) *Haemophilus influenzae* B

f. Psychosocial and behavioral evaluation and counseling, including counseling about high-risk behaviors as well as identification of sexual partners for testing

g. Complete blood count and CD4+ T-lymphocyte count. The **CD4+ count** is the best laboratory indicator of clinical progression, and management strategies are stratified by CD4+ count. Patients with CD4+ counts greater than 500/μL are usually not clinically immunosuppressed.

h. The **purified protein derivative test** and **anergy panel** should be administered to all HIV-positive patients.

(1) HIV may cause cutaneous anergy.

(2) An area of induration larger than 5 mm in HIV-positive patients is considered indicative of TB infection. Preventive therapy with isoniazid should be considered after excluding active TB.

i. **Additional studies** may include chest radiograph, serum chemistry, antibody testing for toxoplasmosis and hepatitis B and C, and RPR.

j. **Antiretroviral therapy** may delay progression to advanced disease. Several antiretroviral agents are used for highly active antiretroviral therapy (HAART). Referral for treatment should be considered for asymptomatic patients with CD4+ counts less than 300/mm³ or symptomatic patients with CD4+ counts less than 500/mm³.

k. *Pneumocystis carinii* **pneumonia (PCP) prophylaxis** with one of the following agents should be given to patients with CD4+ counts less than 200/mm³ or with constitutional symptoms or previous PCP infection:

(1) **Trimethoprim–sulfamethoxazole** one double-strength tablet orally daily

(2) **Aerosolized pentamidine** 300 mg once a month

l. **Nutritional evaluation and counseling**

5. **Pregnancy**. HIV testing should be offered to all pregnant women, and those individuals who are HIV positive should be evaluated as previously described. Without treatment, the risk of transmission to the fetus is 15% to 25%. Breastfeeding increases transmission by an additional 12% to 14%. Neonatal transmission can be decreased to less than 2% with maternal treatment, cesarean delivery, and avoidance of breastfeeding.

B **Human papillomavirus (HPV).** The genital virus in this double-stranded DNA family is responsible for a variety of mucocutaneous genital lesions, affecting both men and women. It is also known to be associated with lower genital tract cancers, especially cervical intraepithelial neoplasia (CIN).

1. **Epidemiology**. More than 20 million people in the United States are infected with HPV. Between 50% and 75% of sexually active men and women acquire HPV at some time in their lives.
   a. The **predominant means of transmission** is through **sexual intercourse**. In women whose sexual partners have obvious genital warts, the risk of contracting warts is 60% to 85%. Incubation time is between 6 weeks and 18 months, with a mean of 3 months.
   b. Recent evidence indicates that **transmission to the fetus may occur**, occasionally causing neonatal and juvenile respiratory papillomatosis. However, the risk is low, occurring in 1 of 1000 fetuses of infected mothers. Potential routes include transplacental, intrapartum, or postnatal. The presence of HPV infection is thus not an indication for cesarean section.
   c. More than 30 types of HPV have been found in genital tract infections.
      (1) HPV types 6 and 11 are the usual causes of visible external warts.
      (2) HPV types 16, 18, 31, 33, and 35 have all been strongly associated with CIN and with external genital squamous intraepithelial neoplasia.

2. **Clinical presentation**. Genital HPV infections are frequently asymptomatic. Lesions include overt anogenital warts (condyloma acuminatum) and dysplastic lesions. Lesions can also be subclinical or latent (not visible to the naked eye). Visual inspection of overt warty disease of the lower genital tract detects obvious lesions, which are often multifocal in distribution.

3. **Diagnosis**
   a. **Direct inspection** discerns overt warts. Their nature can be confirmed by biopsy if any doubt exists.
   b. Approximately 2% to 4% of **Pap smears** demonstrate the pathognomonic cell—the koilocyte (or halo cell). This exfoliated squamous cell has a wrinkled, somewhat pyknotic nucleus surrounded by a perinuclear clear zone or halo. Pap smears with this change are designated as low-grade squamous intraepithelial lesions.
   c. **Colposcopy**, the magnified inspection of lower genital tissues after staining with a weak acetic acid solution, is helpful in detecting latent or associated precancerous lesions caused by HPV. The lesions are flat, small, and acetowhite, with vascular punctation or mosaicism. Histologically, these lesions reveal koilocytosis, acanthosis, and variable nuclear atypia.
   d. Recently, **DNA hybridization techniques** have been used not only to detect HPV, but also to ascertain viral type. Viral typing is becoming an increasingly useful tool in the evaluation of Pap smears with atypical squamous cells of undetermined significance (ASCUS).

4. **Treatment**. Even without treatment, many warts resolve. Therapy does not necessarily eradicate the virus. Treatment of visible warts is aimed at providing symptomatic relief and may reduce, but does not entirely eliminate, the ability of an infected individual to transmit HPV through sexual contact.
   a. **Patient-applied methods**
      (1) Podofilox solution or gel. Patients apply this medication to warts twice daily for 3 days followed by 4 days off for up to four cycles.
      (2) Imiquimod cream. Patients apply this medication to warts three times a week at bedtime and wash it off after 6 to 10 hours. This cream can be used for up to 16 weeks.
   b. **Provider-applied methods**
      (1) Cryotherapy with liquid nitrogen or a cryoprobe
      (2) Podophyllin resin 10% to 25%
      (3) Bichloro- or trichloroacetic acid 80% to 90%
      (4) Surgical excision or ablation

c. **Methods for HPV-related precancerous conditions**
   (1) Loop electrode excision of the transformation zone
   (2) Laser vaporization
   (3) Cryotherapy
   (4) Cone biopsy of the cervix
   (5) Surgical excision of vulvar or vaginal lesions
d. The treatment of **latent HPV infections** without dysplasia is not recommended.
e. Vaccination against several strains of HPV was introduced in the United States in 2006 and this will hopefully decrease infection and subsequent development of cervical intraepithelial neoplasia.

C **Herpes simplex virus (HSV).** HSV-2, a double-stranded DNA virus, is the predominant genital pathogen, although HSV-1 is seen in approximately 13% to 15% of herpetic genital infections. Both these viruses have an affinity for **infecting mucocutaneous tissues of the lower genital tract** and are maintained in pelvic ganglia as a latent reservoir for recurrent herpetic genital infection. Patients with active HSV infection are at increased risk for acquiring HIV when exposed.

1. **Epidemiology.** Seroprevalence studies in the United States showed that 17% of 14- to 49-year-olds tested positive for antibody to type 2 HSV. As many as 50% of affected Americans are unaware that they have HSV. The predominant mode of transmission is sexual intercourse. HSV is responsible for the highly lethal neonatal meningitis in infants delivered through an actively infected lower genital tract. The **incubation time** is between 3 and 7 days.

2. **Clinical presentation.** The most common signs of HSV are recurrent vesiculoulcerative genital lesions. Primary genital herpetic infections are both local and systemic. Vulvar paresthesia precedes the development of multiple crops of vesicular lesions.
   a. **Primary lesions** become shallow, coalescent, painful ulcers in a few days and may last for 2 to 3 weeks. These lesions may be accompanied by severe dysuria with urinary retention, mucopurulent vaginal discharge, painful inguinal adenopathy, generalized myalgias, headaches, and fever.
   b. **Recurrent lesions** are similar but less severe in intensity, duration, and systemic side effects. **Menses** and **stressful life situations** are associated with recurrent outbreaks. Up to 89% of patients have recurrent symptoms. Recurrence is more likely with HSV-2 than HSV-1 infection. Fifty percent of patients report prodromal symptoms of heaviness or tingling prior to recurrent outbreaks.
   c. Infants who come into contact with maternal active infection at birth are at risk for potentially fatal systemic infections. This situation is most likely to occur in infants born to mothers who are having their initial outbreak. When maternal active herpes infection is suspected at term or at the time of labor, cesarean section is generally used as the method of delivery.

3. **Diagnosis. Herpes cultures** obtained from the vesicular fluid or the edge of the ulcerative lesion give the best results. Cultures are also most likely to be positive early in the outbreak. **Cytologic demonstration** of multinucleated epithelial cells with intranuclear inclusions is helpful in the diagnosis. Newer PCR testing has recently been introduced and is thought to be more sensitive than culture. Type-specific antibody to HSV-1 or -2 can be tested for to determine or confirm infection history.

4. **Treatment**
   a. **Primary herpes.** One of the following regimens is appropriate:
      (1) **Acyclovir** 400 mg orally three times daily for 7 to 10 days or 200 mg orally five times daily for 7 to 10 days
      (2) **Famciclovir** 250 mg orally three times daily for 7 to 10 days
      (3) **Valacyclovir** 1 g orally twice daily for 7 to 10 days
   b. **Recurrent herpes.** One of the following regimens is appropriate.
      (1) **Acyclovir** 400 mg orally three times daily for 5 days, 200 mg orally five times daily for 5 days, or 800 mg orally two times daily for 5 days
      (2) **Famciclovir** 125 mg orally twice daily for 5 days
      (3) **Valacyclovir** 1 g orally once daily for 5 days

    c. Frequent recurrence (more than six times per year). Suppressive therapy is used to reduce recurrences by 70% to 80%. Asymptomatic shedding may also be decreased by continuous regimens. One of the following regimens is appropriate.

      (1) Acyclovir 400 mg orally twice daily

      (2) Famciclovir 250 mg orally twice daily

      (3) Valacyclovir 500 mg orally once daily or 1 g orally once daily

D Molluscum contagiosum

1. **Epidemiology.** Molluscum contagiosum is mildly contagious and is caused by a double-stranded DNA poxvirus. The incubation period is several weeks.

2. **Clinical presentation.** This virus creates small (1 to 5 mm), umbilicated papules in the cutaneous genital region of sexually active individuals. It may also affect the nongenital skin.

3. **Diagnosis.** The lesion itself is pathognomonic, but the diagnosis can be confirmed on histologic demonstration of a papule with a hyperkeratotic plug arising from an acanthotic epidermis. There are intracytoplasmic molluscum bodies noted on Wright stain.

4. **Treatment.** The disease is usually self-limited, with spontaneous resolution in 6 to 9 months. Local excision, cryotherapy, electrocautery, and laser vaporization are suitable treatment modalities to decrease the duration of symptoms.

E Hepatitis B virus (HBV)

1. **Epidemiology.** There were approximately 60,000 new infections in the United States in 2004, down from an average of 260,000 in the 1980s. However, approximately 1.25 million chronically infected individuals serve as a reservoir. In the United States, HBV is most commonly transmitted sexually. The disease can also be transmitted by exposure to infected blood. The incubation period is 6 weeks to 6 months. Fifteen to twenty-five percent of those with chronic infection die of liver disease.

2. **Clinical presentation.** HBV infection is symptomatic in adults in about 50% of cases. When symptoms are present, they include jaundice and general malaise. Only 2% to 6% of infected adults become chronically infected, but 90% of infected infants develop chronic infection.

3. **Diagnosis.** Presence of hepatitis B surface antigen (HBsAg) indicates either acute or chronic infection. Presence of hepatitis B surface antibody (anti-HBs) is indicative of immunity, either through prior infection or immunization.

4. **Treatment and prevention.** Supportive treatment is used for acute HBV infection, which is self-limited. Interferon alfa and lamivudine have been used in attempts to treat chronic hepatitis B. Vaccination is the mainstay of prevention. Hepatitis B immune globulin (HBIG) provides post-exposure prophylaxis, and the multidose hepatitis B vaccine gives longstanding immunity.

5. **Pregnancy.** All pregnant women are tested for HBsAg carrier status. When a pregnant woman is identified as a chronic carrier, fetal infection can be prevented by prompt infant immunization and HBIG administration.

V   TRICHOMONIASIS

Of all sexually transmitted protozoal infections, *Trichomonas vaginalis* infection is the most common. This protozoan is responsible for **acute vulvovaginitis.**

A Epidemiology. Approximately 5 million infections are caused by *T. vaginalis* annually in the United States. Infection with this organism accounts for nearly one-third of all office visits for infectious vulvovaginitis. Transmission of this STD is usually by sexual intercourse. Vaginal trichomoniasis has been associated with adverse pregnancy outcomes, but there is no evidence that treatment of asymptomatic women decreases these adverse events.

B Clinical presentation

1. Profuse, yellow-green, malodorous, frothy discharge of low viscosity

2. Vulvar pruritus

3. Vaginal erythema and occasional intense erythematous mottling of the cervix (**strawberry cervix**)

4. Usually asymptomatic male partner

5. Appearance of symptoms usually 5 to 28 days after exposure

6. Infected men are usually asymptomatic but may have nongonococcal urethritis.

C **Diagnosis**

1. Vaginal pH between 5 and 6

2. Inflammatory response and motile, flagellated trichomonads on wet mount preparations, best appreciated when wet mount is promptly viewed. These organisms are twice the size of leukocytes. Diagnosis on wet mount has a 60% to 70% sensitivity.

3. Cultures for *Trichomonas* are available but are usually reserved for resistant cases in which antimicrobial testing can be used.

4. Newer immunochromatic and nucleic probe tests with 83% sensitivity and 97% specificity are available. Positive results on these tests should be interpreted with caution in low prevalence populations.

D **Treatment.**   Therapy using metronidazole in either of the following regimens produces cure rates of greater than 95%. Patients should be counseled to avoid alcohol during treatment with metronidazole and tinidazole because of a possible Antabuse reaction. Sexual partners must be treated to prevent reinfection.

1. **Metronidazole** or **tinidazole** 2 g orally single dose

2. **Metronidazole** 500 mg orally twice daily for 7 days

VI   ECTOPARASITES

This group of STDs includes pediculosis pubis and scabies.

A **Pediculosis pubis** *(Phthirus pubis).*   The **crab louse** is a slow-moving insect approximately 1 mm long. It lays its eggs (**nits**) at the base of hair follicles. After 7 days, nymphs arise from the nits and progress to the adult stage in 2 to 3 weeks. Adult life expectancy of the pubic louse is 30 days.

1. **Epidemiology.** Pediculosis pubis is **highly contagious**. The crab louse can be transmitted through direct sexual contact or through fomites, such as blankets and sheets. Hard, smooth surfaces such as toilet seats are not suitable fomites for the transmission of the crab louse.

2. **Clinical presentation.** Intense vulvar pruritus secondary to an allergic sensitization is the presenting symptom.

3. **Diagnosis.** Identification of the crab louse or nits can be made with a **hand lens inspection** of the hair-bearing pubic region.

4. **Treatment.** The specific treatments listed are not recommended for use in the eye area. When eyelashes are infected, treatment involves application of an occlusive ophthalmic ointment to eyelids two times daily for 10 days. Resistance to treatment a and b below is widespread and retreatment with different agents may be necessary.
   a. **Permethrin** cream, 1%, rinse for 10 minutes
   b. **Pyrethrins with piperonyl butoxide** applied to the affected area and washed off after 10 minutes
   c. **Malathion 0.5%** lotion applied and washed off after 8 to 12 hours. Duration of treatment and odor of medication limits use to treatment failures with the above.
   d. **Ivermectin** 250 μg/kg, repeated in 2 weeks
   e. **Lindane** solution, 1%, applied to infested area for 4 minutes and then washed off. Lindane is contraindicated in pregnancy and lactation and in children less than 2 years of age. Toxicity includes seizures and aplastic anemia and has been reported when exposure exceeded 4 minutes. Use of lindane should be limited to a 4-minute exposure in nonpregnant or lactating adults weighing more than 100 lb and should be reserved for treatment failures with other medications.

    f. Cleaning of all contaminated bedding and clothing is essential. Decontamination by machine washing and heat drying or dry cleaning is warranted.

5. **Follow-up**. Infected individuals should be re-evaluated 1 week after treatment for nits or lice. Retreatment with an alternative regimen is indicated for persistent infestation. All sexual partners within the past month should be treated. Infected patients should be evaluated for other STDs.

B Scabies *(Sarcoptes scabiei).* This mite is 0.4 mm in length. Unlike the crab louse, it can be found anywhere on the skin, where it burrows a 5-mm-long tunnel to lay its eggs. Its life span is approximately 30 days.

1. **Epidemiology**. Scabies can be transmitted by close sexual contact but also by nonsexual contact, such as sharing clothing or bedding.

2. **Clinical presentation**. The predominant symptom is severe, intermittent itching. Hands, wrists, breasts, and buttocks are the most commonly affected sites. With initial infection, sensitization to scabies must occur before pruritus begins. Therefore, it can take several weeks after exposure for symptoms to develop with initial infections. Intense itching can occur within 24 hours of exposure in subsequent infections.

3. **Diagnosis**. Linear burrows are frequently seen with a hand lens. Microscopic slides prepared from scrapings of suspected lesions in mineral oil often demonstrate adult mites, eggs, and fecal pellets.

4. **Treatment**
    a. **Permethrin** cream, 5%, applied to the body from the neck down and washed off after 8 to 14 hours
    b. **Ivermectin** 200 μg/kg, given orally and repeated in 2 weeks
    c. **Lindane** solution, 1%, applied from the neck down and washed off after 8 hours (should not be applied after a bath, when extensive dermatitis is present, in pregnancy or lactation, and in children younger than 2 years of age [see VI A 4 e]). Lindane resistance has been reported in some areas of the world, including the United States. Potential for toxicity also limits its use.
    d. As with pubic lice, **cleaning of all contaminated bedding and clothing** is essential. Decontamination by machine washing and heat drying or dry cleaning is warranted. All close personal or household contacts within the preceding month should be examined and treated.

5. **Follow-up**. The rash and itching associated with scabies can persist for up to 14 days after treatment. If symptoms persist after 2 weeks, reinfection could be present and retreatment should be considered, especially if live mites are observed. Sexual partners and close personal contacts should also be examined and considered for treatment.

Study Questions for Chapter 33

Directions: *Match each description below with the causative agent. Each answer may be used once, more than once, or not at all.*

QUESTIONS 1–5

- [A] Gram-negative diplococcus
- [B] Obligatory intracellular bacteria (subtypes D through K)
- [C] Obligatory intracellular bacteria (L subtypes)
- [D] Gram-negative coccobacillus
- [E] Gram-negative associated with Donovan bodies
- [F] Many species of anaerobic bacteria
- [G] Spirochete
- [H] Retrovirus
- [I] ds-DNA virus (subtypes 6/11 and 16, 18, 35, etc.)
- [J] ds-DNA virus (subtypes 1 and 2)
- [K] ds-DNA virus (poxvirus family)
- [L] Protozoa
- [M] Ectoparasite

1. Papular rash, arthritis, and perihepatic "violin-string" adhesions

2. Vulvar ulcer, marked inguinal lymphadenopathy, diagnosis by complement fixation

3. Congenital infection consisting of nonimmune hydrops, skin rash, and hepatomegaly

4. Presence of lesion associated with prodromal symptoms

5. Vaccine currently available

Directions: *Each of the numbered items or incomplete statements in this section is followed by answers or by completions of the statement. Select the ONE lettered answer or completion that is BEST in each case.*

QUESTIONS 6–9

6. A 22-year-old nulligravid woman presents to you because of a 5-day history of frequent urination and dysuria. She was seen by a doctor 2 days ago and prescribed ampicillin. She has no remarkable medical history. She is sexually active and recently began having intercourse with a new boyfriend. She has no known drug allergies. Today her urinalysis shows the following: 2 squamous cells, 0 nitrites, 18 WBC/hpf, 0 bacteria. Her urine human chorionic gonadotropin (hCG) is negative. The next best step in management is:

- [A] Ceftriaxone
- [B] Trimethoprim–sulfamethoxazole
- [C] Spectinomycin
- [D] Azithromycin
- [E] Observation

7. A 26-year-old woman, gravida 1, para 0, at 14 weeks of gestation, presents to you because of increased vaginal discharge. You perform a wet mount and test for gonorrhea and chlamydia by NAAT. The results of NAAT are positive for chlamydia. The next step in management is (note: TOC = test of cure and RS = rescreen):

- A Azithromycin (patient and partner) + TOC 5 weeks + RS 4 months
- B Doxycycline (patient and partner) + TOC 5 weeks + RS 5 months
- C Ofloxacin (patient and partner) + TOC 4 weeks + RS 4 months
- D Erythromycin (patient and partner) + TOC 3 weeks + RS 4 months
- E Erythromycin (patient and partner) + TOC 2 weeks + RS 3 months

8. A 20-year-old presents to you with a deep, excavating, painless lesion above the clitoris, overlying the pubic bone. Her serum VDRL is positive. A lumbar puncture and analysis of her cerebrospinal fluid also yields a positive VDRL. The best term to describe her lesion is:

- A Condyloma acuminatum
- B Condyloma latum
- C Chancre
- D Gumma
- E Bubo

9. A 17-year-old adolescent presents to your office reporting intense itching "down there." You perform a wet mount and KOH prep but are unable to find anything remarkable. Examination of her pubic hair in the area of the mons with a hand lens reveals several linear lesions and adjacent erythema from self-scratching. Her pregnancy test is negative. The next best step in management is neck-down treatment with:

- A Permethrin 1% for 10 hours + clean toilet seats
- B Permethrin 5% for 10 hours + wash bed sheets
- C Permethrin 5% for 10 minutes + clean toilet seats
- D Lindane 1% for 4 minutes + wash clothing
- E Lindane 1% for 8 hours + wash bed sheets

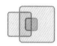

Answers and Explanations

1. **A** [II A 2 f], **2.** **C** [II F 3], **3.** **G** [II B 5], **4.** **J** [IV C 2], **5.** **I** [IV B 4]. Advanced disseminated gonococcal infection can give rise to septic arthritis, rash, and perihepatitis (or Fitz-Hugh-Curtis syndrome). The diagnosis is made by cervical culture for gonorrhea. Lymphogranuloma venereum (LGV) is caused by *Chlamydia trachomatis* serotypes L1 to L3. It consists of genital ulcers; tender, marked inguinal lymphadenopathy (causing distortion of anatomy); and fistula formation in advanced cases. Complement fixation is the test of choice. Untreated congenital syphilis may cause stillbirth, nonimmune hydrops, jaundice, hepatosplenomegaly, and skin rash. With recurrent HSV infection a prodromal paresthesia precedes the appearance of the lesion. Patients are instructed to take the antiviral medication when they notice the prodromal symptoms. A quadrivalent vaccine for HPV types 6, 11, 16, and 18 became available that offers excellent protection from these subtypes of HPV. These subtypes are responsible for the majority of cases of warts and cervical cancers attributed to the HPV virus.

6. The answer is **D** [II B 2]. Symptoms of urethritis (frequency and dysuria) and pyuria ("pus in urine" or many white blood cells in urine) with a negative urine culture in a sexually active woman suggest chlamydial infection. The treatment of choice in a nonpregnant patient is single-dose azithromax or doxycycline. Trimethoprim–sulfamethoxazole can be used for urinary tract infections, although currently it is not the treatment of choice.

7. The answer is **A** [II B 4 and 5 and II A 5]. Although the best studies of management of chlamydia during pregnancy involve an erythromycin base, azithromycin may also be used and is not contraindicated. Both doxycycline and ofloxacin are contraindicated during pregnancy because the former is similar to tetracycline and causes staining of developing teeth, and the latter interferes with cartilage development. The last two answer choices are incorrect because they both perform TOC in less than 4 weeks after treatment. Because nucleic acids test do not test for live organisms, they can remain positive for up to 3 weeks after treatment. Additionally, any treatment used during pregnancy requires TOC and RS.

8. The answer is **D** [III D 2 c]. Neurosyphilis (or tertiary syphilis) is diagnosed by ophthalmic signs in someone whose serum is VDRL positive, or in someone with gummas whose CSF tests positive for VDRL. Condyloma acuminatum (warts) is caused by HPV. Condyloma latum is indicative of secondary syphilis (not tertiary). Painless chancre is a lesion of primary syphilis. Buboes are caused by *Haemophilus ducreyi*, which causes chancroid.

9. The answer is **B** [VI B 4]. Treatment of scabies usually consists of more potent agents, longer duration of treatment, and neck-down treatment in contrast to treatment of lice. Additionally, all bedding and clothing need to be thoroughly washed and decontaminated. Flat, smooth surfaces such as toilet seats are not risk factors for acquisition of scabies or lice. Permethrin 1% is not powerful enough. Lindane 1% for 4 minutes is not long enough. Remember that a positive pregnancy test is a contraindication for treatment with lindane and toxicity limits its use in general.

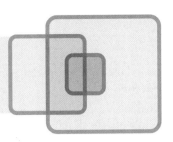

chapter **34**

Pelvic Inflammatory Disease

ANN HONEBRINK

I   INTRODUCTION

Pelvic inflammatory disease (PID) comprises a spectrum of inflammatory diseases of the upper genital tract of women. PID can involve infection of the endometrium (**endometritis**), the oviducts (**salpingitis**), the ovaries (**oophoritis**), the uterine wall (**myometritis**), or portions of the parietal peritoneum (**peritonitis**). PID is usually the result of a sexually transmitted disease (STD) and less often results from iatrogenic causes after instrumentation of the female reproductive tract.

II   DEFINITIONS

A   **Acute PID** refers to the acute symptoms accompanying ascending infection from the cervix to the endometrium, tubes, ovaries, and pelvic peritoneum.

B   **Chronic PID** refers to chronic pelvic pain, often periodic in exacerbation, that can follow an acute episode of PID, a sequela to an inflammatory response to an acute infection in the pelvis. Chronic pelvic infection can also be caused by the more rare pelvic infection with tuberculosis (TB) and actinomycosis.

C   **Silent PID** refers to asymptomatic or mildly symptomatic pelvic infection, which is usually diagnosed when the sequela of tubal damage is found at a later date.

III   EPIDEMIOLOGY

A   **Incidence.**   PID is usually a disease of young women. Peak incidence occurs in women in their late teens and early 20s. The diagnosis is made three times more often in sexually active teens than in young women aged 25 to 29.

  1. Acute PID occurs in 1% to 2% of young, sexually active women annually and is the most common serious infection in women 16 to 25 years of age. Initiation of intercourse at age 15 years results in a one in eight chance of acquiring PID.

  2. Approximately 1 million cases of acute PID occur each year in the United States.

B   **Costs**

  1. Direct and indirect costs of PID and its sequelae are estimated at $4 billion annually.

C   **Medical sequelae** develop in one in four women with acute PID.

  1. **Tubal obstruction** is a sequela of PID and leads to **infertility**. Infertility occurs after acute PID in 6% to 60% of cases, causing more than 100,000 women per year to become infertile. The risk of tubal obstruction depends on the severity and the number of episodes of infection.
      a. After one episode: 11.4%
      b. After two episodes: 23.1%
      c. After three episodes: 54.3%

  2. **Ectopic pregnancy rate** increases six- to 10-fold in women with PID. Approximately 50% of all ectopic pregnancies are thought to result from the tubal damage caused by PID.

3. **Chronic pelvic pain** develops in 20% of women with acute PID. Both chronic pelvic pain and dyspareunia can be sequelae of PID.

4. **Mortality**, although rare, does occur, particularly in neglected cases in which a **ruptured tubo-ovarian abscess** can lead to septic shock and death. In the United States, more than 150 deaths are attributed to PID annually.

D **Sexual activity.** Women who are not sexually active do not contract PID. Conversely, women who are sexually active but use no contraception contract 3.42 cases of PID per 100 woman-years. Frequent sexual activity, early onset of sexual activity, multiple sex partners, and a recent new sex partner are associated with risk for developing PID.

1. **Male condoms,** when used consistently and correctly, are very effective in preventing PID, as well as other STDs. Latex and polyurethane condoms provide greater protection than natural membrane condoms. **Female condoms** are made of polyurethane, and although little data exist regarding their use and PID, they should reduce chance of transmission of STDs and therefore PID.

2. **Oral contraceptives (OCs)** appear to protect users against PID: only 0.91 case of PID per 100 woman-years has been reported among women using the pill. This relationship between the pill and PID may be the result of sexual factors, including:
   a. Decreased menstrual flow
   b. Decreased ability of pathogenic bacteria to attach to endometrial cells
   c. Progestin-induced changes in the cervical mucus that retard the entrance of bacteria. While OC use seems to be protective against the development of PID, OC users are more likely to screen positive for chlamydia.

3. **Other barrier methods of contraception** (e.g., the diaphragm, sponge, and contraceptive foam) also protect against PID. Spermicides may also be bactericidal. However, more recent studies have shown that spermicide use may actually increase HIV transmission during vaginal intercourse. This limits enthusiasm in recommending spermicides for protection against transmission of STDs in general.

4. **Intrauterine devices (IUDs)** have been linked to an increased risk of PID (5.21 cases per 100 woman- years). Infection in this case may be related to insertion rather than a sexually transmitted infection. The risk is confounded by epidemiologic factors: the risk is lower in monogamous, healthy women and increases with a history of STD and sexual promiscuity. Also, currently utilized IUDs are associated with a lower risk than seen with older-model IUDs.

E **Prevention.** The majority of cases of PID are sexually transmitted and are theoretically preventable. Prevention efforts involve:

1. Education of both the public and providers about healthy sexual behaviors to help avoid transmission of infection

2. Screening of individuals at risk for STDs and provision of timely treatment and education to individuals who screen positive to prevent ascending infection

3. Involving male partners in screening, treatment, and prevention programs to prevent further transmission

4. Prompt treatment of PID to prevent tubal sequelae

IV BACTERIOLOGY

Acute PID is usually a **polymicrobial infection** caused by gonorrhea, chlamydia, and organisms that are considered normal flora of the cervix and vagina.

A Causative organisms

1. *Neisseria gonorrhoeae* is a Gram-negative diplococcus. Studies show it is recovered from the cervix in 27% to 80% and the fallopian tubes in 13% to 18% of women diagnosed with PID.

2. *Chlamydia trachomatis* is an obligate intracellular organism. It is recovered from the cervix in 5% to 39% and from the tubes in 0% to 10% of women diagnosed with PID. Antibodies to *C. trachomatis* are found in 20% to 40% of women with a history of PID.

3. *N. gonorrhoeae* and *C. trachomatis* coexist in the same individual in 25% to 40% of cases of PID.

4. Endogenous aerobic bacteria, such as *Escherichia coil, Gardnerella vaginalis, Streptococcus species, Proteus, Klebsiella,* and *Haemophilus influenzae*

5. Endogenous anaerobic bacteria, such as *Bacteroides, Peptostreptococcus,* and *Peptococcus*

6. *Actinomyces israelii,* which is found in 15% of IUD-associated cases of PID, particularly in unilateral abscesses. It is rarely found in women who do not use an IUD.

V PATHOPHYSIOLOGY

When PID occurs, salpingo-oophoritis is usually preceded by cervical infection with gonorrhea and/or chlamydia; infection ascends when an inciting event occurs that allows bacteria to ascend into the uterus and then into the tubal lumen, usually bilaterally. Symptomatic ascending infection follows 10% to 40% of cervical infections with gonorrhoea and chlamydia.

A Inciting events

1. **Menstrual periods**. Degenerating endometrium is a good culture medium and retrograde menstruation encourages ascending infection. In addition, cervical mucus changes during menses allow ascending infection. Two-thirds of acute PID cases begin just after menses.

2. **Sexual intercourse**. Bacteria-laden fluids may be pushed into the uterus, and uterine contractions may assist their ascent.

3. **Iatrogenic events**
   a. Elective abortion
   b. Dilation and curettage or endometrial biopsy
   c. IUD insertion or use
   d. Hysterosalpingography
   e. Chromopertubation at laparoscopy

B Chronology of salpingo-oophoritis.   Infection is usually bilateral, but unilateral infection is also possible, especially in association with an IUD. The **clinical course** is as follows:

1. **Endosalpingitis** develops initially with edema and ultimately proceeds to destruction of luminal cells, cilia, and mucosal folds. Bacterial toxins are most likely to be responsible.

2. Infection spreads to the tubal muscularis and serosa. It also spreads by direct extension to the abdominal cavity through the fimbriated end of the tube.

3. **Oophoritis** develops over the surface of the ovaries, and microabscesses may develop within the ovaries.

4. **Peritonitis** may occur, and upper abdominal infection may result either by direct extension of infection up the abdominal gutters laterally or by lymphatic spread. Development of **perihepatitis** with adhesions and right upper quadrant abdominal pain is known as **Fitz-Hugh-Curtis syndrome**.

5. **Sequelae of PID**
   a. Pyosalpinges (tubal abscesses)
   b. Hydrosalpinges (fluid-filled, dilated, thin-walled, destroyed tubes, usually totally obstructed)
   c. Partial tubal obstruction and crypt formation
   d. Total tubal obstruction and infertility
   e. Tubo-ovarian abscesses
   f. Peritubular and ovarian adhesions
   g. Dense pelvic and abdominal adhesions
   h. Ruptured abscesses, resulting in sepsis and shock
   i. Chronic pelvic pain and dyspareunia

VI DIAGNOSIS

A **Signs and symptoms of PID** are relatively nonspecific. Thus, they produce both a high false-positive rate and a high false-negative rate of diagnosis. Laparoscopic studies have revealed the inadequacy of diagnosing acute PID by means of the usual history and physical examination and laboratory

TABLE 34-1 **Laparoscopic Findings in Patients with False-Positive Clinical Diagnosis of Acute Pelvic Inflammatory Disease**

Laparoscopic Finding	Number of Patients
Acute appendicitis	24
Endometriosis	16
Corpus luteum bleeding	12
Ectopic pregnancy	11
Pelvic adhesions only	7
Benign ovarian tumor	7
Chronic salpingitis	6
Miscellaneous	15
TOTAL	98

Reprinted with permission from Jacobson LJ. Differential diagnosis of acute pelvic inflammatory disease. *Am J Obstet Gynecol* 1980;138:1007.

studies (Table 34-1). In studies using laparoscopic confirmation, the clinical diagnosis of PID only has a two-thirds positive predictive value. In order to prevent sequelae of PID, it is appropriate to maintain a high index of suspicion and low threshold for treatment once other serious causes for symptoms have been ruled out.

B **Clinical criteria for diagnosis**

1. **Minimum criteria for diagnosis**
   a. Lower abdominal tenderness
   b. Uterine or adnexal tenderness
   c. Cervical motion tenderness: lateral motion of the cervix on examination causes pain by putting tension on the adnexa.

2. **Additional criteria.** For women with severe signs, these additional criteria are used to increase the specificity of the diagnosis:
   a. Oral temperature higher than 100.9°F (38.3°C)
   b. Abnormal cervical or vaginal discharge. Mucopurulent cervical discharge with white blood cells (WBCs) seen on wet mount is almost always seen in women with PID. If this finding is not present, other diagnoses should be seriously entertained.
   c. Elevated erythrocyte sedimentation rate (ESR)
   d. Elevated C-reactive protein
   e. Positive test for gonorrhea or chlamydia
   f. Tubo-ovarian abscess seen on ultrasound
   g. Evidence of endometritis on endometrial biopsy
   h. Laparoscopic evidence of PID

C **Differential diagnosis** for PID should include:

1. Ectopic pregnancy

2. Ruptured ovarian cyst

3. Appendicitis

4. Endometriosis

5. Inflammatory bowel disease

6. Degenerating fibroids

7. Spontaneous abortion

8. Diverticulitis

D **Diagnostic techniques**

1. **Cervical Gram stain**. If Gram-negative intracellular diplococci are present, gonorrhea is the presumed diagnosis. However, Gram stain alone misses one-half of the gonorrhea cases. Chlamydia is not diagnosed on Gram stain.

2. **Serum human chorionic gonadotropin (hCG)**. A sensitive pregnancy test is important in the differential diagnosis of pelvic pain to rule out the possibility of ectopic pregnancy. Currently, serum hCG is the test of choice. In the past, approximately 3% to 4% of women admitted with the diagnosis of PID had an ectopic pregnancy.

3. **Ultrasound**. This technique may help define adnexal masses and intrauterine or ectopic pregnancies, especially when a patient has a tender abdomen that does not permit an adequate pelvic examination. This is important for detecting the presence of tubo-ovarian abscesses since antibiotic therapy protocols may be different from PID without tubo-ovarian abscesses. Response to therapy can be measured objectively as pelvic masses and induration regress.

4. **Laparoscopy**. If the disease process is unclear, this technique is the ultimate way to establish the diagnosis.

5. **Culdocentesis**. If purulent fluid is obtained, a culture may assist in antibiotic selection. However, infections may be secondary to another primary process. In addition, the pain associated with this test limits its use.

6. **Blood studies**
   a. **Leukocytosis** is not a reliable indicator of acute PID. Less than 50% of women with acute PID have a WBC count greater than 10,000 cells/mL. Also, it is nonspecific; other infectious causes of symptoms are associated with an elevated WBC count.
   b. An **increased ESR** is a nonspecific finding, but the ESR is elevated in approximately 75% of women with laparoscopically confirmed PID.

7. **Follow-up**. After initiation of appropriate treatment, clinical improvement should be observed in 48 to 72 hours. If no improvement occurs, alternative diagnoses should be considered.

8. **Testing** for HIV and assurance of current Pap smear screening should be offered to all women diagnosed with PID. Additionally, testing for syphilis and hepatitis B should be considered.

VII TREATMENT

A **Empiric treatment** of PID should be given to women with historic risk factors for PID (either sexual activity or instrumentation of the cervix and uterus) if the minimal clinical criteria are met. Treatment of the woman's partner(s) is also critical to prevent reinfection and prevent potential further spread of infection.

B **Individualized treatment** and a **high index of suspicion for infection** are mandatory. Treatment should always include sexual partners. The physician must decide between outpatient management of the woman, with close follow-up in 48 to 72 hours, or hospitalization. **Hospitalization of PID patients** and intravenous antibiotic therapy is indicated in the following scenarios:

1. Until other serious diagnoses are excluded, including appendicitis and ectopic pregnancy

2. If the patient is an adolescent

3. If a pelvic abscess is suspected on examination or ultrasound

4. Severe systemic/peritoneal symptoms including high fever, or signs of peritonitis

5. Inability to tolerate oral outpatient treatment because of vomiting

6. If the patient is pregnant

7. If the patient is unable or unlikely to comply with outpatient therapy and/or 48- to 72-hour follow-up

8. If HIV infection is present

9. If the patient has not responded to outpatient management at 48- to 72-hour follow-up

C **Oral treatment regimens** provide broad coverage for organisms frequently isolated from the genital tracts of women with PID. They are generally appropriate for women who present with milder cases of PID. Select **one** of the following three regimens:

1. **Regimen A**. Use one of the following:
   a. **Ofloxacin** 400 mg orally twice daily for 14 days *or* **levofloxacin** 500 mg orally once daily for 14 days, with or without **metronidazole** 500 mg orally twice a day for 14 days

2. **Regimen B**. Use one of the following:
   a. **Ceftriaxone** 250 mg intramuscular single dose *or* **cefoxitin** 2 g intramuscular single dose with probenecid 1 g orally at the time of injection *or* **other third-generation cephalosporin** *plus* **doxycycline** 100 orally twice daily for 14 days, with or without **metronidazole** 500 mg twice daily for 14 days

D **Parenteral regimens** are generally used in women with more severe PID. Randomized trials have demonstrated the efficacy of both oral and parenteral treatment regimens but have not compared oral and parenteral regimens objectively. Parenteral treatment is generally continued for at least 24 hours after significant clinical improvement has occurred. After this, conversion is made to an oral regimen, which is continued for an additional 10 to 14 days. Regimens are designed to cover both *N. gonorrhoeae* and *C. trachomatis* as well as other commonly isolated organisms.

1. **Regimen A**. Use one of the following:
   a. **Cefotetan** 2 g intravenously every 12 hours *or* **cefoxitin** 2 g intravenously every 6 hours
   b. Plus **doxycycline** 100 mg orally or intravenously every 12 hours. Both the oral and intravenous routes of doxycycline provide similar bioavailability, and considerable pain is usually associated with intravenous administration of doxycycline. Once parenteral therapy is discontinued, oral doxycycline should be continued for a total of 10 to 14 days. Oral clindamycin or metronidazole may be added to doxycycline if an abscess is suspected.

2. **Regimen B**. Use one of the following:
   a. **Clindamycin** 900 mg intravenously every 8 hours *plus* **gentamicin** 2 mg/kg loading dose intravenously or intramuscularly followed by 1.5 mg/kg maintenance dose every 8 hours
   b. When **conversion to oral therapy** takes place, doxycycline 100 mg twice daily or clindamycin 450 mg four times daily can be used. Clindamycin is usually the favored agent when a tubo-ovarian abscess is suspected and doxycycline is favored when chlamydia infection is suspected or confirmed on testing.

3. **Alternative regimens**. Although less data support the use of these regimens, they do have broad-spectrum coverage. Use one of the following:
   a. **Ofloxacin** 400 mg intravenously every 12 hours with or without **metronidazole** 500 mg intravenously every 12 hours
   b. **Levofloxacin** 500 mg intravenously once daily with or without **metronidazole** 500 mg intravenously every 8 hours
   c. **Ampicillin–sulbactam** 3 g intravenously every 6 hours *plus* doxycycline 100 mg intravenously or orally every 12 hours

E Treatment regimens for tubo-ovarian abscess. Since the bacterial flora in tubo-ovarian abscesses is mostly a mixture of Gram-positive, Gram-negative, and anaerobic flora, broad-spectrum antibiotics that cover these organisms should be chosen.

1. **Ampicillin** 2 g intravenously every 4 hours, *plus* **gentamicin** standard dose, *plus* **metronidazole** 500 mg intravenously every 8 hours

2. **Ofloxacin** 400 mg intravenously every 12 hours, *plus* **metronidazole** 500 mg intravenously every 8 hours

3. Single-agent therapy
   a. **Ticarcillin clavulanate** 3.1 g intravenously every 4 hours
   b. **Piperacillin-tazobactam** 4 g/0.5 g intravenously every 8 hours
   c. **Imipenem cilastatin** 500 mg intravenously every 6 hours

F Surgical intervention.   In cases of severe PID, especially when tubo-ovarian abscess is present, consideration should be given to surgical intervention if the patient's condition worsens or fails to improve after around 72 hours of treatment.

1. **Laparoscopy** may be considered for diagnosis and may be followed by laparotomy. Unless a well-defined unilateral abscess allows a unilateral salpingo-oophorectomy, the treatment of choice is a total abdominal hysterectomy, bilateral salpingo-oophorectomy, and drainage of the pelvic cavity. The patient, regardless of age, should be prepared for this possibility before surgery.

2. If an abscess is accessible, then **catheter drainage** may be possible via transvaginal, transabdominal, or transgluteal access.

VIII   **OTHER CAUSES OF PELVIC INFECTION**

A Granulomatous salpingitis

1. **Tuberculous salpingitis** almost always represents systemic TB. The incidence is high in underdeveloped countries and low in developed countries. It usually affects women in their reproductive years, but an increased incidence has been reported among postmenopausal women. Primary genital TB is extremely rare in the United States.
   a. **Physical findings** are variable. Patients usually present with adnexal masses. Induration may be noted in the paracervical, paravaginal, and parametrial tissues. The typical patient is 20 to 40 years of age with known TB and a pelvic mass. Symptoms are related to a family history of TB, low-level pelvic pain, infertility, and amenorrhea.
   b. **Pathology**. Grossly, the uterine tube has a classic "tobacco pouch" appearance—enlarged and distended. The proximal end is closed, and the fimbriae are edematous and enlarged. Microscopically, tubercles show an epithelioid reaction and giant cell formation. Inflammation and scarring are intense and irreversible.
   c. **Treatment** involves the standard regimens for disseminated TB, including isoniazid, rifampin, and ethambutol. Prognosis for cure is excellent, but the outlook for fertility is dismal.

2. **Leprous salpingitis**. The histologic picture is similar to the one for TB, and the two are often difficult to distinguish on a histologic basis. Langerhans giant cells and epithelioid cells are present. Positive cultures are necessary for a diagnosis of TB.

3. **Actinomycosis**. *Actinomycosis israelii*, the causative agent, is pathogenic for humans but not for other mammals. Most gynecologic involvement is infection secondary to appendiceal infection, gastrointestinal tract disorders, or IUD use. A total of 100 cases are reported annually, and the age range of prevalence is about 20 to 40 years.
   a. **Physical findings**. Half the lesions are bilateral and are characterized by adnexal enlargement and tenderness. Presenting symptoms may be confused with those of appendicitis.
   b. **Pathology**. Grossly, there is tubo-ovarian inflammation, as well as copious necrotic material on sections of the tube. The tubal lumen may have an adenomatous appearance. Microscopically, actinomycotic "sulfur" granules are present. Club-like filaments radiate out from the center. A monocytic infiltrate is apparent, and giant cells may be present.
   c. **Treatment**. Therapy is a prolonged course of penicillin.

4. **Schistosomiasis** occurs most commonly in the Far East and Africa.
   a. **Physical findings** are pelvic pain, menstrual irregularity, and primary infertility. The diagnosis is usually made by histopathologic findings.
   b. **Pathology**. Grossly, lesions appear as a nonspecific tubo-ovarian process. Microscopically, the ova or schistosome is seen surrounded by a granulomatous reaction with giant and epidermoid cells. An egg within an inflammatory milieu is a dramatic sight.

5. **Sarcoidosis**. Although rare, sarcoidosis can lead to a granulomatous salpingitis.

6. **Foreign body salpingitis** occurs after the use of non–water-soluble dye material for hysterosalpingography. It may also be secondary to medications placed within the vagina, such as starch, talc, and mineral oil.

B **Nongranulomatous salpingitis** refers to any other bacterial infection, usually of the peritoneal cavity, that can secondarily cause tubal infection, including:

1. Appendicitis
2. Diverticulitis
3. Crohn disease
4. Cholecystitis
5. Perinephric abscess

Study Questions for Chapter 34

Directions: *Each of the numbered items or incomplete statements in this section is followed by answers or by completions of the statement. Select the ONE lettered answer or completion that is BEST in each case.*

1. A 19-year-old woman, whose last menstrual period (LMP) was 32 days ago and who is sexually active, presents to the emergency department reporting a 5-day history of lower abdominal pain. Her vitals are as follows: T = 101°F, BP = 110/75, P = 80, R = 16. Speculum examination reveals purulent exudate at the cervical os, and there is cervical motion tenderness. Bimanual examination is unremarkable for masses but produces severe discomfort. Her quantitative serum hCG = 150 mIU/mL. Urinalysis is normal. Her WBC count is 14,000. An office ultrasound shows a normal-sized, normal-striped uterus and no adnexal masses. The next best step in management of this patient is:

- [A] Repeat serum hCG in 48 hours
- [B] Penicillin G intravenously
- [C] Ampicillin and gentamicin intravenously
- [D] Clindamycin and gentamicin intravenously
- [E] Cefazolin and doxycycline intravenously

2. The most important reason that PID must be recognized and treated promptly is prevention of:

- [A] Pelvic pain syndrome
- [B] Infertility
- [C] Ectopic pregnancy
- [D] Tubo-ovarian abscess
- [E] Pelvic adhesive disease

3. A 17-year-old woman has symptoms suggestive of pelvic inflammatory disease. However, the patient is adamant that she is a virgin. If the signs of PID are present because of inflammation involving the uterus, tubes, and ovaries, the most likely diagnosis is:

- [A] Tuberculosis
- [B] Endomyometritis
- [C] Schistosomiasis
- [D] Appendicitis
- [E] Ectopic pregnancy

QUESTIONS 4–5

A 22-year-old woman, gravida 1, para 0, total abortions 1, presents to the emergency department reporting a 6-day history of lower abdominal pain and purulent vaginal discharge. She denies past medical history or surgery. Her vitals are as follows: T = 102, BP = 118/78, P = 96, R = 14. Her abdomen is without scars, bowel sounds are present, and there is tenderness in the lower pelvic region of the abdomen. However, there is no rebound tenderness or guarding. Her speculum examination reveals white exudate at the external os of the cervix. Bimanual examination reveals severe cervical motion tenderness and uterine tenderness. There is also a fullness in the left adnexa. Her urine hCG is negative, and WBC count = 15,000.

4. The next best step in management is:

- [A] Pelvic ultrasound
- [B] Computed tomography scan
- [C] Quantitative serum β-hCG
- [D] Immediate hospitalization
- [E] Ceftriaxone intramuscularly plus doxycycline orally

5. The most important reason to admit this patient to the hospital is:

A WBC count
B Temperature
C Pelvic examination
D Age of patient
E Patient is unreliable

Answers and Explanations

1. The answer is D [VI D 2]. This patient has acute PID and she happens to be pregnant at the same time. Currently, there are no signs or risk factors for an ectopic pregnancy and with a LMP of 32 days and an hCG = 150, the pregnancy is too early to visualize on ultrasound. Intravenous clindamycin and gentamicin is an appropriate combination for parenteral treatment of PID because this patient is pregnant. This regimen provides anaerobic, aerobic, *N. gonorrhoeae*, and *C. trachomatis* coverage. Penicillin resistance is common in gonorrhea, which makes penicillin alone and the ampicillin and gentamicin combination inappropriate. The use of doxycycline is contraindicated in pregnancy because, like tetracycline, it can stain developing teeth. Resistance to second-generation cephalosporins is increasingly common in endogenous bacteria found in PID as well as gonorrhea.

2. The answer is D [III C]. Untreated PID can lead to formation of tubo-ovarian abscess. Mortality, although rare, does occur, particularly in neglected cases in which a ruptured tubo-ovarian abscess can lead to septic shock and death. In the United States, more than 150 deaths annually are attributed to PID.

3. The answer is D [VI C and Table 34-1]. Inflammation of the tubes and ovaries can be seen in conjunction with any of the conditions listed. The bacterial infection involved in appendicitis can cause secondary tubal infection and is the most likely diagnosis. Patients with false-positive diagnosis of PID were found at laparoscopy to have appendicitis (#1), endometriosis (#2), corpus luteum bleeding (#3), and ectopic pregnancy (#4). Schistosomiasis and tuberculosis are rare in the United States. Endomyometritis usually occurs postpartum, usually as a complication of cesarean section in a patient with prolonged rupture of membranes.

4. A [VI B–D], **5.** C [VI B–D]. Because this patient has symptoms and signs of PID along with an adnexal mass, the next few management steps all depend on an ultrasound examination. You must evaluate for a tubo-ovarian abscess (i.e., adnexal mass on ultrasound) before diagnosing a patient with uncomplicated PID and sending her home on oral treatment. However, if an adnexal mass is seen on ultrasound, it could be either a mass (cyst or tumor) or a tubo-ovarian abscess. Such a patient must be admitted to the hospital and placed on intravenous antibiotics. Surgical exploration should be considered if she does not respond to intravenous antibiotic therapy in 48 to 72 hours. A computed tomography scan is not as useful as an ultrasound in this situation. There is no need for a quantitative hCG when the ultra-sensitive urine hCG (which can detect as low as 5 mIU/mL) is negative. A tubo-ovarian abscess or pelvic abscess may first be appreciated on pelvic examination and can be further evaluated with an ultrasound. The history does not suggest that the patient is unreliable. The other answer choices are not criteria for hospitalization and intravenous antibiotic therapy (although some clinicians may consider her temperature as a reason to hospitalize).

chapter 35

Intimate Partner Violence and Sexual Assault

JANICE B. ASHER

I · RELATIONSHIP VIOLENCE

 Introduction. Relationship violence is the maintenance of power by one intimate partner, usually male, to control another intimate partner, usually female. The **National Center for Injury Prevention and Control (NCIPC) of the Centers for Disease Control and Prevention (CDC)** uses the broad term **intimate partner violence (IPV)** to refer to "actual or threatened physical or sexual violence or psychological and emotional abuse directed to a spouse, ex-spouse, current or former boyfriend or girlfriend, or current or former dating partner." Same-sex partners are probably at the same risk as heterosexual partners.

1. **Frequency**. At the outset, episodes of violence may occur infrequently. Subsequently, they tend to occur more often.

2. **Severity**. Episodes of violence may begin as simple verbal or emotional assaults intended to intimidate and isolate the victim and may then escalate to the intentional infliction of brutal physical injuries.

3. **Role of the physician**. Relationship violence is a major public health concern. Physicians are frequently the only professionals with whom victims of relationship violence come in contact. Physicians have both the opportunity and the responsibility to address domestic violence with all of their female patients.

4. **Public health implications**. Just as inquiry into public health issues such as smoking and alcohol is standard of care for physicians, so is screening adolescent and adult female patients for IPV.

B Epidemiology

1. The CDC reports that 1.5 million women are raped or physically abused by an intimate partner each year.

2. Overall, the lifetime incidence of relationship violence toward women is greater than 25%. More women present for medical care because of battering than the total number who present because of stranger rape, automobile accidents, and mugging.

3. Unfortunately, health care providers usually do not identify abused women, and their abuse-related symptoms are unrecognized. This is true even in cases of acute trauma. In one study, only 13% of women presenting to the emergency department for abuse-related injuries were asked about relationship violence.

C Medical evaluation

1. **Assessment**. Appropriate assessment of relationship violence is much more likely to save time and expense. The time needed to evaluate and treat abuse-related symptoms that are initially unrecognized may be considerable. Moreover, violence assessment is, in itself, a powerful intervention. By routinely asking questions about IPV, physicians are sending important messages: that IPV is common, that it is an area of medical concern, and that the victim of violence can discuss the issue with a physician.

2. **Screening**
   a. **Screening for IPV is standard of care for all adolescent and adult female patients**.
   b. Physicians should practice routine screening of all their female patients for relationship violence because the vast majority of women in abusive relationships do not spontaneously disclose that they are being abused. The primary reason that women give for not mentioning abuse is fear of retaliation by their partners who learn about the disclosure. Women also cite fear of police involvement and feelings of shame and embarrassment.
   c. Relationship violence occurs in **all racial, ethnic, religious, and socioeconomic groups**, and screening for those who fit a certain "profile" may exclude identification of some victims. Studies have shown the value of universal screening to increase the detection rate. The rate is much greater if the physician performs the screening and does not use a self-assessment tool, such as a questionnaire in an office waiting room.
   d. **It is better to inquire about specific behaviors than to use general terms, because the term** *abuse* **means different things to different people. Recommended screening questions include:**
      (1) Are you in a relationship in which you have been hit or physically threatened?
      (2) Are you in a relationship in which you have been forced to have sex?
      (3) Are you afraid of a current or ex-partner?

3. **Clinical picture**. More than 50% of abused women present with such somatic complaints as headache, abdominal pain, pelvic pain, fatigue, shortness of breath, gastrointestinal disturbances, sleep disorders, and other chronic conditions in addition to their physical injuries.

D Physician response

1. After obtaining the victim's history regarding the nature and severity of the abuse, it is important to communicate concern for the patient's safety in a nonjudgmental and compassionate way.

2. An understandable but **dangerous reaction by the physician** is to urge a patient to leave a violent relationship immediately. Abundant data indicate that abused women are most likely to be seriously injured or killed by their partners when they attempt to leave them. It is dangerous for victims to attempt to leave a relationship before they have **formulated a well-developed safety and exit plan.**

3. A physician should focus on concern for the safety of the patient and her children. Safety planning cards are available from local agencies such as women's advocacy groups.

E Documentation.   It is necessary to document patient statements regarding abuse and physical findings associated with battering as part of ensuring patient safety. Such documentation may eventually be useful in a court of law, particularly if custody issues arise. To protect the patient's confidentiality with regard to the abusive partner, documentation of abuse should not appear on the billing diagnosis if the patient's partner will receive insurance information.

1. **Document the abuse in the patient's own words**. For example, "Patient states, 'My husband, John Smith, hit me with his fists,'" is preferable to "history of trauma." Documentation should include the name of the perpetrator and nature of the weapon used. For description of injuries, dated photographs are ideal, but body maps or written descriptions are also acceptable.

2. Whenever possible, **document whether injuries appear recent or old.**

F Follow-up.   **The physician should offer a follow-up visit for the patient.** Once a victim is identified, it is important that a physician offer referral to a relationship violence expert, who may be a hospital-based or community-based social worker, a colleague who is knowledgeable about relationship violence, a local domestic violence advocacy organization, or the **National Domestic Violence Hotline** (1–800–799–SAFE).

II   VIOLENCE IN PREGNANCY

A Introduction.   Violence in pregnancy presents a unique challenge in that there are two victims: mother and fetus. Pregnancy offers physicians a tremendous opportunity for screening and intervention because of the:

      1. Increased availability of medical attention

      2. Desire of pregnant women to ensure a healthy outcome for their infants

B **Epidemiology**

      1. The leading cause of maternal mortality in pregnancy is homicide, and the most likely perpetrator is the woman's partner. More pregnant women die because of relationship violence than of any medical complication of pregnancy. The estimated incidence of relationship violence in pregnancy is 4% to 20%.

      2. Adolescents are overrepresented among abused pregnant women. As many as 29% of pregnant adolescents experience abuse, including sexual abuse and assault.

      3. The single **greatest risk factor** for relationship violence during pregnancy is a **history of violence within the year prior to the pregnancy**. In violent relationships, unintended pregnancy may in itself represent a manifestation of abuse; abused women may not be able to control sexual activity or contraceptive use. Similarly, because abused women cannot necessarily practice "safe" sex, they are also at increased risk for sexually transmitted infections (STDs) during pregnancy.

      4. Several studies have concluded that **violence during the postpartum period is even more common** than during pregnancy. In one study, 90% of women who were battered during pregnancy were abused by their partners within 3 months of delivery.

C **Obstetric complications associated with violence.** Pregnant women in abusive relationships may have limited access to medical care, medications, or even food. Several studies have found that abused pregnant women entered prenatal care significantly later than nonabused pregnant women; restricted access to medical care may explain this result.

      1. An increased incidence of premature delivery, low birth weight, abdominal and vulvar trauma, cesarean section, and pyelonephritis may occur in women who suffer violence during pregnancy.

      2. Abdominal trauma may cause injury to the mother but may also result in serious harm to the fetus, including fetal fractures, dermal scars, and even death.

III   SEXUAL ASSAULT

A **Introduction**

      1. Sexual assault is a form of sexual activity that occurs without the consent of the victim and includes the use of force, implied force, or deception on the part of the assailant.

      2. Physicians play a crucial role in the 48 hours after an assault occurs; they must collect and document evidence properly for use by the police and the courts. Because only a small percentage of women receive emergency medical care or file a police report immediately after an assault, physicians must screen patients for a history of sexual assault to manage symptoms appropriately and to help patients receive aid for potentially devastating emotional sequelae.

      3. Rape may be **broadly defined** as a form of sexual assault in which a bodily orifice is penetrated without consent by a genital organ or object wielded by another person. However, rape may be defined in different ways in various states and countries. For example, some jurisdictions include male rape whereas others (including the FBI) do not.

B **Epidemiology.** Sexual assault is the fastest growing crime in the United States. Of the approximately 1 million sexual assaults that occur each year, two-thirds of incidents are not reported to the police, and two-thirds of these acts are committed by a perpetrator known to the victim. Approximately 25% of females have been victims of sexual assault prior to 18 years of age.

C **Forensic evaluation.** The physical examination has two purposes: **to evaluate injuries and to collect evidence**.

      1. Only trained health care professionals should undertake evidence collection after sexual assault. Improperly collected and poorly handled evidence may negatively affect a victim's criminal case.

         a. If evidence is collected at the clinic site, it is of utmost importance that a chain of custody be established. All evidence must be collected securely, labeled, and sealed, and the physician responsible must know the location of the collected evidence or "rape kit" at all times.

    b. If an appropriately trained clinician is unavailable, or in the absence of an emergency department protocol, referrals to an established sexual assault center, which are designated in most large cities, should be made.

  2. Photographs of external gynecologic injuries should be taken using a 35-mm camera, if possible. Smaller, less obvious contusions, abrasions, and tears are better captured through colposcopic imaging.

D **Documentation.** Medical documentation is an important forensic component in the management of a victim of a violent crime. Because medical documents are considered legal documents, the degree to which the physician accurately describes the care rendered may greatly affect a victim's legal case. The likelihood of rape charges and a resulting conviction are directly related to documentation of injuries.

E **STD evaluation and prophylaxis.** The estimated incidence of STDs resulting from rape is 3.6% to 30%.

  1. Specimens from appropriate sites should be obtained to check for **gonorrhea** (*Neisseria gonorrhoeae*) and **chlamydia** (*Chlamydia trachomatis*). The patient should be offered presumptive treatment for chlamydia and gonorrhea.

  2. Visible vesicles or ulcers may be cultured for **herpes**.

  3. A wet mount of vaginal secretions can be examined for ***Trichomonas*** (as well as for sperm). The absence of sperm does not mean that rape has not occurred. The act of rape is one of forced sexual contact, not necessarily ejaculation.

  4. The patient needs to be advised that seroconversion for **syphilis** and **hepatitis B** takes 6 weeks. All patients who have not received the hepatitis B vaccine should be offered vaccination. **HIV** testing may also be performed at 6 weeks but should be repeated at 3 and 6 months. HIV prophylaxis should be discussed with the patient.

F **Pregnancy evaluation and prophylaxis**

  1. All female rape victims should undergo baseline pregnancy testing and be offered emergency contraception (often referred to as "the morning-after pill"). Emergency contraception greatly reduces the risk of pregnancy when used within 72 hours after intercourse. It may have some effectiveness as long as 5 days after intercourse. Progesterone-only emergency contraception, which has recently become available, is more efficacious and has fewer side effects than estrogen–progesterone preparations.

  2. The only absolute contraindication to emergency contraception is current pregnancy. Physicians may safely offer emergency contraception to women who would not ordinarily be considered good candidates for oral contraception because of concurrent medical problems. Most of the approximately 22,000 pregnancies per year in the United States that result from rape could be prevented if all women who had been raped received emergency contraception within 72 hours of the assault.

G **Follow-up**

  1. In addition to collaborating with the local police, physicians should also offer to refer victims of rape to local victim advocacy agencies, including domestic violence and rape advocacy resources. When available and appropriate, victims' advocates should be present during the initial assault history and during the evidence collection procedure. The additional support offered by these specially trained advocates assists victims during the initial aftermath of the assault and during the longer recovery period.

  2. **Psychological sequelae of rape** may be evident as long as 15 years after the assault. These sequelae include some or all of the features of **posttraumatic stress disorder**, which is chiefly characterized by four symptoms:
    a. Involuntary re-experiencing of the traumatic event through thoughts, nightmares, or flashbacks
    b. Avoidance of activities, including those that were previously pleasurable
    c. Avoidance of circumstances in which the rape occurred

d. A state of increased psychomotor arousal, which may be associated with sleep disturbances and panic attacks

IV ACQUAINTANCE RAPE AND DATING VIOLENCE

A Introduction. Adolescents and young adults are more likely to be victims of sexual assault than women in all other age groups. The prevalence of date rape ranges from 13% to 27% among college women and 20% to 68% among the general adolescent population. In one study, 41% of the women who had been raped stated that they were virgins at the time of the assault.

B Epidemiology. Rape statistics are difficult to obtain because of overall underreporting of sexual assault; it is not surprising that data about the incidence of acquaintance rape are limited.

1. **Association with drugs and alcohol**
   a. As many as 73% of assailants and 55% of victims have used alcohol or drugs immediately before the episode of sexual assault. Alcohol is a disinhibitor, but in itself, it does not cause violence.
   b. Drugs besides alcohol are rapidly gaining prominence in sexual assaults. These include flunitrazepam (Rohypnol), a fast-acting benzodiazepine; ketamine; and γ-hydroxybutyrate and its congeners.
      (1) These drugs are added to the intended victim's drink without her knowledge or consent. In addition to causing disinhibition, one of the effects of such drugs is anterograde amnesia, which makes it difficult to obtain a history of the event.
      (2) Use of these drugs, which may cause symptoms similar to those of alcohol, should be suspected. Certain protocols exist in many emergency departments for urine or blood sample collection to test for the presence of such drugs. In the absence of protocols, the drug manufacturers can be contacted.

2. **Social and cultural factors.** Many cultural stereotypes and values support the notion that date rape simply does not exist or that, if it does, it is justifiable under a variety of circumstances.
   a. The perpetrator (and for that matter the victim) may have grown up in a family, peer group, or culture in which sexual aggression is part of the definition of manhood. Most perpetrators do not consider forceful or coercive sex in the context of a date to be rape.
   b. Many men, as well as women, believe that women are "supposed" to refuse sex and that men are "supposed" to pressure, coerce, or even force them.
   c. Whereas female victims tend to be blamed if they have used alcohol ("it was her own fault") and may even blame themselves, male perpetrators are more likely to be excused ("he would never do that when he's sober").

C Medical evaluation

1. As with other types of rape, the approach to acquaintance rape should include identification and treatment of injuries; prevention of STDs and pregnancy; psychological assessment with appropriate referral for counseling; and, if the patient consents, collection of forensic evidence if the assault has occurred within 72 hours.

2. It is important for the physician to ascertain the victim's level of safety. As in other types of assault in which the victim knows the perpetrator, there may be a high risk of retaliation against the victim for seeking medical care. It is mandatory to review a safety plan with the victim prior to discharge.

D Physician response. The importance of psychological support cannot be overemphasized. The victim is likely to feel traumatized and even ashamed.

1. A compassionate, nonjudgmental response is crucial in helping the victim of rape begin the process of psychological healing.

2. It is crucial to help the patient understand that while she needs to know how to ensure her personal safety as much as possible, she is in no way to blame for a sexual assault. That responsibility rests solely with the perpetrator.

3. It is important to stress to a patient that she can minimize the risk of being the victim of acquaintance rape by not drinking excessive alcohol or by not going to a secluded place with a date. That is by no means the same as saying that if she does not practice these risk reduction behaviors, she is to blame for a rape. The responsibility for a crime always rests with the perpetrator.

E **Prevention.**   The possibility of dating violence, particularly in the context of drugs and alcohol, should be included in routine visits with adolescent patients. This discussion should also include information about STDs, emergency contraception, and long-term contraception. According to the Council on Child and Adolescent Health, such preventive counseling is particularly important at the precollege visit.

Study Questions for Chapter 35

Directions: *Each of the numbered items or incomplete statements in this section is followed by answers or by completions of the statement. Select the ONE lettered answer or completion that is BEST in each case.*

1. A married, 26-year-old woman, gravida 4, para 3, at 30 weeks of gestation, presents to you for routine prenatal care. Her medical history is remarkable for active hepatitis B and moderate asthma. She had an appendectomy 4 years ago. She has no known drug allergies. All of her prenatal labs are in order. Upon measuring her fundus, you notice several bruises in the shape of a long cylindric object on her shins and thighs. What is the best opening question to address relationship violence?

- A "When did your husband beat you?"
- B "Did your husband use a broomstick to beat you?"
- C "Are you afraid of your husband?"
- D "Is your husband physically abusing you with different objects around the house?"
- E "Is your relationship with your husband one that makes you want to hide from him?"

2. A 27-year-old woman, gravida 3, para 2, spontaneous abortions 1, has been beaten many times by her husband. She wants help, but she has not told anyone about what has been happening. The most likely reason that she has not told the physician is:

- A She does not want to talk about the issue
- B She is afraid of breaking up her family
- C It is not a medical problem
- D She is afraid of retaliation by the partner, especially on the children
- E She has deep-rooted masochistic tendencies

3. A woman discloses to her physician that her husband beats her when he is drunk and that she is afraid of him. The physician's main role is to:

- A Help the patient understand why she must leave the relationship immediately
- B Accept that this is a personal issue and not interfere
- C Report the abuse to the National Center for Injury Prevention and Control
- D Involve a social worker
- E Focus on patient safety issues, such as exit plans and copies of important documents

4. Intimate partner violence significantly increases in incidence:

- A After the first year of marriage
- B Shortly after the birth of an infant
- C After one partner retires
- D After a couple's children have left the home
- E In a household where one partner is a homemaker and the other the provider

Answers and Explanations

1. The answer is C [I C 2 c]. The best opening question is the one that is the most general but at the same time addresses the question of domestic violence. Answer choices A, B, and D are too specific and assume too much. Answer choice E is not bad but is not as broad and appropriate as C. All of the following would be good opening questions: (1) Are you afraid of a current or ex-partner? (2) Are you in a relationship in which you have been forced to have sex? (3) Are you in a relationship in which you have been hit or physically abused?

2. The answer is D [I C 2]. A woman fears retaliation by the abusive partner if the partner finds out that she has disclosed the abuse. Abused women are more likely to disclose the abuse to their physicians than to anyone else—but only when asked. The most common reasons women give for staying in abusive relationships are fear of increased violence to themselves and their children if they leave and a lack of safe, affordable housing. A masochistic desire for pain and punishment is unusual. Only two states have mandated reporting laws related to the abuse of competent adults.

3. The answer is E [I D]. Urging a patient to leave a violent relationship immediately, before she has a well-developed safety plan, is fraught with danger for both herself and her children. Physicians should consider domestic violence and its consequences a medical issue of great importance. Details of the abuse should be documented, but the abuse should not be noted in the billing diagnosis if the abusive partner receives billing or insurance-related information. Passing off the patient, to the NCIPC or a social worker, is not the primary role of the physician. Consultation with a social worker can be done after establishing a solid patient–physician relationship and after safety issues have been discussed.

4. The answer is B [II B 4]. The incidence of intimate partner violence is particularly high in the post-partum period. Other life events, such as marriage and retirement, are not associated with an increase in domestic violence. There is an increased incidence of violence when there is a short interpregnancy interval, not when children leave the home. In a homemaker–provider household there may be increased violence depending on the sex of the homemaker and provider, but this is not as significant as the increase in domestic violence in the postpartum period.

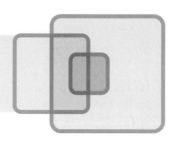

chapter 36

Benign Breast Disease

DAHLIA M. SATALOFF

I **INTRODUCTION**

Most women who present with breast pain, nipple discharge, or breast masses are primarily concerned about the possibility of breast cancer. A careful, thorough history and physical examination are essential to evaluate these conditions. The role of the health care provider must include not only providing evaluation and treatment, but also appropriately communicating the findings and treatment plan to the patient. This includes ensuring that the patient's questions and concerns are addressed. Documentation of these discussions is important.

A **History.** Pertinent aspects of the patient's history include age; age at menarche; parity, including age at first delivery; menopausal status; use and duration of hormone replacement therapy (HRT); history of prior breast biopsy including whether or not atypia was present; personal and family history of cancer, particularly breast (unilateral or bilateral) and ovarian cancer, including age at diagnosis. Paternal family history is equally important to maternal, as breast cancer genetic mutations are autosomal dominant and can be passed down through either side of the family.

B **Physical examination.** Particular attention should be paid not only to palpable lumps, but also to skin changes (such as **dimpling or retraction**) and nipple changes (such as **flattening of the nipple–areolar complex** or **excoriation**). Size discrepancies between the breasts should also be noted. Therefore, it is important to examine the breast in the sitting as well as the supine position. Lymph node–bearing areas in the supraclavicular and axillary regions should be palpated. If clinical evaluation is at all unclear, women should be referred to a breast surgeon.

C **Clinical findings.** Women with benign breast conditions generally present with one of three signs or symptoms: **breast pain, nipple discharge**, or **breast mass**.

II **BREAST PAIN**

Women commonly seek advice from physicians for breast pain (also known as **mastalgia** or **mastodynia**). Breast pain most often occurs in women in the reproductive years (i.e., before menopause). Breast pain is usually associated with benign disease, but that is not uniformly true. Breast cancers can occasionally present with localized pain. The most important aspect of management of breast pain is to rule out an underlying serious abnormality. A careful history and physical examination as well as imaging studies (mammogram or ultrasound) should be performed.

A Types of breast pain

1. **Cyclic mastalgia.** Symptoms of breast pain often occur during the premenstrual or menstrual phases of the menstrual cycle. Pain is usually bilateral but can be unilateral.
   a. **Etiology.** Although this cyclic pattern suggests hormonal involvement, no laboratory tests have confirmed that hormonal variation plays a causal role.
   b. **Treatment**
      (1) **Analgesics**, especially nonsteroidal anti-inflammatory drugs (NSAIDs), are useful in many patients.
      (2) Vitamin E supplementation and a reduction or elimination of caffeine consumption is commonly suggested, and often helpful, although there are no randomized trials demonstrating benefit.

(3) Evening primrose oil has been used with some success.

(4) Danazol (Danocrine) should be reserved for only the most severe cases because of its marked side effect profile (androgenic symptoms such as hirsutism, male pattern baldness, and deepening of the voice) and inconsistent success in reducing symptoms.

(5) Bromocriptine (Parlodel) is also of limited usefulness because of its inconsistent efficacy and potential negative side effects.

(6) Tamoxifen has been used with minimal success; the long-term consequences of its use for breast pain are not clear.

2. Noncyclic mastalgia. This breast pain does not vary with the menstrual cycle.

    a. Etiology. Common noncyclic causes of breast pain are chest wall pain, including costochondritis; trauma; and fibrocystic change.

    b. Treatment. In postmenopausal women who take HRT, reducing the amount of estrogen or discontinuing HRT often remedies breast pain. If the pain is musculoskeletal, a short course of anti-inflammatory agents is indicated. The treatments for cyclical mastalgia (see above) can also be effective in this setting.

3. Breast pain associated with cancer. This type of breast pain is uncommon, and it is more likely to be unilateral and localized.

III   NIPPLE DISCHARGE

A Approximately 3% to 10% of breast complaints involve nipple discharge.

B Etiology. Most nipple discharge is due to a benign cause. The history should include the color of the discharge, whether or not it is spontaneous or elicited, bilateral or unilateral, multiduct or single duct. Physical examination should ascertain the trigger point for the discharge, and whether or not there is an associated mass.

1. Galactorrhea (milky secretions in a woman who is not breastfeeding) is a common cause of noncancerous nipple discharge. It is usually bilateral and multiductal. It is caused by excess production of prolactin due to a pituitary adenoma (prolactinoma) or as a side effect from psychotropic medications (phenothiazines, tricyclic antidepressants) or oral contraceptives.

C Appearance and types of discharge

1. Nipple discharge can be milky, clear, serous, green, purulent, or bloody.

2. Nipple discharge that is surgically significant is unilateral, single duct, and spontaneous. These are usually caused by benign intraductal papillomas, but 10% may be caused by a malignancy.

3. Nipple discharge associated with malignancy can be bloody or clear, is more commonly associated with a mass, and is usually seen in older women.

D Evaluation and treatment

1. Prolactin and thyroid-stimulating hormone (TSH) levels should be evaluated.

    a. Prolactinomas are common benign tumors in the anterior pituitary that produce prolactin. High levels of prolactin are associated with galactorrhea and also menstrual disturbance or amenorrhea in reproductive-aged women. Microadenomas (tumor less than 10 mm) are the most common and are usually associated with an elevated prolactin level. A prolactin level of over 100 ng/mL is usually associated with a pituitary macroadenoma (a tumor greater than or equal to 10 mm). Magnetic resonance imaging (MRI) is recommended to evaluate the pituitary gland when the prolactin level is elevated.

    b. Hypothyroidism causes increased production of prolactin from the anterior pituitary through stimulation by thyroid-releasing hormone (TRH) from the hypothalamus. If the TSH is in the normal range (0.4 to 5 mU/L), then hypothyroidism is not the cause of galactorrhea.

2. A careful evaluation of the patient's **medications** and the side effect profile of each medication is necessary. If the prolactin level is high (or normal), either substituting a drug that does not induce galactorrhea or discontinuing a medication that may be causing galactorrhea should be attempted, if possible.

3. If galactorrhea is not the result of thyroid disease or pituitary adenoma, galactorrhea may respond to treatment with either bromocriptine or cabergoline.

4. The nipple discharge should be tested for the presence of blood (guaiac testing) and if positive, a specimen should be sent for cytology to look for papillary cells.

5. All patients should have a mammogram (usually normal in this setting) and an ultrasound to evaluate the retroareolar ducts for dilation and the presence of an intraductal mass.

6. Patients who give a convincing history of nipple discharge but in whom it cannot be elicited on physical examination should be evaluated radiographically (mammogram and ultrasound). If these studies are normal, consideration should be given to obtaining a breast MRI scan. If that is also normal, patients can be followed. Breast surgical consultation is also advisable.

IV BREAST MASS

Most breast masses are benign. They can be cystic (fluid filled) or solid.

A **Benign breast masses** are more likely to be soft or cystic, have regular borders, and be freely mobile.

B **Malignant breast masses** often exhibit distinct, irregular, and hard edges, but can present with fullness rather than a discreet mass.

C Types of breast masses

1. **Fibrocystic disease or fibrocystic change** (currently the preferred term for this condition). The greatest incidence of fibrocystic change is seen in premenopausal women.
   a. **Clinical manifestations.** Fibrocystic change is characterized by palpable areas of fibrosis and cysts within the breast. Although fibrocystic change was once thought to be a precursor of carcinoma, this belief has been dispelled in the literature. The only risk associated with fibrocystic change is the difficulty that may occur on clinical examination, because carcinomatous lesions may be more difficult to distinguish from the surrounding tissue.
   b. **Treatment.** The most important aspect of treatment is accurate diagnosis. Physical examination and imaging studies should be performed. Repeat examination after the menstrual period can be considered. If questions still exist as to the etiology of the abnormality, breast surgical consultation is advisable.

2. **Cysts.** Cysts are commonly seen in women in the perimenopausal age group.
   a. **Clinical manifestations.** On clinical examination, cysts generally feel rubbery, firm, round, and distinct. Cysts can be tender, especially at the time of menses.
   b. **Evaluation and treatment.** When a suspected breast cyst is palpated on clinical examination, cyst aspiration or ultrasound should be performed to confirm the diagnosis.
      (1) **Aspiration.** Aspiration of a cyst is indicated to establish that a mass is truly a cyst or to relieve pain.
         (a) Fluid aspirated from a benign cyst is likely to be **straw colored or green**. If such fluid is obtained, it **does not require submission** for cytologic evaluation. However, if the fluid obtained is **bloody**, the possibility of carcinoma increases, and the fluid **must be sent for cytopathologic evaluation**. Fluid should also be sent if the lesion does not completely disappear on aspiration (a partially cystic, partially solid mass).
         (b) If the cyst recurs, a second aspiration may be attempted. In this instance, the fluid should be sent for cytologic evaluation. If the cyst recurs a third time, however, surgical removal is recommended. If a clinically suspected breast cyst does not yield fluid on aspiration, then the lesion should be evaluated as a solid breast mass. Imaging studies and a biopsy (fine needle aspiration, core biopsy, or surgical excision) should be obtained.
      (2) **Ultrasound.** Ultrasonic evaluation is useful to confirm that a palpable lesion is cystic or solid.
      (3) **Mammography.** Mammography should be considered if a breast mass is found or if a cystic-appearing lesion yields no fluid on aspiration and is not cystic on ultrasound.

3. **Fibroadenoma**. These benign lesions, most common among women in their 20s and 30s, are well-circumscribed, smooth, freely movable, and distinct. Biopsy is mandatory to rule out carcinoma, even if the clinical appearance is consistent with a fibroadenoma. The clinical impression must be confirmed pathologically. Biopsy can be done by fine needle aspiration cytology, core biopsy, or excisional biopsy.

4. **Sclerosing adenosis**. Sclerosing adenosis is a type of fibrocystic change. This condition is benign, but biopsy is required to distinguish it from carcinoma.

5. **Fat necrosis**. This condition is often identified as an irregular, tender firm mass, without increase in size over time. The cause of fat necrosis is trauma (usually direct injury to the breast). Fat necrosis may mimic carcinoma on mammography and physical examination. Surgical excision may be required to confirm diagnosis.

6. **Mondor disease**. This disease represents thrombophlebitis of the thoracoepigastric vein. This condition can follow trauma (including surgery) or can be idiopathic. The physical examination shows a vertically oriented, often tender cord along the breast, best seen with the patient's arm raised. The condition is benign and self-limited, although treatment with heat and analgesics is helpful.

7. **Duct ectasia**. This condition is seen primarily in perimenopausal and postmenopausal women. Patients report burning, itching, or existence of a pulling sensation in the nipple area, with or without a thick, whitish nipple discharge. In most cases, this condition is benign, but further evaluation is necessary.

Study Questions for Chapter 36

Directions: *Each of the numbered items or incomplete statements in this section is followed by answers or by completions of the statement. Select the ONE lettered answer or completion that is BEST in each case.*

1. A 36-year-old woman, gravida 4, para 4, presents to your clinic because she has had bilateral white-colored nipple discharge for the last 3 months. She breastfed her last baby, but that ended almost 2 years ago. She has no past medical history other than depression, for which she takes a tricyclic anti-depressant. She is married and uses birth control pills for contraception. She has no known drug allergies. Examination of the breasts reveals no discrete masses. When the nipple discharge is placed on a slide and viewed under a light microscope, fat globules are seen that are reminiscent of milk. Which of the following is the next best step in management?

- [A] Obtain a prolactin level
- [B] Schedule a follow-up in 6 weeks
- [C] Collect discharge for cytopathology
- [D] Discontinue antidepressant
- [E] Substitute nonhormonal method of contraception

2. A 30-year-old woman, gravida 2, para 2, presents to your office reporting a mass in her right breast that she just noticed on breast self-examination. She has no medical problems. There is no history of breast or ovarian cancer in her family. Her examination is notable for a 2-cm mass in her right breast that is smooth, mobile, and nontender. Your next step is:

- [A] Reassure her that the mass is benign
- [B] Recommend vitamin E
- [C] Obtain an ultrasound of the mass
- [D] Refer her to a breast surgeon for excision of the mass
- [E] Recommend a mammogram

3. A 60-year-old woman, gravida 3, para 2, spontaneous abortions 1, presents to your clinic reporting brownish red-colored discharge from her left nipple. Her past medical history and medications, respectively, are as follows: diabetes, oral hypoglycemic; hypertension, angiotensin-converting enzyme inhibitor; and major depression, fluoxetine. She is also taking conjugated estrogen with medroxyprogesterone acetate daily. She is allergic to penicillin. She says her mother was diagnosed with ovarian cancer at age 71. What is the next best step in management?

- [A] Mammogram
- [B] Fine needle aspiration (FNA)
- [C] Referral to breast surgeon
- [D] Cessation of hormone replacement therapy
- [E] Ultrasound

4. A 28-year-old woman, gravida 2, para 2, who delivered a healthy female infant 10 days ago, comes to labor and delivery because of a tender breast mass on the right. She is breastfeeding exclusively. On examination of her breasts you note bilateral mild engorgement of the breasts and a tender, firm, linear, and slightly erythematous cord in the lateral aspect of her right breast. What is the next best step in management?

- [A] Observation
- [B] Heat compresses
- [C] Mammogram
- [D] Biopsy
- [E] Dicloxacillin

Answers and Explanations

1. The answer is A [III B–D]. Although a likely cause of this patient's galactorrhea is medication related, it is appropriate to first rule out a pituitary adenoma by checking a prolactin level and, if the level is significantly elevated, then obtaining an MRI to look for an adenoma. Tricyclic antidepressants are associated with elevated prolactin levels, but the MRI will reveal a normal pituitary gland. If a pituitary adenoma is ruled out, then consideration can be made to change the antidepressant to see if the galactorrhea resolves. However, if the depression is difficult to treat, continuing therapy and "living with" the galactorrhea is also an option. There is no need to stop the hormonal contraception at this point. Sending the nipple smear for cytology is not necessary since no red blood cells were seen.

2. The answer is C [IV B 2 b–d]. Although the mass has benign characteristics, it should be fully evaluated. An ultrasound of the mass would be the first step in evaluation. If the lesion is cystic, then aspiration would be indicated. If the lesion is solid, then a mammogram should be considered. Just reassuring the patient that the mass is benign is not appropriate. Vitamin E is a treatment for fibrocystic changes but not a discrete mass.

3. The answer is E [III D]. The first step in management of any breast complaint is a clinical examination of the breast; however, a definitive diagnosis must be obtained, especially since the age of the patient and the bloody nature of the discharge place her at a higher risk of having a malignant breast lesion. The first step is obtaining a mammogram. An ultrasound could be considered if a mass is seen on mammogram. This patient should then be referred to a breast surgeon for further evaluation and probable biopsy. Cessation of hormone replacement therapy should be considered until definitive diagnosis of the condition is made.

4. The answer is B [III D 2–6]. The most likely diagnosis is Mondor disease, or superficial thrombophlebitis of the right thoracoepigastric vein. The other consideration is mastitis commonly seen in lactating women. The key here is the linear tender mass. The best treatment is heat and analgesia. Antibiotics are not necessary because the condition is self-limited. Observation without offering a helpful suggestion is not appropriate.

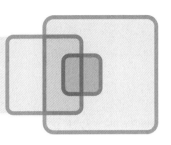

chapter 37

Vulvovaginitis

MICHELLE VICHNIN

INTRODUCTION

Vulvovaginitis is one of the most commonly seen gynecologic problems. A broad spectrum of disorders can produce vulvovaginal symptoms.

VULVOVAGINAL ANATOMY

A **Vulva.** The vulva is made up of the **mons pubis, labia majora and minora, clitoris, and vestibule**; it contains the urinary meatus, vaginal orifice, Bartholin glands (major vestibular glands), ducts of the Skene glands, and minor vestibular glands (Fig. 37-1). The vulva is subject to any conditions that may affect the skin and related structures, including psoriasis, hypersensitivity reactions, and benign and malignant neoplasms.

1. **Anatomy**
   a. The entire vulva is covered by a **keratinized** squamous epithelium.
   b. Hair-bearing regions contain associated hair follicles, sebaceous glands, and apocrine and eccrine sweat glands.
   c. Regions without hair, such as the labia minora and prepuce, contain sebaceous glands but not hair follicles or eccrine and apocrine sweat glands.
   d. The **labia majora** are composed of skin enclosing a variable amount of fat and smooth muscle.
      (1) They extend from the mons anteriorly to the fourchette posteriorly.
      (2) The embryologic homolog in the male is the scrotum.
   e. The **labia minora** are erectile tissue, devoid of fat and composed of skin and vascular and connective tissue.
      (1) They extend from the prepuce two-thirds of the distance of the perineum.
      (2) The embryologic homolog in the male is the floor of the penile urethra.
   f. The **clitoris** is a highly vascular and innervated, erectile organ located between the bifurcating folds of the labia minora.
      (1) It consists of the glans and the body, covered by the prepuce.
      (2) The embryologic homolog in the male is the penis.
   g. The **vestibule** is the space between the labia minora extending from the clitoris to the vaginal introitus. It contains the urethral meatus and the openings of the major and minor vestibular glands as well as the Skene glands.
   h. **Bartholin glands** are the major vestibular glands.
      (1) They lie posterior and lateral to the vaginal introitus.
      (2) The embryologic homolog in the male is the Cowper glands.
   i. **Ducts of the Skene glands** and **minor vestibular glands** are paraurethral structures.
2. **Nerve supply**. The nerve supply to the vulva includes sensory nerves, special receptors, and autonomic nerves to vessels and glands. Symptoms of vulvovaginal disorders are frequently caused by irritation of the sensory nerves of the vulva. The major nerves supplying the vulva include those derived from the pudendal, ilioinguinal, and posterior femoral cutaneous nerves.
   a. The **pudendal nerve** gives rise to the inferior hemorrhoidal nerve, the perineal nerve, and the dorsal nerve of the clitoris.

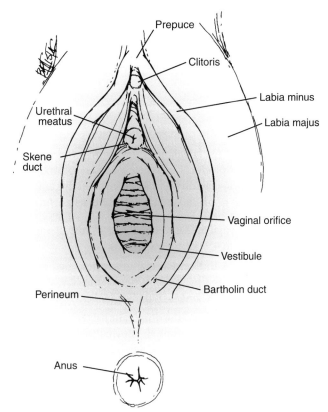

Prepuce

Clitoris

Labia minus

Labia majus

Urethral meatus

Skene duct

Vaginal orifice

Vestibule

Bartholin duct

Perineum

Anus

FIGURE 37–1 Anatomic structures of the vulva.

    b. The **ilioinguinal nerve** gives rise to the anterior labial nerves.

    c. The **posterior femoral cutaneous nerve** gives rise to the posterior labial nerves.

3. Vascular supply. The major blood vessels supplying the vulva derive from the internal pudendal artery, which arises from the internal iliac artery, and the superficial and deep external pudendal arteries, which arise from the femoral artery.

4. Lymphatic supply. The femoral and inguinal lymph nodes receive the lymphatic drainage from the vulva. The superficial inguinal lymph nodes are the initial site of drainage. Many infections or inflammatory conditions of the vulva and distal vaginal wall are accompanied by an increase in lymphatic drainage, resulting in tender lymphadenopathy at this site.

B Vagina. This structure is a hollow cylinder approximately 9 to 10 cm in length. It extends from the introitus to the uterus and lies dorsal to the bladder and ventral to the rectum.

1. Anatomy. The vaginal wall has three layers: the mucosa, muscularis, and adventitia.

    a. The **mucosa** is covered by a stratified, **nonkeratinized**, squamous epithelium.

      (1) It is a mucous membrane that is under the hormonal influence of the ovarian steroids. **Estrogen stimulates** the proliferation and maturation of vaginal epithelial cells, whereas progesterone is inhibitory.

      (2) There are no glandular structures. Endocervical secretions and **transudation of fluid** across the vaginal epithelium provide lubrication.

    b. The **muscularis** is composed of an outer longitudinal and inner circular layer.

    c. The **adventitia** is a strong sheet of connective tissue, condensed anteriorly to form the pubocervical fascia, and fused to the fascial coverings of the pelvic and urogenital diaphragms.

2. Nerve supply. The nerve supply is derived from the lumbar plexus and the pudendal nerve. The pudendal nerve does not have as rich a distribution of fine sensory nerves as the nerves supplying the vulva.

3. Vascular supply. The major vessels supplying the vagina include the vaginal artery, arising from the internal iliac or uterine artery; the azygous artery of the vagina, arising from the cervical branch of the uterine artery; and branches of the pudendal artery. Venous drainage forms a plexus surrounding the vagina, and major vessels follow the arterial course.

4. Lymphatic supply. The lymphatic drainage of the vagina includes a complex anastomotic plexus that involves drainage to the internal iliac, pelvic, sacral, inferior gluteal, anorectal, femoral, and inguinal nodes.

III VAGINAL PHYSIOLOGY

The vaginal ecosystem is a finely balanced environment maintained by a complex interaction among vaginal flora, microbial by-products, estrogen, and host factors. The vagina is **usually resistant to infection** for two reasons: **marked acidity** and a **thick protective epithelium**. Other host factors, such as the immune system, also play a role in vaginal defense mechanisms.

A Microbiology. The vaginal flora play a critical role in vaginal defenses by maintaining the normally acidic pH (3.8 to 4.2) of the vagina.

1. Normally, five to 15 different bacterial species (e.g., group B streptococcus, *Escherichia coli*), both aerobic and anaerobic, inhabit the vagina. The type and number may vary in response to normal and abnormal changes in the vaginal environment.

2. *Lactobacillus acidophilus* is the dominant bacterium in a healthy vaginal ecosystem. Lactobacilli play a critical role in maintaining the normal vaginal environment.
   a. The acidic environment of the vagina is maintained through the production of lactic acid.
   b. Lactic acid and hydrogen peroxide produced by lactobacilli are toxic to anaerobic bacteria in the vagina.

3. **Insults that affect the acidic pH** and lead to a more alkaline environment result in a decrease in lactobacilli, with an overgrowth of pathogenic organisms.

B Host factors

1. **Normal estrogen levels** are necessary for a normal vaginal environment and resistance to infection.
   a. Estrogen stimulates proliferation and maturation of the vaginal epithelium, providing a physical barrier to infection. Conditions associated with decreased estrogen levels are associated with an increase in susceptibility to vaginal infections.
   b. Mature vaginal epithelium provides **glycogen**, necessary for lactobacillus metabolism. If glycogen levels are decreased, lactobacillus counts decrease as well.

2. **Cellular and humoral immunity** plays a role in the normal vaginal defense mechanisms.

C Factors that alter the vaginal environment. Insults that affect the vaginal microbiology, vaginal epithelium, or vaginal pH lead to an increased susceptibility to vaginal infections.

1. **Antibiotics** alter the microbiology of the vagina and can increase the risk of infection.

2. **Hormones** may affect the vaginal epithelium and increase the risk of infection (e.g., decreased estrogen level, increased progesterone level).

3. **Douching or intravaginal medications** can change the vaginal pH or affect the vaginal flora, altering the resistance to infection.

4. **Intercourse** affects the microenvironment of the vagina because semen has an alkaline pH. In addition, intercourse may introduce new organisms into the vagina, thus influencing the microenvironment.

5. **Sexually transmitted diseases (STDs)** affect the microbiology of the vagina, changing the resistance to infection. Other organisms may be the cause of vaginal symptomatology.

6. **Stress, poor diet, and fatigue** probably play a role by affecting microbiology, pH, and the immune system.

7. **Foreign bodies** alter the pH and microbiology of the vagina.

8. Changes in immune function associated with **HIV infection** are associated with recurrent vaginal candidiasis.

IV **DIAGNOSIS**

A thorough history, a physical examination, and judicious use of ancillary tests are critical to attaining the correct diagnosis. The medical history is essential in evaluating the potential causes of vulvovaginal symptoms. The patient's symptomatology is also important.

A **History.** Certain conditions may predispose women to certain types of vulvovaginal infections. Inciting factors may also indicate other causes, such as allergic reactions. Physicians should consider the following factors:

1. **Sexual activity**
   a. Are there complaints of irritation?
   b. What is the relation of the onset of symptoms to intercourse or other sexual activity?
   c. Has the patient engaged in any unusual sexual practices or had new partners?

2. Onset, intensity, and progression of symptoms

3. Recent systemic or local infection

4. Use of antibiotics

5. History of diabetes mellitus

6. Previous vulvovaginal infections

7. Vaginal hygienic practices (e.g., douching)

8. Contraceptive methods

9. Menstrual history

10. Previous treatments; use of self-prescribed medications, herbal remedies, or home remedies

11. Any other factors that may have altered the vaginal environment

B **Symptomatology**

1. **Vulvar symptoms.** The two **most common symptoms** are:
   a. **Burning.** Vulvar irritation or burning is a symptom associated with a variety of disorders, including vulvovaginitis, vulvovestibulitis, and vulvodynia.
   b. **Itching or pruritus.** Vulvar pruritus is a common symptom that may result from vulvovaginitis. Other possible causes include any skin disorder associated with pruritus, including allergic reactions.

2. **Vaginal discharge.** Description of the discharge is crucial to diagnosis and to the differentiation from a normal physiologic finding. Characteristics include:
   a. **Consistency (thick, watery).** A thin, white discharge is often normal.
   b. **Viscosity.** Cervical mucus normally changes during the menstrual cycle. Follicular-phase mucus is normally watery and abundant; postovulatory mucus can be thick and viscous. Patients may observe such changes and report them as abnormal.
   c. **Color.** Normal discharge is usually white to beige. Green, yellow, or brown discharge is usually associated with an infection, a foreign body, or some other abnormality.

3. **Odor.** Description of the odor is useful in establishing a differential diagnosis.
   a. An odor may be present without an associated discharge noticed by the patient.
   b. Complaints of severe, offensive odor occur most often with retained foreign bodies, such as tampons.

V **PHYSICAL EXAMINATION**

A **Pelvic examination** is essential in the management of vulvovaginitis and should consist of a thorough evaluation.

1. Inspection of the **external genitalia** detects gross lesions, edema (and discoloration) of the labia, ulceration, and condylomata. It also rules out pubic lice.

2. The **inguinal area** should be palpated for the presence or absence of lymphadenopathy. Any discoloration should be noted.

TABLE 37–1   Signs, Symptoms, and Diagnosis of Vulvovaginitis

Etiology	Symptoms	Clinical Signs	Diagnostic Method
Monilial vaginitis	Pruritus	Thick white discharge; pH 4.0–4.7	Wet prep or KOH prep (pseudohyphae)
Trichomonas	Malodorous discharge, pruritus	Frothy, copious yellow-green discharge; pH 5.0–7.0	Wet prep (motile trichomonads)
Bacterial vaginosis	Discharge, fishy odor	Thin, gray discharge; pH 5.0–5.5	Wet prep, sniff test (clue cells)
Chlamydia	Discharge	Mucopurulent discharge, cervical erosion	Culture; MicroTrak or Chlamydiazyme
Gonorrhea	Discharge	Cervical discharge	Cervical culture; Gram stain
Genital herpes	Pain	Ulcerative, vulvar vesicles and ulcers	Virus culture, Tzanck prep
Chemical	Discharge	Erythema; may be ulcerative	History and exclusion of other causes
Physiologic	Discharge	No odor or erythema	Wet prep; history, exclusion of other causes; cervical culture

KOH, potassium hydroxide.

B **Speculum examination**, using water as the only lubricant to avoid interfering with specimen collection and culturing, should reveal:

1. **Nature of the vaginal discharge** (e.g., consistency, viscosity, color, and odor)

2. **Evidence of trauma, congenital abnormalities, or characteristic lesions of the vaginal walls** (e.g., "strawberry spots" if *Trichomonas vaginalis* is suspected)

3. **Presence or absence of cervical abnormalities**. A culture of the endocervix detects gonorrhea or chlamydial infection, and a Papanicolaou test (Pap smear) detects carcinoma or infection.

C Laboratory tests

1. When an infectious vaginitis is suspected, **vaginal pH** helps differentiate the various types of infections.

2. A specimen should be obtained for **wet mount preparation**. Microscopic inspection of the vaginal secretions in saline and a 10% potassium hydroxide (KOH) solution is pivotal when diagnosing vaginitis.

3. Occasionally, **cultures** are useful in difficult cases.

VI   VULVOVAGINAL CONDITIONS (see Table 37-1)

Vaginitis is characterized by one or more of the following symptoms: **increased volume of discharge; abnormal color (yellow or green) of discharge; vulvar itching, irritation, or burning; dyspareunia; and malodor**. Vaginitis may be caused by infectious agents (e.g., *Candida, Gardnerella*, and *Trichomonas*) or by atrophic changes. Symptoms of other vulvovaginal conditions, including vulvar dystrophies, vulvar dermatitis, and other skin conditions of the vulva, may be similar to those of vaginitis. Acute herpes simplex genitalis may cause acute vulvar symptoms, necessitating prompt evaluation and treatment.

A **Bacterial vaginosis** is the most common vaginal infection in the United States today. In the past, bacterial vaginitis was known as nonspecific vaginitis and *Gardnerella* vaginitis.

1. **Etiology**
   a. Bacterial vaginosis is a polymicrobial clinical syndrome caused by an **overgrowth of a variety of bacterial species**, particularly **anaerobes**, often found normally in the vagina. Organisms most often involved include *Bacteroides, Peptostreptococcus, Gardnerella vaginalis*, and *Mycoplasma hominis*.

b. The anaerobic bacteria produce enzymes that break down peptides to amino acids and amines, resulting in compounds associated with the discharge and odor characteristic of this infection.

2. **Clinical presentation.** Fifty percent of women with bacterial vaginosis are asymptomatic. In symptomatic patients, the most common presentation is a malodorous, gray discharge.

3. **Diagnosis.** Three of the following four criteria must be present:
    a. The vaginal pH is generally between 5.0 and 5.5.
    b. Wet mount preparations with saline reveal a "clean" background with **minimal or no leukocytes**, an abundance of bacteria, and the characteristic **clue cells**. The clue cells are squamous cells in which coccobacillary bacteria have obscured the sharp borders and cytoplasm.
    c. Application of 10% KOH to the wet mount specimen produces a **fishy odor**, indicating a positive "whiff" test.
    d. A gray, homogenous, malodorous discharge is present.

4. **Treatment.** Therapy is based on the use of agents with anaerobic activity and involves both topical and systemic agents. The combination appears to be 90% effective.
    a. Vaginal preparations
        (1) Intravaginal 2% **clindamycin cream** is used at bedtime for 7 days.
        (2) Intravaginal **metronidazole** is applied once a day for 5 days.
    b. Oral regimens
        (1) Metronidazole may be administered two ways: 500 mg twice daily for 7 days or a single, 2-g dose.
        (2) Clindamycin, 300 mg twice daily for 7 days (may be associated with diarrhea, especially *Clostridium difficile*)
    c. Sexual partners should be treated in cases of repeated episodes of bacterial vaginosis. Routine treatment of partners has not been shown to improve cure rates or lower reinfection rates.
    d. Treatment during pregnancy is critical; data suggest an association of adverse maternal and fetal outcomes with bacterial vaginosis.
        (1) Clindamycin may be used throughout pregnancy.
        (2) Metronidazole may be used after the first trimester.
    e. Patients with recurrences should be screened for STDs.

B *Candida vaginitis* **(candidiasis or moniliasis)** is the second most common vaginal infection in the United States.

1. **Etiology**
    a. The etiologic agent is a yeast (fungi) organism, usually ***Candida albicans***. The organism is a common inhabitant of the bowel and perianal region. Thirty percent of women **may have vaginal colonization and have no symptoms of infection**.
    b. Several factors may lead to symptomatic infection instead of colonization.
        (1) Contraceptive practices (e.g., birth control pills and vaginal spermicides, which influence vaginal pH)
        (2) Use of systemic steroids, which influence the immune system
        (3) Use of antibiotics, which alters the microbiology of the vagina; 25% to 70% of women report yeast infections after antibiotic use. Any antibiotic, particularly a broad-spectrum agent, may play a causative role.
        (4) Tight clothing, panty hose, and bathing suits (yeast thrives in a dark, warm, moist environment)
        (5) Undiagnosed or uncontrolled diabetes mellitus
    c. Another reason for a refractory monilial infection may be **compromised immune status**; with recurrent monilial vaginitis, an HIV test is indicated, along with a fasting serum glucose level.
    d. There has been a recent **increase in the number of infections caused by non-*albicans*** species. Up to 20% of infections may be caused by organisms such as *Candida tropicalis* and *Torulopsis glabrata*. These organisms may be resistant to standard treatment regimens.

2. **Clinical presentation**. Patients with monilial vaginitis characteristically complain of a thick, white discharge and extreme vulvar pruritus. The vulva may be red and swollen.
   a. Symptoms may recur and be most prominent just before menses or in association with intercourse.
   b. Yeast infections may occur more frequently during pregnancy.
   c. Patients with infections caused by *C. tropicalis* and *T. glabrata* may have an atypical presentation. Irritation may be paramount, with little discharge or pruritus.

3. **Diagnosis**. Diagnosis is made by history, physical examination, and microscopic examination of the vaginal discharge in saline and 10% KOH.
   a. On examination, excoriations of the vulva may be noticeable; the vulva and vagina may be erythematous, with patches of adherent cottage cheese–like discharge. Candidal infections of the vulva are characterized by classic **satellite lesions**.
   b. Infection with *C. tropicalis* and *T. glabrata* may not be associated with the classic discharge; discharge may be white-gray and thin.
   c. Vaginal pH may be normal or slightly more basic than normal (4.0 to 4.7).
   d. Wet mount microscopic examination reveals hyphae or pseudohyphae with budding yeast in 50% to 70% of women with yeast infections.
   e. Cultures are not necessary to make the diagnosis except in some cases of recurrent infections.

4. **Treatment**. Many agents are available for the treatment of vulvovaginal candidiasis. These include topical agents, which may be available over the counter (OTC) or by prescription, and oral agents, which are available by prescription only.
   a. **Antifungal intravaginal agents** are administered as suppositories or creams. These drugs are available in three regimens: a single dose, 3-day course, or 7-day course. Agents include butoconazole, clotrimazole, miconazole, tioconazole, and terconazole. **OTC regimens** should be used only by women who have been diagnosed with a yeast infection in the past and are experiencing identical symptoms.
   b. **Oral agents** include fluconazole and ketoconazole.
      (1) **Fluconazole** is available as a single-dose (150 mg) treatment for uncomplicated vaginal candidiasis.
      (2) **Ketoconazole** is used effectively for the treatment of chronic and recurrent candidiasis; a 5% incidence of hepatotoxicity limits more widespread use. The dosing schedule is 200 mg twice a day for 5 days, then 100 to 200 mg daily for 6 months.
   c. **Boric acid capsules intravaginally**, 600 mg for 14 days, may be effective.

5. **Chronic recurrent yeast infections** (5% of women). In most cases, no exacerbating factor can be found; however, the following possibilities should be considered:
   a. Failure to complete a full course of therapy
   b. **HIV infection**. Recalcitrant candidiasis may be a presenting symptom in women with HIV infection. HIV testing should be considered and offered to the patient.
   c. Chronic antibiotic therapy
   d. Infection with a resistant organism such as *C. tropicalis* or *T. glabrata*
   e. Sexual transmission from the male partner
   f. Allergic reaction to partner's semen or a vaginal spermicide
   g. Diabetes. Patients should have a fasting serum glucose level if they have recurrent infections.

C **Trichomonas vaginalis** *vaginitis (trichomoniasis)* is the third most common vaginitis, accounting for 25% of cases.

1. **Etiology**. The motile protozoan *T. vaginalis* is the etiologic agent. The trichomonad can be recovered from 70% to 80% of the male partners of the infected patient; therefore, *Trichomonas* vaginitis is an STD.

2. **Clinical presentation**. *Trichomonas* vaginitis is a multifocal infection involving the vaginal epithelium, Skene glands, Bartholin glands, and urethra.
   a. Unless asked directly, 25% to 50% of women may not report symptoms.
   b. Most women report a discharge that is described as copious, green, and frothy. The discharge may be associated with a foul odor and vulvar irritation or pruritus.

3. **Diagnosis**
   a. **Physical examination**. Classic evidence of trichomoniasis may be seen.
      (1) The characteristic green discharge may be evident.
      (2) Punctation, described classically as the "strawberry cervix," is evident in only 25% of patients.
   b. **Laboratory tests**
      (1) The vaginal pH is usually between 5.0 and 7.0.
      (2) Saline wet mount of the vaginal discharge reveals **numerous leukocytes** and the highly motile, flagellated trichomonads (as many as 75% of cases).
      (3) Cultures are not usually necessary to make the diagnosis. They should be obtained when the diagnosis is suspected but cannot be confirmed by wet mount examination.
      (4) Pap smears may be positive in as many as 65% of cases. Positive Pap smears should be confirmed by wet mount examination because of the high false-positive rate.

4. **Treatment.** Because *Trichomonas* is sexually transmitted, **both partners require therapy**; 25% of women will be reinfected if their partner does not receive treatment.
   a. Vaginal therapy alone is ineffective because of the multiple sites of infection, and **systemic agents are necessary**.
   b. If both partners are treated simultaneously, cure rates of 90% are achieved with treatment with **metronidazole**. Patients should be warned that a disulfiram-like reaction may occur and that they should abstain from alcohol use during treatment.
      (1) The **preferred regimen is 2 g in one dose** because of ease of compliance. As many as 10% of patients may experience vomiting.
      (2) An alternative regimen is 500 mg twice daily for 7 days.
   d. **Resistant cases** may require treatment with intravenous metronidazole. Because resistance is rare, other causes, such as noncompliance of the patient or partner, should be considered.
   e. Metronidazole is **contraindicated for use during the first trimester of pregnancy**. After this time, it can be used to treat *Trichomonas* infections.
   f. Infected patients should be screened for other STDs.

D **Atrophic vaginitis**

1. **Etiology**. Atrophic vaginitis, associated with decreased estradiol levels, is most often seen in postmenopausal women but also may be seen in breastfeeding women. Atrophic changes in the vulvovaginal tissues result from **estrogen withdrawal**; the normal protective thickness of the vaginal epithelium depends on estrogen stimulation.

2. **Clinical presentation**
   a. Without consistent and sufficient estrogen, the vaginal epithelium becomes thin; vulvar structures may atrophy.
   b. The amount of glycogen also decreases, and the pH becomes alkaline.
   c. The vagina is often pale with punctate hemorrhagic spots throughout the vaginal wall. There is an absence of superficial epithelial cells and a predominance of parabasal cells.

3. **Diagnosis**
   a. Atrophic vaginitis must be suspected in hypoestrogenic women who present with leukorrhea, pruritus, burning, tenderness, and dyspareunia.
   b. Physical examination of the vagina reveals atrophic, sometimes inflamed vaginal walls. A discharge may be present.
   c. Vaginal pH is usually greater than 4.5.
   d. Vaginal infection is not identified on a wet mount preparation.

4. **Treatment.** Topical administration of vaginal cream containing estrogen reverses symptoms and tissue changes.
   a. Symptoms respond to short-term therapy but recur on discontinuation.
   b. Changes in tissues require long-term therapy and may not be noticed until after 3 to 4 months of treatment. Proliferation and maturation of the vaginal epithelium, as well as compliance and elasticity of the vaginal wall, are restored.
   c. Therapeutic agents may be systemic or topical.

  (1) Hormone replacement therapy may be given in accordance with a standard regimen.

  (2) Estrogen cream is administered intravaginally every night for up to 2 weeks and then continued once or twice a week to maintain results.

E Vulvar dystrophies

1. **Etiology.** Vulvar dystrophies are dermatologic conditions of the vulvar skin of uncertain etiology. Most frequently seen in postmenopausal women, these conditions often accompany a history of chronic candidal vulvovaginitis. The dystrophies can be:

 a. Hyperplastic when the epithelium is markedly thickened

 b. Atrophic (lichen sclerosus et atrophicus)

 c. A mixture of both

2. **Clinical presentation**

 a. With **hyperplastic dystrophy**, the most common symptom is constant pruritus. Scratching frequently exacerbates the pruritus, creating a vicious cycle.

 b. With **lichen sclerosus**, vulvar burning, pruritus, or chronic soreness associated with "vulvar dysuria" frequently occurs.

3. **Diagnosis. Vulvar biopsy** is ultimately necessary to make the diagnosis, but a preliminary diagnosis can be made based on **physical examination**.

 a. Hyperplastic dystrophy presents as thickened skin ("elephant hide") accompanied by linear excoriations from scratching. Areas of leukoplakia may also be noted.

 b. Lichen sclerosus presents as extremely pale, thin skin, often with subepithelial hemorrhages. In its most severe form, painful contraction of the introitus or clitoral hood is noted. Loss of labial architecture may occur.

4. **Treatment**

 a. Hyperplastic dystrophy responds well to a 6- to 8-week trial of topical fluorinated steroid cream. Chronic therapy may be necessary on an intermittent basis.

 b. Lichen sclerosus. Potent fluorinated steroid creams are the treatment of choice; testosterone was used in the past but is not recommended anymore. Chronic therapy may be necessary as well.

F Traumatic vaginitis

1. **Etiology.** Traumatic vaginitis is usually the result of injury or chemical irritation.

 a. In **adults**, the most common cause of injury to the vagina is a "lost" tampon.

 b. In **pediatric patients**, foreign bodies placed in the vagina serve as sources of infection or trauma (e.g., wads of paper, chewing gum, or paper clips).

 c. Chemical irritation can be secondary to douches, deodorants, lubricants, or topical intravaginal preparations.

2. **Treatment.** Vulvovaginitis resulting from foreign bodies or chemical irritants responds immediately to withdrawal of the causative agent.

G Neoplasia

1. **Etiology.** Malignancies can masquerade for months as vulvar lesions; thus, they are often ignored by patients or mistreated by physicians as irritations or infections.

2. **Diagnosis.** Patients who present with a long-term history of symptoms and treatment failures of vulvar lesions **should undergo biopsy** before receiving further therapy.

3. **Treatment.** Therapy appropriate for the condition described in the pathology report is indicated.

H Herpes simplex genitalis

1. **Etiology**

 a. Herpes genitalis is caused by the herpes simplex virus (HSV), a member of the Herpesviridae family of viruses, which are capable of establishing latent status and causing recurrent disease.

 b. From 70% to 90% of cases of herpes genitalis are caused by HSV type 2 (HSV-2); HSV type 1 (HSV-1) is the etiologic agent in only 13% of cases.

 c. From 60% to 85% of women with antibodies to HSV-2 have never had a recognized genital ulcer.

d. Transmission is through direct contact with an individual who is actively shedding virus from skin or mucous membrane lesions. Often the disease is transmitted by asymptomatic shedding of the virus.

2. Clinical presentation

a. Primary infection

(1) The infection is usually acquired from sexual contact, with symptoms appearing in 2 to 12 days

(2) Primary infection is often associated with systemic, flu-like symptoms (e.g., malaise, myalgias, and headache). Primary symptoms may last from 2 days to 3 weeks. Symptoms may be milder in women with antibodies to HSV-1.

(3) Pain and itching may precede the development of vesicular lesions, which may appear on the labia, perineum, buttocks, urethra, vagina, cervix, and bladder. Cervical involvement is seen in 70% of women with genital involvement.

(4) Vesicles progress to ulcers and may coalesce. Lesions are exquisitely tender. Primary lesions persist for 3 to 6 weeks and usually heal without scarring.

(5) Local symptoms consist of hyperesthesia, burning, itching, dysuria, and (frequently) exquisite pain and tenderness of the vulva. Vulvar pain makes intercourse unbearable and may lead to urinary retention.

(6) Tender inguinal lymphadenopathy may be present.

(7) Viral shedding may persist for 12 days.

(8) Complications include sacral radiculopathy with urinary or fecal retention and aseptic meningitis (rare).

b. Recurrent infection

(1) The dormant herpesvirus resides in the neurons of the sacral ganglia, which supply the areas of cutaneous involvement.

(2) Periodic asymptomatic viral shedding occurs, particularly during the first 6 months after infection.

(3) Recurrences are most frequent during the first year. Frequency of recurrence varies. Some patients never have another outbreak; others have frequent recurrences.

(4) Many women experience prodromal symptoms of itching and burning from 30 minutes to 2 days before an outbreak. Systemic symptoms usually do not occur with recurrences.

(5) Recurrent lesions tend to be less severe and are of shorter duration (3 to 7 days).

3. Diagnosis

a. When typical lesions are present, a presumptive diagnosis of herpes genitalis can be made on physical examination. Thus, **the diagnosis of herpes is a clinical diagnosis.** HSV-2 should be suspected when superficial ulcerations of the vulvovaginal tissues are identified.

b. Viral culture is the **gold standard** by which the diagnosis of HSV infection is made. It requires 48 hours for completion. **Sensitivity** of cultures is **90% if vesicles are present, but only 30% if lesions are crusted.**

c. Cytologic studies and direct identification methods, such as **immunofluorescence**, offer confirmatory evidence of an HSV infection but are only **50% sensitive.**

4. Treatment

a. Local measures used for comfort during the acute outbreak include sitz baths and topical anesthetic creams. The area should be kept clean and dry to avoid secondary infection.

b. Catheterization may be necessary for acute urinary retention.

c. The **antiviral drug acyclovir**, a cyclic purine nucleoside analog, is the first antiviral drug proven to be active against herpesvirus both in vivo and in vitro. It can be applied topically or taken orally for a primary episode of HSV-2 infection. Other antiviral agents are now available.

(1) **Primary HSV outbreak.** Oral antiviral medications decrease the time of viral shedding, the duration of symptoms, and the time to healing in primary herpes outbreaks. Options are:

(a) Acyclovir 400 mg orally three times daily for 7 to 10 days

(b) Valacyclovir 1 g orally twice a day for 7 to 10 days

    (c) Famciclovir 250 mg orally three times a day for 7 to 10 days

    (d) Acyclovir 200 mg orally five times daily for 7 to 10 days

(2) **Recurrent HSV infection**. If oral antiviral medication is started when the recurrence begins, it also decreases duration of viral shedding, time to healing, and local symptoms.

    (a) Acyclovir 400 mg three times daily for 3 to 5 days

    (b) Acyclovir 800 mg three times daily for 2 days

    (c) Valacyclovir 500 mg orally twice daily for 3 days

    (d) Famciclovir 125 mg orally twice daily for 3 to 5 days

(3) **Suppressive therapy**. Studies have shown that oral acyclovir decreases the frequency of recurrences by as much as 75%. Therapy is discontinued annually, and frequency of recurrences is documented. Treatment is restarted as indicated.

    (a) Acyclovir 400 mg twice daily. Suppressive therapy has been approved for up to 6 years.

    (b) Famciclovir 250 mg twice daily

    (c) Valacyclovir 500 mg to 1 g once daily. Valacyclovir therapy for suppression has been approved for up to 1 year.

Study Questions for Chapter 37

Directions: *Match each word or statement below with the most specific anatomic site. Each answer may be used once, more than once, or not at all.*

- A Labia majora
- B Labia minora
- C Clitoris
- D Vestibule
- E Prepuce
- F Bartholin gland
- G Skene gland
- H Pudendal
- I Ilioinguinal
- J Posterior femoral cutaneous
- K External pudendal
- L Cervical

1. Embryologic homolog in the male is the floor of the penile urethra

2. Embryologic homolog in the male is the Cowper gland(s)

3. Contains sebaceous glands but not hair follicles or sweat glands; is a paired structure

4. Source of vaginal lubrication during intercourse

5. Azygous artery of the vagina

Directions: *Each of the numbered items or incomplete statements in this section is followed by answers or by completions of the statement. Select the ONE lettered answer or completion that is BEST in each case.*

6. A 23-year-old woman, gravida 2, para 1, at 10 weeks of gestation, presents to your office and reports increasing yellow vaginal discharge that has an odor. A vaginal smear reveals clue cells. She denies pruritus. She does not have any significant medical history or allergies to medication. The next step in management of this patient is:
   - A Oral metronidazole
   - B Vaginal metronidazole
   - C Oral clindamycin
   - D Vaginal clindamycin
   - E Oral fluconazole

7. A 25-year-old woman, gravida 1, para 1, presents to your office reporting four recurrent yeast infections within the last 2 months. You perform a wet mount and a 10% KOH prep and confirm presence of many pseudohyphae and absence of clue cells or leukocytes. She is not pregnant, is not on birth control, and has not been sexually active for 7 months. What is the next step in management of this patient?
   - A Screen for STDs
   - B Long-term oral ketoconazole
   - C Boric acid capsules intravaginally
   - D Screen for HIV
   - E Random glucose level

Match each of the statements below with the best word(s). Each answer may be used once, more than once, or not at all.

- [A] Bacterial vaginosis
- [B] Moniliasis
- [C] Trichomoniasis
- [D] Herpes simplex
- [E] Atrophic vaginitis
- [F] Lichen sclerosus
- [G] Hyperplastic dystrophy
- [H] Traumatic vaginitis

8. A 19-year-old woman complains of increasing discharge and odor. Her pH is 5.5, and wet mount reveals lack of leukocytes and protozoa.

9. A 24-year-old woman who is 2 months postpartum and is breastfeeding reports itching and dyspareunia. Speculum examination reveals pale, dry vaginal walls.

10. A wet mount shows a predominance of cells with large nuclei (parabasal cells).

Answers and Explanations

1. B [II A 1 e2], **2.** F [II A 1 h2], **3.** B [II A 1 c], **4.** L [II B 1 a2], **5.** L [II B 3]. The embryologic homolog of the labia minora in the male is the floor of the penile urethra. The embryologic homolog of the Bartholin glands in the male is the Cowper glands. Although both the labia minora and the prepuce contain sebaceous glands but not hair follicles, only the labia minora (plural) is a paired structure (i.e., there are two labium majus [singular]). Because the vagina does not contain any glandular structures, the cervical secretions and transudation of fluid from vessels across the vaginal epithelium provide lubrication during intercourse. The azygous artery of the vagina arises from the cervical branch of the uterine artery.

6. The answer is B [VI A 4 d2]. Oral metronidazole is contraindicated in the first trimester; thus, the intravaginal preparation is preferred. Although clindamycin can be used throughout pregnancy, it is not the initial recommended agent for treatment of bacterial vaginosis because it is not as effective. Azithromycin may be used for treatment of chlamydia.

7. The answer is D [VI B 4 c]. Patients with recurrent or recalcitrant fungal infection may be immunocompromised. Therefore, HIV testing is indicated. Screening for diabetes is also indicated, but this is done with a fasting glucose level, not a random glucose. Treatment with boric acid and long-term treatment with oral ketoconazole may be indicated, but evaluating her for an immunocompromised state is the first step.

8. A [VI A 3], **9.** E [VI D 1], **10.** E [VI D 2]. The only discharges that have a pH higher than 4.2 are bacterial vaginosis, trichomoniasis, and atrophic vaginitis. Trichomoniasis is unlikely because there are no protozoa on wet mount and there is a paucity of leukocytes. Atrophic vaginitis is unlikely in a young woman who is not estrogen deprived. Absence of superficial epithelial cells and a predominance of parabasal cells are typical of atrophic vaginitis due to estrogen deficiency.

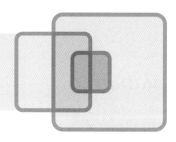

chapter 38

Disorders of the Pelvic Floor

LILY ARYA

I   INTRODUCTION

A Epidemiology

1. Urinary incontinence affects women five times more often than men.

2. From 10% to 25% of women 25 to 64 years of age and as many as 40% of women older than 65 years of age suffer from some form of urinary incontinence.

3. As many as 50% of all parous women have pelvic support defects, and 10% to 20% seek care for pelvic organ prolapse (POP).

4. In the United States, women have a lifetime risk of urinary incontinence or POP that requires surgical treatment of approximately 10%.

5. The true prevalence of fecal incontinence is unknown, but the disorder is estimated to affect as many as 10% of women older than 64 years of age.

6. Thirty percent of women with urinary incontinence also have fecal incontinence.

B Anatomy of the pelvic floor   (Fig. 38-1). The pelvic organs rest on the pelvic floor muscles and are held in place with the help of the endopelvic fascia.

1. The pelvic floor is made up of the **levator ani** and coccygeus muscles. The levator ani has three parts, including the puborectalis and pubococcygeus (also referred to as the pubovisceral muscle) and iliococcygeus muscles.
    a. These muscles, which create a hammock-like sling between the pubis and coccyx, are attached laterally along the pelvic sidewalls.
    b. The levator ani muscle is tonically contracted, providing a firm shelf posteriorly to support the pelvic contents and aiding with urinary and fecal continence.

2. **Endopelvic fascia** is a loose network of connective tissue, small vessels, lymphatics, and nerves, which surrounds and supports the pelvic organs and the vagina. Thickenings of the endopelvic fascia are known as ligaments (e.g., the uterosacral and cardinal ligaments, rectovaginal and vesicovaginal fascia).

3. The **vagina** is attached at three levels. The apex is supported by the cardinal and uterosacral ligaments. The midvagina is supported by the attachment of the vagina to the levator ani at the arcus tendineus fascia pelvis (white line). The lower vagina is supported by its attachment to the perineal membrane and the perineal body. Normal vaginal attachments help to keep the pelvic organs (i.e., the uterus, bladder, and rectum) in place.

C Innervation of the pelvic floor and its functions

1. The levator ani is innervated by sacral nerve roots (S2 to S4). This muscle group is tonically stimulated to contract, providing constant support to the pelvic organs.

2. Bladder filling and voiding functions are controlled by closely coordinated autonomic and somatic pathways.
    a. **Autonomic nervous system**
        (1) **Sympathetic** (thoracolumbar) nerves promote urine storage by **relaxing the bladder (detrusor) muscle** and contracting smooth muscle in the bladder neck and urethra. These nerves are inhibited during voiding.

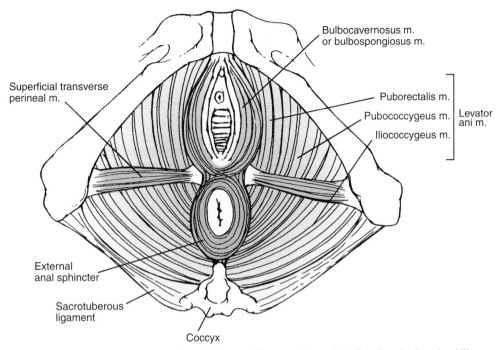

FIGURE 38–1 Levator ani muscles from below. The levator ani has several parts, including the pubovisceral and iliococcygeus muscles. m., muscle.

(2) **Parasympathetic** (sacral) nerves cause the detrusor muscle to contract. They are stimulated during micturition.

b. The **somatic nervous system** controls the striated external urethral sphincter and levator ani muscle through the pudendal nerve and the sacral nerve roots (S2 to S4). Inhibition of these nerves causes relaxation of the bladder outlet and pelvic floor, which must occur during voiding.

c. The **central nervous system (CNS)** provides voluntary control and modification of micturition and defecation reflexes.

II PELVIC ORGAN PROLAPSE (also called pelvic relaxation)

Such prolapse or protrusion of pelvic structures into the vaginal canal results from weakening or damage to pelvic support structures.

A Risk factors

1. Vaginal childbirth may damage or weaken pelvic support structures. This damage may be direct injury to the muscle and fascia of the pelvis or indirect weakness of the muscles caused by neurologic injury.

2. Obesity, chronic cough, and chronic constipation may cause increased intra-abdominal pressures, increasing the risk of POP.

3. Increasing age is associated with an increased risk of POP.

4. A genetic predisposition for POP may exist in some women.

B Terminology

1. **Cystocele** is protrusion of the bladder behind the anterior vaginal wall. This represents failure of support at the midvagina anteriorly.

2. **Uterine prolapse** is descent of the uterus into the lower part of the vagina or through the vaginal opening.

TABLE 38-1   The Halfway Grading System for Pelvic Organ Prolapse*

Grade	Level of Prolapse
1	No prolapse
2	Descent halfway to the hymen
3	Descent to the hymen
4	Descent halfway past the hymen
5	Maximum possible descent for each site

*Descent of the most dependent portion of the prolapse is graded during maximal straining.

3. **Vaginal vault prolapse** is descent of the vaginal apex after hysterectomy. Uterine prolapse and vaginal prolapse represent failure of apical support of the vagina.

4. **Enterocele** is protrusion of small bowel behind the upper vaginal wall into the vaginal canal.

5. **Rectocele** is protrusion of the rectum behind the posterior vaginal wall. This represents failure of the midvaginal support posteriorly.

6. **Relaxed or widened vaginal outlet**. This represents failure of support of the lower vagina.

C **Symptoms.**   Mild forms of POP are often asymptomatic. Advanced forms of POP may cause difficulty with urination or defecation. Associated symptoms may include:

1. **Bulge of tissue** protruding through the vaginal opening

2. Pelvic or vaginal **pressure**, especially after prolonged standing

3. Dyspareunia

D **Evaluation**

1. Prolapse is diagnosed on **pelvic examination**, performed in the lithotomy and standing positions.

2. The severity of prolapse may be classified according to systems that describe the location and severity of POP.
   a. Halfway system (Table 38-1)
   b. Pelvic Organ Prolapse Quantification (POP-Q)

E **Treatment.**   Asymptomatic POP does not require treatment.

1. **Pelvic floor muscle (Kegel) exercises** may improve symptoms caused by mild forms of prolapse.

2. **Pessaries** are devices placed in the vagina that support prolapse.

3. **Surgery** for POP aims to relieve symptoms and to restore normal anatomic relationships. The surgical procedure and approach (abdominal or vaginal) is tailored to the particular type of POP present.
   a. **Hysterectomy** for uterine prolapse
   b. **Anterior repair, paravaginal repair** for cystocele
   c. **Posterior repair** for rectocele
   d. **Enterocele repair**
   e. **Vaginal vault suspension (sacrospinous suspension)**
   f. **Perineorrhaphy** for relaxed vaginal outlet.

III   **URINARY INCONTINENCE**

A Types

1. **Stress urinary incontinence (SUI)** is the loss of urine that occurs with increased abdominal pressure, such as coughing or straining. SUI is the result of loss of **anatomic support of the urethrovesical junction** or **urethra**. It most commonly occurs following pelvic floor muscle and nerve damage that resulted from childbearing.

    a. Urethral hypermobility is the most common form of SUI and usually follows child birth injury to urethral support. The SUI occurs because the urethra can no longer be compressed against the vagina during raised intra-abdominal pressure.

    b. Intrinsic urethral sphincteric deficiency is less common and is caused by a weakened urethral sphincter. Severe SUI develops even with minimal exertion. Risk factors are scarification from prior anti-incontinence surgery and aging.

2. Urge incontinence is defined by the symptom of urine loss that occurs when the patient experiences urgency, or a strong desire to void. This type of incontinence is often accompanied by symptoms of urinary frequency, urgency, and nocturia. Urge incontinence includes the following subtypes:

    a. Detrusor overactivity (DO) (previously called detrusor instability), or overactive bladder, is caused by involuntary detrusor contractions. Its cause is usually unknown.

    b. Neurogenic DO is involuntary detrusor contractions associated with a neurologic disorder (e.g., stroke, spinal cord injury, or multiple sclerosis). It is a common cause of incontinence in elderly and institutionalized women.

3. Overflow incontinence occurs because of underactivity of the detrusor muscle. This form of incontinence is associated with retention of urine. The bladder does not empty completely, and "dribbling" of urine occurs.

4. Extraurethral sources of urine include genitourinary fistulas, which may be congenital or follow pelvic surgery or radiation. These typically cause continuous leaking of urine.

B Evaluation

1. A **detailed history** is essential and should include:

    a. Urinary symptoms, including the presence of voiding frequency, nocturia, urgency, precipitating events, and frequency of loss. A voiding diary allows the patient to document voiding frequency and incontinence episodes during a specific period.

    b. Previous urologic surgery

    c. Obstetric history, including parity, birth weights, and mode of delivery

    d. CNS or spinal cord disorders

    e. Use of medications, including diuretics, antihypertensives, caffeine, alcohol, anticholinergics, decongestants, nicotine, and psychotropics

    f. Presence of other medical disorders (e.g., hypertension or hematuria)

2. Physical examination may detect:

    a. Exacerbating conditions, such as chronic obstructive pulmonary disease, obesity, or intra-abdominal mass

    b. Hypermobility of the urethra

    c. POP

    d. Neurologic disorders

3. Diagnostic tests

    a. A midstream urine specimen is collected for **urinalysis** or **culture and sensitivity**. Infection may aggravate urinary incontinence.

    b. Postvoid residual urine volume should be measured (by ultrasound or catheterization) after the patient has voided. Typically, the postvoid residual urine volume is less than 50 to 100 mL.

    c. The **Q-tip test** is an indirect measure of the urethral axis. A Q-tip is inserted into the urethra with the patient in the lithotomy position. If the Q-tip moves more than 30 degrees from the horizontal with straining, **urethral hypermobility** is present.

    d. Urodynamic testing, including a cystometrogram and voiding studies, may be useful for demonstrating the type of incontinence present. These tests measure pressures within the bladder and abdomen during bladder filling and emptying. Urodynamic testing is indicated for complex cases of urinary incontinence such as mixed incontinence (presence of two or more kinds of incontinence in the same patient) or in patients with incontinence and retention of urine.

4. Cystoscopy is performed in some patients to examine the bladder and urethral mucosa for abnormalities such as diverticula or neoplasms.

C **Treatment.** Therapy depends on the underlying diagnosis.

1. **Treatment of exacerbating factors** such as excess weight, chronic cough, or constipation may improve SUI.

2. **Pelvic muscle rehabilitation** may be helpful for both SUI and DO.
   a. Kegel exercises
   b. Vaginal cones
   c. Biofeedback
   d. Electrical stimulation

3. **Pessaries**, other intravaginal devices, and urethral plugs and inserts are useful conservative therapies for SUI.

4. **Drug therapy** is the mainstay of treatment for DO but is of limited value in treating SUI.
   a. **Antispasmodic agents** (oxybutynin and tolterodine) are highly effective and are the most commonly prescribed treatments for DO. However, they cause side effects, such as dry mouth and constipation, in about 25% of patients.
   b. **α-Adrenergic stimulating agents** (e.g., pseudoephedrine, imipramine) increase smooth muscle contraction in the urethral sphincter and may decrease SUI symptoms.
   c. **Estrogens** (systemic or vaginal) improve irritative bladder symptoms such as urgency and dysuria in postmenopausal women but do not significantly improve urinary leakage. Hormone replacement therapy does not reduce the incidence of urinary symptoms in post-menopausal women.

5. **Surgery** is extremely effective in the treatment of SUI. It is rarely helpful for DO and is generally reserved only for intractable cases.
   a. **Injection of bulking agents** around the urethra is a minimally invasive procedure to treat SUI resulting from intrinsic urethral sphincteric deficiency. Collagen, the bulking agent currently used most commonly, provides a temporary (3 to 12 months) cure or improvement rates ranging from 50% to 70%. They are generally indicated for patients unable to tolerate major surgery.
   b. **Retropubic urethropexy** elevates the urethra and bladder neck by fixing the paraurethral connective tissues to the pubis. The most common type of retropubic operation performed is the **Burch** procedure, which suspends the vaginal fascia lateral to the urethra to the iliopectineal line (Cooper ligament). Burch procedures are most successful in patients who have SUI associated with urethral hypermobility, resulting in long-term cure rates of 75% to 90%. Postoperative complications are uncommon but may include urinary retention and new DO. The procedures may be performed via an abdominal incision or laparoscopically.
   c. **Transvaginal needle procedures** stabilize the bladder neck by anchoring vaginal tissue to the rectus fascia or symphysis pubis. These procedures have lower long-term cure rates than retropubic operations and suburethral slings and are now not generally performed.
   d. **Suburethral sling procedures**, which place various biologic and synthetic materials under the urethra, appear to affect treatment by partially obstructing the urethra during times of increased intra-abdominal pressure. Sling procedures differ according to the type of material and the sling fixation points used; however, they all have high cure rates (80% to 90%). Sling procedures are more effective than retropubic operations in patients with **intrinsic urethral sphincteric deficiency**. Complications of sling procedures may include infection and ulceration (especially with the use of synthetic grafts) and **urinary retention**.

IV FECAL INCONTINENCE

The involuntary loss of stool or gas is a socially embarrassing disorder. Symptoms of fecal incontinence are often not reported to physicians.

A Pathophysiology

1. Fecal continence depends on stool consistency and volume, colonic transit time, rectal compliance, and innervation and function of the anal sphincter and pelvic floor.

2. Gastrointestinal and neurologic disorders may result in fecal incontinence.

3. Obstetric injuries to the pelvic floor, as well as denervation injuries related to childbirth or chronic straining, are the most common cause of fecal incontinence in women.

B Symptoms

1. Fecal urgency

2. Incontinence of flatus

3. Incontinence of stool

C Evaluation. A detailed history and examination, including a vaginal and rectal examination, are essential. Useful tests for determining the etiology of fecal incontinence may include anal ultrasound, anal manometry, and pelvic floor nerve conductance studies.

D Treatment. Therapy may include behavioral modification, pharmacologic agents, biofeedback, and surgery.

Study Questions for Chapter 38

Directions: *Each of the numbered items or incomplete statements in this section is followed by answers or by completions of the statement. Select the ONE lettered answer or completion that is BEST in each case.*

1. A 60-year-old woman, gravida 5, para 4, spontaneous abortions 1, has been treated with vaginal estrogen therapy, various pelvic muscle rehabilitation therapies, and pessaries for symptoms of pelvic prolapse without incontinence for the past 2 years. She desires definitive therapy. She has no past medical history other than hypertension, for which she takes hydrochlorothiazide. All of her children were delivered vaginally. On pelvic examination, vaginal mucosa is pink and moist. The anterior vaginal wall prolapses up to the hymenal ring on Valsalva. When the anterior vagina is supported with half of the speculum, the uterus and cervix prolapse past the hymenal ring as well. There is no stress incontinence when the urethrovesical junction is supported and the cystocele reduced. The uterus is normal in size, contour, and consistency. The sacral neurologic examination is unremarkable. A urine culture is sent. The next best step in management of this patient is:

- A Electrical stimulation of pelvic musculature
- B Abdominal hysterectomy and anterior repair
- C Vaginal hysterectomy and anterior repair
- D Vaginal hysterectomy, anterior repair, and suburethral sling
- E Burch retropubic urethropexy and anterior repair

2. A 32-year-old woman, gravida 3, para 3, just delivered a viable female infant weighing 4000 g via cesarean section for nonreassuring fetal heart rate pattern. She received intrathecal (spinal) anesthetic and narcotic for pain relief during the procedure. Her Foley catheter is left in place for several hours after the cesarean section. This will prevent:

- A Stress incontinence
- B Urge incontinence
- C Overflow incontinence
- D Bypass incontinence
- E Postoperative urinary tract infection

3. A 56-year-old woman, gravida 2, para 2, who reports leaking urine when she coughs and exercises, is diagnosed with genuine stress urinary incontinence. A regimen of Kegel exercises does not improve her symptoms, and she desires more definitive treatment. Her doctor recommends laparoscopic retropubic urethropexy. When discussing the risks and benefits of the laparoscopic Burch procedure, the doctor should mention:

- A Low short-term cure rates
- B 60% long-term cure rates
- C Risk of urinary retention
- D Alternative of drug therapy
- E Risk of graft infection and ulceration

4. A 67-year-old woman, gravida 3, para 3, presents to your office reporting incontinence. She tells you that she voids almost 40 times during the day and has several episodes of nocturia. She says she feels like voiding two to three times an hour and that when she makes it to the bathroom, only small amounts of urine are voided. Her past medical history is remarkable for mild asthma, for which she takes albuterol. Her previous gynecologist also placed her on estrogen patch, estrogen vaginal cream, and intravaginal progesterone tablets. She had a cholecystectomy 20 years ago and she is allergic to penicillin. Her BP = 130/80 mmHg, P = 80 bpm, height = 5 feet 4 inches, weight = 230 lb. On physical examination you notice pink, moist vaginal epithelium with mild cystocele and well-supported proximal urethra. The next best step in management of this patient is:

- **A** Urinalysis
- **B** Tolterodine
- **C** Pseudoephedrine
- **D** Pessary
- **E** Suburethral sling

5. A 55-year-old Caucasian woman, gravida 3, para 3, who delivered all of her children by scheduled cesarean sections (prior to initiation of labor), has mild pelvic organ prolapse. She had her last period 3 years ago and since that time has been on estrogen patches and progesterone vaginal tablets for treatment of hot flushes and vaginal dryness. She has no chronic medical problems but is on antibiotic therapy for acute bronchitis. Her family history is significant for osteoporosis diagnosed at an earlier age than average in her mother, two sisters, and grandmother. The strongest risk factor for pelvic relaxation in this patient is:

- **A** Parity
- **B** Age
- **C** Hormone status
- **D** Genetic
- **E** Cough

Answers and Explanations

1. The answer is C [II E 3]. The patient has uterine prolapse and cystocele, and conservative treatment (pelvic muscle rehab, pessary, and estrogen) has failed. Therefore, the next best treatment is surgical. Cystocele can be cured with anterior repair. Uterine prolapse can be cured with a hysterectomy. Because the anterior repair is performed vaginally, it makes sense to do the hysterectomy vaginally as well (if there are no contraindications) so as to have only one incision site and faster recovery. A suburethral sling is unnecessary for this patient because, in the clinical scenario, "there is no stress incontinence when the urethrovesical junction is supported and the cystocele reduced." Electrical stimulation is a form of pelvic muscle rehabilitation that has been tried and failed.

2. The answer is C [III A 3]. Intrathecal anesthetics and narcotics block nerve impulses to and from the bladder. When the bladder becomes distended with urine, the afferent impulses cannot be transmitted, and therefore the bladder detrusor muscle is underactive. This results in overdistension of the bladder and overflow incontinence. The risk of urinary tract infection is increased with placement of a Foley catheter.

3. The answer is C [III C 4,5]. The laparoscopic Burch has similar cure rates as the nonlaparoscopic Burch. The short- and long-term cure rates are very high (about 90%). The main complication of a retropubic urethropexy is the small risk of urinary retention, which depends on how tight paraurethral tissue is approximated to the Cooper ligament. This can be measured subjectively by the size of the dimple produced on the upper lateral fornices of the vagina. Only urge incontinence is effectively treated with drug therapy. Graft infection and ulceration is a risk of suburethral sling procedures.

4. The answer is A [III B 3a]. Although the clinical scenario is almost definitely urge incontinence, you must rule out urinary tract infection (UTI) because it may mimic symptoms of urgency. Once UTI is ruled out, you may begin therapy with tolterodine or oxybutynin. Pessary and suburethral slings are not as useful for detrusor overactivity as they are for stress incontinence.

5. The answer is D [II A]. The cause of POP is multifactorial. Genetics determine the subtype and density of collagen and connective tissue that a person inherits. Parity is not a risk factor in this patient because she has not had any vaginal deliveries and all of her cesarean sections were performed prior to initiation of labor. Nonchronic coughing (as in acute bronchitis) is not a risk factor for POP. This patient is only 55 years old; therefore, her age is not as large a determinant of her pelvic relaxation as in a woman who is 85 years old. This patient has been on hormone replacement since menopause; therefore, the tissues derived from the urogenital sinus have been stimulated adequately and continuously with estrogen.

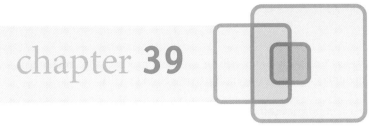

chapter 39

Pelvic Malignancies

CHRISTINA S. CHU

I. CERVICAL CANCER

Cervical cancer is the most preventable gynecologic cancer because of the Pap test. George Papanicolaou developed a method of identifying abnormal cells in exfoliative cytology in the 1920s and published his work in the 1940s. Pap test screening is now an integral part of health care in the United States. In some developing countries, where Pap smears are not routinely performed, cervical cancer remains the most common cause of cancer death in women.

A. Epidemiology and etiology

1. **Frequency peaks** between 45 and 60 years of age.

2. **Increased incidence** is related to:
   a. First intercourse at a young age
   b. Marriage or conception at a young age
   c. Multiple sexual partners
   d. Cigarette smoking. By-products of cigarette smoke are concentrated in cervical mucus and have been associated with a depletion of the cells of Langerhans, which are macrophages that assist in cell-mediated immunity.
   e. High-risk sexual partners (e.g., those whose previous sexual partners developed precancerous or cancerous conditions of the cervix or penis)
   f. Immunosuppression (e.g., from HIV infection or medications to maintain immunosuppression for organ transplantation)

3. **Infectious associations**
   a. **Human papilloma virus (HPV)**, a nonenveloped double-stranded DNA virus, is responsible for the vast majority of cases of cervical cancer. Incorporation of the E6 and E7 open reading frames into the cervical cell genome is associated with progression to invasive disease.
      (1) There are over 100 types of the HPV virus. Not all are associated with cervical cancer.
      (2) HPV is detected in more than 95% of cervical cancers and precancers. It is also detected in 50% of vaginal cancers/precancers, over 50% of vulvar cancers/precancers, 50% of penile cancers, and over 70% of anal cancers.
      (3) About 30 to 40 types of HPV are associated with anogenital infection.
      (4) Of these, about 15 to 20 types are considered oncogenic, and include types 16, 18, 31, 33, 35, 39, 45, 51, 52, and 58.
      (5) Nononcogenic types include types 6, 11, 40, 42, 43, 44, and 54. Of these, types 6 and 11 are most often associated with genital warts.
      (6) By age 50, at least 80% of women in the United States will have acquired a genital HPV infection. Among women under the age of 25, the prevalence is as high as 46%.
      (7) Fortunately, about 70% to 80% of HPV infections are transient and cleared by the immune system within 1 to 2 years.
   b. **Herpes simplex virus-2 (HSV-2)**. HSV-2 DNA and messenger RNA sequences have been found in cervical cancer cells and may increase the likelihood of HPV infection.

B. Preinvasive cervical disease

1. **Pap test screening**. The **cervical transformation zone (TZ)** is the site of most **squamous preinvasive and invasive neoplasms**. The TZ undergoes a transformation from mucus-secreting

glandular cells to non–mucus-secreting squamous cells in a normal process called **metaplasia** (change in growth). **Active metaplasia** is most susceptible to infection by HPV.

   a. Types of Pap smears

     (1) A **traditional Pap smear** is performed using a wooden spatula to wipe cells from the surface of the cervix and a brush to wipe cells from the endocervical canal. The cells are smeared onto a slide that is fixed and stained for cytologic evaluation.

     (2) A **liquid cytology** method (e.g., Thin Prep, AutoCyte) is commonly used to create a Pap test that is easier to evaluate. The specimen is collected by wiping cells from the cervix and endocervix. The cells are then suspended in liquid, which is processed to remove blood, mucus, and debris. The remaining concentrated suspension of cells is used to create a stained slide for evaluation. The specimens collected in this fashion can also be used to identify HPV subtypes, providing information that may help assess risk in a patient with a progressing lesion.

   b. Efficacy of cytologic screening programs

     (1) **Invasive carcinoma of the cervix** is usually preceded by a spectrum of **preinvasive disease**, which can be detected cytologically (e.g., with the Pap test). Detection and simple local treatments of preinvasive cervical disease can prevent invasive cancer.

     (2) **Regular cervical cancer screening programs** have demonstrated a significant decrease in mortality from cervical cancer. Unscreened populations can have as high as a 10-fold or greater increase in mortality from cervical cancer.

   c. Frequency of cervical cytologic screening

     (1) Screening should be initiated within 3 years of the onset of sexual activity or by age 21 years.

     (2) Women with high-risk factors (see I A 2) should be screened annually.

     (3) Women over the age of 30 with low-risk factors and three consecutive negative annual Pap tests can be screened every 2 to 3 years at the discretion of the physician.

     (4) Women over the age of 70 with three or more normal Pap tests in a row in the previous decade may consider discontinuation of Pap testing at the discretion of the physician.

     (5) Women who have had a total abdominal hysterectomy (with removal of the cervix) and no history of cervical cancer or dysplasia may discontinue Pap test screening.

   d. Evaluation of the abnormal Pap test. The **Bethesda System** uses descriptive terms that correlate with histology. This analysis includes:

     (1) A statement regarding the adequacy of the sample

     (2) A general categorization statement (optional)

     (3) A descriptive diagnosis regarding benign or reactive changes, low- or high-grade intraepithelial lesions (LSILs or HSILs), glandular cell abnormalities, or the presence of malignant cells

2. Further diagnosis with colposcopy. The Pap test carries a false-negative rate of 15% to 40% for invasive cancers, and colposcopy provides a more definitive diagnosis. This technique involves using magnification to inspect the TZ after applying a 3% to 5% acetic acid solution. Biopsies are performed of abnormal-appearing epithelium. Colposcopically directed biopsies carry an accuracy of 85% to 95%. **Endocervical curettage** is performed in conjunction with colposcopy to rule out dysplasia within the canal that is not visualized.

3. Treatment. Therapeutic recommendations are based on colposcopic biopsy.

   a. Low-grade lesions can be treated surgically or followed conservatively. Although there is a 70% incidence of regression, there is a 15% incidence of progression to a high-grade abnormality.

   b. Destruction or excision of the TZ may be performed using the following methods:

     (1) **Cold knife conization** is the gold standard because a pathologic specimen with clean margins is obtained. This procedure is performed in the operating room using a scalpel. It is recommended in the following circumstances:

       (a) Significant dysplastic lesions with either a nonvisualized component or a positive endocervical canal curettage

       (b) High-grade lesions that do not correlate with colposcopic findings

       (c) Premalignant or malignant glandular cell abnormalities

     (2) **Loop excision** is commonly called a loop electrosurgical excision procedure (LEEP) or large loop excision of transformation zone (LLETZ). This procedure is easily performed in the office with local anesthesia. A hot metal loop is used to excise a wedge of cervical tissue. Disadvantages include a cautery artifact at the margin of the specimen and a limited biopsy size because of lack of general anesthesia or size of the metal loop.

(3) **Cryotherapy** involves freezing the cervix in the office. It has the disadvantages of yielding no tissue for pathologic evaluation and potential scarring.

(4) **Laser vaporization** or **laser conization** is also performed at some centers.

c. **Cure rates** for preinvasive disease after one treatment range from 85% to 95%. Repeat treatment of the adequately evaluated persistent lesion results in a cure rate of 95%.

d. The risk of premalignant lesions persisting or recurring is 5% to 15%. Of these lesions, 85% are detected within 2 years of the initial treatment. **Follow-up** should include:

(1) Cytologic evaluation every 3 to 6 months for the first year posttreatment

(2) Repeat colposcopic evaluation for persistent or recurrent abnormalities

(3) Hysterectomy for patients who have persistent severe lesions despite repeated conservative local destructive techniques

C Microinvasive carcinoma of the cervix. Much controversy surrounds the exact definition of "early" invasive cancer of the cervix. A commonly adopted definition in the United States is a depth of invasion less than or equal to 3 mm, lesion width of less than or equal to 7 mm, and no evidence of lymphatic or vascular space involvement.

1. **Diagnosis** can be made only by means of a thoroughly examined cone biopsy specimen.

2. The **incidence of pelvic lymph node metastases** is less than 4%.

3. The treatment of choice is **total abdominal hysterectomy**, although cervical conization with negative margins may be used in women who wish to preserve fertility.

4. The **cure rate** is 95%.

D Invasive carcinoma of the cervix

1. **Symptoms**
   a. Postcoital or irregular bleeding is the most common symptom.
   b. Malodorous, bloody discharge; sciatica; leg edema; and deep pelvic pain are seen in advanced disease.

2. **Histology**. Squamous carcinomas (80%) and adenocarcinoma (15%) account for most invasive cervical cancer. There appears to be no difference in survival rates between women with these two groups of cancer when the lesions are matched for grade, size, and stage. Rare tumors of the cervix include small cell carcinomas, sarcomas, and lymphomas.

3. **Staging** (Table 39-1). Staging is **clinical** and does not change after surgery. Assessment for staging is based on cervical biopsies, physical examination, radiologic imaging of the kidneys and

---

TABLE 39-1 Staging System for Cervical Cancer

Stage I: Carcinoma is confined to cervix
  Stage IA: Microscopic tumors ≤5 mm deep or ≤7 mm wide
  Stage IA1: Invasion ≤3 mm in depth and ≤7 mm in width
  Stage IA2: Invasion >3 mm and ≤5 mm in depth, and ≤7 mm in width
  Stage IB: All other cases of stage I
Stage II: Carcinoma extends beyond cervix but not onto pelvic sidewall. Cancer extends into vagina but not lower third
  Stage IIA: No obvious parametrial involvement
  Stage IIB: Obvious parametrial involvement
Stage III: Carcinoma extends to pelvic sidewall. On rectal examination, there is no cancer-free space between tumor and pelvic sidewall. Tumor extends to lower third of vagina. All cases of hydronephrosis and nonfunctioning kidney should be included in stage III diagnoses unless another cause for these conditions can be found
  Stage IIIA: Tumor extends to lower third of vagina, with no extension to pelvic sidewall
  Stage IIIB: Extension onto pelvic sidewall, hydronephrosis, or nonfunctioning kidney
Stage IV: Carcinoma extends beyond true pelvis or clinically involves mucosa of bladder or rectum
  Stage IVA: Spread to mucosa of bladder or rectum
  Stage IVB: Spread beyond true pelvis

ureters to identify hydronephrosis caused by tumor extension, proctoscopy, cystoscopy, and chest radiography.

4. **Treatment**. Therapeutic measures are governed by the patient's age and general health and by the clinical stage of the cancer. Primary modalities include surgery and radiotherapy. Chemotherapy is commonly used as a radiation sensitizer.

   a. **Surgery**. This modality may be considered for patients with stage I or IIA disease. Typically, a **radical hysterectomy** with para-aortic and pelvic lymphadenectomy is performed. This procedure involves en bloc removal of the uterus, cervix, upper third of the vagina, parametrium, and uterosacral and uterovesical ligaments. In addition, the lymphatic nodes of the lower para-aortic, common iliac, and pelvic regions are removed en bloc. Very select cases may be treated with **radical trachelectomy** (radical removal of the cervix, upper vagina, and parametria) in order to preserve fertility. This procedure may be considered in carefully selected women with small tumors (stage IA2 to IB1) who strongly desire to retain the ability to attempt childbearing. A permanent cerclage must be placed at the time of the procedure to maintain competence of the lower uterine segment during pregnancy.

      (1) **Comparable cure rates** between surgery and radiotherapy are the rule in the treatment of early-stage disease. The best treatment of very bulky cervical cancers, which appear to be limited to the cervix, is still debated, but will usually be multimodal.

      (2) The **ovaries may be preserved with** surgical treatment, allowing for continued hormonal function in premenopausal women.

      (3) **Five-year survival rates with surgery** alone range from 75% to 100% for stage IA and IIA patients, depending on operative findings. Postoperative radiation with or without chemotherapy may improve survival in some cases.

   b. **Radiotherapy**. This treatment modality may be used for **all stages of cervical cancer**, either for curative or palliative intent. A series of randomized trials in the 1990s solidified the role of **chemotherapy** as an effective radiation **sensitizer**. Currently, chemotherapy, usually weekly intravenous cisplatin, is **included in most situations in which radiation therapy is used**.

      (1) Primary treatment usually involves **external beam radiotherapy (EBRT)** to the pelvis followed by intracavitary treatment or **brachytherapy**.

      (2) EBRT may be extended to include the para-aortic lymph nodes if they are involved or are at high risk for occult involvement.

      (3) Radiotherapy may be administered **after radical hysterectomy** for high-risk patients, including those with positive surgical margins, lymph–vascular space involvement, and disease within lymph nodes.

      (4) **Five-year survival rates with radiotherapy alone** are comparable for survival with surgery alone for stages IA and IIA disease.

      (5) For advanced-stage disease localized to the pelvis, 5-year survival varies from 50% to 80%. For metastatic disease out of the pelvis, survival is less than 15%.

5. **Follow-up**. Approximately 35% of patients with invasive cervical cancer are estimated to have persistent or recurrent disease. Most of these (85%) have a recurrence of disease within 3 years of the initial treatment.

   a. **Frequent checkups** are mandatory in the first 3 years. Evaluations include pelvic examinations, careful palpation of nodal groups, Pap smears, and radiologic imaging.

   b. **Suspicious signs and symptoms** include a persistent cervical or vaginal mass, unilateral leg edema, hydronephrosis, pelvic or sciatic pain, vaginal discharge, and palpable supraclavicular or groin nodes.

6. **Treatment of recurrent disease**. Treatment depends on whether recurrent disease is confined to the pelvis or is distant.

   a. **Pelvic confined**

      (1) Of **patients treated primarily with surgery**, 25% are saved after recurrence of the disease with pelvic radiotherapy.

      (2) In **patients treated primarily by radiotherapy** and in whom extensive presurgical and intraoperative evaluations reveal no evidence of metastatic tumor, partial or total **pelvic exenteration** (e.g., en bloc removal of the uterus, cervix, vagina, parametrium, bladder,

and rectum) is appropriate. This surgery often involves colostomy, urinary diversion, and vaginal reconstruction. It can be curative in up to 70% of cases.
   b. **Distant recurrence**. These patients are usually treated with chemotherapy. Cures are exceedingly rare, and response rates are variable and of limited duration. Radiotherapy can be used for the palliation of painful metastases.

E **Prevention of cervical cancer**

1. **Secondary prevention** of cancer involves detection of dysplastic lesions (i.e., by Pap testing and colposcopy) and then intervention to treat the precancerous areas before they become cancer.

2. **Primary prevention** of cervical cancer focuses on prevention of HPV infection.
   a. One HPV vaccine is currently approved by the Food and Drug Administration (FDA) for the prevention of HPV infection. Another is nearing approval.
   b. The approved vaccine covers HPV types 6, 11, 16, and 18. HPV 16 and 18 account for 70% of all cervical cancers, adenocarcinoma in situ, severe cervical dysplasia (CIN3), and moderate and severe vulvar and vaginal dysplasia. HPV 16 and 18 are also responsible for 50% of moderate cervical dysplasia (CIN2). Together, these four types are responsible for 90% of cases of genital warts.
   c. The approved vaccine appears to be over 95% effective in preventing HPV 16– and 18–related cervical cancer.
   d. This vaccine is currently approved for girls and young women ages 9 to 26, though additional data are being collected on its effectiveness in women of older ages.
   e. The vaccine is effective at preventing primary infection with the types of HPV virus included, but does not appear to be effective treatment for pre-existing infections. An individual who has been infected with one of the four included types may still benefit and develop immunity to the other strains included in the vaccine.

II ENDOMETRIAL CANCER

This disease is the most common gynecologic malignancy and the most curable.

A **Epidemiology**

1. **Incidence**. Endometrial cancer will eventually affect 2% to 3% of women in the United States.

2. **Risk factors**. Increased risk of endometrial cancer has been associated with factors related to prolonged or increased estrogen exposure without the controlling effects of adequate progestin or progesterone. Conditions associated with excess estrogen include:
   a. **Early menarche**
   b. **Late menopause**
   c. **Obesity** resulting in increased conversion of androstenedione to estrone in fat cells. Women who are more than 50 lb overweight have a 10 times higher risk of developing endometrial cancer over normal-weight individuals.
   d. **Polycystic ovary syndrome (PCOS) with chronic anovulation** is associated with an increase in estrogen production and lack of progesterone production. Ovulation is suppressed by a complex mechanism involving androgens and insulin in the ovary. As a result, production of progesterone (a potent "antiestrogenic" hormone) is suppressed, leaving the endometrium exposed to unopposed estrogen. Unopposed stimulation of the endometrium by estrogen leads to endometrial hyperplasia (a premalignant lesion) and endometrial carcinoma. Since over 50% of women with PCOS are obese, peripheral conversion of androgens to estrogens in fat increases the amount of estrogen available to stimulate the endometrium in these women.
   e. **Exogenous unopposed estrogen**. A significant correlation exists between use of exogenous estrogen and endometrial cancer when estrogen therapy is administered without the protective effects of a progestin.
   f. **Tamoxifen**. This agent acts as an antiestrogen in the breast but stimulates the endometrium similarly to estrogen, resulting in an increased risk of endometrial cancer (relative risk of 7).

The therapeutic benefit in appropriately selected women with breast cancer outweighs this risk.

    g. Estrogen-secreting tumors. Granulosa and theca cell ovarian tumors produce active estrogen and have been associated with a 25% incidence of a concurrent endometrial carcinoma.

    h. Other factors. A history of breast and ovarian cancers is associated with an increased risk of a concomitant endometrial carcinoma. In addition, a history of hypertension and diabetes mellitus is associated with an increased risk of endometrial carcinoma, although these factors may be related to obesity.

  3. The **Lynch II syndrome**, also called **hereditary nonpolyposis colorectal cancer syndrome**, is an autosomal dominant–inherited predisposition to developing cancer. Endometrial cancer is the second most common cancer in women of Lynch II families. It is recommended that affected women consider prophylactic hysterectomy when childbearing is complete.

  4. Factors associated with **decreased risk** are smoking, high parity, and use of oral contraceptives. Endometrial cancer that occurs in the absence of estrogenic risk factors is rare and often has a worse prognosis with more aggressive cell types and early metastases.

  B **Endometrial hyperplasia**, which may be a precursor to endometrial carcinoma

    1. Types of endometrial hyperplasia are classified based on the extent of endometrial gland crowding and on cellular atypia.

      a. Simple hyperplasia without atypia is associated with a 1% risk of progression to cancer. For simple hyperplasia with atypia, the risk is 8%.

      b. Complex hyperplasia without atypia is associated with a 3% risk of progression to cancer. For complex hyperplasia **with atypia, the risk is 29%.**

    2. The **diagnosis of endometrial hyperplasia** must be established with adequate sampling of the endometrium in any woman with abnormal bleeding who is older than 35 years of age.

    3. Treatment of endometrial hyperplasia

      a. Young women desiring fertility may be treated with 3 to 6 months of progestin therapy, followed by a repeat endometrial sampling.

      b. Proper sampling of the endometrium of **perimenopausal and postmenopausal women** with dilation and curettage (D&C) to ensure proper diagnosis is essential.

        (1) For hyperplasia without atypia, initial treatment is **conservative**: 3 to 6 months of progestin therapy followed by a repeat endometrial sampling.

        (2) Hysterectomy is recommended for women with complex atypical hyperplasia and for women with persistent hyperplasia after treatment with a progestational agent.

  C Endometrial carcinoma

    1. Symptoms. The most common symptom of endometrial carcinoma is irregular menses or post-menopausal bleeding. Any woman older than 35 years of age with heavy menses or bleeding throughout the month should have an endometrial biopsy.

    2. Age. The median age for endometrial cancer is 61 years. The largest number of patients is between 50 and 59 years of age.

    3. Histology. The **principal histologic subtype** of endometrial carcinoma is **endometrioid adenocarcinoma** (75% to 85%). The remaining subtypes include mucinous, papillary serous, clear cell, and squamous carcinoma. **Papillary serous and clear cell** subtypes are associated with a lower survival rate. Histologic differentiation correlates with depth of myometrial penetration, pelvic and periaortic lymphatic metastases, and overall 5-year survival.

    4. Staging is based on surgical findings (Table 39-2).

    5. Diagnosis and staging evaluation

      a. D&C. This procedure is the definitive method of diagnosis. However, an **office biopsy** may yield a diagnosis without the additional need for a D&C.

      b. Preoperative workup should include a chest radiograph. A computed tomography (CT) scan or other imaging studies of the abdomen and pelvis are optional.

    6. Treatment. A surgical staging evaluation includes total abdominal hysterectomy, bilateral salpingo-oophorectomy, peritoneal cytology (e.g., washings of the pelvis and abdomen), and omentectomy.

TABLE 39–2 **Staging System for Endometrial Carcinoma**

Stage I: Confined to uterus
 Stage IA: Tumor limited to endometrium
 Stage IB: Tumor invades less than one-half of the myometrium
 Stage IC: Tumor invades more than one-half of the myometrium
Stage II: Involvement of cervix
 Stage IIA: Endocervical glandular involvement
 Stage IIB: Cervical stromal invasion
Stage III
 Stage IIIA: Tumor invades serosa or adnexa, or positive peritoneal cytology
 Stage IIIB: Vaginal metastases
 Stage IIIC: Metastases to pelvic or para-aortic nodes
Stage IV: Mucosal involvement of bladder or rectum or extension beyond true pelvis
 Stage IVA: Tumor invades bladder or bowel mucosa
 Stage IVB: Distant metastases, including inguinal lymph nodes

For all stages, the degree of differentiation is noted. G1, G2, G3.

Intraoperative evaluation of the depth of uterine invasion may be performed by a pathologist. Sampling of **nodes from the pelvic and para-aortic regions** is recommended for patients with poorly differentiated cancer, tumor invasion through more than half of the uterine wall, or cervical extension of tumor. Some experts recommend sampling the lymph nodes in all cases because of the uncertainty associated with intraoperative frozen section.

   a. **Low-risk patients** comprise those with **stage IA, grade 1 or 2 carcinomas**. This group of tumors has few poor prognostic features. Surgery (total abdominal hysterectomy and bilateral salpingo-oophorectomy) alone is usually considered adequate treatment. Disease-free survival rate is 96%.

   b. **Intermediate-risk patients** are those with **grade 3 tumors, stage IB, IC, IIA, or IIB,** and **positive peritoneal cytology with less than one-third myometrial invasion** and **no other extrauterine spread**. These patients may be offered pelvic irradiation, vaginal cuff irradiation, or hormonal therapy. Patients with full surgical staging (negative pelvic and para-aortic lymph nodes) may also forgo adjuvant radiation therapy.

   c. **High-risk patients** include those with **adnexal spread, node metastases, outer one-third myometrial invasion**, or **grade 3 tumors with any invasion**. Adjuvant radiotherapy and/or chemotherapy may be beneficial.

   d. **Stage IV carcinomas**. Treatment in these patients must be individualized. In most instances, treatment programs involve surgery with adjuvant chemotherapy or hormonal therapy.

   e. **Recurrent disease**. Treatment for recurrent disease must be individualized, depending on the extent and site of recurrence, hormone receptor status, and patient's health. Treatment programs may include exenterative procedures, radiotherapy, chemotherapy, and hormonal therapy.

III   EPITHELIAL OVARIAN CANCER

This is cancer arising from the epithelial surface of the ovary. Epithelial ovarian cancer accounts for 90% of ovarian cancers. It is the most difficult gynecologic cancer to diagnose because symptoms are nonspecific. The remaining 10% of ovarian cancers, classified as "nonepithelial ovarian cancers," arise from the ovarian germ cells, or sex cord and stromal cells; for a detailed description, see IV.

A Epidemiology

   1. **Incidence**. The incidence begins to increase in the fifth decade and continues to increase until the eighth decade. Ovarian cancer is the **leading cause of death attributable to gynecologic cancers in the United States**. Approximately 1 in 70 women (1.7%) will contract ovarian cancer.

   2. **Risk factors**
      a. **Family history** of ovarian cancer is the strongest risk factor for the disease; however, **most ovarian cancer is not familial**.

      (1) The risk is 4% to 5% if one relative is affected.

      (2) The risk is 7% if two relatives are affected.

  b. Mutations in autosomal dominant tumor suppressor genes, BRCA1 and BRCA2, which are located on chromosomes 17 and 13, respectively, are identified in 5% to 10% of patients with ovarian cancer.

      (1) These genes account for most cases of familial breast ovarian cancer and confer an increased risk of ovarian cancer. The penetrance of the genes is variable but may confer a risk of 20% to 50%.

      (2) Approximately 2% of Ashkenazi Jews are carriers of mutations in one of these genes. **Familial breast ovarian cancer syndrome** should be suspected if multiple family members have breast and ovarian cancer, if the age of onset of cancers is early, if multiple primary sites of cancer are noted in one patient, or if male breast cancer occurs in the family (likely BRCA2 mutation).

  c. Low parity and infertility are risk factors associated with excess ovulation, which, in turn, may be an irritant to the ovary, increasing the propensity for cancer development.

3. Use of **oral contraceptives** is correlated with a **decreased risk** of ovarian cancer. Whether this is a marker for fertility rather than an independent protective factor is unclear.

4. Preventive measures include **prophylactic oophorectomy**, which should be offered to high-risk patients. These patients still have a 2% risk of developing primary peritoneal carcinoma, a cancer that is histologically identical to ovarian carcinoma but arises from the epithelial surfaces of the abdomen and pelvis. In women with BRCA1 or BRCA2 mutations, prophylactic oophorectomy should be strongly considered in the late 30s; it not only decreases the risk of ovarian cancer, but also decreases the risk of breast cancer. Older women having pelvic surgery should consider prophylactic oophorectomy even if they are not considered high risk.

B Diagnosis

1. Ovarian cancer usually produces **nonspecific symptoms** until the disease is advanced. In more than 70% of cases, the ovarian disease has spread beyond the pelvis before the diagnosis is made.

  a. Abdominal distention caused by ascites is often the presenting complaint.

  b. Lower abdominal pain, a pelvic mass, and weight loss are additional features.

2. Early diagnosis of ovarian cancer is rare, but it may be identified on bimanual pelvic examination or using radiologic imaging studies.

3. There is **no reliable screening test**.

  a. Although **CA-125 levels** are elevated above the normal range in more than 85% of patients with advanced ovarian cancer, these levels should not be used for screening purposes because of the high number of false-negative and false-positive results. This is especially true in early disease when screening would be of most benefit.

  b. Pelvic ultrasound is helpful in characterizing the size and architecture of the adnexal mass. Approximately 95% of ovarian cancers are larger than 5 cm. Multicystic and solid components and free fluid in the cul-de-sac are ultrasonic features suggestive of ovarian carcinoma. Ultrasound screening combined with CA-125 testing has not been shown to improve early detection rates, even in high-risk patients.

  c. For lack of better strategy for screening, many physicians offer annual or biannual testing with **physical examination, CA-125, and transvaginal ultrasound to patients with a family history of ovarian cancer.**

4. Abdominopelvic CT scan, barium enema, and **chest radiography** are helpful in the evaluation of disease in women suspected of having ovarian cancer.

C Staging. Surgical findings are used to stage ovarian cancer (Table 39-3). More than 60% of patients have stage III or IV disease at the time of diagnosis.

D Predominant histologic types

1. Serous tumors account for 40% of ovarian carcinomas.

2. Mucinous tumors account for 10% of ovarian carcinomas.

TABLE 39–3   Staging System for Ovarian Cancer

Stage I: Limited to ovaries
    Stage IA: Limited to one ovary; no ascites containing malignant cells; no tumor on external surface of ovary; capsule intact
    Stage IB: Limited to both ovaries; no ascites containing malignant cells; no tumor on external surface of ovary; capsule intact
    Stage IC: Tumor either stage IA or IB but with ascites containing malignant cells, tumor on surface of one or both ovaries, or rupture of tumor capsule
Stage II: Involvement of one or both ovaries with pelvic extension
    Stage IIA: Extension or metastases to uterus or tubes or both
    Stage IIB: Extension to other pelvic tissues
    Stage IIC: Tumor either stage IIA or IIB but with ascites containing malignant cells, tumor on surface of one or both ovaries, or rupture of tumor capsule
Stage III: Involvement of one or both ovaries with peritoneal metastases outside pelvis or superficial liver metastases or retroperitoneal nodes containing cancer
    Stage IIIA: Tumor limited to pelvis with negative nodes but microscopic seeding of peritoneum
    Stage IIIB: Peritoneal implants ≤2 cm in diameter with negative nodes
    Stage IIIC: Implants >2 cm in diameter or positive retroperitoneal or inguinal nodes
Stage IV: Involvement of one or both ovaries with distant metastases; this can include positive pleural effusion and intrahepatic metastases

---

    3. Endometrioid tumors account for 10% of ovarian carcinomas.

    4. Clear cell carcinoma, which is more common in Asia, accounts for 6% of ovarian carcinomas. These cancers appear to be more resistant to chemotherapy than serous, mucinous, and endometrioid ovarian carcinomas.

    5. Small cell ovarian cancers are rare and have a poor prognosis.

    6. Borderline ovarian tumors (also called "ovarian carcinoma of low malignant potential") account for 15% of epithelial malignancies. This distinct type of ovarian carcinoma has the potential to metastasize but not to invade tissues. The cell type may be papillary serous or mucinous. With surgical debulking, most of these cancers are curable. The average age at diagnosis is 48 years. Patients with these tumors have higher survival rates, and most are diagnosed in stage I.

  E Clinical course of ovarian carcinoma

    1. The **initial spread** of ovarian carcinoma is to adjacent peritoneal surfaces, omentum, and retroperitoneal lymph nodes.

    2. Extra-abdominal and intrahepatic metastases occur late in the disease and only in a small percentage of cases.

    3. Bowel obstruction occurs as a terminal event and results from massive serosal involvement.

  F Treatment.   A combination of surgery and chemotherapy is necessary.

    1. Goals of surgery are to determine the extent of the disease through **staging** and to remove or **debulk** as much tumor as possible. Surgery may include the following:
      a. Exploratory laparotomy through a vertical abdominal incision, allowing a thorough evaluation of the upper abdomen
      b. Peritoneal washings from the pelvis and upper abdomen
      c. Inspection of all peritoneal and diaphragmatic surfaces
      d. Excision of pelvic and para-aortic lymph nodes
      e. Omentectomy
      f. Debulking tumor with the goal of leaving behind as little residual disease as possible

    2. Ovarian cancer is extremely sensitive to chemotherapy. However, this cancer has a tendency to recur.
      a. Taxane (such as paclitaxel or docetaxel) **and platinum** (such as carboplatin or cisplatin) chemotherapy are currently the standard treatment for all patients with ovarian cancer who

have a tumor of stage IB or greater. Patients with stage IA grade 1 or 2 cancers may forgo chemotherapy. Patients with advanced disease that has been optimally debulked may benefit from a combination of intraperitoneal and intravenous chemotherapy.

b. Side effects of paclitaxel include neuropathy, alopecia, myelosuppression, neuropathy, hypersensitivity reaction, and bradycardia.

c. Side effects of carboplatin include nausea and vomiting, myelosuppression, and constipation.

G Recurrent ovarian cancer. Though 70% of ovarian cancer responds to initial surgery and chemotherapy, most patients recur. Recurrent ovarian cancer can only very rarely be cured. Treatment is mainly palliative and usually consists of treatment with chemotherapy. Occasionally, patients may benefit from additional debulking surgery. With time, ovarian cancer develops chemotherapy resistance. Because advanced ovarian cancer usually recurs and 5-year survival in stage III disease is only 20%, patients should be encouraged to enroll in clinical trials using novel treatments.

IV NONEPITHELIAL OVARIAN CANCER

This form of ovarian cancer arises from the germ cells and sex cord–stromal cells of the ovary. These rare cancers account for less than 10% of ovarian tumors. Staging is the same as for epithelial ovarian cancer (see Table 39-3). Treatment consists of surgical staging or debulking, occasionally followed by chemotherapy as detailed for each cancer subtype.

A Germ cell tumors. Benign germ cell tumors, called mature cystic teratomas, or "dermoids," account for 25% to 30% of ovarian neoplasms. Malignant germ cell tumors are believed to arise from primitive germ cells in the ovary. These cancers represent 5% of all ovarian malignancies but account for more than two-thirds of all malignant ovarian neoplasms in women younger than 20 years of age. When disease is limited to one ovary, it is appropriate to **leave the uterus and other ovary in place**, as long as a complete staging, including pelvic and para-aortic lymph node dissection, is performed.

1. **Dysgerminomas.** Histologically, the undifferentiated germ cells present as sheets of uniform polyhedral cells. There is a characteristic lymphocytic infiltrate within delicate fibrous septa. Other characteristics of dysgerminomas include the following:
   a. They are the **most common malignant germ cell tumor**, accounting for approximately 40% of this type of tumor.
   b. Ninety percent of dysgerminomas are found in women younger than 30 years of age.
   c. The propensity for lymphatic invasion is great.
   d. Syncytiotrophoblasts in the tumor occasionally secrete detectable amounts of human chorionic gonadotropin (hCG).
   e. Bilateral tumors occur in more than 20% of cases; 50% of these are macroscopic.
   f. Tumors are exquisitely sensitive to chemotherapy, and the cure rate approaches 95%.

2. **Immature teratomas.** Histologically, a mixture of differentiated fetal tissue representing three germinal layers is present. Usually the immature element is **neural tissue**. Immature teratomas are further characterized by the following:
   a. They account for 20% of all germ cell tumors.
   b. Tumors are rarely bilateral, although 10% of patients have a benign dermoid in the contralateral ovary.
   c. Prognosis is excellent. Adjuvant chemotherapy is recommended for most patients. Patients with low-grade, stage I disease may be followed with surgery alone.

3. **Endodermal sinus tumors or yolk sac tumors.** The classic histologic finding is the **Schiller-Duval body**, a central vessel lined with columnar cells. Endodermal sinus tumors are further characterized by the following:
   a. They account for 20% of all germ cell tumors.
   b. The **median age of patients** with endodermal sinus tumors is 19 years.
   c. Tumors are rarely bilateral.
   d. α-Fetoprotein (AFP) is detectable in the serum of most patients and acts as a tumor marker.

    e. All patients should receive postoperative chemotherapy.

    f. In patients with complete surgical excision of tumor prior to chemotherapy, survival is 96%. Survival with incomplete resection is 55%.

  4. Embryonal carcinomas. The histologic appearance of undifferentiated embryonal tissue consists of solid sheets of anaplastic cells with abundant clear cytoplasm, hyperchromatic nuclei, and numerous mitotic figures. Embryonal carcinoma is further characterized by the following:

    a. This rare cancer occurs in young females; the **median age of patients** with embryonal carcinoma is 15 years.

    b. Tumors elaborate both AFP and hCG. These trophic hormones may be responsible for precocious puberty in prepubertal girls.

    c. Most often, tumors are unilateral with explosive growth tendencies, leading to large tumor masses and acute abdominal pain. Tumors are rarely bilateral.

    d. Surgery and chemotherapy result in cures for approximately one-third of patients.

  5. Nongestational choriocarcinomas. These primary tumors must be distinguished from metastatic disease to the ovary from gestational choriocarcinomas. The histologic appearance is that of atypical to highly anaplastic cytotrophoblastic and syncytiotrophoblastic elements. These tumors are further characterized by the following:

    a. This rare cancer usually occurs in women of reproductive age.

    b. Tumors are rarely bilateral.

    c. hCG is detectable in the serum of most patients and acts as a tumor marker.

    d. Tumors can present as a pelvic mass and precocious puberty in prepubertal girls.

    e. Treatment with surgery and chemotherapy results in 80% survival.

  6. Polyembryonal cancer. This cancer has the histologic appearance of embryoid bodies in various states of development. This tumor is further characterized by the following:

    a. This rare cancer usually occurs in women of early reproductive age.

    b. Tumors are rarely bilateral.

    c. hCG and AFP are often detectable in the serum of patients and act as a tumor marker.

  7. Mixed germ cell tumors. Approximately 10% of germ cell tumors are composed of two or more subtypes of cancer. Treatment and prognosis are based on the most severe element.

B **Sex cord–stromal neoplasms.** The sex cord cells are granulosa cells and the male homolog, the Sertoli cells. Stromal cells include theca cells, Leydig cells, and fibroblasts. Tumors arising from these cells often produce estrogens and androgens. Granulosa cells, Sertoli cells, and theca cells are usually estrogenic. Leydig cells and specific steroid cells are usually androgenic.

  1. Juvenile granulosa cell tumors that occur in premenarchal women induce abnormal bleeding and breast development. Early-stage disease is curable with surgery, but the prognosis for disease spread beyond the ovary is poor.

  2. Adult granulosa cell tumors have the following characteristics:

    a. They are bilateral in less than 5% of cases.

    b. Tumors vary in size from microscopic to tumors that fill the abdomen.

    c. Tumors are characterized histologically by **Call-Exner bodies** (e.g., rosettes or follicles of granulosa cells, often with a central clearing).

    d. Ninety percent of cases present as stage I disease and are usually curable. More advanced stage disease is prone to recurrence, often many years after initial treatment.

  3. Sertoli-Leydig cell tumors or arrhenoblastoma are rare tumors of mesenchymal origin.

    a. Their usual endocrine activity is androgenic.

    b. Defeminization is the classic feature of the androgen-secreting tumors, including breast and uterine atrophy, which is followed by masculinization, including hirsutism, acne, receding hairline, clitoromegaly, and deepening of the voice. Prognosis is based on the extent of differentiation.

C **Gonadoblastomas.** These tumors are composed of **germ cells and stromal cells.** They occur in **dysgenic ovaries** commonly present in individuals with a Y chromosome or fragment because of a mosaic genotype (46,X/46,XY) or testicular feminization (46,XY with androgen insensitivity).

Both ovaries are usually affected, and it is recommended that these individuals undergo prophylactic bilateral oophorectomy. **Dysgerminomas** or occasionally other germ cell malignancies occur in 50% of patients with gonadoblastomas.

V VAGINAL CANCER

A **Squamous cell carcinomas.** These cancers are usually located in the upper half of the vagina. They are the most common histologic type.

1. **Symptoms**
   a. The most common symptom is **vaginal discharge**, which is often bloody.
   b. Because of the **elasticity of the posterior vaginal fornix**, tumors may be large before they are symptomatic.

2. **Age**. This rare, malignant cancer occurs in women between 35 and 70 years of age.

3. **Lymphatic spread**. The upper vagina is drained by the common iliac and hypogastric (internal iliac) nodes, whereas the lower vagina is drained by the regional lymph nodes of the femoral triangle.

4. **Staging** (Table 39-4)

5. **Treatment**. Treatment is primarily by radiotherapy. Large carcinomas of the vault or vaginal walls are treated initially with external radiation; this shrinks the neoplasm so that local radiation therapy will be more effective. Occasionally, vaginal cancer is amenable to primary surgical excision or to excision with a radical hysterectomy and upper vaginectomy.

6. **Five-year survival rates**
   a. **Stage I:** 80% to 90%
   b. **Stage II:** 60%
   c. **Stage III:** 40%
   d. **Stage IV:** 0%

TABLE 39–4   Staging System for Vaginal Cancer

Stage I: Limited to vaginal mucosa
Stage II: Involvement of subvaginal tissue but no extension onto pelvic sidewall
Stage III: Extension onto pelvic sidewall
Stage IV: Extension beyond true pelvis or involvement of mucosa of bladder or rectum

B **Diethylstilbestrol (DES)-related adenocarcinoma (clear cell carcinoma).** DES was used in the 1940s through the early 1970s in high-risk pregnancies (e.g., diabetes, habitual abortion, and threatened abortion) to prevent miscarriage. In all documented cases of genital tract abnormalities, maternal DES use began before the 18th week of pregnancy.

1. **Age**
   a. The mean age for development of clear cell adenocarcinoma of the vagina is 19 years for patients with a history of DES exposure.
   b. The risk for development of these carcinomas through the age of 24 years in DES-exposed women has been calculated to be between 0.14 and 1.4 per 1000.

2. **Characteristics of clear cell carcinoma**
   a. Approximately 40% of the cancers occur in the cervix, and the other 60% occur primarily in the upper half of the vagina.
   b. The **incidence of lymph node metastases** is high—about 16% in stage I and 30% or more in stage II.

3. **Treatment**
   a. If the cancer is confined to the cervix and the upper vagina, radical hysterectomy and upper vaginectomy with pelvic lymphadenectomy and ovarian preservation are recommended.

b. Advanced tumors and lesions involving the lower vagina are treated more appropriately by radiation, which should include treatment of the pelvic nodes and parametrial tissues.

4. Prognosis. Five-year survival rates are better than those for the squamous tumors of the cervix and upper vagina, probably because of earlier detection.

VI VULVAR CARCINOMA

A Epidemiology. Factors associated with vulvar carcinoma include the following:

1. A history of vulvar condylomata or granulomatous venereal disease

2. A history of vulvar Paget disease

3. A history of vulvar carcinoma in situ

4. A history of cervical or vaginal cancer

5. More than 50% of the patients are between the ages of 60 and 79 years. Fewer than 15% are younger than 40 years of age.

B Etiology. Little is known about causal factors in vulvar carcinoma. Recently, HPV types 16 and 18 have been detected in squamous cancer of the vulva.

C Symptoms. Recognition of a lesion is often accompanied by a delay in diagnosis because of either self-treatment by the patient or lack of recognition by the treating physician. Vulvar cancer usually presents with:

1. A history of chronic **vulvar irritation** or soreness

2. A **visible lesion on the labia**, which is often painful or pruritic

D Histology. Squamous carcinoma comprises 90% of these tumors. The remaining 10% consist of malignant melanoma, basal cell carcinoma, and sarcoma. The Bartholin gland may give rise to vulvar adenocarcinoma.

E Patterns of spread

1. Local expansion involves the contiguous structures of the urethra, vagina, perineum, anus, rectum, and pubic bone.

2. Lymphatic spread follows the lymphatic drainage pattern of the vulva, which includes superficial inguinal nodes, deep femoral groups, and pelvic nodes.

3. Hematogenous spread occurs in the advanced or recurrent cases.

F Diagnosis. Incisional or excisional biopsy of the suspect lesion under local or general anesthesia confirms the diagnosis.

G Pretreatment evaluation. Clinical assessment of tumor size (T), nodes (N), and metastases (M) and surgical staging are appropriate (Table 39-5).

H Treatment. Surgical treatment is individualized.

1. T1 lesions (tumor 2 cm or smaller in size)
  a. Radical local excision of the lesion with a 1-cm margin laterally and a depth down to the inferior fascia is indicated when:
     (1) Biopsy of the tumor reveals a depth of invasion of less than 1 mm.
     (2) Tumor is unifocal.
     (3) Remaining vulva is normal.
  b. No groin dissection is necessary.

2. T2 and early T3 tumors without suspect inguinal nodes
  a. Radical vulvectomy may be partial or total, depending on the size and location of the lesion.
  b. Bilateral inguinal and femoral lymphadenectomy may be warranted. Ipsilateral inguinal and femoral lymphadenectomy may be considered when the lesion is well lateralized.

TABLE 39–5   Clinical Assessment and Staging System for Vulvar Carcinoma

Assessment
Tumor size (T)
T1: Tumor ≤2 cm in size that is confined to vulva
T2: Tumor >2 cm in size that is confined to vulva
T3: Tumor of any size that spreads to urethra, vagina, perineum, or anus
T4: Tumor of any size that infiltrates bladder and rectal mucosa or is fixed to bone
Node (N)
N0: No regional nodes palpable
N1: Unilateral regional lymph node metastases
N2: Bilateral regional lymph node metastases
Metastases (M)
M0: No metastases
M1: Distant metastases, including pelvic nodes

Staging
Stage I: T1 N0 M0
Stage II: T2 N0 M0
Stage III: T3 N0 M0; T3 N1 M0; T1 N1 M0; or T2 N1 M0
Stage IVA: T1 N2 M0; T2 N2 M0; T3 N2 M0; or T4, any N, M0
Stage IVB: Any T, any N, M1

3. **Tumors with disease in inguinal nodes** are treated with lymphadenectomy. If there are more than two histologically positive nodes, external beam radiation is administered to the groin and pelvis.

4. **Advanced disease.** Individualized treatment may include surgery, radiation, and chemotherapy. Pelvic radiotherapy is recommended for patients with involved nodes. Survival is poor.

Study Questions for Chapter 39

Directions: *Match the statement below with the best system. Each answer may be used once, more than once, or not at all.*

QUESTIONS 1–2

A Brain
B Ureter
C Liver
D Intestine
E Spleen

1. Advanced cervical cancer can affect this structure by extension and pressure effects

2. Advanced ovarian cancer often affects this structure by spread and encroachment

3. HPV is associated with the development of cervical, vaginal, vulvar, and anal cancers. Which of the following statements is true?

A HPV types 16 and 18 are detected in over 95% of cases of cervical cancer
B The quadrivalent vaccine that is currently approved for prevention of HPV infection is over 95% effective in preventing HPV 16– and 18–related cervical cancers
C By age 50, 46% of women in the United States will have acquired a genital HPV infection
D HPV types 6 and 11 are oncogenic and therefore are most often associated with genital warts
E 95% of HPV infections are transient and will be cleared within 1–2 years

4. A 40-year-old woman, gravida 1, para 1, presents to you because she wants to decrease her risk of ovarian cancer via a prophylactic oophorectomy. She has no chronic medical problems except obesity. Her gynecologic history is remarkable for first sexual intercourse at age 15 years, four sexual partners in her entire life, and breastfeeding of her only child. Her Pap smear has shown exposure to HPV. She had infertility and conceived her only child with in vitro fertilization, and subsequently was taking birth control pills. She smokes one pack per week (for the last 10 years) and has an occasional drink with her husband. Her family history is remarkable for breast cancer in her mother and maternal grandmother and ovarian cancer in her maternal aunt. The most significant risk factor for developing ovarian cancer is her:

A Family history
B HPV
C Low parity
D Birth control pills
E Smoking

5. A 23-year-old woman, gravida 1, para 0, spontaneous abortions 1, has undergone colposcopy for evaluation of a high-grade lesion found on Pap smear. The squamocolumnar junction was visible in its entirety, and the endocervical curettage was normal. A directed biopsy of the cervix revealed a 1-mm focus of invasion. The next best step in management is:

A Radical trachelectomy
B Cryotherapy of cervix (Cryo)
C Cold knife conization of cervix (CKC)
D Simple hysterectomy and bilateral salpingo-oophorectomy (TAH-BSO)
E Radical hysterectomy (Rad Hyst)

QUESTIONS 7–11

Directions: *Match the statement below with the histology. Each answer may be used once, more than once, or not at all.*

A Squamous
B Serous
C Mucinous
D Endometrioid
E Clear
F Small
G Papillary serous
H Dysgerminoma
I Teratoma
J Endodermal sinus
K Choriocarcinoma
L Sertoli-Leydig
M Gonadoblastoma
N Melanoma

6. Most common histology for cervical cancer

7. Subtype of endometrial cancer with very poor prognosis; is also type of borderline ovarian tumor

8. Most common malignant germ cell tumor

9. Uncommon, aggressive vulvar cancer that is known as the most common cancer to metastasize to the placenta

10. Most common endometrial cancer

Answers and Explanations

1. B [Table 39-1], **2. D** [Table 39-3, III E 3]. Cervical cancer extends laterally toward the pelvic sidewall and can encroach on the ureter resulting in hydronephrosis (stage IIIB). However, ovarian cancer spreads out over the peritoneal surface and implants on the peritoneum and intestinal wall. This can eventually lead to bowel obstruction.

3. The answer is B [I A 3 a]. The approved quadrivalent vaccine appears to be over 95% effective in preventing HPV 16– and 18–related cervical cancer. HPV 16 and 18 account for 70% of all cervical cancers, adenocarcinoma in situ, severe cervical dysplasia (CIN3), and moderate and severe vulvar and vaginal dysplasia. HPV 16 and 18 are also responsible for 50% of moderate cervical dysplasia (CIN2). Nononcogenic types include types 6, 11, 40, 42, 43, 44, and 54. Of these, types 6 and 11 are most often associated with genital warts. By age 50, at least 80% of women in the United States will have acquired a genital HPV infection. Among women under the age of 25, the prevalence is as high as 46%. Within 1–2 years 70% of all HPV infections are cleared by the body's immune system.

4. The answer is A [III A 2, 3]. The family history of ovarian cancer is the strongest risk factor for developing ovarian cancer, especially if it is a first-degree relative. The familial breast ovarian cancer syndrome that is usually associated with an autosomal dominant mutation in the BRCA1 and BRCA2 genes should be suspected when multiple breast and ovarian cancers occur in one family. Mutations in these genes account for 5% to 10% of all cases of ovarian cancer. Oral contraception is associated with a decreased risk of ovarian cancer. HPV is associated with cervical, not ovarian, cancer. Low parity is a risk factor for ovarian cancer but is not the strongest risk factor here. Smoking is associated with many types of cancers but does not have a large relative risk in ovarian cancer.

5. The answer is C [I C 1]. The diagnosis of microinvasive cervical cancer can be made only by thorough examination of a cone biopsy specimen. If the diagnosis of microinvasion is confirmed, further treatment may involve a simple hysterectomy only. An endometrial biopsy is not necessary for further evaluation of HSIL. Cryotherapy is not a good option because it may not completely destroy the microinvasive lesion (therefore no cure) and it does not provide a pathologic specimen for further evaluation of the lesion. In this patient, a TAH-BSO is not the best initial step here because she has no children and is still of childbearing age. A radical trachelectomy would allow preservation of fertility in this patient, but first the diagnosis of microinvasive cancer needs to be confirmed by cone biopsy. A radical hysterectomy is too radical of a procedure for a microinvasive lesion. It is not without complications.

6. A [I D 2], **7. G** [II C 3 and III D 6], **8. H** [IV A 1], **9. N** [VI D], **10. D** [II C 3]. The most common histologic type of cervical cancer is squamous cell carcinoma (80%), followed by adenocarcinoma (15%). Papillary serous subtypes of endometrial carcinoma are associated with increased aggressiveness and low survival. However, papillary serous carcinoma of the ovary is a borderline ovarian tumor that can be treated with surgical debulking. Most of these cancers are curable. Dysgerminomas are the most common malignant germ cell tumors. Ninety percent are found in women younger than 30 years of age. These tumors are exquisitely sensitive to chemotherapy. The most common histology for vulvar carcinoma is squamous cell carcinoma (90%). Melanomas are uncommon vulvar cancers, but they are aggressive and tend to metastasize to distant locations (such as the placenta and brain). The principal histologic subtype of endometrial carcinoma is endometrioid adenocarcinoma (75% to 85%).

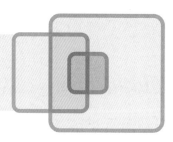

chapter 40

Medicolegal Considerations in Obstetrics and Gynecology

LUIGI MASTROIANNI, JR.

I INTRODUCTION

Law defines modes of behavior among the members of a society and the groups within a society, such that conflicting interests may be resolved in a civilized fashion. Medicine is one such group. In medicine, the law permeates, defines, and regulates the relationship between the physician and patient, the physician and hospital, and the physician and society. Moreover, legal issues dealing with access to medical care and consumer demands regarding health care are dominant in public policy discussions. Obstetrics and gynecology is at the cutting edge of these matters because the field involves the most critical aspects of life: conception, reproduction, and pregnancy. Thus, it is important for the student of medicine to understand, in a preliminary fashion, the legal issues that involve the practice of obstetrics and gynecology.

II MALPRACTICE

A **Definition.** Malpractice is **professional misconduct** whereby a physician departs from the standards of care through a lack of skill, a lack of knowledge, or a lack of judgment in carrying out professional duties.

B **Elements of negligence**

1. **Duty**. A physician has a particular duty or obligation to the patient. A **physician–patient relationship** exists when a patient comes to a physician, who agrees to undertake her care. It is a form of **implied contract**. In this relationship, a physician must act:
   a. In accordance with standards established or accepted by a reasonable fraction of the profession practicing in a given area
   b. As a reasonable physician, taking reasonable care of a patient and not taking unreasonable risks

2. **Breach of duty**. A physician who fails to act in accordance with professional norms has departed from the standard of care and has committed a breach of the duty owed to the patient. This breach must be substantiated by the testimony of an expert.

3. **Causation**. The breach of duty owed must be the proximate cause of a patient's injury for a malpractice action to exist.

4. **Damages**. Actual loss, injury, or damage must have occurred, although pain and suffering is a common accompaniment.

C **Recovery.** The patient or plaintiff must prove that it is more probable than not that the elements of negligence are satisfied (**preponderance of evidence**) to recover compensation for the damage incurred.

III PRECONCEPTION ISSUES

A constitutional right of privacy protects an individual's procreative choice from government intrusion. The **right to use contraception** was the earliest right to reproductive freedom (*Griswold v Connecticut*, 1965).

A Hormonal contraceptives

1. Most lawsuits regarding hormonal contraceptives are **product liability** cases against the manufacturer.
   a. The general rule is that a manufacturer must provide patients with a written warning of all untoward side effects.
   b. A physician must inform patients of the possible side effects and explain the alternative methods of contraception. All of these discussions must be documented.

2. A physician has a duty to:
   a. Perform a thorough physical examination
   b. Perform relevant laboratory examinations
   c. Warn patients of possible adverse side effects
   d. Closely monitor patients in whom side effects develop

B **Intrauterine devices (IUDs)** have been in the past the center of legal and medical controversy since the Dalkon Shield was recalled in 1974.

1. All IUDs, except for the Mirena (hormone-containing device) and the ParaGard (a copper-containing device), have been withdrawn by the manufacturers because of litigation costs. Most lawsuits have been product liability cases, with claims that the IUD has caused:
   a. Uterine and pelvic infections
   b. Infertility
   c. Uterine perforation
   d. Ectopic pregnancy

2. A physician has a duty to:
   a. Inform patients of the risks involved with IUD insertion and use
   b. Explain alternative methods of contraception and their risks
   c. Perform a physical examination
   d. Perform a Papanicolaou (Pap) test and cervical cultures
   e. Examine patients in 3 months after insertion of an IUD and yearly thereafter

3. Since reintroduction of the copper-containing IUD (ParaGard) in 1988 with its recommendations on patient selection and informed consent, there has been no successful litigation.

C Sterilization. This surgical procedure is undertaken for the express purpose of eliminating reproductive capacity.

1. **Voluntary sterilization**
   a. **Public hospitals** cannot refuse to perform sterilization procedures because it would abridge a woman's reproductive right of privacy.
   b. **Private physicians and hospitals** may, however, decline to perform this procedure on moral grounds.
   c. **Federal funding regulations** require that a Department of Health and Human Services consent form be signed 30 to 180 days before surgery. Consent cannot be obtained if the patient is:
      (1) Younger than 21 years of age
      (2) In labor
      (3) Under the influence of alcohol or drugs
      (4) Mentally incompetent
      (5) Having an abortion. Federal regulation is such that to qualify for federal funding, tubal ligation and abortion cannot be performed at the same time because the federal government will not fund abortion.
   d. A physician has a duty to inform patients that:
      (1) The operation will result in sterility
      (2) The procedure should be looked upon as permanent
      (3) There are alternative forms of contraception
      (4) There is no guarantee of sterility; pregnancy occurs at a rate of 15 to 20 per 1000 cases over 10 years, with ectopic pregnancy being the main concern

IV GENETIC COUNSELING

Five percent of all newborns are born with a congenital disorder.

A Routine genetic screening

1. Legislation requires **phenylketonuria** and **hypothyroid** testing in newborns.

2. Testing for **cystic fibrosis** should be discussed and offered at the preconceptional and/or prenatal visit.

3. There are centers for voluntary **screening of sickle cell disease, homocystinuria, galactosemia, Tay-Sachs**, and **maple syrup urine disease**.

4. Prenatal **maternal serum α-fetoprotein** (MSAFP) or **multiple marker** (MSAFP, human chorionic gonadotropin, and estradiol) testing to determine the risk of neural tube defects and Down syndrome is routinely recommended for all women, including those younger than 35 years of age.

B Couples may consider genetic counseling before conception to determine if they have an increased risk of having a child with a birth defect, syndrome, or other inherited genetic conditions. Counseling is recommended when there is a family history of birth defects, mental retardation, or genetic disorders, such as muscular dystrophy, cystic fibrosis, or hemophilia.

C **Particular problems** of which a physician must be aware include the following:

1. **Teratogens**
   a. Rubella
   b. Phenytoin
   c. Alcohol
   d. Tobacco
   e. Illicit drugs (e.g., cocaine)

2. **Autosomal dominant disorders**
   a. Neurofibromatosis
   b. Hereditary familial polyposis

3. **Autosomal recessive disorders**
   a. Cystic fibrosis
   b. Infantile polycystic kidney disease
   c. Congenital deafness
   d. Tay-Sachs disease
   e. Thalassemia

4. **X-linked disorders**
   a. Duchenne muscular dystrophy
   b. Hemophilia

D **Referral to a genetic counselor** is appropriate for pregnant women if there is:

1. A genetic or congenital abnormality in a family member

2. A family history of a genetic problem

3. Abnormal development in a previous child

4. Mental retardation in a previous child

5. Maternal age 35 years or older

6. Specific ethnic background suggestive of a genetic abnormality (e.g., Tay-Sachs disease in Ashkenazi Jews, among others)

7. Exposure to drugs or teratogens

8. A history of three or more spontaneous abortions

E **Amniocentesis** or chorionic villus sampling must be offered to pregnant women if there is:

1. Maternal age 35 years or older

2. A history of multiple miscarriages

3. A family history of genetic disease

4. An abnormal MSAFP

V TERMINATION OF PREGNANCY

A | Right of privacy. A woman's right to abortion falls within a right of privacy interpreted by the U.S. Supreme Court to exist within the Constitution. This right was upheld in *Roe v Wade*, 1973.

B | Trimester model

1. **During the first trimester**, the decision to abort is a decision that is strictly between a woman and her physician.

2. **During the second trimester**, the state may impose regulations reasonably related to a woman's health.

3. **After the second trimester or after the fetus is viable**, the state may regulate abortion, except when necessary to preserve a woman's health.

C | State restrictions. Since *Roe v Wade* in 1973, the time of the abortion decision, states have formulated many laws to limit a woman's access to abortion. For example, in ***Planned Parenthood v Casey***, 1992, the U.S. Supreme Court upheld a **Pennsylvania** statute.

1. **Restrictions on elective abortion imposed by the Pennsylvania statute, which was upheld**
   a. Physicians are required to discuss the nature, risks, and alternatives to abortion, as well as the gestational age of the fetus.
   b. A 24-hour waiting period is required between the time this information is given and the time the abortion is performed.
   c. Either parental consent or, alternatively, judicial bypass if parental consent is denied, is required for a minor.

2. The Supreme Court struck down the provision of the statute that required spousal notification.

VI REPRODUCTIVE TECHNOLOGIES

Techniques in reproductive medicine have created a change in society's concept of the family. Examples include artificial insemination by husband or donor; in vitro fertilization and embryo transfer (IVF-ET); and other assisted reproductive techniques, including gamete or zygote intrafallopian transfer, intracytoplasmic spermatozoa injection (ICSI), donor oocytes, donor embryos, and embryo freezing. A child may be born with as many as five parents: a genetic father, a social father, a genetic mother, a gestational mother, and a social mother. These technologies create legal issues of inheritance, legitimacy, adultery, confidentiality, the status of residual embryos, "parental" responsibilities for a child's diseases and defects, and the legal status and rights of each "parent."

A | Artificial insemination

1. **Definition.** Placement of a husband's semen (artificial insemination by husband [AIH]) or a donor's semen (donor insemination [DI]) into the female genital tract is called artificial insemination.

2. **Consent of the husband.** When the husband of a child's mother consents to DI, the husband assumes the same legal right and obligations as a natural parent, including:
   a. The duty to support the child
   b. The right to visitation in case of divorce

3. **Right to privacy.** Given the U.S. Supreme Court's recognition of a right to privacy, when a single woman requests DI, a public institution providing these services cannot abridge this woman's right to privacy and, thus, would logically have to provide this service; however, a private practitioner could choose not to provide this service.

4. **A physician has a duty to explain** that there is:

    a. No guarantee of pregnancy

    b. A possibility of birth defects that may be attributable to unknown recessive genes of the donor

    c. Little chance of sexually transmitted disease (STD) transmission because of screening and the quarantined freeze preservation of semen

  5. Liability may arise when:

    a. A physician has not adequately screened a donor for genetic defects or STDs, including HIV

    b. A husband's consent has not been obtained

B In vitro fertilization

  1. Definition. In IVF, sperm and ova are obtained and incubated outside the body, and the resulting conceptus is implanted into a uterus.

  2. Legal concepts

    a. When a husband provides sperm and a wife provides an ovum, traditional family principles apply. This is similar to AIH.

    b. When a donor provides sperm and a wife provides an ovum, legal concepts of DI and adoption apply.

    c. When the ovum comes from a female donor and is fertilized and then transferred into another woman's uterus, the legal relationships that arise are complex and not clearly formulated. The essential question is whether genetic material, a contractual relationship, or carrying and giving birth determine the claim of motherhood.

C Gestational carrier

  1. Definition. When a female partner is incapable of carrying a pregnancy, a couple enters into a contract with another woman (a gestational carrier), who agrees to receive an embryo fertilized with the partner's spermatozoa, and to relinquish her rights to the child. In exchange, she receives payment for medical care, lost wages, and hospitalization.

  2. Problems arising with the gestational carrier

    a. Gestational carrier develops maternal feelings toward the infant and refuses to give the child/children up.

    b. Gestational carrier decides not to honor the contract and terminate the pregnancy.

    c. Gestational mother exposes the fetus to teratogens or addicting drugs.

    d. The infant is defective, and the contractive couple decides not to accept it.

    e. There is a multiple gestation.

D Embryo freezing

  1. Definition. Embryo freezing entails preservation by cryopreservation of unused fertilized ova for future implantation.

  2. Problems

    a. Concerns have been raised as to the propriety of eugenic considerations and commercialism.

    b. The destruction of unused embryos has been deemed unethical by some critics.

    c. If the parents die, the rights and obligations of frozen embryos have yet to be decided.

    d. If the embryos are donated, then the donated embryo may carry genetic disorders of the biologic parents of which the adoptive parents are unaware.

VII   BIRTH-RELATED SUITS

A Wrongful conception

  1. Definition. Conception is deemed wrongful if it arises after:

    a. Failed sterilization

    b. Ineffective prescription of contraception

    c. Failure to diagnose pregnancy in a timely fashion

    d. Unsuccessful abortion

  2. Liability arises secondary to a physician's negligence, resulting in the birth of an unplanned child. Negligence is based on:

    a. Improper performance of a sterilization procedure or an abortion

    b. Failure to ascertain the success of the procedure

    c. Failure to inform the woman about the possibility of procedural failures

B Wrongful birth and wrongful life

1. **Wrongful birth** is an action brought by parents of a child, alleging that a child with a congenital defect was born because of negligent genetic counseling. Thus, a physician has failed to:

    a. Recognize a genetic problem

    b. Recognize a condition that places a fetus at risk for a genetic problem

    c. Inform the mother of the ability to detect genetic problems and to offer termination

2. **Wrongful life** is an action similar to wrongful birth. However, the **child brings suit against the physician**, alleging that no life at all would have been preferable to life with a congenital defect.

VIII   BIRTH INJURY

A Definition. A birth injury results when an obstetrician's neglect results in injury to a child (e.g., birth trauma, brain damage, or neurologic damage).

B **Alleged negligence** may arise from a failure to:

1. Monitor fetal heart rate adequately

2. Assess the degree of risk of a pregnancy

3. Perform expedient delivery to avoid perinatal asphyxia that leads to brain damage

4. Monitor a pregnancy adequately

5. Use obstetric forceps or vacuum extraction properly

6. Recognize possible macrosomia and the potential for shoulder dystocia and resulting Erb palsy

C Brain damage. Current studies indicate that it is impossible to isolate a single cause of brain dysfunction. The National Institutes of Health has stated that:

1. **Mental retardation is multifactorial**, resulting from a combination of genetic, biochemical, viral, and developmental factors, and is not necessarily related to birth trauma.

2. **Severe mental retardation and epilepsy** are possibly associated with birth asphyxia but only when accompanied by cerebral palsy, which is associated with prematurity, intrauterine growth retardation, and birth asphyxia.

IX   INFORMED CONSENT

A General definition. "Every human being of adult years and sound mind has a right to determine what shall be done with his/her own body" (*Schloendorff v Society of New York Hospital*, 1914).

B Negligence theory of consent. To sue successfully under this theory, the patient or plaintiff must show that:

1. A physician was under a duty to disclose an adequate amount of material information.

2. A physician disclosed an inadequate amount of material information.

3. The patient agreed to therapy based on this inadequate information.

4. The patient was harmed.

5. If the significant information had been given, the suggested therapy would have been refused

C **Disclosure rules** establish the appropriate standard of care in obtaining informed consent. States differ as to which standard is applicable.

1. **Majority rule.** A physician needs to disclose only information that a reasonable physician would disclose and need not disclose information that would not customarily be disclosed. This rule operates from the physician's point of view.

2. **Minority rule.** A physician needs to disclose only information that a reasonable patient in similar circumstances would wish to know to make a reasonable decision.

D General guidelines in obtaining informed consent

1. A physician must obtain a patient's informed consent before treating her.

2. A physician must provide information concerning the probable benefits, risks, and nature of the suggested diagnostic or therapeutic interventions.

3. A physician must provide an explanation of reasonable alternatives to the recommended intervention and the consequences of no intervention.

4. Information must be:
   a. What a reasonable practitioner would reveal under similar circumstances
   b. What a reasonable patient would consider significant under similar circumstances

E **Exceptions to informed consent** include the following:

1. If a risk is not reasonably foreseeable, it need not be disclosed.

2. Disclosure may be partial if full disclosure would be detrimental to a patient's best interest.

3. If the danger is commonly known, it can be assumed that the patient knows of the danger.

4. The patient may request not to be told of risks.

5. If the risk concerns improperly performing an appropriate procedure, it need not be disclosed.

6. In an emergency, where delay would result in death or serious injury and where a patient is unable to reflect and give an informed decision, informed consent is not required.

7. If a patient is declared either generally or specifically incompetent, informed consent cannot legitimately be obtained.

F Procedure for obtaining informed consent.   Informed consent is a process by which a physician imparts information to a patient who, by virtue of this information, may intelligently decide whether to submit to and participate in the physician's proposed intervention. Thus, the physician must do the following:

1. Discuss the need for the intervention.

2. Discuss the intervention honestly and explain it in layman's terms along with the reason for its necessity.

3. Explain the risks inherent in the procedure.

4. Explain alternatives and the probable result of no intervention.

5. Allow the patient to ask questions.

6. Document the conversation, listing the major risks and alternatives presented.

7. Explain that it is the patient's right to know a reasonable amount about the proposed intervention and that this right is being forfeited if she refuses to discuss the intervention. Document this discussion.

8. Inform the patient about the risks and the recovery time.

9. Refrain from altering records.

10. Personally obtain the consent, not relegating this duty to a nurse or staff member.

Study Questions for Chapter 40

Directions: *Each of the numbered items or incomplete statements in this section is followed by answers or by completions of the statement. Select the ONE lettered answer or completion that is BEST in each case.*

1. It is important for a physician to _____ when counseling a couple who wishes artificial insemination.

- [A] Explain that divorce absolves the husband from child support
- [B] Explain that there is no guarantee of pregnancy if protocol is followed
- [C] Explain that, with screening, birth defects are not possible
- [D] Explain that transmission of STDs is very likely
- [E] Explain that a divorce excludes the husband from access to the child

2. An obstetrician is called at home by a woman who is in labor. Although she has never been to see the obstetrician for a prenatal visit, she would like him to deliver her infant. The obstetrician refuses to attend to her because he is in the middle of dinner. She subsequently delivers a healthy infant at home. If this woman sues the physician for negligence, which of the following would be his best defense?

- [A] Labor is not a disease, so it was not necessary to attend to this pregnant woman
- [B] Because the woman did not come for prenatal visits, she is not entitled to a physician
- [C] Because the woman gave birth to a healthy infant, no harm was done
- [D] The physician never accepted the woman as his patient
- [E] The patient was contributorily negligent in not calling the physician long in advance of active labor

3. A gynecologist has a longstanding relationship with a patient. The woman becomes pregnant but does not inform her gynecologist of her pregnancy and is not scheduled to see him until the next annual visit. One Saturday she calls to report nausea and vomiting but is unable to reach her physician, who is on vacation and has left no other physician to take care of his patients. Three months later the patient goes into preterm labor and delivers a premature infant. The infant ultimately dies 1 month later. In a lawsuit, which of the following statements is the physician's best defense?

- [A] No physician–patient relationship existed
- [B] The physician did not breach any duty owed to the patient
- [C] The premature delivery and fetal death was unrelated to the physician's time on vacation
- [D] A premature infant is not a viable human being
- [E] The woman has not suffered any injuries

4. A 34-year-old woman, gravida 1, para 1, delivers a boy with Tay-Sachs disease. Eight years later, she and her husband obtain the services of a lawyer and sue the physician, alleging that he was remiss in genetic counseling, and because of this, a child with an irreversible neurologic disease had to be brought into the world. The best term to describe this lawsuit is:

- [A] Wrongful birth
- [B] Wrongful conception
- [C] Wrongful life
- [D] Medical malpractice
- [E] Wrongful counseling

Answers and Explanations

1. The answer is B [VI A 2, 4, 5]. The couple who wishes artificial insemination by donor (AID) must be told of the risks of acquiring birth defects due to unknown recessive genes of the donor. There is no guarantee of pregnancy. Even though there is little risk of sexually transmitted disease because of screening and quarantined freeze preservation of semen, there is no guarantee against that transmission. It is essential that the husband give his consent because, in doing so, he is accepting all responsibility for the child born through the donor insemination process. In addition to that responsibility, in case of divorce, the husband maintains his right to visitation and is responsible for child support.

2. The answer is D [II B 1–4]. For a physician to be sued for negligence, the plaintiff must clear four hurdles. These are (1) that a duty existed; (2) that the duty was breached; (3) that, because of the breach of duty, harm was directly caused; and (4) real damage occurred. In this case, no physician–patient relationship existed because the physician refused to help a person who was not his patient. Although it might be argued that it would have been morally correct for the physician to attend to this woman, the law does not recognize a duty to rescue. A physician–patient relationship must be entered into voluntarily and cannot be coerced on either part.

3. The answer is C [II B 1–4]. Although the physician was negligent in not having another physician cover for him while he was on vacation, his negligence did not proximately cause his patient's ultimate injury. Any relationship between the physician's negligence of not being present and the patient's premature delivery 3 months later is too remote to establish causation. Because a premature infant was born and lived for 1 month, it is a human being and a legal entity that can maintain a lawsuit. Also, the mother can maintain a lawsuit apart from her infant.

4. The answer is A [VII B 1]. Wrongful birth actions are brought by the parents of a child with a congenital defect, alleging that a physician was remiss in genetic counseling, and because of this, a defective child was allowed to be born. In general, these cases have been successful, especially in cases where testing would have been easy, such as in prenatal testing for Tay-Sachs disease. Wrongful life actions that are brought by a child, alleging that no life would have been better than life with congenital defects, have generally been unsuccessful. Compensation prior to these injuries, however, may be granted on negligence theory. In cases involving wrongful conception (namely, parents seeking compensation for a normal child resulting from a failed sterilization), willingness to compensate has been low. In cases in which the resulting child was abnormal, medical expenses for the care of the infant have been granted. Important to the determination of wrongful conception is documentation of whether the mother was informed of the possibility of failure of the sterilization procedure. There is no such term as "wrongful counseling." Medical malpractice is an umbrella term, and it does not specifically describe this clinical scenario.

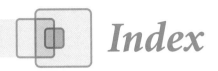

Index

Page numbers in *italics* denote figures; those followed by "t" denote tables.

Abdominal circumference, 148
Abdominal distention, 430
Abdominal ectopic pregnancy, 287–288
Abdominal hysterectomy, 425
Abdominal incision, cesarean birth, 125
Abdominal pain, 288
Abdominal pregnancy, 287
Abdominopelvic CT scan, 430
Ablation, endometrial, 254
Abnormal labor patterns, 106t
Abnormal uterine bleeding, 247–257, 333
  absent ovulation, 247
  anovulation, causes of, 249
  chronic bleeding, 247
  contraceptive use/pregnancy, 251
  current bleeding history, 251
  diagnosis, 251–252
  diagnostic procedures, 252
  differential diagnosis, 248t
  dilation and curettage, 252
  endocrine abnormalities, 247
  endometrial biopsy, 252
  estrogen breakthrough bleeding, 247
  etiology, 249–251
  gynecologic examination, 251
  history, 251
  hormonally related bleeding, 250
    estrogen withdrawal bleeding, 250
    progesterone breakthrough bleeding, 250
  hysteroscopy, 252
  infrequent bleeding, 247
  infrequent ovulation, 247
  laboratory studies, 251–252
    androgen profile, 252
    coagulation profile, 252
    complete blood count, 251
    pregnancy test, 251
    prolactin, 252
    thyroid-stimulating hormone, 252
  medical history, 251
  medical therapy, 253–254
    desmopressin, 254
    GnRH agonists, 253
    nonsteroidal anti-inflammatory drugs, 253
  medication history, 251
  menstrual history, 251
  normal menstrual cycle, 247–248
    length, 247
    physiology of, 248–249
    regularity, 247
    volume/duration, 248
  oligomenorrhea, 251
  organic causes, 250–251
  pathophysiology, 249
    endometrium, 249
    estrogen stimulates endometrium, 249
    spiral arteries, 249
    unopposed estrogen, 249
    unopposed estrogen stimulation, 249
  physical examination, 251
  postovulatory estrogen-progesterone withdrawal, 248
    corpus luteum, 248–249
    endometrial proliferation, 248
    estrogen, 248
    progesterone/estrogen, 249

  sonohysterography, 252
  structural causes, 247
  surgical therapy, 254
    D&C, 254
    endometrial ablation, 254
    hysterectomy, 254
  treatment, 252–254
    estrogens, 253
    hormonal therapy, 252–253
    oral contraceptive therapy, 253
    progestins, 252
  ultrasonography, 252
  visualization of endometrial cavity, 252
Abortion, 132–135
  classification, 132
  etiology, 132
  incidence, 132
  incomplete abortion, 132
  induced abortion, 133–135
  inevitable abortion, 132
  maternal mortality, 135
  missed abortion, 132
  spontaneous abortion, 132
  threatened abortion, 132
Abruptio placentae, 22, 92–93, 164
  clinical presentation, 92
  cocaine, 92
  complications, 93
  definition, 92
  diagnosis, 93
  etiology, 92
  fetal heart rate monitoring, 93
  history of, 92
  incidence, 92
  laboratory tests, 93
  management, 93
  maternal hospitalization, 93
  maternal hypertension, 92
  maternal trauma, 92
  pathophysiology, 92
  premature contractions, 93
  rupture of membranes, 92
  smoking, 92
  sudden decompression, 92
  thrombophilia, 92
  tocolytic drugs, 93
  ultrasound, 93
  uterine fibroids, 92
Absence of labor, chorioamnionitis, 159
Absent ovulation, 247
Abuse. *See* Physical abuse; Sexual abuse
Acanthosis nigricans, 232
Acidemia, 111
Acidosis, 118
Acne, 231–232
Acquaintance rape, 390–391
  epidemiology, 390
  medical evaluation, 390
  physician response, 390–391
  prevention, 391
Acrocentric chromosomes, 308
ACTH. *See* Adrenocorticotropic hormone
Actin, 98
Actinomycosis, 381
Active phase of labor, 105, 112
Activin, 208
Acute pyelonephritis, 179–180

Acute systemic pyelonephritis, high-risk pregnancy, 51
Acute urethritis, 179
Acyclovir, 409
Adenomas, 218
Adenomyosis, 282
Adenyl cyclase, 206
Adequate antibiotic therapy, 76
Adhesiolysis, 300
Adhesions
  intrauterine, 222
  pelvic, 281
Adnexal masses, 282
Adolescent patient, 316–329
  adolescent, 324–326
  adrenal tumors, 320
  amenorrhea, 325–326
  androgen insensitivity syndrome, 320–321
  androgenic substances, 320
  androgens, childhood ingestion, 320
  congenital adrenal hyperplasia, 320
  contraception, 326
  delayed puberty, 324
  dysfunctional uterine bleeding, 324–325
  ectopic ureter, with vaginal terminus, 319
  genitalia, external, developmental defects of, 320–321
  Kallmann syndrome, 325
  labial agglutination, 317–318
  lichen sclerosus et atrophicus, 316–317
  maternal virilizing tumor, 321
  neoplasms, 318–319
  normal puberty, 321
  ovarian tumors, 319
  pediatric patient, 316
    congenital anomalies, 319
  precocious puberty, 323
  prolapsed urethra, 318
  pubertal development, 321–324
  rectal examination, 316
  sexual abuse, 326
  Swyer syndrome, 325
  Tanner staging, 322t
    normal breast development, *322*
    normal pubic hair development, *323*
  trauma, 317
  true hermaphroditism, 321
  Turner syndrome, 325
  21-hydroxylase defect, 320
  vaginal discharge, 318
  vaginal ectopic anus, 319
  vaginal tumors, 318
  vulvovaginal lesions, 316–318
Adrenal gland, pregnancy, 15
Adrenal hyperplasia, 230
Adrenal tumors, 320
Adrenarche, 321
Adrenocorticotropic hormone, 6
Adult granulosa cell tumors, 433
Afterpains, puerperium, 25
Age, high-risk pregnancy, 43
AIS. *See* Androgen insensitivity syndrome
Albumin, 239
Alcohol use in pregnancy, 81–83
  fetal alcohol syndrome, 82
  high-risk pregnancy, 43
  history of, in antepartum care, 38

Alcohol use in pregnancy, (*Cont.*)
  screening, high-risk pregnancy, 44t
  teratogenesis, 82
  teratology, 71, 82
  threshold, 83
Allen-Masters peritoneal defects, 272
Alpha-fetoprotein, 442
  elevated, 59t
  maternal, 57
Alpha-methyldopa, 165
Alpha-thalassemia, 60, 182
Alprazolam, 212
Ambiguous genitalia, developmental defects
      with, 320–321
Amenorrhea, 215–225, 227, 325–326, 334
  adenomas, 218
  androgen insensitivity syndrome, 219
  aromatase enzyme activity, 217
  Asherman syndrome, 219
  categories, 215–216
  classification, 215–219
  clinical evaluation, 219–220
  clomiphene, 222
  combined hormone replacement
      therapy, 221
  craniopharyngioma, 218
  differential diagnosis, *216*
  estrogen replacement therapy, 221
  eugonadotropic amenorrhea, 218–219,
      222–223
  hirsutism, 222
  hypergonadotropic amenorrhea, 216,
      220–221
  hypogonadotropic amenorrhea, 217,
      221–223
  infection, 219
  laboratory evaluation, *221*
  management, 220–223
  normal menstrual cycle, 215
  ovarian drilling, 222
  in pregnancy, 19
  serum human chorionic gonadotropin, 219
  17α-hydroxylase deficiency, 217
Amino acids, fetal requirements, 12
Aminophylline, 184
Amniocentesis, 63–64, 190–191
Amnioinfusion, 118
Amnion, 12
Amniotic fluid, 12, 22, 62–63
  lecithin, *22*
  sphingomyelin, *22*
Amniotic membranes, 12
  amnion, 12
  chorion, 12
  membranes, 12
Amniotomy, 105
Ampicillin, 380
Ampicillin-sulbactam, 380
Anaerobes, 404
Analgesia for labor, 141–143
Androgen insensitivity syndrome, 219,
      320–321
Androgen-producing neoplasm, 231
Androgen-producing tumors, 241
Androgen-receptor blockers, 243
  cyproterone acetate, 243
  flutamide, 243
  spironolactone, 243
Androgen synthesis, 207
Androgenic drug exposure, 241
Androgenic substances, 320
Androgens, 229, 238–239, 331–332
  childhood ingestion, 320
  excess, 296

Androstenedione, 332
Anemia, 180–182
  acquired anemias, 180
  hereditary anemias, 180–182
  high-risk pregnancy, 50
Anencephalic fetuses, 6
Anencephaly, 6
Anergy panel, 366
Anesthesia, 139–147, 168
  cardiac, 139–140
  central nervous system, 141
  cesarean birth, 125
  cesarean birth anesthesia, 143–144
    epidural anesthesia, 144
    general anesthesia, 144
    postoperative analgesia, 144
    spinal anesthesia, 143–144
  gastrointestinal changes, 140
  hematologic changes, 140
  labor analgesia, 141–143
    combined spinal epidural analgesia, 142
    epidural analgesia, 141–142
    intravenous analgesia, 143
    regional blocks, 143
  obstetric pain neuropathways, 141
    first stage of labor, 141
    second stage of labor, 141
  physiologic changes, pregnancy, 139–141
  renal, 141
  reproductive tract, 141
  respiratory system, 140
Aneuploidy
  screening for, 36, 51
Anorexia nervosa, 217, 325
Anovulation, 296
  causes of, 249
Anovulatory cycles, 331, 333
Antagonists, 165
Antepartum bleeding, 89–97
  abruptio placentae, 92–93
    clinical presentation, 92
    cocaine, 92
    complications, 93
    diagnosis, 93
    etiology, 92
    fetal heart rate monitoring, 93
    history of, 92
    incidence, 92
    laboratory tests, 93
    management, 93
    maternal hospitalization, 93
    maternal hypertension, 92
    maternal trauma, 92
    pathophysiology, 92
    premature contractions, 93
    rupture of membranes, 92
    smoking, 92
    sudden decompression, 92
    thrombophilia, 92
    tocolytic drugs, 93
    ultrasound, 93
    uterine fibroids, 92
  APT test, 94
  back pain and, 93
  beta-mimetic tocolytics, 93
  bloody show, 93
  cervical pathology, 94
  consumptive coagulopathy, 93
  couvelaire uterus, 93
  fetal maternal hemorrhage, 93
  hemorrhage, 91
  hemorrhagic shock, 93
  magnesium sulfate, 93
  maternal shock, 91

  painless, 89
  placenta accreta, 91
  placenta previa, 89–92
    advanced maternal age, 89
    Asian/African ethnicity, 89
    cesarean birth, 90
    clinical presentation, 89
    delivery, 90
    diagnosis, 90
    etiology, 89
    examination, 90
    expectant management, 90
    fetal complication, 91–92
    fetal morbidity, 92
    incidence, 89
    management, 90–91
    marginal previa, 89
    maternal complication, 91–92
    maternal morbidity, 91–92
    multiparity, 89
    partial previa, 89
    preterm delivery, 92
    previous cesarean birth, 89
    previous dilation, curettage, 89
    smoking, 89
    transabdominal ultrasound, 90
    transvaginal ultrasound, 90
    ultrasound, 90
    uteroplacental relationships, *91*
    variations of, *90*
  prostaglandin inhibitors, 93
  renal failure, 93
  uterine rupture, 94
  vaginal delivery, 93
  vaginal infections, 94
  vaginal lacerations, from trauma, 94
  vasa previa, rupture of, 93–94
Antepartum care, 32–41
  alcohol, 38
  aneuploidy screening, 36
  antepartum tests, 33t
  blood pressure, 37
  caffeine, 38
  Caldwell-Moloy classification, pelvic
      types, *35*
  calories, 37
  Chadwick sign, 34
  clinical pelvimetry, 34
  coitus, 38
  complete obstetric history, 33–34
  date of confinement, calculating, 32–33
  diagonal conjugate, 34
    variations in length, *35*
  dietary composition, 37
  domestic violence screening, 34
  exercise, 37
  family health history, 34
  fetal heart tones, 37
  first-trimester screening, 36
  flu shot, 38
  glucose, urine dip, 37
  gynecologic history, 34
  initial prenatal blood work, 36
  initial visit, 33–34
  integrated screening, 36
  integrated screens, 36
  lifestyle modifications, 37–38
  maternal weight, 37
  mean duration of pregnancy, 32
  medical history, 34
  medications, 38
  milestones, 37
  Naegele's rule, 33
  nutrition, 37

patient history, 33–34
pelvic types, 35–36
peripartum tests, 33t
physical examination, 34–36
preconception care, 32
prior pregnancy
   complications, 34
   information, 34
protein, urine dip, 37
QUAD screening, 36
screening, 34–36
screening, options for, 36
sequential screening, 36
sequential screens, 36
smoking, 38
social history, 34
subsequent prenatal visits, 36–37
substance abuse screening, 34
surgical history, 34
travel, 37
ultrasound, 33
uterine size, 37
weight gain, 37
Antepartum tests, 33t
  in antepartum care, 33t
Antibiotic therapy, 317, 402
Antibody screening, 50
Antifungal intravaginal agents, 406
Antigens, maternal sensitization, 192
Antihypertensive therapy, 165, 168
  alpha-methyldopa, 165
  antagonists, 165
  labetalol, 165
  nifedipine, 165
Antiphospholipid antibody syndrome, 312
Antiphospholipid syndrome, 309
Antiretroviral therapy, 366, 409
Antispasmodic agents, 418
Antral follicle, 298
  oogenesis, 208
Appendicitis, 280
APS. *See* Antiphospholipid syndrome;
       Autoimmune polyglandular
       syndrome
APT test, antepartum bleeding, 94
Aromatase enzymes, 217, 332
Aromatase inhibitors, 273
Aromatic ring, steroid hormones, 6
Arrhenoblastoma, 73, 433
Arterial blood gas analysis, 187
Artificial insemination, 443–444
Asherman syndrome, 219, 222
  or intrauterine adhesions, 222
Asphyxia, 111
Assisted reproductive technology, 303
  gamete intrafallopian transfer, 303
  ICSI, 303
  IVF, 303
  preimplantation genetic diagnosis, 303
  zygote intrafallopian transfer, 303
Asthma, 184
Asymptomatic bacteriuria, 179, 336
  high-risk pregnancy, 51
Atrophic vaginitis, 407–408
Autoimmune disorders, high-risk
     pregnancy, 48
Autoimmune polyglandular syndrome,
     high-risk pregnancy, 48
Autonomic nervous system, 278
Autosomal dominant disorders, 442
Autosomal recessive disorders, 60, 442
Azithromycin, 360–362
Azoospermia, 301
AZT. *See* Zidovudine

Back pain, antepartum bleeding, 93
Bacterial sexually transmitted diseases,
     358–363
  bacterial vaginosis, 362
  chancroid, 361
  chlamydia, 360–361
  gonorrhea, 358
  granuloma inguinale, 361
  lymphogranuloma venereum, 362
  Thayer-Martin culture medium, 359
Bacterial vaginosis, 362, 404–405
Barium enema, 430
Barrier contraception methods, 346–347
  cervical caps, 347
  condoms, 346
  diaphragms, 347
  spermicides, 346–347
  vaginal sponges, 347
Bartholin glands, 400
Barton forceps, 129
Basal body temperature
  monitoring of, 297
  in natural family planning, 354
BBT. *See* Basal body temperature
Before, during, or after labor and delivery,
    169
Benign breast disease, 394–399
  benign breast masses, 396
  breast masses, 396–397
    types of, 396–397
  breast pain, 394–395
  clinical findings, 394
  discharge, 395
  etiology, 395
  evaluation, 395–396
  malignant breast masses, 396
  nipple discharge, 395–396
  noncyclic mastalgia, 395
  patient history, 394
  physical examination, 394
  treatment, 395–396
Benign breast masses, 396
Beta-mimetic tocolytics, antepartum
    bleeding, 93
Beta-thalassemia, 60
Bicornuate uterus, 312
Bilateral hilar adenopathy, 185
Bilirubin, 64
Bilirubin in amniotic fluid, 190
Biologic functions, hormones
    characteristics, 2
Biometry, 62
Biophysical profile, 63
Birth injury, 445
  alleged negligence, 445
  brain damage, 445
Birth-related suits, 444–445
  wrongful birth, 445
  wrongful conception, 444–445
  wrongful life, 445
Bishop scoring system, 151t
Bleeding
  abnormal, 247, 249–250
  absent ovulation, 247
  anovulation, causes of, 249
  antepartum, 89–97
  chronic bleeding, 247
  contraceptive use/pregnancy, 251
  current bleeding history, 251
  diagnosis, 251–252
  diagnostic procedures, 252
  differential diagnosis, 248t
  dilation and curettage, 252
  endocrine abnormalities, 247

endometrial biopsy, 252
estrogen breakthrough bleeding, 247
etiology, 249–251
gynecologic examination, 251
history, 251
hormonally related bleeding, 250
  estrogen withdrawal bleeding, 250
  progesterone breakthrough
    bleeding, 250
hysteroscopy, 252
infrequent bleeding, 247
infrequent ovulation, 247
laboratory studies, 251–252
  androgen profile, 252
  coagulation profile, 252
  complete blood count, 251
  pregnancy test, 251
  prolactin, 252
  thyroid-stimulating hormone, 252
medical history, 251
medical therapy, 253–254
  desmopressin, 254
  GnRH agonists, 253
  nonsteroidal anti-inflammatory
    drugs, 253
medication history, 251
menstrual history, 251
normal menstrual cycle, 247–248
  length, 247
  physiology of, 248–249
  regularity, 247
  volume/duration, 248
oligomenorrhea, 251
organic causes, 250–251
pathophysiology, 249
  endometrium, 249
  estrogen stimulates endometrium, 249
  spiral arteries, 249
  unopposed estrogen, 249
  unopposed estrogen stimulation, 249
physical examination, 251
postovulatory estrogen-progesterone
    withdrawal, 248
  corpus luteum, 248–249
  endometrial proliferation, 248
  estrogen, 248
  progesterone/estrogen, 249
in pregnancy, 21–22
puerperium, 26
sonohysterography, 252
surgical therapy, 254
  D&C, 254
  endometrial ablation, 254
  hysterectomy, 254
treatment, 252–254
  estrogens, 253
  hormonal therapy, 252–253
  oral contraceptive therapy, 253
  progestins, 252
ultrasonography, 252
visualization of endometrial cavity, 252
Blood coagulation factors, puerperium, 26
Blood count, 50
Blood flow to uterus, 6
Blood pressure. *See* Hypertension in
    pregnancy
Blood type, high-risk pregnancy, 50
Bloody show, 93. *See also* Bleeding
Boric acid capsules intravaginally, 406
Bowel movement, fetal, 22
Bowel obstruction, 431
BPP. *See* Biophysical profile
Bradycardia, 112
Braxton Hicks contractions, 21

Breach of duty, 440
Breast cancer, 351–352
Breast changes, in pregnancy, 19
Breast masses, 394, 396–397
    types of, 396–397
Breast pain, 394–395
    with cancer, 395
Breastfeeding, counseling on drug use, 85
Breech presentation, 23–24, *25*
    Piper forceps, 128
Brow presentation, *24*

CA-125, 271
Caffeine use
    in antepartum care, 38
    high-risk pregnancy, 44
CAH. *See* Congenital adrenal hyperplasia
Calcium supplementation, 212
Caldwell-Moloy classification, pelvic types, *35*
Call-Exner bodies, 433
Calorie intake, antepartum, 37
cAMP. *See* Cyclic adenosine monophosphate
Cancer chemotherapy, teratology, 72
Candida albicans, 405
Candida vaginitis, 405. *See also* Candidiasis;
    Moniliasis
Candidiasis, 405
Cannabinoids, use in pregnancy, 82
Carboplatin, side effects of, 432
Cardiac disease, high-risk pregnancy, 47
Cardiac system changes in pregnancy,
    139–140
Cardiovascular changes, puerperium, 26
Cardiovascular complications, from drug
    use, 83
Cardiovascular disease, 230, 336, 351
Cardiovascular lesions, 75
Cardiovascular system, 165
    fetal, 13–14
Catheter drainage, 381
Causation, 440
CD4+ count, 366
Cefotetan, 380
Cefotoxitin, 380
Cefoxitin, 380
Ceftriaxone, 361, 380
Cellular atypia, 260
Cellular leiomyomas, 260
Cellulitis, in pregnancy, 82
Central nervous system, 325, 336
    changes in pregnancy, 141
Central precocious puberty, 323
Cephalic presentations, fetus, 23
Cerclage, 312
Cervical cancer, 351, 423, 426
    Bethesda System, 424
    epidemiology, 423
    invasive carcinoma of cervix, 425
    microinvasive carcinoma of cervix, 425
    preinvasive cervical disease, 423–425
    prevention of cervical cancer, 427
    staging, 425t
Cervical caps, 347
Cervical cerclage, 130–132
    abdominal placement, 131
    McDonald technique, 131, *131*
    Shirodkar technique, 131
    success rate, 132
Cervical changes in pregnancy, 19
Cervical cytologic screening, 424
Cervical dilation, *105*
Cervical gram stain, 379
Cervical insufficiency, 49–50
Cervical pathology, 94

Cervical pregnancy, 287
Cervical secretions, natural family planning,
    354–355
Cervical transformation zone, 423
Cervix
    changes in labor, 101
    digital examination, 159
    dilation, 101, *105*
    effacement, 101
    effacement of, 101
    high-risk pregnancy, 49
    invasive carcinoma, 425
    microinvasive carcinoma, 425
    strawberry, 370
Cesarean birth, 123–127
    abdominal incision, 125
    anesthesia, 125, 143–144
        epidural anesthesia, 144
        general anesthesia, 144
        postoperative analgesia, 144
        spinal anesthesia, 143–144
    antacids, 125
    cesarean hysterectomy, 126
    classic incision (Sanger), 124
    complications, 126
    considerations, 127
    contraindications, 127
    contraindications to labor, 124
    delivery, 125
    dystocia, 124
    emergency procedure, 126
    endomyometritis, 126
    high-risk pregnancy, 46
    incidence, 123, 126
    indications, 123–124
    informed consent, 125
    low transverse (Kerr), 124
    low vertical (Sellheim or Krönig), 124
    orientation, 124
    patient preparation, 125
    perinatal mortality, 123
    placenta previa, 90
    polymicrobial, 126
    preoperative hematocrit, 125
    prerequisites, 127
    primary cesarean births, 123
    procedure, 125–126
    prophylactic antibiotics, 125–126
    repeat cesarean birth, 123
    rupture, risk of, 126
    surgical techniques, 125
    thromboembolic disorders, 126
    types of operations, 124–125
    urinary tract infection, 126
    uterine incision, 125
    uterine rupture, future pregnancies, 126
    vaginal birth after, 126
    wound closure, 125
    wound infection, 126
CGB, Cortisol–binding globulin
Chadwick sign, 19, 34
Chancre, 363
Chancroid, 361
Changes specific to labor, 183
Chemical nature, hormones, 1
Chemotherapy, 426
Chest radiography, 430
Chickenpox, 76
Chlamydia, 360–361, 389
Chlamydia testing, 50
Chocolate cysts, 272
Cholesterol, 4
Chorioamnionitis, 22, 159
Choriocarcinoma, 199

Chorion, 12
Chorionic sac, 20
Chorionic villus sampling, 64
Chromosomal abnormalities, 63
    prenatal diagnosis, 56–57
Chromosomal inversions, 309
Chronic hypertension, 163–165
    effects on fetus, 164
    effects on mother, 164
    high-risk pregnancy, 47
Chronic pelvic pain, 270, 376
Chronic PID, 282
Chronic recurrent yeast infections, 406
Chronic uterine bleeding, 247
Cimetidine, 243
Ciprofloxacin, 361–362
Classic forceps, 129, *129*
Clear cell carcinoma, 431, 434–435
Cleft lip, 73
Cleft palate, 73
Clindamycin, 362, 380
Clinical pelvimetry, high-risk pregnancy, 49
Clitoris, 400
Clomiphene, 222
Clomiphene citrate, 297
Clue cells, 362, 405
CMV. *See* Cytomegalovirus
CNS. *See* Central nervous system
Coagulation profile, 262
Coagulation system, 166
Coagulative necrosis, 260
Cocaine use, 81, 83–84
    abruptio placentae, 92
    cardiovascular effects, 83
    dopamine reuptake, 83
    norepinephrine reuptake, 83
    pharmacologic effects, 83
    tachycardia, 83
    teratology, 72
    uterine contractions, 83
    vasoconstriction, 83
Coelomic epithelium, metaplasia of, 269
Coital problems, infertility and, 302
    fertile days, 302
    history, 302
    regular coitus, 302
Color Doppler ultrasound, 280
Colposcopy, 367, 424
Combination oral contraceptives, 211, 242,
    350–352
    composition, 350
    controversies, 350–351
    efficacy, 350
    mode of action, 350
    new preparations, 352
    noncontraceptive benefits, 352
    puerperium, 26
Complete breech, fetus, 24
Complications of pregnancy, 26–27
Condoms, 346
Condyloma latum, 363
Confinement date, calculating, 32–33
Confirmation of pregnancy, 20
Congenital adrenal hyperplasia, 320
Congenital anomalies, 47, 223
Congenital heart defects, 57
Congenital heart disease, 73
Congenital malformations, 57, 70
    baseline rate, 56
    prenatal diagnosis, 57
Congenital rubella syndrome, 75
Consent, 443
Consumptive coagulopathy, 93
    antepartum bleeding, 93

Contemporary pregnancy tests, 2
Contraception, 326, 346–357
  barrier methods, 346–347
    cervical caps, 347
    condoms, 346
    diaphragms, 347
    spermicides, 346–347
    vaginal sponges, 347
  combination oral contraceptive pills,
      350–352
    composition, 350
    controversies, 350–351
    efficacy, 350
    mode of action, 350
    new preparations, 352
    noncontraceptive benefits, 352
  contraceptive vaginal ring, 352–353
  copper-impregnated IUD, 354
  efficacy, 346
  emergency contraception, 353–354
  intrauterine devices, 347–349
    advantages, 348
    contraindications, 348
    disadvantages, 348
    efficacy, 348
    mode of action, 348
    pregnancy-related issues, 348–349
    types, 348
  mifepristone, 354
  morning-after pill, 353
  natural family planning, 354–355
    advantages, 355
    basal body temperature, 354
    cervical secretions, 354–355
    disadvantages, 355
    efficacy, 355
    fertility awareness, 354
    menstrual calendar calculations, 354
  progestin-only methods, 349–350
    implantable progestin, 350
    injectable progestin, 349
    minipill, 349
    mode of action, 349
    progestin-only IUD, 350
  right to use, 440
  surgical sterilization, 355
  transdermal patch, 353
  Yuzpe contraception method, 353
Contraceptive vaginal ring, 352–353
Contractions in pregnancy, 21
Contraindications to labor, 124
Copper-impregnated IUD, 348, 354
Cord compression, correction of, 118
Cordocentesis, 190
Cornual resection, 290
Corpus luteum, 3–4, 248
  oogenesis, 210
Corticosteroid, 243
Cortisol, 242
Cortisol-binding globulin, in pregnancy, 1
Cortisol secretion, fetus, 23
Counseling, genetic, 442–443
  amniocentesis, 442–443
  particular problems, 442
  referral to genetic counselor, 442
  routine genetic screening, 442
Couvelaire uterus, antepartum bleeding, 93
Crab louse, 370
Craniopharyngioma, 218
Crowning, 105
Culdocentesis, 379
Cushing syndrome, 231, 241
Cyclic adenosine monophosphate, 206
Cyproterone acetate, 243

Cystic fibrosis, 442
  genetic screening, 59–60
  screening, 301
Cystitis, 179
Cystocele, 415
Cystoscopy, 417
Cysts, 396
Cytomegalovirus
  high-risk pregnancy, 48
  teratology, 75

Damages, for negligence, 440
Danazol, 273
Darkfield examination, 363
Dating pregnancy, 20
Dating violence, 390–391
  epidemiology, 390
  medical evaluation, 390
  physician response, 390–391
  prevention, 391
D&C. *See* Dilation and curettage
Decreased ovarian reserve, 296, 298
  estradiol, 298
  markers, 298
  treatment, 298–299
Deep vein thrombosis, 186–187
Delayed puberty, 218, 324
Delivery, 98–110, 123–138
  operative vaginal, 127–130
  vaginal, operative, 127–130
Delivery of shoulders, 105
Depressants, use in pregnancy, 82
Depression, 278
  high-risk pregnancy, 48–49
Desmopressin, 254
Detoxification from drugs, in pregnancy, 84
Detrusor overactivity, 417
DHT. *See* Dihydrotestosterone
Diabetes, 72–73, 175–177, 230, 233
  fetal glucose levels, 175
  first trimester, 176
  follow-up, 177
  gestational diabetes, 175, 177
  glucose metabolism, effect of pregnancy
    on, 175
  high-risk pregnancy, 47–49
  management, 176–177
    preexisting diabetes, 176
    prior to conception, 176
  method of delivery, 176
  phosphatidylglycerol, 176
  preexisting, effect on pregnancy, 175–176
  risk factors, 177
  screening, 177
  second trimester, 176
  shoulder dystocia, 176
  third trimester, 176
  timing of delivery, 176
  universal screening, 177
Diabetogenic effect, human placental
    lactogen, 3
Diagonal conjugate, 34
  variations in length, *35*
Diaphragms, 347
Dietary composition, antepartum, 37
Dihydrotestosterone, 239
Dilation, cervix, 101
Dilation and curettage, 252, 254, 289
  with hysteroscopy, 333
Dilation curve, nulliparous labor, *100*
Dilation of cervix, 101
Dimpling or retraction, 394
Discharge, nipple, 395–396
Disclosure rules, 445

Disorders of androgen excess, 218
Disorders of androgen synthesis, 222
Disorders of outflow tract or uterus, 219
Diverticulitis, 280
DNA, abnormalities in, 57
Documentation, sexual assault, 389
Domestic violence
  screening, 34
Domestic violence, high-risk pregnancy, 44
Donor oocytes, 299
Donor sperm, 302
Douching, 402
Doxycycline, 360, 362–363, 380
Drug use, high-risk pregnancy, 43
DUB. *See* Dysfunctional uterine bleeding
Duct ectasia, 397
Duration of pregnancy, 32
Duty, legal, 440
Dysfunctional labor patterns, 105
Dysfunctional uterine bleeding, 324–325,
    333
Dysgenic ovary, 433
Dysgerminomas, 432, 434
Dysmenorrhea, 210–211, 270, 280, 324, 352
  clinical aspects, 210
  management, 211
  physiology, 211
Dyspareunia, 270, 336, 341
Dyspnea of pregnancy, 184
Dystocia, 124

Ecchymoses, 317
Eclampsia, 46, 163
Ectoparasites, 370–371
  pediculosis pubis, 370
  scabies, 371
Ectopic pregnancy, 44, 279, 287–293, 349,
    352, 376
  abdominal pain, 288
  artificial reproductive techniques, 288
  complications, 291
  cornual resection, 290
  diagnosis, 288–290
    diagnostic tests, 288–290
    differential diagnosis, 288
    physical examination, 288
  dilation and curettage, 289
  etiology, 287–288
  fertility, 291
  follow-up, 291
  hCG testing, 290
  human chorionic gonadotropin, 289
  intrauterine device, 288
  laparoscopy, 290
  laparotomy, 290
  linear salpingotomy, 290
  location, 287
    abdominal, 287
    cervical, 287
    heterotopic, 287
    ovarian, 287
    tubal, 287
  medical treatment, 291
  methotrexate treatment, 291t
  oophorectomy, 290
  operative laparoscopy, 290
  pelvic inflammatory disease, 287
  pregnancy status, 288
  prevalence, 287
  prognosis, 291
  recurrence, 291
  salpingectomy, 290
  serum progesterone levels, 290
  smoking, 288

Ectopic pregnancy, (*Cont.*)
  surgery, 290
  symptoms, 288
  transvaginal ultrasound, 288
  treatment, 290–291
  treatment algorithm, *289*
  tubal surgery, 287
  vaginal bleeding, 288
Ectopic tubal gestation, 279
Ectopic ureter, with vaginal terminus, 319
Education, regarding high-risk pregnancy, 42
Effacement of cervix, 101
Elective abortion. *See* Induced abortion
Elective cesarean birth, high-risk pregnancy, 52
ELISA. *See* Enzyme-linked immunosorbent
    assay
Embryo, 20
  freezing, 444
  implantation, 5
  transfers, 303
Embryonal carcinomas, 433
Emergency contraception, 353–354
Emergency procedure, 126
Empiric fertility treatment, 300
End-organ disease, 166
  baseline evaluation for, 165
Endocervical curettage, 424
Endocrine changes, 1
Endocrine disorders, 297
Endocrine tests for pregnancy, 19
Endocrinology of pregnancy, 1–10, 15
  circulating estrogens, increased levels of, 1
  cortisol-binding globulin, 1
  estrogen synthesis, late pregnancy, 5
  estrogens, 607
    biological activities, 6–7
      anencephalic fetuses, 6
      blood flow to uterus, 6
      end-of-gestation, 6
      lactation, 7
      low-density lipoprotein, uptake
        by placenta, 6
      maternal heart disease, 182
      parturition, 6
      placental sulfatase deficiency, fetus
        with, 6
      reduced maternal estriol levels, 7
      stimulates, 6
    chemical nature, 6
      aromatic ring, steroid hormones, 6
      estradiol, 6
      estriol, 6
      estrone, 6
    fetal adrenal glands, role of, 6
    placental estrogens, androgen
      precursors, 6
    production, 6
      fetal adrenal cortex, 6
      fetal liver, 6
      placenta, 6
    secretory patterns, 6
      adrenocorticotropic hormone, 6
      anencephaly, 6
      estriol, 6
      placental sulfatase deficiency, 6
    source, 6
  female fetus, 1
  fetus, 1
  hormone characteristics, 1–2
    biologic functions, 2
    chemical nature, 1
    fetus, 1
    mother, 1
    placenta, 1

progesterone deficiency, 2
  protein hormones, 1
  secretion patterns, 2
  source, 1–2
  steroids, 1
human chorionic gonadotropin, 1–3
  biologic functions, 3
    clinical uses, 3
    corpus luteum, 3
    fetal testicular testosterone, 3
    multiple marker screen, 3
    with trophoblastic neoplasia, 3
    viability of pregnancy, assessment, 3
  chemical nature, 2
  secretion patterns, 2
    contemporary pregnancy tests, 2
    high levels, 2
    low levels, 2
    serum hCG assays, 2
    urine hCG assays, 2
  source, 2
human placental lactogen, 1, 3
  biologic function, 3
    clinical use, 3
    diabetogenic effect, 3
    increased insulin levels, 3
    insulin-directed glucose, 3
    maternal free fatty acids, 3
    plasma insulin, 3
  chemical nature, 3
  human chorionic somatomam-
    motropin, 3
  secretory patterns, 3
  source, 3
male fetus, 1
placenta, 1
progesterone, 4–5
  21-carbon steroid, 4
  biologic functions, 5
    fetus rejection prevention, 5
    implantation of embryo, 5
    mifepristone, 5
    myometrium, 5
    support pregnancy, 5
  cholesterol, 4
  corpus luteum, 4
  fetal adrenal cortex, 4
  fetal liver, 4
  placenta, 4
  pregnenolone, 4
  progesterone sources, 4
  secretory patterns, 4–5
    late pregnancy, 5
  steroid-forming glands, 4
progesterone synthesis, late pregnancy, 5
prolactin, 4
  biologic function, 4
    mammary glands, lactation, 4
  chemical nature, 4
  secretory patterns, 4
  source, 4
  protein hormones, 1
  thyroid-binding globulin, 1
Endodermal sinus tumors, 432
Endometrial ablation, 254
Endometrial biopsy, 252, 262
Endometrial cancer, 333, 340, 351–352,
    427–429
  endometrial carcinoma, 428–429
  endometrial hyperplasia, 428
  epidemiology, 427
  staging, 429t
Endometrial cavity, visualization of, 252
Endometrial glands, 205

Endometrial hyperplasia, 230, 428
  diagnosis of, 428
  treatment of, 428
Endometrial neoplasia, 333, 335
Endometrioid adenocarcinoma, 428
Endometrioid tumors, 431
Endometriomas, 272, 300
Endometriosis, 269–277, 281–282, 299
  Allen-Masters peritoneal defects, 272
  aromatase inhibitors, 273
  CA-125, 271
  chocolate cysts, 272
  chronic pelvic pain, 270
  coelomic epithelium, metaplasia of, 269
  conservative surgery, 274
  danazol, 273
  diagnosis, 271–272
  differential diagnosis, 271
    gastrointestinal system, 271
    gynecologic causes, 271
    musculoskeletal system, 271
    urinary system, 271
  distant sites, 271
  dysmenorrhea, 270
  dyspareunia, 270
  endometriomas, 272
  etiology, 269–270
  genetic influences, 269
  gonadotropin-releasing hormone
    agonists, 273
  hematogenous spread, 269
  history, 271
  incidence, 269
  infertility, 270
  infertility and, 300
    diagnosis, 300
  laparoscopy, 272
  markers, 271
  medical therapy, 272–274
  oral contraceptives, 273
  ovulation, 270
  pain, 269–270
  pelvic examination, 271–272
  pelvic imaging, 272
  radical surgery, 274
  retrograde menstrual flow, 269
  surgical therapy, 274
  symptoms, 270–271
  tethering effect, 271
  treatment, 272–274
  uterosacral ligaments, 271
Endometritis, 375
Endometrium, abnormal uterine
    bleeding, 249
Endomyometritis, 126
Endopelvic fascia, 414
Endosalpingitis, 377
Enlargement of abdomen in pregnancy, 19
Enterocele, 416
  repair, 416
Enteroviruses, teratology, 77
Environmental risks
  high-risk pregnancy, 44
  teratology, *68*
Enzyme deficiencies, 217
Enzyme-linked immunosorbent assay, 366
Epilepsy, 445
  teratology, 73
Episiotomy, 105–106t, 127
Epithelial ovarian cancer, 429–432
  clinical course, 431
  diagnosis, 430
  epidemiology, 429–430
  predominant histologic types, 430–431

recurrent ovarian cancer, 432
staging, 430–431t
treatment, 431
Ergonovine, 107
Erythromycin, 362–363
Estradiol, 6, 205, 220, 331, 340
Estriol, 6, 58
Estrogen, 205, 249, 335, 340, 418, 607
abnormal uterine bleeding, 253
biological activities, 6–7
anencephalic fetuses, 6
blood flow to uterus, 6
end-of-gestation, 6
lactation, 7
low-density lipoprotein, uptake
by placenta, 6
maternal heart disease, 182
parturition, 6
placental sulfatase deficiency,
fetus with, 6
reduced maternal estriol levels, 7
stimulates, 6
breakthrough bleeding, 247, 249
chemical nature, 6
aromatic ring, steroid hormones, 6
estradiol, 6
estriol, 6
estrone, 6
circulating, in pregnancy, increased
levels of, 1
excess, manifestations of, 333
fetal adrenal glands, role of, 6
oogenesis, 207
placenta, 11
placental estrogens, androgen precursors, 6
production, 6, 249
fetal adrenal cortex, 6
fetal liver, 6
placenta, 6
two-cell hypothesis, 207, *207*
replacement, 221, 274
secretory patterns, 6
adrenocorticotropic hormone, 6
anencephaly, 6
estriol, 6
placental sulfatase deficiency, 6
source, 6
withdrawal, 407
bleeding, 250
Estrogen-secreting tumors, 428
Estrone, 6, 331, 333
Ethambutol, 186
Eugonadotropic amenorrhea, 218–219,
222–223
Evaluation of patients in preterm labor,
155–156
Exogenous unopposed estrogen, 427
External genitalia, 403
External ultrasound device, 112

Face presentation
delivery, *102*
fetus, *24*
Factor V Leiden, 351
False labor, 101
Family health history, in antepartum
care, 34
Family planning, 346–357. *See also*
Contraception
natural, 354–355
Fat necrosis, 397
Fatigue, in pregnancy, 19
Fecal incontinence, 418
evaluation, 419

pathophysiology, 418–419
symptoms, 419
treatment, 419
Federal funding regulations, 441
Female athlete triad, 217
Female condoms, 346, 376
Female fetus, endocrine system, 1
Ferriman-Gallwey scoring system, 232
Fertility awareness, natural family planning,
354
Fertilization, *in vitro*, 299, 311–312, 444
Fetal adrenal cortex, 4, 6
Fetal adrenal glands, role of, 6
Fetal alcohol syndrome, 44, 71
Fetal anatomic survey, 61
Fetal aneuploidy, genetic screening, 58–59
Fetal cortisol levels, 98
labor, 98
Fetal echocardiography, 63
Fetal glucose levels, 175
Fetal head, extension of, 104
in labor, 104
Fetal heart rate, 111
patterns
accelerations, *114*
baseline FHR, 112
contractions, 114
early decelerations, *115*
FHR accelerations, 114
FHR decelerations, 114
FHR variability, 112–113
interpretation of, 112–117
late decelerations, *116*
mild variable decelerations, *115*
minimal variability, *113*
moderate variability, *113*
moderate variable deceleration, *116*
severe variable deceleration, *116*
tracings, 117–118
further assessment of fetal well-being, 118
nonreassuring FHR patterns, 117
reassuring FHR patterns, 117
women with nonreassuring FHR
patterns, 117–118
Fetal heart tones, 37
Fetal hypoxia
normal fetal oxygenation, 111
pathophysiology of, 111
Fetal liver, 4, 6
Fetal lung maturity, 64
Fetal monitoring, 111–122
heart rate, 117–118
accelerations, *114*
baseline FHR, 112
continuous monitoring, 112
contractions, 114
early decelerations, *115*
FHR accelerations, 114
FHR decelerations, 114
FHR variability, 112–113
further assessment of fetal well-being, 118
intermittent FHR auscultation, 112
interpretation of, 112–117
late decelerations, *116*
mild variable decelerations, *115*
minimal variability, *113*
moderate variability, *113*
moderate variable deceleration, *116*
nonreassuring FHR patterns, 117
reassuring FHR patterns, 117
severe variable deceleration, *116*
types of, 112
women with nonreassuring FHR
patterns, 117–118

hypoxia
normal fetal oxygenation, 111
pathophysiology of, 111
intrapartum, 111–122 (*See also*
Intrapartum fetal monitoring)
oxygen saturation monitoring, 118–119
Fetal mortality, 47
Fetal movement, in pregnancy, 19
Fetal oxygen saturation monitoring, 118–119
Fetal oxygenation, 111
Fetal rejection prevention, 5
Fetal scalp blood sampling, 118
Fetal scalp electrode, 112
Fetal skin sampling, 64
Fetal testicular testosterone, 3
Fetal transfusion, 191
Fetal viability, 21
Fetal well-being, 63
Fetoplacental unit, access to, 70
Fetus, 12–15, 21. *See also* Fetal
amino acids, 12
amniotic fluid, 12, 22
amniotic membranes, 12
amnion, 12
chorion, 12
membranes, 12
bowel movement, 22
cardiovascular system, 13–14
cortisol secretion, 23
endocrine system, 1
gastrointestinal system, 14
glucocorticoids, 23
glucose, 12
growth/development, 22–23
growth hormones, 12
human chorionic somatomammotropin, 12
human placental growth hormone, 12
human placental lactogen, 12
insulin, 12
insulin-like growth factors I/II, 12
heart beat, identification of, 20
hematologic system, 14–15
hemodynamics, 13
hemodynamics in utero, *13*
hemoglobin dissociation curves, fetal,
maternal, *15*
hyperbilirubinemia, 14
immune system, 15
lie, 23
longitudinal lie, 23
oblique lie, 23
transverse lie, 23
lung maturation, 23
lung maturity, 22–23
meconium, 14
organ systems, 13–15
adrenal gland, 15
endocrine system, 15
hemoglobin, 15
thyroid gland, 15
oxygen, 12
phosphatidylglycerol, 22
physiology, 11–18
placenta, 11–12
function, 11–12
estrogen, 11
gas exchange, 11
growth factors, 12
immunology, 12
mother-to-fetus nutrient
transfer, 11
peptides, 12
progesterone, 11

Fetus, (*Cont.*)
  proteins, 12
  secretion, 11
  metabolism, 12
  structure, 11
    to fetal blood, 11
    from maternal blood, 11
    placental cotyledons, 11
    villa, 11
  presentation, 23–24
    breech presentation, *25*
    breech presentations, 23–24
    brow presentation, *24*
    cephalic presentations, 23
    complete breech, 24
    face presentation, *24*
    frank breech, 24
    incomplete breech, 24
    vertex presentation, *23*
  renal system, 14
  requirements, of 12
  respiratory distress syndrome, 22
  respiratory system, 14
  status, 21–24
  status of, 21–24
  ultrasonographic recognition, 20
  umbilical cord, 12
    umbilical arteries, 12
    umbilical vein, 12
  viability, 21
  weight, 22
FHR. *See* Fetal heart rate
Fibroadenoma, 397
Fibrocystic disease, 396
Fibroids, 49, 300, 336
Finasteride, 243
First stage of labor, 99–100, 104–105, 141
  pain neuropathways, 141
First trimester, 20–21, 61, 443
  maternal infection, 50
  screening, 36, 51
  signs/symptoms, 20–21
  ultrasound, 61
FISH, 63
Fishy odor, 405
Fitz-Hugh-Curtis syndrome, 377
5α-reductase, 239
Flu shot, in antepartum care, 38
Fluoxetine, 212
Flutamide, 243
Folic acid deficiency, 180
Follicle-stimulating hormone, 205, 220,
        297, 330–332
  receptors for, 206
Forceps deliveries
  Barton forceps, 129
  classic forceps, 129, *129*
  classification of, 128
  Kielland forceps, 129
  low forceps, 129
  midforceps, 129
  outlet forceps, 129
  Piper forceps, 129
  planes of pelvis, *128*
  specialized forceps, 129, *130*
Forceps delivery, 127–130
Foreign body salpingitis, 382
Forensic evaluation, sexual assault,
        388–389
Fragile X syndrome, prenatal diagnosis,
        57–58
Frank breech, fetus, 24
Free fatty acids, in pregnancy, 3
FSH. *See* Follicle-stimulating hormone

Galactorrhea, 395
Galactosemia, 217, 442
Gamete intrafallopian transfer, 303
Gap junctions, 99
Gas exchange, placenta, 11
Gastrointestinal changes in pregnancy, 140
Gastrointestinal system, fetal, 14
GBS. *See* Group B streptococcus
Genetic amniocentesis, 63
Genetic counseling, 56, 442–443
  amniocentesis, 442–443
  congenital malformations, baseline rate, 56
  particular problems, 442
  prenatal diagnosis, 56
  referral to genetic counselor, 442
  routine genetic screening, 442
  screening, 56
Genetic screening, 58–60
  cystic fibrosis, 59–60
  fetal aneuploidy, 58–59
  hemoglobinopathies, 60
  neural tube defects, 59
  Tay-Sachs disease, 60
Genitalia, external, developmental defects of,
        320–321
Gentamicin, 380
Germ cell
  origin, 319
  tumor, 432
German measles, 50, 74–75
Gestational age *vs.* fundal height, *20*
Gestational carrier, 444
Gestational diabetes, 175, 177
  screen, 51
Gestational hypertension, 163
Gestational sac. *See* Chorionic sac
Gestational trophoblastic disease, 178, 196–204
  benign GTD, 196
  gestational trophoblastic tumor, 196,
        199–201
    abortion/ectopic pregnancy, after, 200
    characteristics, 199–200
    classification, 200t
    diagnosis, 200
    future fertility, 201
    management, 200
    metastatic disease, 200
    metastatic GTT, 201
    molar pregnancy, after evacuation of,
        200
    nonmetastatic GTT, 200
    poor-prognosis metastatic GTT, 201
    recurrence rates, 201
    workup, 200
  GTT, 196
  hydatidiform mole, 196–199
    birth control, 199
    clinical classification, 197t
    clinical features, 197–198
    complete mole, 196–197
      partial mole, comparison of, 198t
    diagnostic studies, 198
    dilation and suction curettage, 199
    diploid complete hydatiform mole,
        chromosomal origin, *197*
    follow-up of complete or partial molar
        pregnancy, 199
    future fertility, 199
    hCG, 199
    histologic features, 196–197
    malignant potential, 197, 199
    molar pregnancies, management of, 198
    normal pregnancy, 199
    origin, 196–197

partial mole, 197
physical examination, 199
prophylactic chemotherapy, 199
risk of developing GTT, 199
second molar pregnancy, risk of, 199
triploid partial hydatidiform mole,
        chromosomal origin, *198*
hydatiform mole, 196
incidence, 196
Gestational trophoblastic tumor, 196, 199–201
  abortion/ectopic pregnancy, after, 200
  characteristics, 199–200
  classification, 200t
  diagnosis, 200
  future fertility, 201
  management, 200
  metastatic disease, 200
  metastatic GTT, 201
  molar pregnancy, after evacuation of, 200
  nonmetastatic GTT, 200
  poor-prognosis metastatic GTT, 201
  recurrence rates, 201
  workup, 200
GIFT. *See* Gamete intrafallopian transfer
Glomerular endotheliosis, 166
Glucocorticoids, 184
  fetus, 23
Glucose
  fetal requirements, 12
  metabolism, 175
  urine dip, in antepartum care, 37
Glycogen, 402
GnRH. *See* Gonadotropin-releasing
        hormone
Gold standard, 279, 409
Gonadal agenesis (46,XX karyotype), 217
Gonadal dysgenesis, 217, 325–326
Gonadotropin-releasing hormone, 206, 300
  agonists, 243, 273
  amplitude/frequency, 206
  characteristics, 206
  down-regulation, 206
  gonadotropin production, 206
  pulsatile manner, 206
  secretion, 206
Gonadotropins, 206–207, 242, 303
Gonorrhea, 358, 389
  culture, 50
Gram stain, 359
Granuloma inguinale, 361
Granulomatous salpingitis, 381–382
Granulosa cell membrane, 206
Granulosa cells, 206
Graves disease, 178
Gravida, 33
Group B streptococcus, 52
Growth factors, placenta, 12
Growth hormones, fetal, 12
  human chorionic somatomammotropin, 12
  human placental growth hormone, 12
  human placental lactogen, 12
  insulin, 12
  insulin-like growth factors I/II, 12
Growth spurt, 321
GTD. *See* Gestational trophoblastic disease
GTT. *See* Gestational trophoblastic tumor
Gynecologic history, in antepartum care, 34

Habitual abortion, 132
Haemophilus influenzae, 185
Hair changes, 336
Hair removal techniques, 242
  bleaching, 242
  depilatories, 242

eflornithine HCl, 242
electrolysis, 242
laser, 242
shaving, 242
tweezing, 242
waxing, 242
Hair types, 238
lanugo, 238
terminal, 238
vellus, 238
Hallucinogens, use in pregnancy, 82
Hb S. *See* Sickle hemoglobin
hCG. *See* Human chorionic gonadotropin
Headaches, 334
Heart beat, fetal, identification of, 20
Heart defects, 57
Heart disease, 73, 182–183
diagnosis during pregnancy, 183
incidence in pregnancy, 182
management, 183
maternal, 182
Heart rate monitoring. *See* Fetal monitoring
Hegar sign, 19
HELLP syndrome, 163
Hematologic changes in pregnancy, 140
Hematologic system, fetal, 14–15
Hematomas, 317
Hemodynamics in utero, *13*
Hemoglobin, fetal, 15
Hemoglobin A, 60
Hemoglobin A₂, 60
Hemoglobin dissociation curves, fetal,
maternal, *15*
Hemoglobin F, 60
Hemoglobinopathies, genetic screening, 60
Hemolysis, elevated liver enzymes, low
platelets. *See* HELLP
syndrome
Hemorrhagic shock, antepartum bleeding, 93
Hepatic system, fetal, 14
Hepatitis, in pregnancy, 82
Hepatitis B, 51, 369, 389
high-risk pregnancy, 48
Hepatocellular adenoma, 351
Hermaphroditism, 321
Heroin
teratology, 72
use in pregnancy, 85
Herpes simplex, 75, 368, 389, 423
genitalis, 408–410
high-risk pregnancy, 48
Herpes zoster, 76–77
Heterotopic pregnancy, 287
High-risk pregnancy
acute systemic pyelonephritis, 51
advice for patient, 42
age, 43
alcohol abuse screening, 44t
alcohol use, 43
anemia, 50
antibody screen, 50
asymptomatic bacteriuria, 51
autoimmune disorders, 48
autoimmune polyglandular syndrome, 48
caffeine use, 44
cardiac disease, 47
cervical insufficiency, 49–50
cervix, 49
cesarean birth, 46
chronic hypertension, 47
clinical course, 50
clinical pelvimetry, 49
congenital anomalies, 47
continuous assessment is necessary, 47

cytomegalovirus, 48
depression, 48–49
diabetes, 47–49
domestic violence, 44
drug use, 43
ectopic pregnancy, 44
education, 42
elective cesarean birth, 52
elevated maternal serum alpha-
fetoprotein, 51
empiric plan, 52
environmental risks, 44
fetal alcohol syndrome, 44
fetal growth and development, 47
fetal mortality, 47
first trimester, maternal infection in, 50
first-trimester screening programs, 51
hepatitis B virus, 48
herpes simplex virus, 48
HIV, 48
hydrops, 48
hypertension, pregnancy-induced, 46
identification, 42–55
immunization, 50–51
infectious diseases, 48
infertility, history of, 47
initial prenatal visit, 43–49, 45t
alcohol abuse screening, 44t
general history, 43–44
medical history, 47–49
medications, 49
obstetric history, 44–47
physical abuse during pregnancy, 45t
spontaneous preterm delivery, risk
determination, 46t
T-ACE questionnaire, 44t
laboratory studies, 50–52
aneuploidy, screening for, 51
antibody screen, 50
blood type, 50
chlamydia testing, 50
complete blood count, 50
gestational diabetes screen, 51
gonorrhea culture, 50
group B streptococcus, 52
HBV testing, 51
HIV testing, 51–52
neural tube defects, screening for, 51
pap smear, 51
rubella titer, 50
sickle-cell screen, 52
syphilis test, 50
urinalysis, 51
large infant, 45
leiomyomata, 49
leukocytosis, 51
management of risk, 52
maternal death, 42
maternal mortality, 42
microcytosis, 50
minor ailments, 42
multipara, 44
neonatal morbidity, 47
neural tube defect, 51
noxious chemicals, 44
nullipara, 44
obesity, 49
parity, 44
parvovirus infection, 48
past obstetric history, 52t
perinatal death, 45
perinatal mortality, 42
perineum, 49
physical examination, 49–50

evaluation of uterus, 49–50
general examination, 49
pelvic examination, 49
preconception care, 43
preterm delivery, 44
prevention, 42
previous cesarean birth, 46
pulmonary disease, 47
pulmonary embolism, 42
radiation, 44
reassurance, 42
renal disease, 47
Rh sensitization, 50
risk assessment, 52
screening, 42
second-trimester pregnancy loss, 44–45
socioeconomic status, 43
substance abuse, 43–44
support, 42
systemic lupus erythematosus, 48
thromboembolic disease, 48
thyroid disease, 48
tobacco use, 43
TORCH, 48
toxoplasmosis, 48
underweight, 49
uterine anomalies, 50
vagina, 49
varicella zoster virus infection, 48
vulva, 49
zidovudine, 52
Hirsutism, 222, 231–232, 234–235, 238–246,
352
3α-androstanediol glucuronide, 239
5α-reductase, 239
albumin, 239
androgen-receptor blockers, 243
cyproterone acetate, 243
flutamide, 243
spironolactone, 243
androgens, 238–239
antiandrogens, 234
cimetidine, 243
combination hormonal contraceptives,
242
combined hormonal contraception, 234
corticosteroid, 243
diagnosis, 239–242
differential diagnosis, 240–241
androgen-producing tumors, 241
androgenic drug exposure, 241
Cushing syndrome, 241
idiopathic hirsutism, 240
incomplete androgen insensitivity,
241
metabolic syndrome, 240
nonclassic adrenal hyperplasia, 240
pituitary disorders, 241
polycystic ovary syndrome, 240
Y-containing mosaics, 241
dihydrotestosterone, 239
drug ingestion, 240
ethnic background, 240
etiology, 238
family history, 240
finasteride, 243
free testosterone, 239
gonadotropin-releasing hormone
agonists, 243
hair removal techniques, 242
bleaching, 242
depilatories, 242
eflornithine HCl, 242
electrolysis, 242

Hirsutism, (*Cont.*)
  laser, 242
  shaving, 242
  tweezing, 242
  waxing, 242
  hair types, 238
    lanugo, 238
    terminal, 238
    vellus, 238
  hirsutism, 238
  history, 239–240
  history of infertility, 240
  hypertrichosis, 238
  idiopathic ovarian-related hirsutism, 242
  insulin-sensitizing agents, 243
  ketoconazole, 243
  laboratory evaluation, 241–242
    cortisol, 242
    gonadotropins, 242
    serum 17-OHP, 241
    serum 3α-AG, 242
    serum androstenedione, 241
    serum DHEAS, 241
    serum testosterone, 241
    testosterone levels, 241
    thyroid-stimulating hormone, 242
  local trauma, 240
  mechanical hair removal, 234
  medroxyprogesterone acetate, 243
  menstrual cycles, 240
  new hair follicles, preventing, 242
  onset, 239
    abrupt, 240
    gradual, 240
  ovarian tumors, removal of, 242
  sex hormone-binding globulin, 239
  testosterone, 238–239
  total testosterone, 239
  treatment, 242–243
  virilization, 238, 240
  virilizing process, arresting, 242
History, 220
HIV, 365, 389
  high-risk pregnancy, 48
  testing, 51–52
Homocystinuria, 442
Hormonal contraceptives, 441
Hormonal fluctuation, manifestations of, 333–334
Hormonal therapy, abnormal uterine bleeding, 252–253
Hormonally related bleeding, 250
  estrogen withdrawal bleeding, 250
  progesterone breakthrough bleeding, 250
Hormone characteristics, 1–2
Hormone therapy, 220–221, 335, 339–341
Hot flashes, 334, 336–337. *See also* Vasomotor symptoms
hPL. *See* Human placental lactogen
Human chorionic gonadotropin, 58, 196–198, 289–290
  in pregnancy, 1–3, 19
    biologic functions, 3
      clinical uses, 3
      corpus luteum, 3
      fetal testicular testosterone, 3
      multiple marker screen, 3
      with trophoblastic neoplasia, 3
      viability of pregnancy, assessment, 3
    chemical nature, 2
    secretion patterns, 2
      contemporary pregnancy tests, 2
      high levels, 2

low levels, 2
  serum hCG assays, 2
  urine hCG assays, 2
source, 2
Human chorionic gonadotropin assays, 2
Human chorionic somatomammotropin, 12
  in pregnancy, 3
Human papilloma virus, 367, 423
Human placental growth hormone, 12
Human placental lactogen, 12
  in pregnancy, 1, 3
    biologic function, 3
      clinical use, 3
      diabetogenic effect, 3
      increased insulin levels, 3
      insulin-directed glucose, 3
      maternal free fatty acids, 3
      plasma insulin, 3
    chemical nature, 3
    human chorionic somatomam-motropin, 3
    secretory patterns, 3
    source, 3
Humoral immunity, 402
Hydatidiform mole, 196–199
  birth control, 199
  clinical classification, 197t
  clinical features, 197–198
  complete mole, 196–197
    partial mole, comparison of, 198t
  diagnostic studies, 198
  dilation and suction curettage, 199
  diploid complete hydatiform mole, chromosomal origin, *197*
  follow-up of complete or partial molar pregnancy, 199
  future fertility, 199
  hCG, 199
  histologic features, 196–197
  malignant potential, 197, 199
  molar pregnancies, management of, 198
  normal pregnancy, 199
  origin, 196–197
  partial mole, 197
  physical examination, 199
  prophylactic chemotherapy, 199
  risk of developing GTT, 199
  second molar pregnancy, risk of, 199
  triploid partial hydatidiform mole, chromosomal origin, *198*
Hydronephrosis, 319
Hydrops, high-risk pregnancy, 48
Hydroureter, 319
Hyperandrogenic drugs, 231
Hyperandrogenism, 227–229
Hyperbilirubinemia, 14
Hyperemesis gravidarum, 19
Hypergonadotropic amenorrhea, 216, 220–221
Hypergonadotropic hypogonadism, 324
Hypermenorrhea, 334
Hyperoxia, maternal, 117
Hyperplasia, 428
Hyperplastic dystrophy, 408
Hyperprolactinemia, 296
Hyperreflexia, 167
Hypertension in pregnancy, 46, 163–174
  antepartum management, 165
  antihypertensive management, 165
  chronic hypertension, 163–165
    effects on fetus, 164
    effects on mother, 164
  eclampsia, 163
  gestational hypertension, 163

HELLP syndrome, 163
preeclampsia, 163, 165, 169
  antepartum treatment, 167
  clinical signs, 167
  delivery, 167
  edema, 167
  future hypertension, 169
  hyperreflexia, 167
  hypertension, 167
  intrapartum management, 168
  laboratory findings, 167
  magnesium, 168t
  management, 167–169
  pathophysiology, 165–167
  postpartum management, 168–169
  prevention, 169
  prognosis, 169
  rate of occurrence, 165
  recurrence, 169
  risk factors, 165
  route of delivery, 167
  severe, criteria for, 164t
  treatment, 169
severity, 164t
Hyperthermia, teratology, 72
Hypertrichosis, 238
Hypogonadotropic amenorrhea, 217, 221–223
Hypogonadotropic hypogonadism, 324–325
Hypothalamic amenorrhea, 296
Hypothalamic-pituitary-ovarian axis, 296
Hypothyroidism, 178, 222, 296, 442
Hypoxemia, 111
Hypoxia, 111, 113
Hysterectomy, 199, 254, 264, 416, 425–426
  cesarean, 126
Hysterosalpingography, 262, 299, 310
Hysteroscopy, 252, 262, 300, 310, 312, 341

ICSI, 303
Identification of high-risk pregnancy, 42–55
Idiopathic hirsutism, 240, 242
Ilioinguinal nerve, 401
Imipenem cilastatin, 381
Immune globulin, 63–64
Immune system, fetal, 15
Immunization, high-risk pregnancy, 50–51
Immunofluorescence, 409
Imperforate anus, rectovaginal communication, 319
Imperforate hymen, 325
Implanon, 350
Implantable progestin, 350
Implied contract, 440
In labor and postpartum, 183
In vitro fertilization, 299, 311–312, 444
Inborn errors of metabolism, 57
Incomplete abortion, 132
Incomplete androgen insensitivity, 241
Incomplete breech, fetus, 24
Incontinence
  fecal, 418
    evaluation, 419
    pathophysiology, 418–419
    symptoms, 419
    treatment, 419
  urinary, 416–418
    evaluation, 417
    treatment, 418
    types, 416
Increased incidences of abortion and premature labor, 261
Induced abortion, 133–135
Induction of labor, 22, 133, 150

Inevitable abortion, 132
Infection
  puerperal, 27
    fever, 27
    pelvic infections, 27
    urinary tract infections, 27
  teratology, 74–77
Infectious complications of drug use, 83
Infectious diseases, high-risk pregnancy, 48
Infertility, 230, 270, 295–306, 375
  assisted reproductive technology, 303
    gamete intrafallopian transfer, 303
    ICSI, 303
    IVF, 303
    preimplantation genetic diagnosis, 303
    zygote intrafallopian transfer, 303
  causes, 295
  coital problems, 302
    fertile days, 302
    history, 302
    regular coitus, 302
  decreased ovarian reserve, 298
    estradiol, 298
    markers, 298
    treatment, 298–299
  endometriosis, 300
    diagnosis, 300
  with endometriosis, 270
  history of, 47
  incidence, 295
  male factor infertility, 301–302
    diagnosis, 301
  ovulatory dysfunction, 296–298
    diagnosis, 296
    etiology, 296
    treatment, 297
  preconception counseling, 296
  treatment, 295–296, 302
  tubal factor, 299
    diagnosis, 299
    treatment, 299
    tubal disease, 299
  unexplained infertility, 302
    diagnosis, 302
  uterine/vaginal outflow tract
      abnormalities, 299–300
    diagnosis, 299–300
    treatment, 300
    uterine factor, 299
    vaginal outflow tract, 299
  Y chromosome microdeletion, 301
Influenza A, 185
Informed consent, 445–446
  cesarean birth, 125
  exceptions to, 446
  guidelines in obtaining, 446
  obtaining, 446
Infrequent bleeding, 247
Infrequent ovulation, 247
Inguinal area, 403
Inguinal nodes, 436
Inhibin, 58, 208, 331
Initial prenatal blood work, in antepartum
    care, 36
Initial prenatal visit, high-risk pregnancy,
    43–49, 45t
  alcohol abuse screening, 44t
  general history, 43–44
  medical history, 47–49
  medications, 49
  obstetric history, 44–47
  physical abuse during pregnancy, 45t
  spontaneous preterm delivery, risk
      determination, 46t

Initial visit, in antepartum care, 33–34
Injectable progestin, 349
Inner ear problems, 75
Insemination, intrauterine, 302
Insulin, 12
  resistance, 229, 233
Insulin-dependent diabetes mellitus, 311
Insulin-directed glucose, in pregnancy, 3
Insulin-like growth factors I/II, 12
Insulin levels, in pregnancy, 3
Insulin-sensitizing agents, 243
Integrated screening, in antepartum care, 36
Interstitial cystitis, 282
Intimate partner violence, 386–393. *See also*
    Relationship violence
Intrapartum fetal monitoring, 111–122
  heart rate, 111, 117–118
    accelerations, *114*
    baseline FHR, 112
    continuous monitoring, 112
    contractions, 114
    early decelerations, *115*
    FHR accelerations, 114
    FHR decelerations, 114
    FHR variability, 112–113
    further assessment of fetal well-being, 118
    intermittent FHR auscultation, 112
    interpretation of, 112–117
    late decelerations, *116*
    mild variable decelerations, *115*
    minimal variability, *113*
    moderate variability, *113*
    moderate variable deceleration, *116*
    nonreassuring FHR patterns, 117
    reassuring FHR patterns, 117
    severe variable deceleration, *116*
    types of, 112
    women with nonreassuring FHR
        patterns, 117–118
  hypoxia
    normal fetal oxygenation, 111
    pathophysiology of, 111
  oxygen saturation monitoring, 118–119
Intrauterine adhesions, 222
Intrauterine devices, 288, 347–349, 376, 441
  advantages, 348
  contraindications, 348
  disadvantages, 348
  efficacy, 348
  mode of action, 348
  pregnancy-related issues, 348–349
  types, 348
Intrauterine growth retardation, 75
Intrauterine pressure catheter, 114
Intravenous immunoglobulin, 313
Intravenous use of drugs, 83
Intrinsic urethral sphincteric deficiency, 418
Involution of uterus, puerperium, 25
Ionizing radiation, teratology, 68–69
  acute high dose, 68–69
  chronic low dose, 69
  radioactive iodine, 69
IPV. *See* Intimate partner violence
Iron deficiency anemia, 180, 352
Ischemia, 210
Isoimmunization, 188
IUD. *See* Intrauterine devices
IUPC. *See* Intrauterine pressure catheter
Ivermectin, 370–371
IVF, 300, 302–303
IVIG. *See* Intravenous immunoglobulin

Jarisch-Herxheimer reaction, 364
Juvenile granulosa cell tumors, 433

Kallmann syndrome, 218, 325
Karyotype, 63
KEEPS. *See* Kronos Early Estrogen
    Prevention Study
Kegel exercise, 416
Ketoconazole, 243
Kidney, glomerular endotheliosis, 166
Kielland forceps, 129
Klebsiella pneumoniae, 185
Kleihauer-Betke, 189
Kronos Early Estrogen Prevention Study, 340

Labetalol, 165
Labia, 435
  agglutination, 317–318
  majora, 336, 400
  minora, 336, 400
Labor, 22, 98–110
  abnormal labor patterns, 106t
  actin, 98
  active phase, 105, 112
  amniotomy, 105
  anesthesia, 141–143
    combined spinal epidural analgesia, 142
    epidural analgesia, 141–142
    intravenous analgesia, 143
    regional blocks, 143
  cervical dilation, *105*
  changes of cervix, 101
  dilation, 101
  dilation curve, nulliparous labor, *100*
  dilation of cervix, 101
  dysfunctional labor patterns, 105
  effacement of cervix, 101
  engagement, 102–104
  episiotomy, 106t
  external rotation, 104
  face presentation, *102*
  false labor, 101
  fetal cortisol levels, 98
  fetal head, extension of, 104
  first stage of, pain neuropathways, 141
  first stage of labor, 104–105
  gap junctions, 99
  induction of, 22, 133, 150
  internal rotation, 104
  lacerations, birth canal, 107
    first-degree lacerations, 107
    fourth-degree lacerations, 107
    second-degree lacerations, 107
    third-degree lacerations, 107
  latent phase, 105
  left occiput anterior position, *103*
  myometrial physiology, 98–99
  myometrium, physiology of, 99
  myosin, 98
  occiput, 101–102
  occiput anterior, 102
  occiput posterior, 102
  occiput presentation, 101–104, *102*
  occiput transverse, 101
  oxytocin stimulation, 98
  pain of contractions, 101
  placental separation, 106
  premature, 21
  progesterone withdrawal, 98
  prostaglandin release, 98
  ruptured membranes, 104
      (*See also* Preterm labor)
    ferning, 104
    nitrazine test, 104
    pooling, 104
  second stage of, pain neuropathways, 141
  second stage of labor, 105

Labor, (*Cont.*)
  spontaneous vaginal delivery, 105
  stages, 99–101
    first stage, 99–100
    second stage, 100–101
    third stage, 101
  stages of labor, third stage, 106–107
  tocolytic agents
    complications of, 99t
    contraindications to, 100t
  true labor, 101
    vs. false labor, 101t
  uterine contractions, 101
    characteristics of, 101
  uterine hemostasis, 106–107
  uterine smooth muscle, contraction of, 98
Lacerations, birth canal, 107
  first-degree lacerations, 107
  fourth-degree lacerations, 107
  second-degree lacerations, 107
  third-degree lacerations, 107
Lactation, 7, 27–28
  continued prolactin production, 28
  initiation of, 28
  initiation of lactation, 28
  let-down reflex, 28
  mastitis, 28
  nursing, 28
  oxytocin, 28
  physiology, 27–28
  prolactin, 28
  puerperium, 26
  stimulates milk production, 28
Lactobacillus acidophilus, 402
Lactogen, placental, 3
  biologic function, 3
    clinical use, 3
    diabetogenic effect, 3
    increased insulin levels, 3
    insulin-directed glucose, 3
    maternal free fatty acids, 3
    plasma insulin, 3
  chemical nature, 3
  human chorionic somatomammotropin, 3
  secretory patterns, 3
  source, 3
Laparoscopy, 279–280, 290, 299–300, 303,
    379, 381
Laparotomy, 290
Large infant, high-risk pregnancy, 45
Late pregnancy
  estrogen synthesis, *5*
  progesterone synthesis, *5*
LDL. *See* Low-density lipoprotein
Lecithin, in amniotic fluid, *22*
Left occiput anterior position, *103*
  labor/delivery, *103*
Left occiput posterior position, 102
Left occiput transverse position, 101
Leiomyomas, 258–268, 299
  classification, 259–260
  cytogenetic studies, 258
  degenerative changes, 260
  etiology, 258
  GnRH agonists, 263
  hormones, 258
  local factors, 258
  location classification, 259
  management, 262–263
  pathology, 259–260
  signs, 261
  surgery, 263–265
  symptoms, 260–262
  treatment, 262–265
  uterine myomata, *259*

Leiomyomata, high-risk pregnancy, 49
Leprous salpingitis, 381
Let-down reflex, 28
Leukocytes, paternal, 313
Leukocytosis, 379
  high-risk pregnancy, 51
  puerperium, 26
Levator ani, 414, *415*
Levofloxacin, 380
LGV. *See* Lymphogranuloma venereum
LH. *See* Luteinizing hormone
Liability, 444
Lichen sclerosus, 316–317, 408
Lie of fetus, 23
Liley graph, 190, *191*
Lindane, 370–371
Linear salpingotomy, 290
Lipid levels, 233
Liver, 166
  tumor, 351
Lochia, 25
Lochia alba, 25
Lochia rubra, 25
Lochia serosa, 25
Longitudinal lie, fetus, 23
Low-density lipoprotein, uptake by
    placenta, 6
Low-energy high-frequency sound waves, 60
Low forceps, 129
Lung maturity, fetus, 22–23
Luteal-phase endometrial biopsy, 297
Luteinizing hormone, 205, 229, 331
  receptors, 206–207
Lymphogranuloma venereum, 362
Lynch II syndrome, 428
Lytic enzymes, 249

Maculopapular rash, 363
Magnesium sulfate, antepartum bleeding, 93
Magnetic resonance imaging, 262, 310
Majority rule, 445
Male condoms, 346, 376
Male factor infertility, 301–303
  diagnosis, 301
Male fetus, endocrine system, 1
Malformations
  congenital, 57, 70
Malignant breast masses, 396
Malmström vacuum extractor, 129
Malpractice, 440
  elements of negligence, 440
  recovery, 440
Maple syrup urine disease, 442
Marijuana use
  teratology, 72
  use in pregnancy, 85
Mastalgia, 394
  cyclic, 394–395
  noncyclic, 395
Mastitis, 28
Mastodynia, 394
Maternal estriol levels, reduced, 7
Maternal heart disease, 182
Maternal medical disorders, teratology, 72–74
Maternal mortality, high-risk pregnancy, 42
Maternal serum alpha-fetoprotein, high-risk
    pregnancy, 51
Maternal virilizing tumor, 321
Maternal weight, in antepartum care, 37
McDonald technique, cervical cerclage,
    131, *131*
Meconium, 14
Medial episiotomy, 105, 127
Medical complications of pregnancy,
    175–195

anemia, 180–182
  diabetes, 175–177
  heart disease, 182–183
  pulmonary disease, 183–186
  Rh isoimmunization, 188–192
  seizure disorders, 188
  thromboembolic disease, 186–187
  thyroid disease, 177–178
  urinary tract infection, 179–180
Medical history, in antepartum care, 34
Medicolegal issues, 440–448
  birth injury, 445
    alleged negligence, 445
    brain damage, 445
  birth-related suits, 444–445
    wrongful birth, 445
    wrongful conception, 444–445
    wrongful life, 445
  disclosure rules, 445
  genetic counseling, 442–443
    amniocentesis, 442–443
    particular problems, 442
    referral to genetic counselor, 442
    routine genetic screening, 442
  informed consent, 445–446
    exceptions to, 446
    guidelines in obtaining, 446
    obtaining, 446
  malpractice, 440
    elements of negligence, 440
    recovery, 440
  negligence theory of consent, 445
  preconception issues, 440–441
    hormonal contraceptives, 441
    intrauterine devices, 441
    sterilization, 441
  reproductive technologies, 443–444
    artificial insemination, 443–444
    embryo freezing, 444
    gestational carrier, 444
    in vitro fertilization, 444
  termination of pregnancy, 443
    right of privacy, 443
    state restrictions, 443
    trimester model, 443
Mediolateral episiotomy, 105, 127
Medroxyprogesterone acetate, 243
Megaloblastic anemia, 180
Menarche, 322, 427
Mendelian abnormalities, prenatal
    diagnosis, 57
Menometrorrhagia, 248, 251, 324
Menopause, 330–345, 427
  clinical manifestations of, 335–339
  endocrinology, 332
  health risk assessment, 341
  lifestyle in, 342
  ovarian function, 331–332
  physiology of, 331–333
  premature menopause, 332–333
  premature ovarian failure, 332–333
  screenings, 341–342
Menorrhagia, 248, 251, 260, 334
Menstrual calculations, natural
    family planning, 354
Menstrual cycle, 205–215, 240
  androgen synthesis, 207
  body temperature, *209*
  changes, 333
  estrogen production, two-cell hypothesis,
    207, *207*
  follicle-stimulating hormone receptors,
    206
  follicular phase, 205
  gonadotropin-releasing hormone, 206

amplitude/frequency, 206
  characteristics, 206
  down-regulation, 206
  gonadotropin production, 206
  pulsatile manner, 206
  secretion, 206
gonadotropins, 206–207
hormonal correlates, *209*
length of cycle, 205
luteal phase, 205
luteinizing hormone receptors,
      206–207
mean duration, 205
menstruation, 210
  clinical problems, 210–212
  dysmenorrhea, 210–211
    clinical aspects, 210
    management, 211
    physiology, 211
    ischemia, 210
  premenstrual syndrome, 211
    clinical manifestations, 211
    epidemiology, 211
    etiology, 211
    premenstrual dysphoric disorder, 211
  normal, 247–248
    length, 247
    regularity, 247
    volume/duration, 248
oogenesis, 207–210, *208*
    antral follicle, 208
    corpus luteum, 210
    estrogen, 207
    ovulation, 209–210
    preantral follicle, 207
    preovulatory follicle, 208
    primordial follicle, 207
  ovulation, 205
Mental retardation, 445
Metabolic acidosis, 111
Metabolic syndrome, 230, 240
Metformin, 235
Methadone, use in pregnancy, 85
Methotrexate, 291t
Metronidazole, 362, 370, 380, 407
Metroplasty, 312
Metrorrhagia, 248, 334
Microcytic anemia, 182
Microcytosis, high-risk pregnancy, 50
Midforceps, 129
Mifepristone, 5, 354
Minipill, 349
Minority rule, 445
Miscarriage, 132
Miscarriage, recurrent, 132
Missed abortion, 132
Mittelschmerz, 279
Mixed germ cell tumors, 433
Molluscum contagiosum, 369
Mondor disease, 397
Moniliasis, 405
Mood disturbance, 334
Morning-after pill, 353
Morning sickness of pregnancy, 19
Mother, endocrine system, 1
MSAFP, 58–59
Mucoid discharge, 318
Mucopurulent cervicitis, 360
Mucosa, 401
Multipara, 33
  high-risk pregnancy, 44
Mumps, teratology, 77
Muscularis, 401
Mycoplasma pneumoniae, 185
Myocardial infarction, 351

Myomectomy, 264
Myometrial physiology, 98–99
Myometritis, 375
Myometrium
  atrophy, 336
  physiology of, 99
  in pregnancy, 5
Myosin, 98

NAAT. *See* Nucleic acid amplification test
Naegele's rule, 20, 33
National Domestic Violence Hotline, 387
Natural family planning, 354–355
  advantages, 355
  basal body temperature, 354
  cervical secretions, 354–355
  disadvantages, 355
  efficacy, 355
  fertility awareness, 354
  menstrual calendar calculations, 354
Nausea, in pregnancy, 19
NCAH. *See* Nonclassic adrenal hyperplasia
Negligence, elements of, 440
Negligence theory of consent, 445
Neonatal morbidity, 47
Neoplasia, 351, 408
Neural tube defect, 57
  genetic screening, 59
  high-risk pregnancy, 51
  screening for, 51
Neurologic complications of drug use, 83
Neuropathologic changes, 75
Neurosyphilis, 364
Nicotine, 85. *See also* Tobacco
Nifedipine, 165
Night sweats, 334
Nipple discharge, 394–396
Nitrazine test, ruptured membranes
      in labor, 104
Nits, 370
Nonclassic adrenal hyperplasia, 240
Noncyclic mastalgia, 395
Nonepithelial ovarian cancer, 432–434
  germ cell tumors, 432
  gonadoblastomas, 433
  sex cord-stromal neoplasms, 433
  staging, 434t
Nongestational choriocarcinomas, 433
Nongranulomatous salpingitis, 382
Nonlactating women, puerperium, 26
Nonpolyposis colorectal cancer
      syndrome, 428
Nonsteroidal anti-inflammatory drugs, 253,
      272, 335
Normal menstrual cycle, 247–248
  length, 247
  physiology of, 248–249
  regularity, 247
  volume/duration, 248
Normal pregnancy, 19–31. *See also*
      Pregnancy
  clinical evidence, 19–20
  complications, 26–27
  confirming diagnosis, 20
  diagnosis, 19–20
  fetal presentation, 23–24
  fetal status, 21–24
    growth/development, 22–23
    lie of fetus, 23
  first trimester, 20–21
  fundal height *vs.* gestational age, *20*
  lecithin, in amniotic fluid, *22*
  mastitis, 28
  nursing, 28
  physiology, 27–28

pregnancy dating, 20
presumptive symptoms, 19
puerperium, 25–27
  physiology, 25–26
second trimester, 21
sphingomyelin, in amniotic fluid, *22*
third trimester, 21
Normal puberty, 321
Norplant, 350
Noxious chemicals, high-risk pregnancy, 44
NSAIDs. *See* Nonsteroidal anti-inflammato-
      ry drugs
Nuchal translucency, 58
Nucleic acid amplification test, 359–360
Nulligravida, 33
Nullipara, high-risk pregnancy, 44
Nulliparous labor, dilation curve, *100*
Nursing newborn, 28
Nutrient transfer, placenta, 11

Obesity, 165, 230, 232, 234, 332, 351, 427
  high-risk pregnancy, 49
Oblique lie, fetus, 23
Obstetric conjugate, 34
Obstetric history, in antepartum care, 33–34
Obstetric ultrasound, 56–66
Occiput, 101–102
Occiput anterior position, 102
Occiput posterior position, 102
Occiput presentation, labor/delivery,
      101–104, *102*
Occiput transverse position, 101
Ocular defects, 75
Ofloxacin, 360, 380
Oligo-ovulation, 296
Oligohydramnios, 115
Oligomenorrhea, 205, 227, 247, 251
^{125}I radioisotope scanning, 187
Oocytes, donor, 299
Oogenesis, 207–210, *208*
  antral follicle, 208
  corpus luteum, 210
  estrogen, 207
  ovulation, 209–210
  preantral follicle, 207
  preovulatory follicle, 208
  primordial follicle, 207
Oophorectomy, 290, 430
Oophoritis, 375, 377
Opiates, use in pregnancy, 82
Oral contraceptives, 211–212, 280,
      376, 430
  abnormal uterine bleeding, 253
Oral glucose tolerance test, *233t*
Ortho Evra patch, risks of, 353
Osteopenia, 338
Osteoporosis, 337–338
Outlet forceps, 129
Ovarian aging, 298
Ovarian androgens, 331
Ovarian cancer, 351–352, 430–431
  epithelial, 429–432
    clinical course, 431
    diagnosis, 430
    epidemiology, 429–430
    predominant histologic types, 430–431
    recurrent ovarian cancer, 432
    staging, 430–431t
    treatment, 431
  low malignant potential, 431
  nonepithelial, 432–434
    germ cell tumors, 432
    gonadoblastomas, 433
    sex cord-stromal neoplasms, 433
    staging, 434t

Ovarian drilling, 222
Ovarian estrogen production, 332
Ovarian failure, 326
Ovarian hyperthecosis, 231
Ovarian pregnancy, 287
Ovarian stromal tissue, 331–332
Ovarian torsion, 280
Ovarian tumors, 319, 431
    removal of, 242
Overflow incontinence, 417
Ovulation, 205
    infrequent, 247
    oogenesis, 209–210
    puerperium, 26
Ovulatory dysfunction, 296–298
    diagnosis, 296
    etiology, 296
    treatment, 297
Oxygen, fetal requirements, 12
Oxygenation, 111, 117
Oxytocin, 107, 199
    lactation, 28
    stimulation, 98

Paclitaxel, side effects of, 432
Pain, 280
    of contractions, 101
    with endometriosis, 269–270
    neuropathways
        obstetric, 141
            first stage of labor, 141
            second stage of labor, 141
            second stage of labor, 141
    pelvic, 278–286 (*See also* Pelvic pain)
    perception of, 278
    referred, 279
    symptoms, 281
Pap test, 367, 423–424
    high-risk pregnancy, 51
Paracrine factors, 258
Paravaginal repair, 416
Parental genetic abnormalities, 311–312
Parity, 33
    high-risk pregnancy, 44
Parturition, 6
Parvovirus
    high-risk pregnancy, 48
    teratology, 77
Past obstetric history, high-risk pregnancy, 52t
Paternal blood type, 189
Paternal leukocytes, 313
Patient history, in antepartum care, 33–34
PCP. *See* Phencyclidine; *Pneumocystis carinii*
    pneumonia
PDD. *See* Premenstrual dysphoric disorder
Pediatric gynecology, 316–329, 408
    adolescent, 316, 324–326
    adrenal tumors, 320
    amenorrhea, 325–326
    androgen insensitivity syndrome, 320–321
    androgenic substances, 320
    androgens, childhood ingestion, 320
    congenital adrenal hyperplasia, 320
    contraception, 326
    delayed puberty, 324
    dysfunctional uterine bleeding, 324–325
    ectopic ureter, with vaginal terminus, 319
    genitalia, external, developmental defects
        of, 320–321
    Kallmann syndrome, 325
    labial agglutination, 317–318
    lichen sclerosus et atrophicus, 316–317
    maternal virilizing tumor, 321
    neoplasms, 318–319

normal puberty, 321
ovarian tumors, 319
pediatric patient, 316
    congenital anomalies, 319
precocious puberty, 323
prolapsed urethra, 318
pubertal development, 321–324
rectal examination, 316
sexual abuse, 326
Swyer syndrome, 325
Tanner staging, 322t
    normal breast development, *322*
    normal pubic hair development, *323*
trauma, 317
true hermaphroditism, 321
Turner syndrome, 325
21-hydroxylase defect, 320
vaginal discharge, 318
vaginal ectopic anus, 319
vaginal tumors, 318
vulvovaginal lesions, 316–318
Pediculosis pubis, 370
Pedunculated, 259
Pelvic adhesions, 281
Pelvic examination, 262, 403
Pelvic floor, 414–422
    anatomy, 414
    fecal incontinence, 418
        evaluation, 419
        pathophysiology, 418–419
        symptoms, 419
        treatment, 419
    innervation, 414–415
    levator ani muscles, *415*
    muscle exercise, 416
    pelvic organ prolapse, 415–416
        evaluation, 416
        halfway grading system, 416t
        risk factors, 415
        symptoms, 416
        terminology, 415
        treatment, 416
    urinary incontinence, 416–418
        evaluation, 417
        treatment, 418
        types, 416
Pelvic infections, puerperal, 27
Pelvic inflammatory disease, 280, 282, 287,
    299, 352, 375–385
    acute, 375
    bacteriology, 376–377
        causative organisms, 376–377
    chronic, 375
    chronology of salpingo-oophoritis, 377
    clinical criteria, 378
    costs, 375
    diagnosis, 378–379
    diagnostic techniques, 379
    differential diagnosis, 378–379
    empiric treatment, 379
    epidemiology, 375–376
    Fitz-Hugh-Curtis syndrome, 377
    granulomatous salpingitis, 381–382
    incidence, 375
    inciting events, 377
    individualized treatment, 379–380
    laparoscopy, 378t
    medical sequelae, 375–376
    nongranulomatous salpingitis, 382
    oral treatment regimens, 380
    parental regimens, 380
    pathophysiology, 377
    prevention, 376
    sexual activity, 376

silent, 375
surgical interventions, 381
symptoms, 378
treatment, 379–381
tubo-ovarian abscess, 380–381
Pelvic lymph node, 425
Pelvic magnetic resonance image, 300
Pelvic malignancies, 423–439
    cervical cancer, 423
        Bethesda System, 424
        epidemiology, 423
        invasive carcinoma of cervix, 425
        microinvasive carcinoma of cervix, 425
        preinvasive cervical disease, 423–425
        prevention of cervical cancer, 427
        staging, 425t
    endometrial cancer, 427–429
        endometrial carcinoma, 428–429
        endometrial hyperplasia, 428
        epidemiology, 427
        staging, 429t
    epithelial ovarian cancer, 429–432
        clinical course, 431
        diagnosis, 430
        epidemiology, 429–430
        predominant histologic types, 430–431
        recurrent ovarian cancer, 432
        staging, 430–431t
        treatment, 431
    nonepithelial ovarian cancer, 432–434
        germ cell tumors, 432
        gonadoblastomas, 433
        sex cord-stromal neoplasms, 433
        staging, 434t
    vaginal cancer, 434–435
        diethylstilbestrol-related
            adenocarcinoma, 434–435
        squamous cell carcinomas, 434
    vulvar carcinoma, 435–436
        clinical assessment, 436t
        diagnosis, 435
        epidemiology, 435
        etiology, 435
        histology, 435
        patterns of spread, 435
        pretreatment evaluation, 435
        staging, 436t
        symptoms, 435
        treatment, 435–436
Pelvic muscle, rehabilitation, 418
Pelvic organ prolapse, 415–416
    evaluation, 416
    halfway grading system, 416t
    risk factors, 415
    symptoms, 416
    terminology, 415
    treatment, 416
Pelvic pain, 270, 278–286, 376
    acute, 278–280
    adenomyosis, 282
    adnexal masses, 282
    anatomy of, 278–279
    causes, 280t
    character, 279
    chronic, 278, 280–282
        causes of, 281t
    chronic PID, 282
    depression, 278
    differential diagnosis, 279–283
    dysmenorrhea, 280
    ectopic pregnancy, 279
    endometriosis, 281–282
    evaluation, 279
    gastrointestinal disorders, 280

imaging, 279
laparoscopy, 279
location, 279
menstrual cycle relationship, 279
neuroanatomy, 278–279
nongynecologic causes, 282–283
    gastrointestinal, 283
    musculoskeletal, 283
    psychological, 283
    urologic, 282
onset, 279
ovarian torsion, 280
parasympathetic nerve fibers, 279
pelvic adhesions, 281
pelvic inflammatory disease, 280
pelvic magnetic resonance imaging, 279
pelvic ultrasound, 279
physiology of, 279
    referred pain, 279
    splanchnic pain, 279
recurrent, 280–282
ruptured ovarian cyst, 279
severity, 279
sexual abuse, 278
sexual dysfunction, 278
substance abuse, 278
sympathetic nerves, 278
treatments, 283
tubo-ovarian abscess, 282
urologic causes, 280
Pelvic relaxation, 415–416
Pelvic types, in antepartum care, 35–36
Pelvic ultrasound, 300, 430
Pelvimetry, 34
    high-risk pregnancy, 49
Penicillin-allergic pregnant patients, 364
Penicillin desensitization, 364
Peptides, placenta, 12
Percutaneous umbilical blood sampling, 64
Perihepatitis, 377
Perimenopause, 330, 428
    clinical manifestations, 333–335
    endocrinology, 331
    menstrual cycles, 331
    ovarian function, 330
    physiology of, 330–331
Perinatal asphyxia, 111
Perinatal mortality, 42, 45, 164
    high-risk pregnancy, 42
Perineorrhaphy, 416
Perineum, high-risk pregnancy, 49
Peripartum tests, 33t
Peripheral precocious puberty, 323
Peripheral testosterone levels, 332
Peritoneum, 272
Peritonitis, 375, 377
Permethrin, 370–371
Pessaries, 416, 418
Phencyclidine
    teratology, 72
    use in pregnancy, 82
Phenylketonuria, 442
    teratology, 73
Phosphatidylglycerol, fetus, 22
Phthirus pubis, 370
Physical abuse, 386–393
    documentation, 387
    epidemiology, 388
    follow-up, 387
    medical evaluation, 386–387
    National Center for Injury Prevention and
        Control, 386
    National Domestic Violence Hotline, 387
    obstetric complications, 388

physician response, 387
    violence in pregnancy, 387–388
Physical examination, high-risk pregnancy,
        49–50
    evaluation of uterus, 49–50
    general examination, 49
    pelvic examination, 49
Physician, duty to explain, 443–444
Physician-patient relationship, 440
PID. *See* Pelvic inflammatory disease
Piper forceps, 129
    in breech delivery, 128
Piperacillin-tazobactam, 381
Pituitary disorders, 218, 241
Pituitary suppression, 303
Pituitary tumors, 222
PKU. *See* Phenylketonuria
Placenta, 4, 6, 11–12
    accreta, 91
    endocrine changes, 1
    endocrine system, 1
    function, 11–12
        estrogen, 11
        gas exchange, 11
        growth factors, 12
        immunology, 12
        mother-to-fetus nutrient transfer, 11
        peptides, 12
        progesterone, 11
        proteins, 12
        secretion, 11
    metabolism, 12
    previa, 22, 89–92
        advanced maternal age, 89
        Asian/African ethnicity, 89
        cesarean birth, 90
        clinical presentation, 89
        delivery, 90
        diagnosis, 90
        etiology, 89
        examination, 90
        expectant management, 90
        fetal complication, 91–92
        fetal morbidity, 92
        incidence, 89
        management, 90–91
        marginal previa, 89
        maternal complication, 91–92
        maternal morbidity, 91–92
        multiparity, 89
        partial previa, 89
        preterm delivery, 92
        previous cesarean birth, 89
        previous dilation, curettage, 89
        smoking, 89
        transabdominal ultrasound, 90
        transvaginal ultrasound, 90
        ultrasound, 90
        uteroplacental relationships, *91*
        variations of, *90*
    structure, 11
        to fetal blood, 11
        from maternal blood, 11
        placental cotyledons, 11
        villa, 11
Placental abruption, 92–93
Placental cotyledons, 11
Placental estrogens, androgen precursors, 6
Placental separation, 106
Placental site trophoblastic tumor, 199
Placental sulfatase deficiency, 6
    fetus with, 6
Planes of pelvis, *128*
Planned Parenthood v. Casey, 443

Plasma insulin, in pregnancy, biologic
        function, 3
Plasma protein A, pregnancy-associated, 58
Plasma volume expansion, 183
Plastic cup extractor, 130
Platinum, 431
Pneumocystis carinii pneumonia, 366
Pneumonia, 184
Polycystic ovary, 218, 222, 227–237, 240,
        249, 310, 326, 427
    acanthosis nigricans, 232
    acne, 231–232
    amenorrhea, 227
    androgen production, 229
    biochemical hyperandrogenism, 228
    candidate genes, 228–229
    clinical hyperandrogenism, 227
    diabetes, 233
    diagnosis, 232
    differential diagnosis, 228t, 230–231
        androgen-producing neoplasm, 231
        Cushing syndrome, 231
        hyperandrogenic drugs, 231
        nonclassic adrenal hyperplasia, 230
        ovarian hyperthecosis, 231
    etiology, 228–229
    evaluation, 231–234
    Ferriman-Gallwey scoring system, 232
    genetic studies, 228
    health consequences, 230
        cardiovascular disease, 230
        diabetes, 230
        endometrial hyperplasia, 230
        infertility, 230
        metabolic syndrome, 230
        obesity, 230
    hirsutism, 231–232, 234–235
        antiandrogens, 234
        combined hormonal contraception, 234
        mechanical hair removal, 234
    history, 231–232
    hyperandrogenism, 227, 229
    infertility treatment, 235
    insulin resistance, 229, 233
    laboratory testing, 232–234
    lipid levels, 233
    luteinizing hormone, increased, 229
    menstrual cycle frequency, 231
    menstrual irregularities, 227
    menstrual irregularity, 234
    metabolic correction, 235
        metformin, 235
        thiazolidinediones, 235
    obesity, 232, 234
    oligomenorrhea, 227
    oral glucose tolerance test, *233t*
    pathophysiology, 229
    polycystic ovaries, 228
    Rotterdam criteria, 227–228
    theca cells, androgens from, 229
    treatment, 234–235
Polyembryonal cancer, 433
Polyhydramnios, fetal malformations with, 63t
Polymenorrhea, 205, 247
Polymicrobial infection, 376
Polyps, 300
Posterior femoral cutaneous nerve, 401
Postmenopause, 330
Postovulatory estrogen-progesterone with-
        drawal, 248
    corpus luteum, 248–249
    endometrial proliferation, 248
    estrogen, 248
    progesterone/estrogen, 249

Postpartum hemorrhage, 26, 261
Postpill amenorrhea, 218
Postterm pregnancy, 148–153
    abdominal circumference, 148
    anencephaly, 149
    antenatal testing, 149–150
    biophysical profile, 149–150
    biophysical profile score, 150t
    biparietal diameter, 148
    Bishop scoring system, 151t
    clinical significance, 149
    congenital primary fetal adrenal
        hypoplasia, 149
    contraction stress test, 149
    crown-rump length, 148
    date of confinement, estimated, 148
    etiology, 148–149
    femur length, 148
    fundus, 148
    gestational age, determining, 148
    induction of labor, 150
    intrapartum management, 150
    management, 149–151
    Naegele's rule, 148
    nonstress test, 149
    perinatal mortality rate, 149
    placental sulfatase, 149
    previous postterm pregnancy, 149
    quickening, 148
    reactive test, 149
Posttraumatic stress disorder, 389
Postvoid residual urine volume, 417
Powder-burn lesion, 272
PPH. *See* Postpartum hemorrhage
Preantral follicle, oogenesis, 207
Precocious puberty, 323
Preconception care, 32
    high-risk pregnancy, 43
Preconception counseling, 296
Preconception issues, 440–441
    hormonal contraceptives, 441
    intrauterine devices, 441
    sterilization, 441
Preeclampsia, 46, 163, 165, 167–169
    antepartum treatment, 167
    with chronic hypertension, 163
    clinical signs, 167
    delivery, 167
    edema, 167
    future hypertension, 169
    hyperreflexia, 167
    hypertension, 167
    intrapartum management, 168
    laboratory findings, 167
    magnesium, 168t
    management, 167–169
    pathophysiology, 165–167
    postpartum management, 168–169
    prevention, 169
    prognosis, 169
    prophylaxis, 168
    rate of occurrence, 165
    recurrence, 169
    risk factors, 165
    route of delivery, 167
    severe, criteria for, 164t
    treatment, 169
Pregnancy, 1–10, 20–22, 221–222
    abdominal, 287
    cervical, 287
    clinical evidence, 19–20
    complications, 26–27
    confirming, 20
    confirming diagnosis, 20

dating, 20
diagnosis, 19–20
    presumptive symptoms, 19
ectopic, 287–293 (*See also* Ectopic
        pregnancy)
    etiology, 287–288
    prevalence, 287
endocrinology, 1–10
    cortisol-binding globulin, 1
    estrogen synthesis, late pregnancy, 5
    estrogens, 607
        biological activities, 6–7
            anencephalic fetuses, 6
            blood flow to uterus, 6
            end-of-gestation, 6
            lactation, 7
            low-density lipoprotein, uptake by
                placenta, 6
            maternal heart disease, 182
            parturition, 6
            placental sulfatase deficiency, fetus
                with, 6
            reduced maternal estriol levels, 7
            stimulates, 6
        chemical nature, 6
            aromatic ring, steroid hormones, 6
            estradiol, 6
            estriol, 6
            estrone, 6
        fetal adrenal glands, role of, 6
        placental estrogens, androgen
            precursors, 6
        production, 6
            fetal adrenal cortex, 6
            fetal liver, 6
            placenta, 6
        secretory patterns, 6
            adrenocorticotropic hormone, 6
            anencephaly, 6
            estriol, 6
            placental sulfatase deficiency, 6
        source, 6
    female fetus, 1
    fetus, 1
    hormone characteristics, 1–2
        biologic functions, 2
        chemical nature, 1
        fetus, 1
        mother, 1
        placenta, 1
        progesterone deficiency, 2
        protein hormones, 1
        secretion patterns, 2
        source, 1–2
        steroids, 1
    human chorionic gonadotropin,
            2–3
        biologic functions, 3
            clinical uses, 3
            corpus luteum, 3
            fetal testicular testosterone, 3
            multiple marker screen, 3
            with trophoblastic neoplasia, 3
            viability of pregnancy,
                assessment, 3
        chemical nature, 2
        secretion patterns, 2
            contemporary pregnancy
                tests, 2
            high levels, 2
            low levels, 2
            serum hCG assays, 2
            urine hCG assays, 2
        source, 2

    human placental lactogen, 1, 3
        biologic function, 3
            clinical use, 3
            diabetogenic effect, 3
            increased insulin levels, 3
            insulin-directed glucose, 3
            maternal free fatty acids, 3
            plasma insulin, 3
        chemical nature, 3
        human chorionic somatomam-
            motropin, 3
        secretory patterns, 3
        source, 3
    male fetus, 1
    placenta, 1
    progesterone, 4–5
        21-carbon steroid, 4
        biologic functions, 5
            fetus rejection prevention, 5
            implantation of embryo, 5
            mifepristone, 5
            myometrium, 5
            support pregnancy, 5
        cholesterol, 4
        corpus luteum, 4
        fetal adrenal cortex, 4
        fetal liver, 4
        placenta, 4
        pregnenolone, 4
        progesterone sources, 4
        secretory patterns, 4–5
            late pregnancy, 5
        steroid-forming glands, 4
    progesterone synthesis, late pregnancy, 5
    prolactin, 4
        biologic function, 4
            mammary glands, lactation, 4
        chemical nature, 4
        secretory patterns, 4
        source, 4
    protein hormones, 1
    thyroid-binding globulin, 1
fetal presentation, 23–24
fetal status, 21–24
    growth/development, 22–23
    lie of fetus, 23
first trimester, 20–21
    signs/symptoms, 20–21
heterotopic, 287
hypertension in, 163–174 (*See also*
        Hypertension)
loss, 132, 307–315
mastitis, 28
medical complications, 175–195
    anemia, 180–182
    diabetes, 175–177
    heart disease, 182–183
    pulmonary disease, 183–186
    Rh isoimmunization, 188–192
    seizure disorders, 188
    thromboembolic disease, 186–187
    thyroid disease, 177–178
    urinary tract infection, 179–180
normal, 19–31
    fundal height *vs.* gestational age, *20*
    lecithin, in amniotic fluid, *22*
    sphingomyelin, in amniotic fluid, *22*
nursing, 28
ovarian, 287
physiologic changes, 139–141
physiology, 27–28
postterm, 148–153 (*See also* Postterm
        pregnancy)
    abdominal circumference, 148

anencephaly, 149
antenatal testing, 149–150
biparietal diameter, 148
clinical significance, 149
congenital primary fetal adrenal
        hypoplasia, 149
crown-rump length, 148
date of confinement, estimated, 148
etiology, 148–149
femur length, 148
fundus, 148
gestational age, determining, 148
management, 149–151
Naegele's rule, 148
perinatal mortality rate, 149
placental sulfatase, 149
previous postterm pregnancy, 149
quickening, 148
pregnancy dating, 20
presumptive symptoms, 19
puerperium, 25–27
physiology, 25–26
rate, 350
recurrent loss, 311–312 (*See also*
        Recurrent pregnancy loss)
rupture of membranes, 22
second trimester, 21
signs/symptoms, 21
second trimester, complications, 21
substance abuse in, 81–88
alcohol, 81
alcohol use, 82–83
    fetal alcohol syndrome, 82
    teratogenesis, 82
    threshold, 83
behaviors, 82
breastfeeding, counseling on, 85
cannabinoids, 82
cardiovascular complications, 83
cellulitis, 82
cocaine use in pregnancy, 83–84
    cardiovascular effects, 83
    dopamine reuptake, 83
    norepinephrine reuptake, 83
    pharmacologic effects, 83
    tachycardia, 83
    uterine contractions, 83
    vasoconstriction, 83
counseling, 85
dependence, 81
depressants, 82
detoxification, 84
hallucinogens, 82
hepatitis, 82
heroin, 85
infectious complications, 83
intravenous use, 83
laboratory studies, 85
marijuana, 85
methadone, 85
multidisciplinary approach, 85
neurologic complications, 83
occurrence rates, 81
opiates, 82
overdose, 84
phencyclidine, 82
psychoactive substances, 82
sexually transmitted diseases, 83
signs of, 82
stimulants, 82
tobacco, 85
treatment, 84–85
termination, 133 (*See also* Abortion)
induction of labor, 133

progesterone antagonists, 134
surgical evacuation, 133
third trimester, 21
complications, 21
tubal, 287
violence in, 387–388
Pregnenolone, 4
Preimplantation diagnosis, 64, 303, 311–312
Premature birth, 349
Premature labor, 21, 261
Premature menopause, 330
Premature ovarian failure, 217
Prematurity, 164
Premenstrual dysphoric disorder, 211
Premenstrual syndrome, 211
clinical manifestations, 211
epidemiology, 211
etiology, 211
premenstrual dysphoric disorder, 211
Prenatal diagnosis, 56–66
genetic counseling, 56
genetic screening, 58–60
indications for, 56–58, *58*
    abnormal maternal serum alpha-
            fetoprotein, 57
    chromosomal abnormalities, 56–57
    congenital malformations, 57
    fragile X syndrome, 57–58
    mendelian abnormalities, 57
obstetric ultrasound, 56–66
techniques, 60–64
    amniocentesis, 63–64
    chorionic villus sampling, 64
    fetal echocardiography, 63
    ultrasound, 60–63, *62*
Preovulatory follicle, oogenesis, 208
Preponderance of evidence, legal burden, 440
Presentation of fetus, 23–24
breech presentation, *25*
breech presentations, 23–24
brow presentation, *24*
cephalic presentations, 23
complete breech, 24
face presentation, *24*
frank breech, 24
incomplete breech, 24
vertex presentation, *23*
Presumptive symptoms of pregnancy, 19
Preterm delivery, 44
Preterm labor, 154–162
adjunctive therapy, 158
antibiotics, 158
corticosteroids, 158
diagnosis, 156
epidemiology, 154
evaluation, 155–156
fetal assessment, 158
    fetal well-being, 158
    ultrasound, 158
history, 155
indicated preterm birth, 154
indomethacin, 157
magnesium sulfate, 156
management, 156–158
nifedipine, 157
physical examination, 155–156
    digital cervical examination, 156
    fetal heart rate, 156
    speculum examination, 155
    urine specimen, 156
prevention, 155
progesterone, secondary prevention
        with, 155
refractory preterm labor, 158

risk factors, 154–155
cocaine use, 154
infection, 155
maternal medical history, 154–155
obstetric conditions, 155
obstetric history, 154
sociodemographic factors, 154
tobacco smoking, 154
uterine conditions, 154
spontaneous preterm birth, 154
tocolysis, 156–157
tocolytic therapy, contraindications
        to, 157
Preterm premature, rupture of membranes,
        158–159
absence of labor, 159
chorioamnionitis, 159
digital examination of cervix, avoiding,
        159
intrauterine infection, 158
management, 159
nonreassuring fetal heart rate testing, 159
Preventing, 242
Previous cesarean birth, high-risk
        pregnancy, 46
Primary amenorrhea, 215
Primary cesarean births, 123
Primary infertility, 295
Primipara, 33
Primiparity, 149
Primordial follicle, oogenesis, 207
Prior pregnancy
complications, 34
information, 34
Private physicians and hospitals, 441
Product liability, 441
Professional misconduct, 440
Progesterone, 4–5, 297, 312, 331
21-carbon steroid, 4
biologic functions, 5
    fetus rejection prevention, 5
    implantation of embryo, 5
    mifepristone, 5
    myometrium, 5
    support pregnancy, 5
breakthrough bleeding, 250, 253
cholesterol, 4
corpus luteum, 4
deficiency, in pregnancy, 2
fetal adrenal cortex, 4
fetal liver, 4
placenta, 4, 11
pregnenolone, 4
progesterone sources, 4
secretory patterns, 4–5
    late pregnancy, 5
steroid-forming glands, 4
withdrawal, 98
Progesterone-only contraceptives,
        puerperium, 26
Progestin
abnormal uterine bleeding, 252
Progestin-containing intrauterine device,
        341
Progestin-impregnated IUD, 348
Progestin-only contraception methods,
        349–350
implantable progestin, 350
injectable progestin, 349
minipill, 349
mode of action, 349
progestin-only IUD, 350
Progestin-only IUD, 348, 350
Progestogen, 334, 340

Prolactin, 220, 297
  in pregnancy, 4
    biologic function, 4
      mammary glands, lactation, 4
    chemical nature, 4
    secretory patterns, 4
    source, 4
Prolapsed urethra, 318
Prolonged second stage of labor, 128
Prophase, 207
Prophylactic antibiotics, 126
Prostaglandin, 107, 211, 280
  inhibitors, antepartum bleeding, 93
  release, 98
  synthetase inhibitors, 211, 280
Protein, urine dip, in antepartum care, 37
Protein hormones, in pregnancy, 1
Proteinuria, 163
Prothrombin G20210A mutation, 351
Pseudocapsule, 259
Psychoactive substance, use in pregnancy, 82
Psychotropic drug use, teratology, 74
Pubarche, 321
Puberty
  central precocious, 323
  delayed, 218, 324
  development, 321–324
  normal, 321
  peripheral precocious, 323
  precocious, 323
Public hospitals, 441
Pudendal nerve, 400
Puerperium, 25–27
  afterpains, 25
  blood, 26
  blood coagulation factors, 26
  cardiovascular changes, 26
  combination oral contraceptives, 26
  complications, 26–27
  family planning, 26
  fever, 27
  involution of uterus, 25
  lactating mothers, 26
  lactating women, 26
  leukocytosis, 26
  lochia, 25
  lochia alba, 25
  lochia rubra, 25
  lochia serosa, 25
  menstruation, 26
  nonlactating mothers, 26
  nonlactating women, 26
  ovulation, 26
  pelvic infections, 27
  physiology, 25–26
  postpartum hemorrhage, 26
  progesterone-only contraceptives, 26
  puerperal infection, 27
  renal system, involutional changes, 25–26
  urinary tract infections, 27
Pulmonary angiogram, 187
Pulmonary disease, 183–186
  asthma, 184
  dyspnea of pregnancy, 184
  Haemophilus influenzae, 185
  high-risk pregnancy, 47
  Influenza A, 185
  Klebsiella pneumoniae, 185
  Mycoplasma pneumoniae, 185
  physiologic changes with pregnancy, 183
  pneumonia, 184
  sarcoidosis, 185
  tuberculosis, 185–186
Pulmonary embolism, 42, 187

Pulmonary hypertension, 182
Purified protein derivative test, 366
Pyelonephritis, 179–180
Pyelonephritis, high-risk pregnancy, 51
Pyuria, 360

Q-tip test, 417
QUAD screening, 36
Quickening, fetal, 19

R-R wave intervals, consecutive, 112
Radiation, 426
  high-risk pregnancy, 44
  teratology, 69
    doses, 70t
Radioactive compounds, 44
Rape, 388
  psychological sequelae, 389
RDS. *See* Respiratory distress syndrome
Real-time ultrasonography, 187
Reassurance, with high-risk pregnancy, 42
Recreational drugs, teratology, 71
Rectal examination, 316
Rectocele, 416
Recurrent miscarriage, 132
Recurrent pregnancy loss, 132, 307–315
  age, 307
  anatomic causes, 309–310
  antiphospholipid antibody syndrome, 312
  antiphospholipid syndrome, 309
  bicornuate uterus, 312
  cerclage, 312
  chromosomal inversions, 309
  congenital anomalies, 308
  diagnosis, 310
  endocrinologic factors, 310–311
  etiology, 308–311
    general population, 307–308
  genetic/parental chromosomal
      abnormality, 308
  hormonal conditions, 308
  hysteroscope, 312
  incidence, 307
  insulin-dependent diabetes mellitus,
      311
  intravenous immunoglobulin, 313
  metroplasty, 312
  parental genetic abnormalities,
      treatments, 311–312
  paternal leukocytes, 313
  polycystic ovarian syndrome, 310
  preimplantation genetic diagnosis,
      311–312
  progesterone, 312
  Robertsonian translocation, 308–309
  RPL evaluation overview, 311
  structural anomalies, uterus, 308
  thrombophilias, 311
  treatment, 311–313
  unicornuate uterus, 312
  uterine didelphys, 312
  uterine septums, 312
  in vitro fertilization, 311–312
  workup for, 133
Recurrent yeast infections, 406
Referred pain, 279
Refractory preterm labor, 158
Relationship violence, 386–393
  documentation, 387
  epidemiology, 388
  follow-up, 387
  medical evaluation, 386–387
  National Center for Injury Prevention
      and Control, 386

National Domestic Violence Hotline, 387
  obstetric complications, 388
  physician response, 387
  violence in pregnancy, 387–388
Removal of Y-containing gonads, 221
Renal changes in pregnancy, 141
Renal disease, high-risk pregnancy, 47
Renal failure, antepartum bleeding, 93
Renal function, 166–167
  glomerular changes, 166
  renin-angiotensin-aldosterone system, 166
  tubular changes, 166
Renal system
  fetal, 14
  puerperium, involutional changes, 25–26
Renin-angiotensin-aldosterone system, 166
Repeat cesarean birth, 123
Reproductive technologies, 443–444
  artificial insemination, 443–444
  embryo freezing, 444
  gestational carrier, 444
  in vitro fertilization, 444
Reproductive tract, changes in pregnancy, 141
Requirements of fetus, 12
Resistant ovary syndrome, 217
Respiratory distress syndrome, fetus, 22
Respiratory system
  changes in pregnancy, 140
  fetal, 14
Restriction fragment length polymorphisms, 64
Retrograde menstrual flow, 269
Retropubic urethropexy, 418
Rh isoimmunization, 188–192
  criteria, 189
  epidemiology, 188–189
  prevention, 189
  Rh-negative
    sensitized pregnant woman, 189–192
    unsensitized pregnant woman, 189
Rh sensitization, high-risk pregnancy, 50
Rifampin, 186
Right occiput posterior position, 102
Right occiput transverse position, 101
Right to privacy, 443
Robertsonian translocation, 308–309
Rotterdam criteria, polycystic ovary syn-
      drome, 227–228
RU486. *See* Mifepristone
Rubella
  syndrome, 75
  teratology, 74–75
  titer, 50
Rupture of membranes, 104
  ferning, 104
  in labor, 104
    ferning, 104
    nitrazine test, 104
    pooling, 104
  nitrazine test, 104
  pooling, 104
  preterm premature, 158–159
    absence of labor, 159
    chorioamnionitis, 159
    digital examination of cervix, avoiding,
        159
    intrauterine infection, 158
    management, 159
    nonreassuring fetal heart rate testing, 159
Ruptured ovarian cyst, 279
Ruptured tubo-ovarian abscess, 376

Sacrospinous suspension, 416
Saline sonohysterography, 310
Salpingectomy, 290

Salpingitis, 375
Salpingo-oophoritis, 377
Sarcoidosis, 185, 382
Sarcoma botryoides, 318
Sarcoptes scabiei, 371
Satellite lesions, 406
Scabies, 371
Scalp stimulation test, 118
Schiller-Duval body, 432
Schistosomiasis, 381
Sclerosing adenosis, 397
Second stage of labor, 100–101, 105, 112, 141
    pain neuropathways, 141
Second trimester, 21, 61, 443
    complications, 21
    pregnancy loss, 44–45
    signs/symptoms, 21
    ultrasound, 61
Secondary amenorrhea, 215
Secondary dysmenorrhea, 280, 324
Secondary infertility, 295
Secretion patterns, hormones, 2
Seizure disorders, 188
    effects of pregnancy on, 188
    effects on pregnancy, 188
    management, 188
Seizure prophylaxis, 168
Semen. *See* Sperm
Sequential screening, in antepartum care, 36
Sertoli-Leydig cell tumors, 433
Serum 17-OHP, 241
Serum 3α-AG, 242
Serum alpha-fetoprotein, abnormal
            maternal, 57
Serum androstenedione, 241
Serum DHEAS, 241
Serum hCG assays, 2
Serum human chorionic gonadotropin, 219
Serum pregnancy tests, 20
Serum progesterone, 290, 297
Serum testosterone, 241
17α-hydroxylase deficiency, 217
Severity, 164t
Sex hormone-binding globulin, 239, 332
Sex steroids, 206
Sexual abuse, 278, 317, 326
Sexual assault, 388–390
    documentation, 389
    follow-up, 389
    forensic evaluation, 388–389
    pregnancy evaluation, 389
    prophylaxis, 389
    STD evaluation, prophylaxis, 389
Sexual dysfunction, 278
Sexually transmitted diseases, 83, 358–374, 402
    bacterial sexually transmitted diseases,
            358–363
        bacterial vaginosis, 362
        chancroid, 361
        chlamydia, 360–361
        gonorrhea, 358
        granuloma inguinale, 361
        lymphogranuloma venereum, 362
        Thayer-Martin culture medium, 359
    control, 358
    ectoparasites, 370–371
        pediculosis pubis, 370
        scabies, 371
    evaluation, 389
    evaluation, prophylaxis, 389
    syphilis, 363–365
        clinical presentation, 363
        Darkfield examination, 363
        diagnosis, 363–364

epidemiology, 363
    follow-up, 365
    Jarisch-Herxheimer reaction, 364
    treatment, 364
    treatment, 358
    trichomoniasis, 369–370
        clinical presentation, 369–370
        diagnosis, 370
        epidemiology, 369
        treatment, 370
    viral sexually transmitted diseases, 365
        hepatitis B virus, 369
        herpes simplex virus, 368
        HIV, 365
        human papillomavirus, 367
        molluscum contagiosum, 369
SHBG. *See* Sex hormone-binding globulin
Shirodkar technique, cervical cerclage, 131
Shoulder pain, 279
Sickle cell
    anemia, 180
    screen, 52, 60, 442
    trait, 181
Sickle cell-hemoglobin C disease, 181
Sickle cell-thalassemia disease, 181
Sickle hemoglobin, 60
Sleep disturbance, 334
Small cell ovarian cancers, 431
Smoking, effects of, 38, 184, 288
    abruptio placentae, 92
    placenta previa, 89
Social history, in antepartum care, 34
Socioeconomic status, high-risk pregnancy, 43
Sonohysterography, 252, 300, 333, 341
Sources of hormones, 1–2
Specialized forceps, 129, *130*
Spectrophotometry, 190
Speculum examination, 404
Sperm, 196, 301
    donor, 302
Spermicides, 346–347
Sphingomyelin, in amniotic fluid, *22*
Spiral arteries, abnormal uterine bleeding, 249
Spiral computed tomography scan, 187
Spironolactone, 243
Splanchnic pain, 279
Spontaneous abortion, 132, 349
Spontaneous vaginal delivery, 105
Squamocolumnar function, 336
Stable severe preeclampsia, 167
Stages of labor, 99–101
    first stage, 99–100
    second stage, 100–101
    third stage, 101, 106–107
State restrictions, 443
Status asthmaticus, 184
STDs. *See* Sexually transmitted diseases
Sterilization, 441
    surgical, 355
    voluntary, 441
Steroid-forming glands, 4
Steroids, in pregnancy, 1
Stimulants, use in pregnancy, 82
Stimulators, 211
Strawberry cervix, 370
Streptomycin, 186
Stress, 218, 402
Stress urinary incontinence, 416
Stroke, 351
Stromal cells, 433
Structural defects, teratology, 68
    deformations, 68
    disruptions, 68
    malformations, 68

Submucous leiomyomas, 261
Substance abuse
    screening, 34
Substance abuse in pregnancy, 43–44, 81–88
    alcohol, 81
    alcohol use, 82–83
        fetal alcohol syndrome, 82
        teratogenesis, 82
        threshold, 83
    behaviors, 82
    breastfeeding, counseling on, 85
    cannabinoids, 82
    cardiovascular complications, 83
    cellulitis, 82
    cocaine use in pregnancy, 83–84
        cardiovascular effects, 83
        dopamine reuptake, 83
        norepinephrine reuptake, 83
        pharmacologic effects, 83
        tachycardia, 83
        uterine contractions, 83
        vasoconstriction, 83
    complications, 83–84
    counseling, 85
    dependence, 81
    depressants, 82
    detoxification, 84
    hallucinogens, 82
    hepatitis, 82
    heroin, 85
    infectious complications, 83
    intravenous use, 83
    laboratory studies, 85
    marijuana, 85
    methadone, 85
    multidisciplinary approach, 85
    neurologic complications, 83
    occurrence rates, 81
    opiates, 82
    overdose, 84
    phencyclidine, 82
    psychoactive substances, 82
    sexually transmitted diseases, 83
    signs of, 82
    stimulants, 82
    tobacco, 85
    treatment, 84–85
Suburethral sling procedures, 418
SUI. *See* Stress urinary incontinence
Suit against physician, by child, 445
Support, with high-risk pregnancy, 42
Surgical ablation, 300
Surgical history, in antepartum care, 34
Surgical sterilization, 355
Swyer syndrome, 325
Syphilis, 363–365, 389
    clinical presentation, 363
    congenital, 363
    Darkfield examination, 363
    diagnosis, 363–364
    epidemiology, 363
    follow-up, 365
    Jarisch-Herxheimer reaction, 364
    teratology, 76
    test, 50
    treatment, 364
Systemic lupus erythematosus, high-risk
            pregnancy, 48
Systemic pyelonephritis, high-risk
            pregnancy, 51

T-ACE questionnaire, 44t
Tachycardia, 112
Tamoxifen, 427

Tanner staging, 322t
   normal breast development, *322*
   normal pubic hair development, *323*
Taxane, 431
Tay-Sachs disease, 442
   genetic screening, 60
TBG. *See* Thyroid-binding globulin
Teratogens, 68–77, 187, 442
Teratology, 67–80
   adequate antibiotic therapy, 76
   administration of teratogen, 67
   alcohol, 71, 82
   animal research, 70–71
   cancer chemotherapy, 72
   cardiovascular lesions, 75
   categories of structural defects, *69*
   chickenpox, 76
   cleft lip, 73
   cleft palate, 73
   cocaine, 72
   congenital heart disease, 73
   congenital malformations, 70
   congenital rubella syndrome, 75
   cytomegalovirus, 75
   developmental stage at exposure, 67
      lowered susceptibility, 67
      maximum susceptibility, 67
      resistant period, 67
   diabetes mellitus, 72–73
   diagnostic radiation, 69
   dose effect, 69
   dose threshold, 71
   enteroviruses, 77
   environmental influences, *68*
   epidemiologic studies, 71
   epilepsy, 73
   fetal alcohol syndrome, 71
   fetoplacental unit, access to, 70
   genetic susceptibility, 67
   heroin, 72
   herpes simplex virus type 2, 75
   herpes zoster, 76–77
   human research, 71
   hyperthermia, 72
   hypothyroidism, 73
   infections, 74–77
   inner ear problems, 75
   intrauterine growth retardation, 75
   ionizing radiation, 68–69
      acute high dose, 68–69
      chronic low dose, 69
      radioactive iodine, 69
   malformations, 73
   marijuana, 72
   maternal medical disorders, 72–74
   medications, 70–72
   mumps, 77
   neuropathologic changes, 75
   ocular defects, 75
   parvovirus B19, 77
   phencyclidine, 72
   phenylketonuria, 73
   psychotropic drug use, 74
   radiation, doses, 70t
   recreational drugs, 71
   rubella virus, 74–75
   structural defects, 68
      deformations, 68
      disruptions, 68
      malformations, 68
   syphilis, 76
   teratogenic agents, 68–77
   teratogenic drugs, 71
   thalidomide, 70

thrombophilic disorders, 74
   time of exposure, 69
   toxoplasmosis, 75–76
   varicella zoster virus, 76–77
   virilizing tumors, 73
Teratomas, 432
Termination of pregnancy, 443
   right of privacy, 443
   state restrictions, 443
   trimester model, 443
Tertiary syphilis, 363
Testicular feminization. *See* Androgen
      insensitivity syndrome
Testosterone, 238–239, 297, 332
   levels, 241, 301
Tethering effect, with endometriosis, 271
Thalassemias, 60, 182
Thalidomide, teratology, 70
Thayer-Martin culture medium, 359
Theca cells, 206, 229
   androgens from, 229
Theca lutein cysts, 197, 199
Thelarche, 321
Thiazolidinediones, 235
Third stage of labor, 101
Third trimester, 21, 61
   complications, 21
   ultrasound, 62–63
Thoracolumbar, 278
Threatened abortion, 132
3α-androstanediol glucuronide, 239
Thromboembolic disorders, 126, 186–187
   diagnosis, 186
   epidemiology, 186
   high-risk pregnancy, 48
   management, 187
   pathophysiology, 186
Thrombophilia, abruptio placentae, 92
Thrombophilias, 311
Thrombophilic disorders, teratology, 74
Thyroid-binding globulin, in pregnancy, 1
Thyroid disease, 15, 177–178
   effects of pregnancy, 177
   Graves disease, 178
   high-risk pregnancy, 48
   hyperthyroidism, 178
   hypothyroidism, 178
Thyroid-stimulating hormone, 220,
      242, 297
Thyroid storm, 178
Ticarcillin clavulanate, 381
Tinidazole, 370
Tobacco use in pregnancy, 43, 85
Tocodynamometer, 114
Tocolysis, 99
Tocolytic agents
   abruptio placentae, 93
   complications of, 99t
   contraindications to, 100t
Topical estrogen, 317, 341
TORCH, 48
Toxoplasmosis
   high-risk pregnancy, 48
   teratology, 75–76
Trachelectomy, 426
Transdermal patch, 353
Transvaginal needle procedures, 418
Transverse lie, fetus, 23
Trauma, 317
Traumatic vaginitis, 408
Treponemal antibody tests, 363
Trichomoniasis, 369–370, 389
   clinical presentation, 369–370
   diagnosis, 370

   epidemiology, 369
   treatment, 370
Trimethoprim-sulfamethoxazole, 362
Trisomy 21, incidence of, 57t
Trophoblastic neoplasia, 3
True hermaphroditism, 321
True labor, 101
   vs. false labor, 101t
TSH. *See* Thyroid-stimulating hormone
Tubal disease, infertility and, 299
Tubal ligation, 299
Tubal obstruction, 375
Tubal pregnancy, 287
Tubal reanastomosis, 299
Tuberculosis, 185–186
Tuberculous salpingitis, 381
Tubo-ovarian abscess, 282, 380–381
Turner syndrome, 216, 325
21-carbon steroid, 4
21-hydroxylase defect, 320

UAE. *See* Uterine artery embolization
Ultrasonography, 262
   in antepartum care, 33
   fetus recognition, 20
   obstetric, 56–66
      during pregnancy, indications, 61
      prenatal, 60–63, *62*
Umbilical cord, 12, 197
   compression, 115, 118
   umbilical arteries, 12
   umbilical vein, 12
Underweight, high-risk pregnancy, 49
Unexplained infertility, 302
   diagnosis, 302
Unicornuate uterus, 312
Unopposed estrogen stimulation, abnormal
      uterine bleeding, 249
Ureterocele, 319
Urethra, 416
Urethral hypermobility, 417
Urethral sphincteric deficiency, 417
Urethritis, 179, 360
Urethrovesical junction, anatomic
      support, 416
Urge incontinence, 417
Urinalysis, high-risk pregnancy, 51
Urinary frequency, 261
Urinary incontinence, 336, 416–418
   evaluation, 417
   treatment, 418
   types, 416
Urinary luteinizing hormone kits, 297
Urinary retention, 261
Urinary symptoms, 417
Urinary tract infection, 126, 179–180
   acute pyelonephritis, 179–180
   acute urethritis, 179
   asymptomatic bacteriuria, 179
   cystitis, 179
   puerperal, 27
Urination, pregnancy and, 19
Urine, extraurethral sources of, 417
Urine hCG assays, 2
Urine pregnancy tests, 20
Urodynamic testing, 417
Urogenital atrophy, 335–336, 341
Uterine anomalies, high-risk pregnancy, 50
Uterine artery embolization, 265
Uterine bleeding, 197–198, 247
Uterine changes in pregnancy, 19
Uterine contractions, 101, 211
   characteristics of, 101
Uterine didelphys, 312

Uterine hemostasis, 106–107
Uterine incision, cesarean birth, 125
Uterine leiomyomas. *See* Leiomyomas
Uterine outflow tract abnormalities, 299–300
   diagnosis, 299–300
   treatment, 300
   uterine factor, 299
Uterine perforation, 348
Uterine polyps, 299
Uterine prolapse, 415
Uterine rupture, 94
Uterine septums, 312
Uterine size, in antepartum care, 37
Uterine smooth muscle, contraction of, 98
Uteroplacental perfusion, decreases in, 164

Vacuum extractor operations, 127–130
   complications, 130
   Malmström vacuum extractor, 129
   maternal complications, 130
   neonatal injury, 130
   plastic cup extractor, 130
Vagina, 401, 414
   cancer, 434–435
      diethylstilbestrol-related
         adenocarcinoma, 434–435
      squamous cell carcinomas, 434
   fornix, 434
   high-risk pregnancy, 49
   infections, 94
   lacerations, from trauma, 94
   physiology, 402
      host factors, 402
      microbiology, 402
      vaginal environment, 402
Vaginal agenesis, 325
Vaginal delivery, operative, 127–130
Vaginal discharge, 318, 403–404, 434
Vaginal ectopic anus, 319
Vaginal outflow tract abnormalities,
      infertility and, 299–300
Vaginal ring, 341
Vaginal sponges, 347
Vaginal tumors, 318
Vaginal vault prolapse, 416
Vaginal vault suspension, 416
Varicella, 185
   vaccine, 185
Varicella zoster virus
   high-risk pregnancy, 48
   teratology, 76–77

Vasa previa, rupture of, 93–94
Vaso-occlusive, 181
Vasoconstriction, 106–107, 249
Vasomotor symptoms, 336–337
VDRL. *See* Venereal Disease Research
      Laboratory
Venereal Disease Research Laboratory, 50
Venography, 187
Venous thromboembolism, 350
Ventilation-perfusion scan, 187
Vertex presentation, fetus, *23*
Viability of pregnancy, assessment, 3
Villa, placenta, 11
Violence
   obstetric complications, 388
   relationship, 386–393
Viral sexually transmitted diseases, 365
   hepatitis B virus, 369
   herpes simplex virus, 368
   HIV, 365
   human papillomavirus, 367
   molluscum contagiosum, 369
Virilization, 238, 240
Virilizing process, arresting, 242
Virilizing tumor
   maternal, 321
   teratology, 73
Vitamin B_{12} deficiency, 180
VMSs. *See* Vasomotor symptoms
Voluntary sterilization, 441
von Willebrand disease, 251
Vulva, 400–401
   anatomic structures, *401*
   biopsy, 408
   carcinoma, 435–436
      clinical assessment, 436t
      diagnosis, 435
      epidemiology, 435
      etiology, 435
      histology, 435
      patterns of spread, 435
      pretreatment evaluation, 435
      staging, 436t
      symptoms, 435
      treatment, 435–436
   dystrophies, 408
   high-risk pregnancy, 49
   irritation, 435
Vulvovaginal anatomy, 400–402
Vulvovaginal conditions, 404–410
Vulvovaginal lesions, 316–318

Vulvovaginitis, 400–413
   atrophic vaginitis, 407–408
   bacterial vaginosis, 404–405
   Bartholin glands, 400
   diagnosis, 403–404t
   herpes simplex genitalis, 408–410
   history, 403
   laboratory tests, 404
   neoplasia, 408
   pelvic examination, 403
   physical examination, 403–404
   speculum examination, 404
   symptomatology, 403
   traumatic vaginitis, 408
   vagina, 401
   vaginal physiology, 402
      host factors, 402
      microbiology, 402
      vaginal environment, 402
   vulva, 400–401
      anatomic structures, *401*
   vulvar dystrophies, 408
   vulvovaginal anatomy, 400–402
   vulvovaginal conditions, 404–410
VZV. *See* Varicella zoster virus

Warfarin, 187
Weight, fetal, 22
Weight gain, antepartum, 37
Whiff test, 362
Widened vaginal outlet, 416
Wound closure, cesarean birth, 125
Wound infection, cesarean, 126
Wrongful birth, 445
Wrongful conception, 444–445
Wrongful life, 445

X-linked disorders, 57, 442
XY genotype, Swyer syndrome. *See* Gonadal
      dysgenesis

Y chromosome microdeletion,
      301
Y-containing mosaics, 241
Yeast infection, 406
Yolk sac tumors, 432
Yuzpe method, 353

Zidovudine, 52
ZIFT. *See* Zygote intrafallopian transfer
Zygote intrafallopian transfer, 303